Principles of
CRITICAL CARE
SECOND EDITION

COMPANION HANDBOOK

NOTICE

Principles of
CRITICAL CARE
SECOND EDITION

COMPANION HANDBOOK

JESSE B. HALL, M.D.
GREGORY A. SCHMIDT, M.D.
LAWRENCE D. H. WOOD, M.D., Ph.D.

Section of Pulmonary and Critical Care Medicine
University of Chicago
Chicago, Illinois

McGRAW-HILL
HEALTH PROFESSIONS DIVISION

New York   St. Louis   San Francisco   Auckland   Bogotá   Caracas
Lisbon   London   Madrid   Mexico City   Milan   Montreal
New Delhi   San Juan   Singapore   Sydney   Tokyo   Toronto

McGraw-Hill

*A Division of The **McGraw·Hill** Companies*

PRINCIPLES OF CRITICAL CARE,
2ND EDITION, COMPANION HANDBOOK

1234567890   DOCDOC   99

ISBN   0-07-026029-X

This book was set in Palatino by York Graphic Services.
The editors were Joseph A. Hefta and Muza Navrozov.
The production supervisor was Richard C. Ruzycka.
The cover was designed by Marsha Cohen/Parallelogram Graphics.
The index was prepared by Tony Greenberg, M.D.
R. R. Donnelly & Sons Company was printer and binder.

This book is printed on acid-free paper.

**Cataloging-in-Publication Data are on file for this title at the Library
of Congress.**

To the many students
who have inspired
our teaching

to our wives for their
limitless patience, and

to Cora Taylor, our secretary,
whose skill, efficiency, and spirit
earn our gratitude daily

CONTENTS

CONTRIBUTORS

This companion to *Principles of Critical Care* consists of brief summaries of chapters of that textbook, each reduced in length and complexity to be readily available as an introductory bedside guide. The original chapters and authors are listed at the end of each synopsis to guide the interested reader to more complete descriptions. The editors are indebted to the original authors for their most excellent and extensive reviews of these topics.

In the preparation of this companion text, the editors were assisted by a superb group of colleagues, each taking responsibility for summarizing a number of the original chapters. These individuals are:

Steven Baker, M.D.
Sangeeta Bhorade, M.D.
Edward Bottei, M.D.
Scott Budinger, M.D.
Shannon Carson, M.D.
Thomas Corbridge, M.D.
Patrick Cunningham, M.D.
Delbert Dorscheid, M.D.
Ivor Douglas, M.D.
Philip Factor, D.O.
Sean Forsythe, M.D.
Yiping Fu, M.D.
Brian Gehlbach, M.D.
Manu Jain, M.D.
Kim Josen, M.D.
Eugene Kaji, M.D.
John P. Kress, M.D.

Pam Kuagoolwongse, M.D.
Anna Lee, M.D.
John McConville, M.D.
Babak Mokhlesi, M.D.
Edward Naurekas, M.D.
Maurice Ndukwu, M.D.
Imre Noth, M.D.
Michael O'Connor, M.D.
David Rubin, M.D.
William Sanders, M.D.
Gregory A. Schmidt, M.D.
Matthew Trunsky, M.D.
Avery Tung, M.D.
Micheal Waldman, M.D.
Lisa Wolfe, M.D.
Sarah Young, M.D.

The editors thank these collaborators for their insights and efforts in the task of condensing such a large amount of information into the book you now hold.

Jesse B. Hall, M.D.
Director of Critical Care Services
Professor of Medicine and of Anesthesia and Critical Care
Section of Pulmonary and Critical Care Medicine
University of Chicago
Chicago, Illinois

Gregory A. Schmidt, M.D.
Director of Academic Programs
Professor of Clinical Medicine and of Clinical Anesthesia
    and Critical Care
Section of Pulmonary and Critical Care Medicine
University of Chicago
Chicago, Illinois

Lawrence D. H. Wood, M.D., Ph.D.
Faculty Dean of Medical Education, University of Chicago
    Pritzker School of Medicine
Professor of Medicine and of Anesthesia and Critical Care
Section of Pulmonary and Critical Care Medicine
University of Chicago
Chicago, Illinois

PREFACE

Critical care has evolved during the last four decades into a discipline combining the clinical scholarships of anesthesia, medicine, and surgery. In editing the second edition of *Principles of Critical Care* (PCC), we encouraged our contributors to describe the differential diagnosis and management of each disease as the intensivist sees the critically ill patient. Written from this perspective, 108 chapters described the diagnosis and management of critical illness and discussed the organization of critical care in 1767 pages. Because the bulk of this book makes it impractical to have it available at all times, the editors, with the help of critical care colleagues and senior critical care fellows, aimed to condense the clinical portions of PCC into this completely revised and updated pocket-sized *Companion Handbook*, which practitioners of critical care carry with them.

The *Companion Handbook, Second Edition*, is meant to provide a brief introduction to, or reminder of, some aspect of critical care which intensivists may require when they cannot consult PCC. Users of the *Companion Handbook* should be warned that such a condensed, streamlined approach to critical illness can magnify several pitfalls intrinsic to critical care. By its very nature, critical care is exciting and attracts physicians having an inclination to action. Despite its obvious utility in urgent circumstances, this proclivity can replace effective clinical discipline with excessive, unfocused ICU procedures. We believe this common approach inverts the stable pyramid of bedside skills, placing most attention on the least informative source of data while losing the rational foundation for diagnosis and treatment. An associated problem is that ICU procedures become an end to themselves rather than a means to answer thoughtful clinical questions. Too often, these procedures are implemented to provide "monitoring," ignoring the fact that the only alarm resides in the intensivist's intellect. Students of critical care benefit from the dictum:

"Don't just do something, stand there—take time to process the gathered data to formulate a working hypothesis concerning the mechanism(s) responsible for each patient's main problem(s) so that the next diagnostic or treatment intervention can best test that possibility." Without this exhortation to thoughtful clinical decision-making, students of critical care are swept away by the burgeoning tools of the ICU toward the unproductive subspecialty: critical care technology. Furthermore, effective critical care is rarely in brilliant, incisive, dramatic, and innovative interventions but most often derives from meticulously identifying and titrating each of the patient's multiple problems toward improvement at an urgent but continuous pace. This conservative approach breeds skepticism toward innovative strategies that are incompletely evaluated, and demands that the goals and adverse effects of traditional therapies be clarified so that the least amount of each intervention is employed to achieve its stated therapeutic goal, all in order to maximize one principle of patient care—"First, Do No Harm."

These several important principles of critical care necessarily get minimized in the *Companion Handbook*, which we consider to complement PCC as a single educational package. Accordingly, we recommend that relevant subjects in the standard textbook be consulted as soon as time permits. To facilitate this consultation, each of the critical illnesses and procedures discussed in the *Companion Handbook* refers to the relevant chapters in PCC. Used in this way, the companion handbook provides students, residents, fellows, and critical care physicians and nurses with quick access to essential information during the initial presentation or rapid evolution of critical illness in most ICU patients.

I. NORMAL BLOOD GAS AND RESPIRATORY GAS EXCHANGE VALUES

Arterial oxygen saturation (Sa_{O_2})	96–100% (.96–1.0)
Mixed venous oxygen saturation ($S\bar{v}_{O_2}$)	>70% (>.7) <80% (<.8)
pH	7.35–7.45
Pa_{CO_2}	35–45 mmHg (4.7–6.0 kPa)
Pa_{O_2}	75–100 mmHg (10.0–13.3 kPa)
Arterial oxygen content (Ca_{O_2})	18–21 mL O_2/dL (vol %)
Alveolar-arterial differences for O_2 (A-aD_{O_2}) at $F_{I_{O_2}}$ = .21	5–25 mmHg
$F_{I_{O_2}}$ = 1.0	<150 mmHg
Shunt fraction ($\dot{Q}S/\dot{Q}T$)	3–8% (.03–.08)
Dead space fraction (V_D/V_T)	<.35
Oxygen consumption ($\dot{V}_{O_2}$)	3–4 mL/kg/min
CO_2 production ($\dot{V}_{CO_2}$)	3–4 mL/kg/min
Oxygen transport ($\dot{Q}_{O_2}$)	12–16 mL/kg/min
Respiratory quotient (RQ)	.7–1.0
Tidal volume (V_T)	6–8 mL/kg
Respiratory rate (f)	8–16/min
Respiratory system static compliance (Cst, rs)	70–100 mL/cmH$_2$O
Respiratory system resistance to airflow (Rrs)	<3 mmH$_2$O/L/s

II. RESPIRATORY PARAMETERS

$$Pa_{CO_2} = \frac{k\dot{V}_{CO_2}}{\dot{V}_A} \qquad = \frac{k\dot{V}_{CO_2}}{(f)(V_T) \times (1 - V_D/V_T)}$$

where f = Breathing frequency
V_T = Tidal volume
V_D/V_T = Dead space fraction
k = 0.863

Dead space fraction $\quad = \dfrac{Pa_{CO_2} - Pe_{CO_2}}{Pa_{CO_2}}$

(V_D/V_T)
where Pe_{CO_2} = partial
pressure of carbon
dioxide in expired gas

Modified alveolar gas $\qquad PA_{O_2} = F_{I_{O_2}}(P_{ATM} - P_{H_2O}) - \dfrac{Pa_{CO_2}}{RQ}$
equation:

Static compliance (Cst,rs) $\quad = \dfrac{V_T}{(Pplat - PEEP)}$

Resistant to airflow (Rrs) $\quad = \dfrac{Ppeak - Pplat}{FLOW}$

Pulmonary capillary $\qquad = ([Hgb] \times 1.39) + PA_{O_2} \times .0031$
content (Cc'_{O_2})

Shunt fraction $(\dot{Q}s/\dot{Q}T)$ $\qquad = \dfrac{Cc'_{O_2} - Ca_{O_2}}{Cc'_{O_2} - C\bar{v}_{O_2}}$

III.   RESPIRATORY GAS TRANSPORT

Oxygen delivery $(\dot{O}_{O_2})$ $= \dot{Q}_T \times Ca_{O_2}$

Aterial oxygen content (Ca_{O_2}) $= 1.39 \times Sa_{O_2} \times [Hgb] + .0031 \times Pa_{O_2}$

Mixed venous oxygen content $(C\bar{v}_{O_2})$ $= 1.39 \times S\bar{v}_{O_2} \times [Hgb] + .0031 \times P\bar{v}_{O_2}$

Arterio-venous oxygen content difference $= Ca_{O_2} - C\bar{v}_{O_2}$

Oxygen consumption $(\dot{V}_{O_2})$ $= \dot{Q}_T(Ca_{O_2} - C\bar{v}_{O_2})$

Extraction fraction $= \dfrac{Ca_{O_2} - C\bar{v}_{O_2}}{Ca_{O_2}}$

Respiratory quotient (RQ) $= \dfrac{\dot{V}_{CO_2}}{\dot{V}_{O_2}}$

CO_2 production $(\dot{V}_{CO_2})$ $= f \cdot V_T \cdot F_{E_{CO_2}}$

O_2 consumption $(\dot{V}_{O_2})$ $= f \cdot V_T \cdot (F_{I_{O_2}} - F_{E_{O_2}})$, when RQ = 1.0

IV CIRCULATORY PARAMETERS AND CALCULATIONS

Systemic systolic pressure (SP)	100–140 mmHg
Systemic diastolic pressure (DP)	60–90 mmHg
Pulse pressure (SP − DP)	30–50 mmHg
Mean arterial pressure (BP, mmHg)	$\dfrac{(SP + 2DP)}{3}$ at normal heart rate
Heart rate (HR)	60–90/min
Stroke volume (SV)	50–100 mL
Stroke index (SI)	SV/body surface area (BSA) = 35–50 mL/m^2
Right atrial pressure (Pra)	2–8 mmHg
Pulmonary systolic pressure	16–24 mmHg
Pulmonary diastolic pressure	5–12 mmHg
Pulmonary pulse pressure	8–15 mmHg
Mean pulmonary artery pressure ($P\overline{p}a$)	9–16 mmHg
Mean pulmonary capillary wedge pressure (Ppw)	5–12 mmHg
Cardiac output ($\dot{Q}T = SV \times HR$)	4–6 L/min
Cardiac index ($CI = \dot{Q}T/BSA$)	2.5–3 L/min/m^2

Systemic vascular resistance

$$SVR = \frac{\overline{BP} - Pra}{\dot{Q}T}$$

10–15 mmHg/L/min
(to convert to c.g.s. units, multiply × 80)
(900–1200 dyne·s/cm^5)

Pulmonary vascular resistance

$$PVR = \frac{Ppa - Ppw}{\dot{Q}T}$$

1.5–2.5 mmHg/L/min
(120–200 dyne·s/cm^5)

$$\text{Venous return (VR)} = \frac{Pms - Pra}{Pvr}$$

4–6 L/min

where PMS = mean systemic pressure — 10–15 mmHg

Rvr = resistance to venous return — 1–2 mmHg/L/min

V. THE INTERNAL MILIEU

Normal Body Water Distribution

Total body water (TBW) in liters	$= 0.6$ (female) $- 0.7$ (male) $\times$ body weight (kg)
Intracellular fluid (ICF)	$= 0.67$ TBW
Extracellular fluid (ECF)	$= 0.33$ TBW
Vascular volume (L)	$= 0.33$ ECF

Normal Electrolyte Concentration Ranges

Na^+	136–146 meq/L
Ka^+	3.5–5.1 meq/L
Cl^-	98–106 meq/L
HCO_3^-	22–26 meq/L
Mg^{2+}	1.3–2.1 meq/L (0.65–1.05 mmol/L)
PO_4^{3-}	2.7–4.5 mg/dL (0.87–1.45 mmol/L)
Ca^{2+}	8.4–10.2 mg/dL (2.1–2.55 mmol/L)
iCa^{2+}	2.24–2.60 meq/L (1.12–1.30 mmol/L)

Calculated osmolality (Osm) =

$$2 \times [Na^+] + \frac{[Glucose]}{18} + \frac{[BUN]}{2.8}$$

Normal = 285–295 mOsm/L

Fractional excretion of sodium

$$FE_{Na} = \frac{[Na^+]urine \times [Cr]serum}{[Na^+]serum \times [Cr]urine}$$

$<1 \rightarrow$ Prerenal
$>1 \rightarrow$ Renal

Anion gap $= [Na^+] - [Cl^-] - [HCO_3^-]$
Normal = 8–12 meq/L

VI.   THE CENTRAL NERVOUS SYSTEM

Glasgow Coma Score

Eye Opening	Spontaneous	4
	To sound	3
	To pain	2
	Never	1
Best motor response	Obeys command	6
	Localizes pain	5
	Flexion (withdraw)	4
	Flexion (abnormal)	3
	Extension	2
	None	1
Best verbal response	Oriented	5
	Confused conversation	4
	Inappropriate words	3
	Incomprehensible sounds	2
	None	1
	Total ranges from	3–15

Principles of
CRITICAL CARE
SECOND EDITION

COMPANION HANDBOOK

Chapter 1 _____

SEVERITY-OF-ILLNESS SCORING SYSTEMS

SHANNON S. CARSON

Over the past two decades, a number of scoring systems have been developed to provide clinicians with standardized means of assessing illness severity in critically ill patients. Most systems do this by providing estimations of survival for groups of intensive care unit (ICU) patients. These systems have proven to be valuable instruments in individual ICUs for assessing quality and planning resource utilization. The ability to make objective comparisons of different groups of ICU patients has also been extremely useful for clinical investigation. These systems have less utility in predicting outcome for individual patients.

Methodology

In general, most of these tools utilize specific physiologic parameters such as vital signs or laboratory values, which are measured on the day of ICU admission. Physiologic variables are chosen based upon predictive value and frequency of routine measurement. Additional variables such as measures of chronic organ dysfunction or admission source may also be included. Variables are weighted according to degree of abnormality, and individual "scores" are obtained from the cumulative weights of abnormal physiologic variables. These scores have a direct correlation to increasing likelihood of death. The physiologic scores may be combined with other variables in logistic regression equations that provide a risk of death for the specific patient. The instruments are validated prospectively in large groups of patients from multiple institutions within a country or from multiple countries. Predictive accuracy of the models is demonstrated by the sensitivity, specificity, and positive and negative predictive values.

1

Discrimination, the ability to correctly separate patients with and without the target outcome, is demonstrated by the area under the receiver operating characteristic (ROC) curve. An area greater than 0.8 suggests good discrimination, and an area of 1.0 is perfect prediction. Calibration, the agreement between the predicted and observed outcomes at all levels of the severity scale, is evaluated using goodness-of-fit statistics.

Frequently Used Severity-of-Illness Scoring Systems

In deciding which scoring system should be used in a given situation, users must consider the population of patients used in the validation of the instrument and make sure that their own patient groups are well represented. The length of time that has passed since the instrument was validated is important. Users should also take into account the convenience, frequency of measurement, and reliability of required variables within their own ICUs. Finally, some instruments have proprietary restrictions that may be prohibitive.

The most frequently cited instrument in the United States is the Acute Physiology and Chronic Health Evaluation (APACHE) II system. This instrument was validated using 5815 patients from 13 different hospitals in the United States. It utilizes 12 physiologic variables as well as age, chronic health measures, and type of admission to determine the APACHE II score, a relative indicator of illness severity. Coefficients corresponding to emergent or nonemergent operative status and diagnosis leading to ICU admission are combined with the APACHE II score in a logistic regression equation to give a predicted mortality. APACHE II did not include patients receiving coronary artery bypass grafting in its validation set.

The authors of the APACHE system revised some variables and increased the number of diagnoses in developing the APACHE III system. APACHE III was validated using 17,440 patients in 40 different U.S. hospitals. The area under the ROC curve for APACHE III for predictions of death made on the first day was 0.9. Risk estimates made on days 2 through 7 of ICU admission can also be obtained with slightly lower discrimination. Use of APACHE III for calculation of predicted mortality is proprietary. Criticisms of APACHE II and III include difficulty in assigning a primary diagnosis to complicated patients with multiple problems and variability in determination of the Glasgow Coma Scale score.

The Mortality Probability Models (MPM II) were validated using 19,124 patients from 12 countries. Variables for MPM II are measured at the time of admission (MPM$_0$) or within the first 24 h of admission (MPM$_{24}$). Burn, coronary care, and cardiac surgery patients were excluded. Areas under the ROC curves were 0.82 for MPM$_0$ and 0.84 for MPM$_{24}$. Systems for estimating mortality 48 or 72 h after admission were developed, but they have lower discrimination. The Simplified Acute Physiology Score (SAPS II) was validated in 1993 using 13,152 patients from 12 countries. Area under the ROC curve for SAPS II was 0.86. Variables for MPM II and SAPS II are outlined in Table 1-1. MPM II and SAPS II do not require a Glasgow Coma Scale score or diagnosis leading to admission.

Rather than using specific physiologic variables, some systems focus on number of organ systems affected—a close parallel to the way many intensivists prognosticate at the bedside. Examples would include the Multiple Organ Dysfunction Score used for surgical patients and the Logistic Organ Dysfunction Score. The Therapeutic Intervention Scoring System (TISS) documents the intensity ICU resources required to manage a patient as a measure of illness severity. This system does not give mortality estimates.

Scoring systems for trauma patients have been developed to assist with triage and for mortality prediction. These systems were developed using general trauma populations from large registries rather than trauma patients specifically requiring ICU care. Some of these systems are described in Table 1-2.

Sources of Bias in Scoring Systems

Error and bias may limit the reproducibility of scoring systems outside the original sample of patients. Not all variables required for a system will always be measured in clinical practice, and this will introduce detection bias. In this instance,

TABLE 1-1   Variables Included in Severity-of-Illness Scoring Systems in Clinical Use

	APACHE II	APACHE III	MPM II_0 ADM	MPM II_{24}, 24 Hours	SAPS II
Age	X	X	X	X	X
Prior treatment location		X			
Type of admission	X	X	X	X	X
CPR prior to ICU admission			X		
Mechanical ventilation			X	X	
Vasoactive drug therapy				X	
Acute diagnoses					
Acute renal failure		X			
Cardiac dysrhythmias		X			
Cerebrovascular incident		X			
Gastrointestinal bleeding		X			
Confirmed infection				X	
Intracranial mass effect			X	X	
Select one of 50 diagnoses	X				
Select one of 78 diagnoses		X			
Physiology					
Temperature	X	X			X
Heart rate	X	X	X		X
Respiratory rate	X	X			
Blood pressure	X	X	X		X
Hematocrit	X	X			
White blood cell count	X	X			X
Albumin		X			
Bilirubin		X			X

(continued on page 5)

Glucose		X			
Serum sodium	X	X			X
Serum potassium	X				X
Serum bicarbonate					X
Blood urea nitrogen		X			X
Creatinine	X	X		X	
Urine output		X		X	X
Pa_{O_2} or $(A-a)D_{O_2}$ or Fi_{O_2}	X	X		X	X
pH and P_{CO_2}	X	X			
Prothrombin time				X	
GCS or modified GCS score	X	X			X
Coma or deep stupor			X	X	
Chronic health status					
AIDS	X	X			X
Immunosuppression	X	X			
Lymphoma	X	X			[a]
Leukemia/mult. myeloma	X	X			[a]
Metastatic cancer		X	X	X	X
Hepatic failure	X	X			
Cirrhosis	X	X	X	X	
Chronic renal insufficiency	X			X	
Chronic heart insufficiency	X				
Chronic respiratory insufficiency	X				

[a] In SAPS II, these two criteria are grouped into one entity called *hematologic malignancy*.

ABBREVIATIONS: APACHE II, Acute Physiology and Chronic Health Evaluation II; APACHE III, Acute Physiology and Chronic Health Evaluation III; MPM II$_0$, Mortality Probability Models II, assessment at ICU admission; MPM II$_{24}$, Mortality Probability Models II, assessment 24 hours after ICU admission; SAPS II, Simplified Acute Physiology Score II; CPR, cardiopulmonary resuscitation; $(A-a) D_{O_2}$, alveolar-arterial oxygen difference; Fi_{O_2}, Fraction of inspired oxygen; GCS, Glasgow Coma Scale; AIDS, acquired immunodeficiency syndrome; mult. myeloma, multiple myeloma.

TABLE 1-2 Characteristics of the Major Trauma Scoring Systems

Name	Purpose and Main Characteristics	Variables Included	Comments
ISS	Description of the severity of injury Anatomic description Blunt trauma	Anatomic variables: 3 highest scoring body regions from the AIS are squared and summed Value 3–75	Developed for MVA (blunt) trauma victims.
TS	Triage Survival probability Physiologic score Blunt and penetrating trauma	Respiratory rate Respiratory effort Systolic blood pressure Capillary refill GCS Range 1–16[a]	Immediately available for triage. Determination of respiratory effort and capillary refill are subjective.
RTS	Triage Survival probability Physiologic score Blunt and penetrating trauma	Respiratory rate Systolic blood pressure GCS Each coded 0–4 Range 0–12[b]	Value of each variable empiric, but weight of variables for probability of survival by regression analysis. Better goodness of fit than TS.

TRISS	Survival probability Considers anatomy, physiology, age, blunt and penetrating trauma	RTS ISS (with revised AIS-85) Age < or > 55 years Blunt/penetrating trauma	Coefficients by regression analysis. Different values for blunt or penetrating trauma.
ASCOT	Survival probability Considers anatomy, physiology, age, blunt and penetrating trauma	RTS Anatomy profile component— ICD/AIS-85 Age (5 subclasses) Blunt/penetrating trauma Set-aside: very severe or very minor injury	More variables for calculation of survival probability. Better performance than TRISS for blunt and penetrating trauma.

[a]A score of 1 is the worst prognosis.
[b]A score of 0 is the worst prognosis.
ABBREVIATIONS: ISS, Injury Severity Score; TS, Trauma Score; RTS, Revised Trauma Score; TRISS, Trauma Score, ISS, age combination index; ASCOT, A Severity Characterization of Trauma; GCS, Glasgow Coma Scale; AIS, Abbreviated Injury Scale; AIS-85, The fifth review of the Abbreviated Injury Scale; ICD, International classification of diseases.

unmeasured variables are assigned normal values, which will underestimate mortality. Many systems require use of the worst physiologic value in 24 hours, which is sometimes difficult to determine. Also, assessment of neurologic function in sedated patients is problematic. Statistical regression techniques often underpredict the likelihood of death in patients with higher illness severity and overpredict the likelihood of death for less severely ill patients. Therefore, hospitals that tend to manage patients at either end of the spectrum may not be fairly represented. The length of time that a patient is critically ill prior to ICU admission, or lead-time differences, can affect mortality. This becomes an issue for patients transferred from another ICU or hospital wards. Finally, rapid correction of severe physiologic abnormalities in the emergency department prior to arrival in the ICU may lead to underestimation of illness severity.

Applications of Severity-of-Illness Measures

Various applications of severity-of-illness scoring systems are outlined in Table 1-3. In clinical trials, severity of illness can be used to characterize the study population for comparison with other studies and one's own practice. The systems are helpful in assessing the success of randomization and in performing stratified randomization. In the administration of an ICU, scoring systems can be used to relate resource utilization to severity of illness or to help assess the effectiveness of changes in personnel, organization, or admission policies. Comparisons of performance with that of other ICUs can be carried out in a more objective manner as long as the validation group for the scoring system represents the different ICUs fairly. In using scoring systems to assess ICU performance, it should be remembered that the systems do not measure quality of life, functional status, or patient satisfaction, nor do they predict long-term outcomes beyond hospital survival.

The use of severity-of-illness scoring systems to guide patient management is controversial. Most instruments were designed and validated using data from patients already admitted to an ICU; therefore using scoring systems to make triage decisions regarding appropriateness of ICU admission

TABLE 1-3 Potential Uses of Severity-of-Illness
Scoring Systems

Uses of scoring systems in randomized, controlled trials (RCTs) and
  clinical research
  To compare different RCTs and clinical studies
  To determine sample size
  To do stratified randomization (a priori subgroups identification;
     stratification for severity of illness)
  To assess success of randomization
  To assess treatment effects in subgroups (post hoc subgroup
    identification)
  To compare study patients with patients in clinicians' practices
Uses of scoring systems for administrative purposes
  To describe resource utilization of ICU
  To describe acuity of illness
  To relate resource utilization to acuity of care
  To guide reimbursement and budget of ICU
Uses of scoring systems to assess ICU performance
  Quality Assurance
    To assess performance of an ICU in general or for specific
     disease category
    To assess performance of an ICU over time
    To compare individual intensivists' performances
    To assess the performance of a therapeutic intervention
  Comparison of ICU performance in different categories of
    hospitals, countries, etc.
  Performance for different ICU administrative characteristics
    (open/closed unit, communication, ICU director task, etc.)
  Effectiveness
Uses of scoring systems to assess individual patient prognosis and
  to guide care
  Triage of patients
  Decisions regarding intensity of care
  Decisions to withhold and withdraw care

---

is not valid. Some trauma scoring systems would be exceptions (see above). Use of scoring systems to guide decisions
regarding withholding and withdrawal of care is problematic
because these instruments were developed to describe illness
severity and predict mortality in groups of patients rather

than individual patients. Although some systems may be more accurate than clinicians in predicting mortality of high-risk patients, the highest precision reported for any instrument is 95% probability of death. This means that 5% of patients in that group would survive. Information from scoring systems may be useful to a clinician or a patient in making difficult decisions regarding care, but only within the context of the individual patient's overall clinical circumstances and the patient's own wishes regarding aggressive care.

For a more detailed discussion, see Chap. 7 in *Principles of Critical Care,* 2d ed.

Chapter 2

CARDIOPULMONARY RESUSCITATION

DELBERT DORSCHEID

The American Heart Association (AHA) provides guidelines for resuscitation of patients in a wide variety of clinical circumstances. As such, these AHA protocols should form the basis of treatment of critically ill patients in cardiopulmonary arrest. However, the AHA algorithms should not be viewed as all-encompassing or inflexible. Rather, an approach that creatively utilizes all the diagnostic and therapeutic modalities readily available in the intensive care unit (ICU) offers the greatest likelihood of successful resuscitation.

General Principles

Cardiopulmonary arrest implies the state of profoundly inadequate tissue perfusion and oxygen delivery such that cell death is imminent. The absolute length of time that any given tissue bed can survive in this condition before irreversible damage results is controversial. Nonetheless, it is clear that unless resuscitated within a very few minutes, the patient who experiences cardiopulmonary arrest is unlikely to survive to discharge. AHA guidelines reccomend early assessment and defibrillation, when indicated, to reestablish adequate circulation and ventilation prior to attending to the airway, breathing, and circulation—the ABCs of resuscitation. In addition to urgent defibrillation, other features of the resuscitation that take precedence over the ABCs are the need to protect the patient from further injury and compression of exsanguinating hemorrhage.

Control of the *airway* and provision of adequate *breathing* are immediate objectives in all patients. This is not to say that every patient must be intubated but rather that immediate assessment of airway and breathing coupled with measures to correct the deficiencies revealed are always the highest priorities. Oral airways, bag-mask ventilation, and noninvasive positive-pressure ventilation are alternatives. Inadequate perfusion can certainly occur in the presence of a "normal" blood pressure. Therefore, assessment of *circulation* should include not only blood pressure and heart rate but also indicators of end-organ perfusion such as the temperature of the extremities, capillary refill, the quality of mentation and level of consciousness, and urine output. An adequate circulating volume is essential and must be swiftly established through the rapid infusion of crystalloid, colloid, or red blood cells (Chap. 24). Unlike many other clinical situations, volume resuscitation of the patient in cardiopulmonary arrest requires the ability to infuse liters of fluid within minutes. Placement of a short, large-bore central catheter is a high priority. AHA guidelines suggest the use of large-bore antecubital vein catheters, but in the critical care setting, venous catheters in the internal jugular or subclavian vein (*not* "triple-lumen" or pulmonary artery catheters, which have multiple small-caliber channels, but a large-bore catheter) are preferred. In addition to hypovolemia, dysrhythmias such as bradycardia or tachycardia or a depressed inotropic state may also explain the circulatory collapse. The dysrhythmias and resuscitation strategies are discussed below. The primary indication for the empiric use of a vasoconstrictor is the absence of appropriate vasoconstriction in the setting of hypotension. Use of these agents in other situations should be considered a temporizing measure only, until the underlying problem can be adequately addressed.

If resuscitation is successful, the level of *disability* must be assessed. This includes a determination of the present neurologic status and how it may compare to previous assessments. Various assessment scales exist, but the Glasgow Coma Scale (Table 2-1) is the most elaborate and is best able to predict the subsequent treatment and outcome. Additional consideration includes the need for ongoing *diagnosis* of the causative cardiac dysrhythmia. This is to ensure the maintenance of the stable patient and to arrive at a definitive therapy. Following is a summary of the major dysrhythmias and the suggested AHA treatment guidelines during the resuscitation phase.

TABLE 2-1   Glasgow Coma Scale

Eye opening points
    4   Spontaneously opens eyes
    3   Opens eyes to verbal command
    2   Opens eyes to painful stimulus
    1   Does not open eyes to pain
Verbal response points
    5   Completely oriented
    4   Confused conversation
    3   Inappropriate words
    2   Incomprehensible sounds
    1   No verbal response
Motor response points
    6   Obeys commands
    5   Localizes to pain
    4   Withdraws to pain
    3   Decorticate posturing
    2   Decerebrate posturing
    1   Flaccid

NOTE: Score = eye opening points + verbal response points + motor response points; total possible points = 15; coma = 8 or less; worst score = 3.

Ventricular Fibrillation/Pulseless Ventricular Tachycardia

Ventricular fibrillation is the most common cause of sudden death and the most amenable to treatment (Table 2-2). The absolute priority in any attempt at resuscitation from ventricular fibrillation or pulseless ventricular tachycardia is defibrillation. Neither cardiopulmonary resuscitation (CPR) nor attempts at intubation should be instituted until failure of the first three defibrillation attempts, assuming that a defibrillator is immediately available. If initial attempts at defibrillation fail, attention should be turned toward optimizing myocardial responsiveness by improving oxygenation, acid-base status, and myocardial perfusion pressure. Correction of hypoxia and acidosis are best accomplished by securing control of the airway and assisting ventilation with 100% supplemental oxygen. Myocardial perfusion pressure (diastolic blood pressure minus right atrial pressure) of at least 15 mmHg appears to be critical for successful defibrillation.

TABLE 2-2   Approach to Ventricular Fibrillation
and Pulseless Ventricular Tachycardia

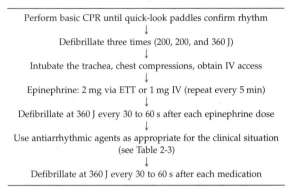

Perform basic CPR until quick-look paddles confirm rhythm
↓
Defibrillate three times (200, 200, and 360 J)
↓
Intubate the trachea, chest compressions, obtain IV access
↓
Epinephrine: 2 mg via ETT or 1 mg IV (repeat every 5 min)
↓
Defibrillate at 360 J every 30 to 60 s after each epinephrine dose
↓
Use antiarrhythmic agents as appropriate for the clinical situation
(see Table 2-3)
↓
Defibrillate at 360 J every 30 to 60 s after each medication

Hence, in addition to the institution of CPR, epinephrine is recommended in an attempt to raise mean arterial pressure. There is evidence, however, that the standard recommended dose of 0.5 to 1.0 mg IV push every 5 min may be grossly inadequate and consideration of much greater doses of epinephrine (up to 0.2 mg/kg) may be appropriate. Present guidelines suggest that a regimen of escalating doses of epinephrine (e.g., 1, 3, and 5 mg every 5 min) can be useful in some resuscitative efforts. A variety of antiarrhythmic agents may be useful when initial defibrillation fails or to stabilize the just-resuscitated patient. The list of candidate drug options is listed in Table 2-3.

Ventricular Tachycardia with a Pulse

The appropriate response to the patient experiencing ventricular tachycardia with a pulse depends on how well the patient is tolerating the dysrhythmia (Table 2-4). Unstable patients, who should be cardioverted at an early stage, include those experiencing chest pain, dyspnea, congestive heart failure (CHF), hypotension, or other evidence of inadequate tissue perfusion. Even then, cardioversion should be attempted

TABLE 2-3   Antiarrhythmic Options for Ventricular
Tachycardia or Fibrillation

---

1. Lidocaine: 1.5 mg/kg for 2 doses (max: 3 mg/kg)—may be
   followed with an infusion of 1 to 4 mg/min.
2. Bretylium: 5 mg/kg IV initially, then 10 mg/kg IV every 5 min up
   to 35 mg/kg—may be followed with an infusion of 1 to 4 mg/min.
3. Magnesium sulfate: 1 to 2 g IV, up to 10 g—may be followed with
   an infusion of 1 to 5 g/h.
4. Procainamide: 17 mg/kg IV given not faster than 30 mg/min—
   may be followed with an infusion of 1 to 4 mg/min.
5. Sodium bicarbonate: 1 to 2 meq/kg IV for patients with cyclic
   antidepressant overdose—may be followed by an infusion to
   maintain serum pH between 7.5 and 7.55.
6. Amiodarone: 150 mg IV over 10 min, followed by an infusion of
   1 mg/min for 6 h, then 0.5 mg/min for 18 h—additional boluses of
   150 mg may be necessary for recurrent VT/VF.

---

in a conscious patient only after sedation with a short-acting
barbiturate or benzodiazepine. For the stable patient the antiarrhythmic medications listed in Table 2-3 are all candidates.

TABLE 2-4   Ventricular Tachycardia with a Pulse

If stable:
    Oxygen, IV access
    Lidocaine, 1 mg/kg bolus
    Lidocaine, 0.5 mg/kg every 8 min until ventricular tachycardia
      has resolved or total 3 mg/kg is reached
    Procainamide, 20 mg/min until ventricular tachycardia is
      resolved or 1 g total is reached
If unstable (chest pain, dyspnea, CHF, hypotension, infarction):
    Oxygen, IV access
    Lidocaine, 1 mg/kg bolus
    (Consider sedation)
    Synchronized cardioversion at 50 J
    Synchronized cardioversion at 100 J
    Synchronized cardioversion at 200 J
    Synchronized cardioversion at up to 360 J
    If recurrent, lidocaine, procainamide, or bretylium
    Repeat cardioversion at previously successful level

TABLE 2-5   Asystole

If possibly ventricular fibrillation, defibrillate
CPR, IV access
Epinephrine, 0.5–1.0 mg IV every 5 min
Intubate when possible
Atropine, 1.0 mg IV, repeat × 1 or 2 in 5 min
(Consider bicarbonate)
Consider pacing

Asystole/Bradycardia

Tables 2-5 and 2-6 detail the AHA algorithms for resuscitating the asystolic or bradycardic patient. There is some evidence that extreme vagal tone can lead to asystole; therefore a fully vagolytic dose of atropine (2 to 3 mg) may be considered as the initial dose rather than the traditional recommendation of 1.0 mg. If no treatable cause is found, the resuscitation effort should be considered futile after 20 min in all cases except hypothermia.

In general, bradycardias require urgent treatment only when they are hemodynamically significant or when ventricular escape ectopy is apparent. In heart block or bradycardia where the QRS is longer than 0.12 ms and likely to be

TABLE 2-6   Bradycardia

If sinus, junctional, 1° AVB,[a] or type I 2° AVB, treat only if signs or
    symptoms present. If type II 2° AVB or 3° AVB, treat even if
    asymptomatic.
Atropine, 0.5 mg–1.0 IV (should be considered safe only if the
    ventricular escape originates high in the conduction fibers,
    junctional)
Repeat atropine every 5 min until total 3.0 mg is reached
External pacemaker
or
Dopamine, 2–20 μg/kg/min or isoproterenol, 2–10 μg/min
Transvenous pacemaker

---

[a]AVB, atrioventricular bradycardia.

originating from low in the conduction tract, the use of atropine should be discouraged due to a possible paradoxical response.

Pulseless Electrical Activity (PEA)

The presence of a complex with a very weak or absent pulse should immediately generate a search for evidence of hypovolemia, hypoxia, pneumothorax, acidosis, pericardial tamponade, and pulmonary embolus. Swift correction of these conditions is essential for successful resuscitation from PEA (Table 2-7). Institution of specific therapeutic interventions, however, may depend upon their availability—e.g., the immediate ability to perform pulmonary arterial embolectomy. In addition, as the goal of resuscitation is the prevention of premature or unnecessary death but not to prolong the act of dying, reflexive institution of all heroic measures in every patient is probably not warranted.

TABLE 2-7   Differential Diagnosis and Therapy of Pulseless Electrical Activity

---

HYPOs
   Hypoxemia—ABCs
   Hypovolemia—volume infusion
   Hypothermia—warming
Circulatory obstruction
   Pericardial tamponade—volume infusion, pericardiocentesis
   Tension pneumothorax—needle or tube thoracostomy
   Pulmonary embolism—thrombolysis, thrombectomy
Primary cardiac
   Massive myocardial infarction—reperfusion
   Acute valvular regurgitation—afterload reduction, surgery
   Myocardial rupture—afterload reduction, pericardiocentesis, surgery
Toxins
   Digitalis—Fab fragments
   Ca^{2+} channel blockers—calcium, glucagon
   β-blockers—glucagon
   Cyclic antidepressants—sodium bicarbonate

Supraventricular Tachycardia

Patients who are hypotensive, experiencing chest pain, or are otherwise seriously threatened by the dysrhythmia should be treated with synchronized cardioversion, using 50 to 350 J, whereas others less seriously threatened can be treated by vagotonic maneuvers or agents such as adenosine, esmolol, and diltiazem; overdrive pacing; and synchronized cardioversion if necessary. Not uncommonly it is unclear whether a tachycardia is supraventricular or ventricular in origin. The unstable patient should be promptly cardioverted in either case. In the stable patient, however, a trial of adenosine (6 mg injected quickly followed by 12 mg if the tachycardia persists) may clarify the site of origin of the tachycardia and in some cases even distupt it.

Miscellaneous Issues

Bicarbonate is frequently administered to patients in cardiopulmonary arrest, often even in the absence of blood gas evidence of acidemia. Recently some have pointed out the lack of efficacy of sodium bicarbonate in cardiac resuscitation. Because of the ease with which carbon dioxide crosses cell membranes compared to the more polar bicarbonate ion, some investigators are concerned about the generation of a paradoxical intracellular acidosis. Therefore routine administration of bicarbonate cannot be recommended.

Calcium is an excellent inotrope in situations of decreased ionized calcium. Such conditions may exist in the patient coming off a bypass pump or receiving massive transfusions, as in the setting of liver transplantation. Additionally, calcium is effective in reversing the vasodilation produced by calcium-channel blockers, such as verapamil. However, there is no evidence that calcium administration improves survival rates during cardiopulmonary resuscitation. In addition, there is concern about the cytotoxic effects of calcium, which could leak into ischemic cells.

Resuscitation in the ICU may at times offer therapeutic modalities not often available on regular hospital wards. Fiberoptic bronchoscopy may be of use for clarifying appropriate endotracheal tube (ETT) placement and patency.

Echocardiography allows rapid assessment of both left and right ventricular filling and function as well as detection of pericardial effusions and assessment of their hemodynamic significance. End-tidal CO_2 monitoring may also allow assessment of ETT positioning as well as the return of cardiac output. Hence, resuscitation in the ICU offers an opportunity for implementation of creative diagnostic and therapeutic approaches.

For a more detailed discussion, see Chap. 8 in *Principles of Critical Care,* 2d ed.

Chapter 3

VASCULAR CANNULATION

PHILLIP FACTOR

Peripheral Venous Cannulation

The peripheral venous system comprises the veins found by palpation or observation in the subcutaneous tissues; they are typically the first choice for vascular access in hemodynamically stable patients. These veins are readily accessible in most patients and can accommodate large-bore catheters that rival central lines in their fluid delivery rates. However, in the setting of hemodynamic compromise, it should be kept in mind that the time from fluid administration to arrival at the right atrium may be unpredictable. Many factors affect peripheral intravenous (IV) site selection, including adequacy of peripheral veins, required duration of cannulation, patient mobility and comfort, planned infusion rate, and catheter size. Infusion of hypertonic solutions and large-bore catheters may prove irritating to the endothelium, leading to discomfort, infusion phlebitis, and increased risk of catheter-related infection. Central venous access may be preferable in these settings. Complications of peripheral venous cannulation include infection (cellulitis, septicemia), vasovagal responses, subcutaneous infiltration and skin necrosis, subcutaneous hematomas, and thrombophlebitis. Catheter care is an extensive subject, but based on a number of studies and the practices at our hospitals, we recommend the following: (1) all peripheral catheters should be changed at intervals of 72 h or less; (2) catheters inserted in emergency situations should be changed as soon as possible; and (3) dressing changes should be performed every 24 to 48 h, preferably by a dedicated IV team.

21

Central Venous Cannulation

Central venous cannulation is preferred over peripheral access for the indications listed in Table 3-1. No absolute contraindication to central venous access can be identified. Other than coagulopathy and recent fibrinolytic therapy, contraindications are site specific (Table 3-2).

GENERAL CONSIDERATIONS

Regardless of the site of method chosen for central venous cannulation, the patient must be well informed and must give appropriate consent; all equipment should be at the bedside and the patient prepositioned. In the absence of externalized cerebral ventricular drains or impending respiratory failure, most patients can tolerate a few moments of reverse Trendelenburg positioning. Supplemental oxygen should be employed in patients at risk for arterial desaturation (e.g., lower lobe pneumonias or placement of sterile drapes over the face). Skin antisepsis should include an iodine-based solution, which should be allowed to air-dry. Sterile technique is required with the placement of any central line. Inexperienced operators should be closely supervised; sedated, mechanically ventilated patients should be considered for physicians in training. Critically ill patients who require central venous

TABLE 3-1   Indications for Central Venous Access

Inadequate peripheral veins
Central venous pressure monitoring (CVP, pulmonary artery
   catheters)
Administration of phlebitic medications (potassium, chemotherapy)
Extremely rapid fluid administration
Cardiopulmonary resuscitation
Intracardiac pacing
Frequent phlebotomies
Long-term intravenous therapy (antibiotics, chemotherapy)
Hemodialysis
Hyperalimentation
Administration of vasoactive drugs

TABLE 3-2   Relative Contraindications to Central Venous Cannulation

General contraindications
   Physician inexperience
   Coagulopathy
   Recent fibrinolytic therapy
   Severe thrombocytopenia
   Inability to identify pertinent landmarks
   Infection or burn at planned catheter entry site
   Uncooperative patient
Subclavian vein
   Upper thoracic trauma
   Compromised pulmonary function (COPD)
   High levels of PEEP
   Coagulopathy
   SVC thrombosis
   Severe electrolyte or acid-base disturbance
Internal jugular vein
   Inability to identify landmarks
   COPD, high levels of PEEP
   Tracheostomy with excessive pulmonary secretions
   SVC thrombosis
Femoral vein
   Absence of femoral pulse
   Vena caval compromise: clot, extrinsic compression, IVC filter
   Local infection at insertion site
   Penetrating abdominal trauma
   Cardiac arrest or low-flow states
   Requirements for patient mobility

ABBREVIATIONS: COPD, chronic obstructive pulmonary disease; PEEP, positive end-expiratory pressure; SVC, superior vena cava; IVC, inferior vena cava.

cannulation are frequently confused or uncooperative. Extreme caution must be exercised to prevent uncontrolled general anesthesia when parenteral sedation is used, especially in patients with compromised cardiopulmonary and neurologic function. Short-acting parenteral benzodiazepines are useful in this setting. Following catheter placement, adequacy of blood return should be reconfirmed. Postprocedure chest x-ray should be used to confirm catheter tip location (ideally 2 to 4 cm above the junction of the right atrium and superior vena cava) and to rule out pneumothorax.

CATHETER SELECTION

Catheter-through-needle devices should be avoided. These cannulation devices require utilization of a larger than necessary needle and confer the additional risk of catheter emboli if the catheter is inadvertently withdrawn through the needle. Readily available catheter-over-needle devices and prepared guidewire kits make this method unnecessary, even in emergency situations. Long-arm catheters are placed via the antecubital veins and advanced into the central venous circulation. These devices are excellent choices for patients with coagulopathies, although advancement of these catheters into the thorax can be difficult. These catheters can occupy the entire lumen of an antecubital vein, leading to venous stasis, endothelial injury, and thrombophlebitis. Until more data regarding use of these catheters are available, long-term use cannot be recommended.

The requirement for long-term indwelling central venous catheters has been met with the development of barium-impregnated silicone rubber (Silastic) catheters (i.e., Hickman, Gorshong, Quinton, Broviac), which can be tunneled beneath the skin prior to entry into a central vein. This type of tunneled catheter has a small Dacron cuff, which is positioned subcutaneously to serve as a mechanical barrier to migration of bacteria along the catheter. These devices require a high level of care, including frequent heparin flushes and dressing changes. Patients can be educated to care for their own catheters, allowing increased independence from health care facilities. Tunneled catheters are not without risk; infection, central vein thrombosis, and thrombotic occlusion of the catheter may occur. Slowed infusion rates or inability to withdraw blood may suggest catheter thrombosis. Administration of streptokinase or urokinase through the catheter may be useful in this setting. Totally implantable catheter devices obviate some of the problems with tunneled catheters. This type of device typically consists of a stainless steel or plastic portal with a self-sealing diaphragm connected to a central catheter. A Huber needle is inserted through the skin to access the device. The subcutaneous location eliminates the need for difficult dressing changes and daily heparin flushes. The reported infection rates are approximately one-third those of externalized, tunneled catheters. Mechanical problems such as occlusion and inability to withdraw blood occur frequently.

The high flows required for dialysis require the placement of large-bore double-lumen catheters into the central venous system. Stiff, large-bore catheters limit patient mobility, are associated with venous perforation, and require frequent replacement. Utilization of flexible silicone rubber catheters with Dacron cuffs (e.g., Quinton Permacath) now allows these catheters to be left in place for prolonged periods pending creation and maturation of an arteriovenous graft or fistula.

Multiple-lumen catheters have supplanted the need for multiple central venous lines. The widespread use of these catheters has preceded adequate study of the risks, costs, and complications. Pending further study, several recommendations regarding their use can be made: (1) they should be used only when peripheral access is inadequate to support multiple lines; (2) the subclavian vein should be the preferred site of insertion; (3) these catheters should not be placed through catheter sheath introducers; (4) a uniform, hospitalwide protocol describing catheter use and care (e.g., frequency of heparin flushes and dressing changes, specific port utilization) should be employed. No specific recommendations can be made regarding duration of cannulation. Routine catheter changes every 5 to 7 days may decrease the incidence of line-related sepsis in some settings but are associated with an increased risk of insertion-related complications (see below).

Catheter sheath introducers are large-bore catheters (8.5F) that were developed to facilitate the placement of pulmonary artery catheters. These short, Teflon-coated catheters are also useful for rapid volume administration (see below). Several problems have been associated with them, including vascular perforation, air embolism, and infection. These catheters are not designed for long-term use (i.e., >72 h) and should not be left in place following restoration of intravascular volume or removal of a pulmonary artery (PA) catheter. If a PA catheter is not inserted into the sheath introducer, it is important that the catheter be occluded with the obturator that is included with the sheath introducer kit to prevent air embolism and bacterial migration. Most sheath introducers are not designed for use with triple-lumen catheters. The inability to secure multilumen catheters to sheath introducers can result in unwanted inward and outward movement, which may track bacteria (or air) into the sheath introducer or lead to migration into the right heart. Certain clinical settings require extremely rapid delivery of volume. Placement of a short, 8.5F sheath introducer into a large central vein (internal jugular, subclavian, or femoral vein) can allow for pressurized delivery rates of up to 1400 mL/min through the side port. Fluid administration rates in these ranges are most likely to be limited by the IV tubing diameter. Use of blood infusion, large-bore trauma tubing, or urologic tubing will reduce this limitation.

Catheter Insertion Techniques

The selection of a site should be guided on the basis of operator experience and clinical situation. The techniques described below utilize the Seldinger techniques of guidewire-directed cannulation. Regardless of site or technique, careful consideration must be given when advancement of the guidewire through the right heart is planned in unstable patients, especially in the presence of profound acid-base, temperature, and electrolyte abnormalities due to the high risk of ventricular arrhythmias. Table 3-2 provides a list of general and site-specific relative contraindications.

INTERNAL JUGULAR VEIN CANNULATION

There are three commonly practiced approaches to cannulation of this vein. The method chosen should reflect prior experience and judgment based on prior experience.

The medial approach (Fig. 3-1C) is a good choice for inexperienced operators. The patient should be supine, in Trendelenburg position, with the head turned slightly to the contralateral side. The needle is advanced through the skin at the apex formed by the junction of the sternal and clavicular heads of the sternocleidomastoid muscle. The needle should

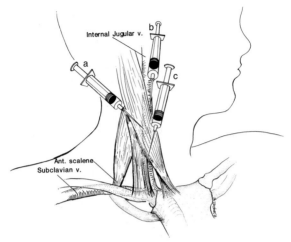

FIGURE 3-1 Internal jugular vein cannulation. Lateral approach (a). Anterior approach (b). Medial approach (c).

be elevated approximately 30 degrees above the neck and directed toward the ipsilateral nipple. The needle should be advanced slowly to a depth not to exceed 2 cm to avoid the common complication of pneumothorax. If this is unsuccessful, the needle should be withdrawn and reduced to an angle of about 15 degrees above the skin. If cannulation is unsuccessful after a total of five attempts, alternative approaches should be pursued.

The anterior approach (Fig. 3-1*B*) requires that the needle be inserted through the skin lateral to the carotid pulse, along the medial border of the sternocleidomastoid at the level of the inferior margin of the thyroid cartilage. As with the median approach, the needle should be held 30 degrees above the neck and advanced no more than 2 or 3 cm toward the ipsilateral nipple. If this is unsuccessful, the angle between the syringe and skin may be reduced.

With the lateral approach (Fig. 3-1*A*), the needle is advanced through the skin where the external jugular vein crosses the lateral margin of the sternocleidomastoid muscle, typically about 4 cm above the sternoclavicular joint. Unlike the case in the other internal jugular approaches, the needle should be advanced toward the contralateral nipple to a depth that should not exceed 3 to 4 cm. This approach has an increased risk of carotid artery puncture but less risk of pneumothorax.

SUBCLAVIAN VEIN CANNULATION

As with the internal jugular vein, three commonly used infraclavicular approaches are available for cannulation of the subclavian vein. Several supraclavicular approaches have also been described but are rarely practiced and are associated with significant risk of pneumothorax. For subclavian vein cannulation, the patient should be supine and in the Trendelenburg position. A small towel placed between the scapulae will help open up the sternoclavicular angle and improve access for the infraclavicular approaches. Of the infraclavicular approaches, the medial approach is most commonly used (Fig. 3-2C). An entrance site 1 cm below and lateral to the junction of the medial one-third and distal two-thirds of the clavicle is selected. The needle should be advanced through the skin at a 15-degree angle above the chest wall and directed toward the suprasternal notch. If difficulty advancing the needle behind the clavicle is encountered, direct posterior pressure on the needle at the skin insertion site will help keep it in a plane parallel to the chest wall and limit entry into the thoracic cavity while allowing passage behind the clavicle. The needle should be advanced no more than 4 cm. If necessary, the needle should be retracted and redirected in more inferior and superior directions. Once the vein is cannulated, the bevel of the needle should be rotated toward the right atrium to facilitate guidewire placement.

The lateral approach (Fig. 3-2A) is similar to the medial except that the entrance site is at the junction of the lateral one-third and medial two-thirds of the clavicle. The risks of subclavian artery puncture and brachial plexus injury limit the utility of this route, although it may be good for patients with narrow sternoclavicular angles. The middle approach (Fig. 3-2B) employs an entrance site midway between the medial and lateral approaches. Insertion technique is otherwise the same.

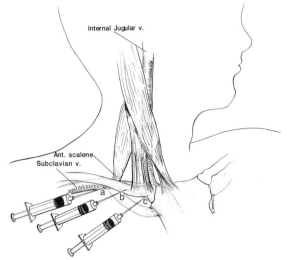

FIGURE 3-2 Subclavian vein cannulation, infraclavicular approaches. Lateral approach (a). Middle approach (b). Medial approach (c).

FEMORAL VEIN CANNULATION

The extrathoracic location of this vessel makes it an excellent choice for cannulation in patients with coagulopathies or those who are at extreme risk for pneumothorax or ventricular arrhythmias. Recent data also indicate that common iliac vein pressures obtained from femorally inserted catheters are accurate reflections of central venous pressure. When these catheters are properly cared for, short-term infection rates are similar to those with internal jugular and subclavian catheters. The femoral vein should be cannulated 1 to 3 cm below the inguinal ligament immediately medial to the femoral arterial pulse. The needle should be advanced in a direction parallel to the arterial pulse. Difficulty with guidewire insertion may be due to needle advancement into or through the posterior wall of the vein; withdrawal of the needle and lowering the syringe to the skin may obviate this problem. Poor delivery of medications to the right atrium has been observed in low-cardiac-output states, making this site a poor choice for use during cardiac arrests.

AXILLARY VEIN CANNULATION

This uncommon site can be used to access the central circulation. In severely burned patients, it may be the only available site for cannulation. Cannulation is achieved by inserting a needle inferior to the axillary artery in the apex of the axilla and advancing it in a direction parallel to the axillary artery. Rotation of the head toward the entrance site may reduce the incidence of cephalad malpositioning of the catheter tip. This site is associated with a low risk of pneumothorax and is useful when pulmonary artery catheterization is planned. No data regarding infection risk are available to permit the development of guidelines for duration of use.

EXTERNAL JUGULAR VEIN CANNULATION

Although the external jugular vein is not truly a central vein, its junction with the subclavian vein may occasionally allow for guidewire advancement into the central venous circulation.

Complications of Central Venous Cannulation

The complications of central venous cannulation are listed in Table 3-3. Pneumothoraxes due to central venous cannulation do not always require tube thoracostomy. Chest tubes should be placed in patients with hemodynamic or respiratory compromise (e.g., tension pneumothorax) or nonresolving pneumothoraxes. Uncomplicated pneumothoraxes (i.e., no pleural fluid) can be treated with small-diameter chest tubes attached to one-way valves (thoracic vents). Catheter embolism is typically associated with the use of catheter-through-needle devices. Removal of these emboli can present a difficult clinical challenge. Snares have been developed to facilitate their removal. The sudden onset of mental status changes, hypoten-

TABLE 3-3   Complications of Central Venous Cannulation

Pneumothorax
Catheter or guidewire embolism
Catheter knotting
Air embolism
Central vein thrombosis
Arrhythmias
Myocardial or central vein perforation
Cardiac tamponade
Infection (local or systemic)
Hydrothorax
Hematoma
Myocardial perforation
Phrenic nerve, brachial plexus damage
Subcutaneous emphysema or fluid infiltration
Arterial puncture and/or laceration
Catheter malposition
Thoracic duct laceration

---

sion, and rash (livedo reticularis of the upper extremities) should suggest the diagnosis of air embolism. A churning, "cogwheel" murmur may be heard. This complication can occur with any form of IV access. Patients should be placed in the left lateral decubitis position. Successful aspiration of air from the right ventricle has been reported using large-bore central lines. Central vein thrombosis occurs in 20 to 70 percent of chronically cannulated patients and is often asymptomatic. Diagnosis is based on clinical suspicion, reduced catheter flow rates, and signs of venous obstruction. Venography is the diagnostic procedure of choice, although Doppler ultrasound and iodine-125 fibrinogen scanning are also useful. Fibrinolytics can be useful in symptomatic patients; rarely, surgical thrombectomy is required. Arrhythmias occur frequently with the passage of central lines into the right ventricle. Patients with preexisting left bundle branch block may be at risk for complete heart block if the right bundle becomes injured during catheter placement. Empiric pacemaker placement is not necessary; however, a transcutaneous pacemaker should be available if required. Central venous and right ventricular perforations are unusual but not rare complications of central venous cannulation. Perforation typically occurs with the use of stiff catheters that are advanced too far into the central circulation. New pleural fluid collections or x-ray signs of a mediastinal hematoma should suggest the diagnosis if the perforation is above the pericardium. Right ventricular or superior vena cava (SVC) perforation typically presents as cardiac tamponade and is usually fatal. Cautious advancement of a pliable catheter can prevent this problem. The distal portion of the central catheter should be 2 to 4 cm above the junction of the right atrium and SVC, and the catheter tip should lie parallel to the cannulated vessel, not perpendicular to its wall.

In general, if catheter-related infection is suspected and the entry site appears clean, the catheter can be changed over a guidewire pending the results of blood and quantitative catheter-tip cultures. If the catheter-tip culture yields more than 15 colony-forming units (CFU) and the blood culture is positive for the same organism, catheter-related sepsis is likely. Positive catheter cultures (>15 CFU) and negative blood cultures indicate catheter infection. Catheter-related sepsis requires that the line be removed and a new insertion site selected. Tunneled catheter-related infections present a more challenging problem. Many cases of sepsis related to these lines can be treated with parenteral antibiotics. The catheter should be removed if signs of septicemia persist (>3 to 5 days) despite appropriate antibiotics, if spetic emboli appear, or if the catheter tunnel is infected. Successful treatment of fungal catheter infections is unlikely and should prompt removal of the catheter. Persistent bacteremia following catheter removal in the presence of documented central vein thrombosis suggests the diagnosis of catheter-related septic central vein thrombosis. This condition can be treated medically with antibiotics and anticoagulation.

Arterial Cannulation

Arterial pressure monitoring has become commonplace in critical care settings due to improvements in the function and availability of bedside pressure monitoring devices and the increased use of arterial blood gases. Arterial lines can be used for infusion of fluids and nonvasoactive medications in emergency settings. Because of its peripheral and accessible location, the radial artery is the first choice for most patients. The axillary, dorsalis pedis, and femoral arteries are used less often. When used in appropriately selected patients however, they have complication rates similar to those of radial artery cannulation. The use of end arteries (e.g., the brachial artery) is not recommended due to the high risk of limb-threatening ischemia.

The overall complication rate of arterial catheterization is difficult to determine but appears to rise with underlying coagulopathy, hypotension, underlying peripheral vascular disease, duration of cannulation, placement by cutdown, number of cannulation attempts, and the ratio of catheter-to-artery diameter. The three primary complications of note are bleeding, infection, and distal limb ischemia. Other less frequent complications are site-related and include peripheral nerve damage (especially to the radial nerve), arteriovenous fistulas, pseudoaneurysm formation, air embolism, cerebral embolism, retroperitoneal hemorrhage, and peritoneal perforation.

RADIAL ARTERY CATHETERIZATION

No absolute contraindication to radial artery cannulation can be offered other than absence of ulnar collateral flow. Patients with Raynaud's phenomenon, thromboangiitis obliterans, and other large vessel vasculitides should be considered carefully prior to catheter placement. Some 15 to 20 percent of patients have inadequate collateral circulation to the hand; thus Allen's test should be performed in all patients prior to attempts at cannulation of the radial artery. Return of normal color to the fingers should occur within 7 s; longer than 14 s should definitely be considered abnormal. The limitations of this bedside maneuver are of note; thus ultrasonic flow analysis of the arterial supply should be employed whenever possible.

The patient should be prepared by mildly dorsiflexing the wrist over a small towel or roll of gauze and the fingers should be gently taped down to prevent motion in the area. Following antiseptic treatment and administration of local anesthesia, the arterial pulse beneath the carpal ligament should be delineated. A 20- to 22-gauge tapered-tip catheter should be advanced through the skin at a 45-degree angle until blood return is observed. The catheter angle should then be reduced to 15 to 20 degrees and the needle advanced 1 to 2 mm further into the lumen of the vessel. Blood return should be reconfirmed prior to sliding the catheter over the needle into the artery without further advancement of the needle. At no time should the needle be redirected while the tip is beneath the skin. Penetration of both sides of the vessel is not uncommon; thus, withdrawal of the catheter by 1 to 2 mm may be required to reestablish blood return prior to catheter advancement. Flush solutions should not be administered in an effort to "float" the catheter into place. Guidewire-through-catheter devices are available and have been shown to improve cannulation success rates. Following insertion, the catheter should be sutured to the skin.

FEMORAL ARTERY CATHETERIZATION

The large caliber of this vessel makes it a good choice for cannulation and pressure monitoring. Significant atherosclerosis at the insertion site or in the aorta, the absence of arterial pulsation, and severely compromised blood flow to the ipsilateral leg are contraindications to cannulation of this vessel. The femoral artery should be approached as described for femoral venous cannulation using a 4- to 6-in. 18-gauge catheter and the Seldinger technique. Short catheters intended for peripheral arterial cannulation should not be used.

DORSALIS PEDIS ARTERY CATHETERIZATION

This superficial artery is occasionally the only available site for peripheral arterial cannulation and is a reasonable alternative to radial arterial cannulation. Collateral circulation in the foot can be assessed by simultaneously compressing both the posterior tibial and dorsalis pedis arteries. The patient then wiggles his or her toes to produce blanching and the posterior tibial artery is released. Although the utility of this test has not been established, normal skin color should return within 10 s.

Cannulation of this vessel is similar to that of the radial artery. The distance of this vessel from the central circulation may make this an unreliable pressure monitoring site, especially in patients on vasoactive medications. Pressure in this vessel reflects the sum of the intravascular distending pressure; reflected waveforms created by vessel wall's recoil and systolic (not mean) pressure may be 15 to 20 mmHg above lower extremity cuff pressures. Cannulation of this vessel is associated with increased risk of thrombosis as compared with other sites.

AXILLARY ARTERY CATHETERIZATION

While this vessel can be difficult to access, its significant collateral circulation, proximal location, and large lumen make it a resonable choice for pressure monitoring. Cannulation is achieved by palpating the artery in the apex of the axilla. An 18-gauge catheter should be advanced into the artery parallel to its course. Retrograde flow into the cerebral circulation with excessive use of pressurized flushing systems is a greater possibility with this vessel than with the radial artery. Retrograde flow has been associated with cerebral embolism and brain abscess.

Care and Maintenance of Catheters

Care of central venous catheters has been the focus of extensive study. Utilization of catheters designed for long-term use, frequent inspection of the insertion site for signs of inflammation (every other day coupled with dressing changes), line and dressing care by a dedicated IV team, and limitation of central line manipulation can limit the incidence of line-related sepsis. Differing conclusions regarding duration of cannulation, necessity of routine line changes, and the use of guidewire exchanges have been reported. The recent development of antibiotic-impregnated catheters has further complicated interpretation of prior studies of catheter use. The current protocol in our intensive care unit (ICU) incorporates the use of heparin-coated catheters impregnated with silver sulfadiazene and chlorhexidine. A recent randomized, prospective study has reported that these catheters are associated with decreased incidence of catheter related infections. Our protocol does not mandate routine central line changes. Rather, in patients with new unexplained fever or signs of sepsis, the catheter is promptly changed a single time over a guidewire. A subsequent line change or an erythematous-appearing entrance site requires insertion at a new site. In addition to this policy, we use a chlorhexidine skin prep and avoid transparent/semiocclusive dressings. The entrance site is covered with sterile gauze that is taped over the edges only.

Substantial data exist to suggest that the incidence of infection with PA catheters and sheath introducers rises significantly after 3 days of use. This is likely due to migration of bacteria through the sheath introducer. Thus, these catheters should be changed at 72-h intervals. A single study has reported that semiocclusive dressings do not increase the risk of catheter infection after 72 h of use with sheath introducers. However, this study did note increased entrance-site colonization rates when these dressings are used, and colonization has been shown to be a predictor of subsequent catheter infection. Thus, use of these dressings should be avoided.

Infection of arterial catheters is uncommon owing to the high rates of blood flow in peripheral arteries. Thus, few data are available to guide management of these devices. Local infection rates must be taken into account in deciding whether to implement routine changes of these catheters. If possible, small-gauge catheters (22 gauge) should be used to prevent thrombosis and/or obstruction of peripheral arteries, which may be associated with increased catheter infection rates. Additionally, these catheters should be inserted under sterile conditions, much as in the insertion of central venous lines. Placement of these catheters is acutely ill patients is frequently impeded by low blood pressures and vasoconstriction, requiring multiple passes through the skin. The operator should consider changing to a fresh catheter after three passes through the skin so as to prevent tracking of bacteria into the artery. If routine arterial line changes are felt necessary, it is possible to change these catheters over a guidewire following inflation of a blood pressure cuff proximal to the insertion site. However, no data are available to support this, and the potential risk of guidewire-induced injury to the endothelium should make this an alternative to placement in a new location. If semiquantitative cultures are available, routine catheter tip culture shoud be considered.

Alternative Approaches for Vascular Access

The extensive venous channels within the corpora cavernosa of the penis allow for its use as a short-term venous access site. An 18- to 20-gauge needle can be inserted into one of the corpora. Drainage rates averaging 13.4 mL/s have been reported. Utilization of this route in emergency settings is untested. Placement of a steel needle (16 to 20 gauge) into the marrow of the ribs or sternum in adults can allow for infusion rates in excess of 100 mL/h. Hypertonic and strongly alkaline solutions should be avoided. The theoretical risk of fat or cortical bone emboli has not been substantiated by clinical reports.

Subcutaneous infusions of small amounts of fluids and medications can be used when other routes are unavailable. Excessive delivery of fluids can result in impairment of blood supply to the skin, with subsequent necrosis and sloughing. Subcutaneous administration of medications (e.g., epinephrine, terbutaline, insulin, herparin) is well documented to be safe. Absorption may be unreliable in patients with circulatory collapse.

Certain drugs can be administered via an endotracheal tube or directly into the peritoneum in emergency situations. Diazepam, atropine, lidocaine, isoproterenol, epinephrine, naloxone, and terbutaline have all been used endotracheally in the absence of intravascular access. Dosages require modification (e.g., double the usual epinephrine dose) to counterbalance reduced and delayed absorption.

Chapter 4

FLUID THERAPY AND BLOOD PRODUCTS

IMRE NOTH

Despite years of experience, choice of fluids for resuscitation of critically ill patients remains an area of active controversy among physicians. Colloids and crystalloids are the primary means of fluid replacement.

Colloids

Albumin, a protein produced in the liver, provides the major oncotic activity of the blood. Normal synthesis ranges from 120 to 200 mg/kg per day. One-third to one-half is present in the intravascular space.

Serum albumin is prepared in 5% and 25% solutions for therapeutic use. A 5% solution has osmotic and oncotic properties roughly equivalent to those of plasma. These agents would be ideal for treatment of patients who are both hypovolemic and hypoproteinemic. Albumin's oncotic properties make it useful in edematous patients in order to return extravascular fluid to the intravascular space, with the understanding the infused albumin redistributes relatively rapidly to the extravascular space. Patients with liver failure and congestive heart failure may receive albumin with furosemide in order to allow urinary excretion of fluid overload.

Plasma protein fraction (PPF) is a mixture of albumin and alpha, beta, and gamma globulins. Although primarily albumin, PPF can be associated with allergic reactions (as can albumin preparations themselves, rarely) with significant hypotension. Since PPF offers no additional advantage to albumin alone, it is not recommended for use.

Dextran is an effective synthetic colloid with similar usage to albumin. It is renally excreted with a clearance rate of

60% within 12 hours of use. Significant side effects limiting its use include decreased renal perfusion, dextran-induced renal failure, antithrombotic activity, and anaphylaxis.

Hetastarch is a synthetic colloid closely resembling glycogen. Its half-life is significantly longer than that of albumin and approaches 2 weeks. Side effects include coagulopathy; decreased fibrinogen; decreased platelets; prolongation of PT, PTT, and thrombin time; and anaphylaxis. It has the advantage of being much less expensive than albumin.

Crystalloids

The primary crystalloid preparations used in critically ill patients are normal saline, Ringer's lactate, or variants of these solutions. Hypotonic solutions are not indicated in treating hypovolemia and should be used primarily for specific problems such as decreasing sodium concentration when treating hypernatremia and other free water deficit states. Normal saline and Ringer's lactate solutions are basically isotonic solutions. These will equilibrate between the intravascular, intracellular and interstitial spaces. Only 25% of infused isotonic crystalloid will remain in the intravascular space after one hour. A dilutional decrease of the hematocrit occurs with the early part of crystalloid administration and corrects a little, as some of the intravascular volume is lost to the interstitial space. Ringer's lactate and normal saline may be used interchangeably in the treatment of hypovolemia, shock, and oliguria.

Hypertonic solutions may be useful in certain instances for volume expansion, as in burn patients, in order to reduce total water load and hence edema. Caution must be exercised, as severe electrolyte and osmolality abnormalities may develop. Slow infusion rates and reducing intravenous fluid concentrations appropriately, in accord with carefully monitored serum sodium levels, help to circumvent these problems.

Central pontine myelinolysis or osmotic demyelination syndrome may occur when severe hyponatremia is corrected too rapidly or to an excessive level of serum sodium.

It carries a mortality of 20 to 50%. Clinical presentation includes rapid progressive paresis and pseudobulbar symptoms of dysphagia and dysarthria. Other common symptoms include reflex changes, extraocular muscle palsies, seizures, tremor, and incontinence.

Whole Blood

Whole blood is primarily indicated in treating hemorrhagic shock. Equivalent resuscitation of hemoglobin, hematocrit, and volume status in the absence of a coagulopathy can be achieved with red blood cells and crystalloid solutions. Transfusion of one unit of whole blood will provide 1.0 g/dL hemoglobin or a 3% elevation in hematocrit in the absence of active bleeding.

Red Blood Cells

Removal of 200 to 250 mL of plasma from whole blood results in "packed" red blood cells (PRBC). A unit of PRBCs will provide the same increase in hemoglobin and hematocrit as a unit of whole blood. With the addition of glycerol, PRBCs may be frozen for storage. When required, the blood is thawed to 37°C and washed of glycerol; it should be transfused within 24 hours. Indications for PRBC transfusion include major trauma with bleeding; shock secondary to blood loss, intraoperative blood loss > 750 mL or 15% of total blood volume, and anemia.

Platelets

Bleeding time is normal if the platelet count is greater than $100,000/\mu L$ and platelet function is intact. Prophylactic platelet transfusion is typically indicated at $20,000/\mu L$ or less. In stable patients, even lower values may be tolerated. Transfusions may be warranted in active bleeding with platelet counts below $50,000/\mu L$. Platelet transfusions are usually not effective in patients with rapid platelet destruction, such as idiopathic thrombocytopenic purpura (ITP), drug-related thrombocytopenia, thrombotic thrombocytopenic purpura (TTP), or hemolytic uremic syndrome (HUS). Transfusion may not be effective in hypersplenism, fever, sepsis, disseminated intravascular coagulation (DIC), or in the presence of platelet antibodies.

Single-donor platelet packs contain at least 5.5×10^{10} platelets per microliter in 50 mL plasma. Individual packs may be pooled for easier administration. One pack should increase platelet count by 5,000 to $10,000/\mu L$. Packs may also be "concentrated" by removing the plasma to avoid adverse reactions. Platelets stored at room temperature are more effective for prophylactic treatment, whereas patients with active bleeding might benefit most from platelets stored at 4°C.

Platelet packs contain white blood cells (WBCs) and RBCs. ABO-incompatible plasma in platelet packs may cause a positive direct antiglobulin test and occasionally, hemolysis and diminished platelet survival. In patients who develop HLA antigens, single-donor HLA-matched packs may be beneficial. Single-donor plateletpheresis products equal about six units of random-donor platelets in 300 mL of plasma.

Granulocytes

Granulocyte transfusions are a consideration in febrile neutropenic patients (<500 neutrophils per microliter) with a good chance of bone marrow recovery. Granulocytes must be stored at room temperature and transfused within 24 hours. Side effects include chills and fever; allergic reactions are common. Granulocytapheresis products should be HLA-matched as well as ABO-compatible. Severe pulmonary insufficiency has been reported as a side effect of transfusion. This risk is increased when amphotericin B is being coadministered. Transfusion should be administered slowly to minimize pulmonary side effects.

Plasma

Plasma is indicated for patients with coagulation factor deficiencies from bleeding, thrombotic thrombocytopenic purpura (TTP), hemolytic uremic syndrome (HUS), or for those who require rapid reversal of vitamin K deficiency or warfarin overdose. Fresh frozen plasma (FFP) is separated from freshly drawn whole blood. One milliliter supplies one unit of coagulation factor activity. FFP should not be chosen over crystalloid or colloid for volume expansion. FFP should be ABO-compatible, but cross-matching is not required.

Liquid plasma is separated from whole blood up to 5 days after expiration. It contains stable coagulation factors, but factors V and VIII are diminished as compared with FFP. Cryoprecipitate forms when FFP is thawed. This portion contains von Willebrand factor, factor VIII, fibrinogen, factor XIII, and fibronectin. Infusion of large amounts can cause hyperfibrinogenemia. Factor concentrates allow the delivery of large quantities of clotting factors in small volumes.

Leukocyte-Poor, Washed Blood Products and Irradiated Blood Products

Patients may become alloimmunized to antigens present on the cell membranes of leukocytes, platelets, or plasma substances. Transfusion of blood products in these patients may result in fevers, allergic reactions, anaphylactic reactions, or noncardiogenic pulmonary edema. Leukocyte-poor products are indicated in such patients. This may be achieved by centrifugation, saline washing, or microaggregate blood filters. Patient groups that are preemptively treated with leukocyte-poor products include bone marrow transplant recipients and others who may require long-term platelet transfusions in an attempt to delay alloimmunization. Disadvantages of saline washing include risk of bacterial contamination, shorter half-life, and partial loss of product. Microaggregate filters circumvent these drawbacks but are unable to remove plasma.

A radiation dose of 15 to 50 Gy prevents replication in 85 to 95% of the lymphocytes present in various blood products, thus reducing the possibility of graft-versus-host disease in recipients at risk for this complication. Indications for irradiated products include patients with graft-versus-host disease

(GVHD), those with congenital immune deficiencies, and recipients of bone marrow transplants.

Emergency Transfusion

Complete transfusion workup requires 30 to 45 minutes. Emergencies therefore may require whole-blood administration without full type and cross-match. Blood tubes and requests should have identification numbers. Most hemolytic transfusion reactions occur from ABO incompatibility secondary to clerical errors. Group O, Rh-negative PRBCs can be given if immediate transfusion is needed. Transfusion can be hastened with a pressure cuff around the unit of blood.

Massive Transfusion

Replacement of the patient's entire blood volume over a 24-hour period or less defines massive transfusion and is associated with several potential complications (Table 4-1). Aging RBC products have potassium ions released from the RBCs; patients with shock, acidosis, and renal insufficiency may be at risk for iatrogenic hyperkalemia. Cold blood products may contribute to hypothermia. Transfusions also offer a significant volume challenge, and frequent assessment of patients

TABLE 4-1   Potential Complications
of Massive Transfusion

Dilutional effects
   Thrombocytopenia
   Coagulopathy
Consequences of prolonged blood storage
   Hyperkalemia (in renal impairment)
   Left shift of the oxyhemoglobin dissociation relationship
     (temporary)
Miscellaneous
   Hypothermia
   Volume overload
   Metabolic alkalosis
   Hypocalcemia

---

receiving substantial blood products is required in order to detect volume overload. *Most importantly, massive transfusion is often accompanied by coagulation abnormalities, and frequent monitoring and administration of FFP, platelets, or other constituents should be anticipated.*

Disease Transmission

The risk of disease transmission by transfusion is estimated as follows: for HIV, 1 in 493,000 per transfused unit; for hepatitis B, 1 in 63,000; and for hepatitis C, 1 in 103,000. Most reactions due to contaminating organisms are caused by endotoxin produced in cold-growing gram-negative bacteria such as *Pseudomonas, Citrobacter, Escherichia coli,* and *Yersinia.* High fever, shock, hemoglobinuria, disseminated intravascular coagulation, and renal failure characterize these types of transfusion reactions. If bacterial contamination is suspected, transfusion should be discontinued and the blood unit inspected for purple color, clots, or hemolysis. Treatment includes appropriate antibiotics and supportive measures.

Red Cell–Related Transfusion Reactions

Acute hemolytic transfusion reaction can lead to intravascular hemolysis. Frequently rapid, it can lead to shock, acute renal failure, or bleeding. In the event that intravascular hemolysis is suspected, the following steps should be taken:

1. Stop infusion.
2. Check labels, forms, and patient identification.
3. Monitor urine output.
4. Maintain urine output >100 mL/h.
5. Check BP and treat shock if present.
6. Initiate reaction workup; notify and send unused blood bag and freshly drawn blood samples to the blood bank.
7. Perform baseline and follow-up laboratory studies:

   a. Blood urea nitrogen, creatinine, and electrolytes
   b. PT, PTT, fibrinogen, platelet count, fibrin degradation products, D-dimer

    c. Hemoglobin and hematocrit
    d. Urinalysis for hemoglobinuria
    e. Plasma or serum evaluation for hemoglobinemia
    f. Baseline and serial serum bilirubin

8. Consider whole blood or plasma exchange, dialysis, or heparin therapy (for DIC).
9. Give compatible blood transfusions if clinically indicated.

For a more detailed discussion, see Chaps. 20 and 62 in *Principles of Critical Care,* 2d ed.

Chapter 5

VASOACTIVE DRUGS

SANGEETA BHORADE

The use of vasoactive medications in the intensive care unit (ICU) may be lifesaving. However, if they are not used with proper indication in a specific clinical situation, these medications may not be helpful and may even be harmful to the critically ill patient. These drugs are discussed in the context of the four most common syndromes in which vasoactive medications are used: (1) left ventricular dysfunction, (2) acute right heart syndrome, (3) renal augmentation/perfusion, and (4) sepsis syndrome and septic shock.

There are several important considerations prior to starting treatment with vasoactive medications. Addressing the underlying condition and identifying any correctable factors prior to the initiation of vasoactive drugs are of utmost importance in the treatment of any of the above disorders. In addition, supportive therapies, such as mechanical ventilation, may be just as effective in certain situations as vasoactive drugs. Last, attention to the specific actions of these medications may be helpful in selecting an appropriate drug. The receptor selectivity of five commonly used agents in the ICU is presented in Table 5-1. In addition, general information about each medication including dosage ranges is presented in Table 5-2.

Vasoactive medications should be used to maintain perfusion to the brain, kidney, myocardium, and gastrointestinal tract. While blood pressure is one measure of global perfusion, it generally is not a good measure of individual organ perfusion. Adequate regional perfusion may be monitored by assessing end-organ function such as mental status, electroencephalogram (ECG), and cardiac enzymes suggestive of myocardial ischemia/infarction, urine output, BUN and creatinine levels, and evidence of lactic acidosis. Newer monitoring techniques—including gastric tonometry and laser Doppler flowmetry—may also assist in assessing regional

TABLE 5-1 Summary of Pharmacologic Receptor Selectivity for Commonly Used Adrenergic Drugs

Catecholamine	DA-1	β_1	β_2	α_1	α_2
Dopamine[a]	$1+$[b]$-4+$	$0-3+$	$0-2+$	$0-3+$	$0-1+$
Dobutamine	0	$3+$	$1+$	$0-1+$	0
Norepinephrine	0	$2+$	$1+$	$3+$	$3+$
Epinephrine	0	$3+$	$3+$	$3+$	$3+$
Isoproterenol	0	$3+$	$3+$	0	0

[a]Dopamine's pharmacologic effects are very much dose related and somewhat variable between patients. Low doses (~1–3 μg/kg/min) stimulate primarily the DA-1 and DA-2 receptors; high doses (>20–50 μg/kg/min) produce mostly α-adrenergic stimulation.
[b]Relative degree of stimulation on 1- to 4-point scale.

perfusion, thus providing a more rational approach to the use of vasoactive drugs.

Most vasoactive medications are started at a relatively low dose (see Table 5-2) with titration upward as dictated by the clinical situation. Continuous reassessment of the patient's clinical state is important with regard to dosing changes, substitution of one medication for another, and the addition of second agent, if necessary. Last, weaning the patient from vasoactive drugs is frequently difficult and attention must be focused on the patient's underlying condition.

Left Ventricular Dysfunction

In general, appropriate therapy in patients with left ventricular (LV) dysfunction requires the institution of a positive inotropic agent that alters preload and afterload favorably without provoking myocardial ischemia.

DOBUTAMINE

Dobutamine (DBT) is a synthetic catecholamine with positive inotropic effects and minimal vasoactive properties, making it an ideal drug in the treatment of LV dysfunction. By augmenting cardiac output, DBT may decrease preload and afterload, resulting in decreased ventricular filling pressures

TABLE 5-2 Vasoactive Drugs for Shock

Drug	Indication	Receptor/Target	Dose Range	Adverse Effects
Amrinone	LVD	PDE inhibition	5–20 μg/kg/min after 0.75 mg/kg bolus	Thrombocytopenia, arrhythmias, hepatic dysfunction
Angiotensin II	Sepsis	Arteriolar smooth muscle		Unknown
Dobutamine	LVD, ARHS	$\beta_1 > \beta_2$	0.05–1.6 mg/kg/min	Tachycardia, arrhythmias
Dopamine	LVD? (<10 μg/kg/min)	$\beta_1 > \alpha > DA > \beta_2$	2–20 μg/kg/min	Tachycardia, arrhythmias, tissue ischemia
Epinephrine	Anaphylactic shock, cardiac arrest	α, β	5–20 μg/min	Tachycardia, arrhythmias, tissue ischemia
Nitric oxide (NO)	ARHS	Vascular smooth muscle	2–70 ppm inhaled	Methemoglobinemia, NO_2 accumulation
Nitroglycerin	LVD	Vascular smooth muscle	5–500 μg/kg/min	Methemoglobinemia, HA, flushing, tachycardia
Nitroprusside	LVD, HTN crisis	Vascular smooth muscle	0.5–8 μg/kg/min	Cyanide, thiocyanate toxicity
Norepinephrine	ARHS	$\alpha > \beta_1$	0.1–1.0 μg/kg/min	Tissue ischemia
Prostacyclin	ARHS	Vascular smooth muscle	4–5 ng/kg/min	Systemic hypotension
Prostaglandin E1	ARHS	Vascular smooth muscle	0.1–1.0 mg/kg/min	Systemic hypotension
Vasopressin	Sepsis	V receptors	0.01–0.04 U/min	Unknown

ABBREVIATIONS: LVD, left ventricular dysfunction; ARHS, acute right heart syndrome; HTN, hypertensive.

and arterial vasodilation, respectively. Typically cardiac output and oxygen delivery increase by one-third with DBT infusion while blood pressure remains unchanged. Of note, downregulation of β_1 adrenergic receptors may result in tachyphylaxis, a progressive decline in effectiveness with prolonged use. If blood pressure falls during the administration of DBT, administration of intravenous fluids to restore preload as well as decreasing the dose may be necessary. This drug is generally well tolerated, with minimal problems related to tachycardia and, rarely, arrhythmias.

AMRINONE

Amrinone is a phosphodiesterase inhibitor that increases the availability of intracellular cyclic adenosine monophosphate (cAMP), resulting in positive inotropic and vasodilatory properties. The effect of this agent has not been found to be superior to that of DBT and thus is a second-line agent that should be used in cases where dobutamine has been ineffective or contraindicated. Because of the different mechanisms of action, amrinone may augment the effect of DBT on cardiac output. Although the oral form of this medication was deemed unsafe and taken off the market, the intravenous form has relatively few side effects; these include thrombocytopenia, hypotension, and arrhythmias.

ISOPROTERENOL

Isoproterenol is a powerful inotropic and chronotropic agent whose actions are mediated via the activation of β_1 and β_2 receptors. However, the powerful effects of this medication may cause significant myocardial ischemia and vasodilation, often resulting in hypotension and decreased blood flow to vital organs. Currently, this medication is best reserved for the treatment of hemodynamically significant bradycardia, although often, in these cases, a transvenous or external pacemaker is preferable.

DOPAMINE

Dopamine (DA) is an endogenous catecholamine and neurotransmitter. When it is administered exogenously, dopamine has several pharmacologic effects depending upon the dose that is administered. Its positive inotropic actions start at doses as low as 2 to 5 μg/kg per min via the activation of β_1-adrenergic receptors, although its predominant effect at this dose is activation of dopaminergic receptors in the renal, splanchnic, and cerebral circulations (see below). When higher doses are given (5 to 10 μg/kg per min), the β_1-receptor agonist activity persists and cardiac output may increase. However, the inotropic effects of DA are clearly inferior to those of DBT. As the dose of DA increases (10 to 20 μg/kg per min), the α_1-receptor agonist effects increase, resulting in significant vasoconstriction of both systemic and pulmonary circulations, which may be detrimental in patients with LV dysfunction. Dose-related tachycardia and arrhythmias are side effects of DA.

NITROGLYCERIN

Nitroglycerin relaxes vascular smooth muscle and is a general vasodilator. Nitroglycerin is a precursor to nitric oxide (NO), also known as endothelium-derived relaxing factor (EDRF). NO is initially formed by nitroglycerin in the endothelial cell and then diffuses out of the endothelium and into smooth muscle, where it causes smooth muscle dilation via the formation of cyclic guanosine monophosphate (cGMP). Nitroglycerin may decrease LV filling pressures by venodilation in doses up to 40 μg/min and may increase cardiac output through arterial vasodilation at doses greater than 200 μg/min. Side effects—including severe headaches, flushing, tachycardia, and the development of methemoglobinemia—as well as difficulties with the administration of the drug, usually limit its clinical use unless the patient has ongoing myocardial ischemia.

NITROPRUSSIDE

Nitroprusside is a nonspecific vasodilator that is most commonly used in treating severe hypertension. However, it may have some use in patients with LV dysfunction. Some of the advantages of nitroprusside include its rapid onset of action (1 to 2 minutes), a short elimination time (2 to 3 minutes in patients with normal renal and liver function), and ease of administration. However, nitroprusside toxicity may be alarming and warrants careful monitoring. This toxicity is related to cyanide, the breakdown product of nitroprusside, which is then metabolized by the liver to the less toxic thiocyanate, which is cleared by the kidneys. Toxicity is the result of accumulation of either cyanide or thiocyanate and is dependent upon the total administered dose of the drug. The initial signs and symptoms of toxicity (restlessness, mental confusion, hyperreflexia, and metabolic acidosis) are not easily recognized early in the course of critically ill patients. Initial efforts to minimize toxicity include infusion of hydroxycobalamine or thiosulfate. If toxicity is suspected, nitroprusside should be discontinued and a cyanide and/or thiocyanate level obtained. Medications used to treat nitroprusside toxicity—including hydroxycobalamine, sodium nitrite, sodium thiosulfate, and methylene blue—should be used with caution, as they are also associated with adverse effects.

Acute Right Heart Syndromes

Acute right heart syndromes are typically caused by any disorder (e.g., massive pulmonary embolism or acute lung injury) associated with an acute rise in right ventricular (RV) afterload, which, in turn, may lead to RV dilation and dysfunction. As RV cavity pressures rise and systemic arterial (and, therefore, coronary) pressure falls, the RV may become ischemic, heightening the degree of dysfunction and precipitating a vicious cycle leading to RV failure, shock, and death. RV infarction resembles other right heart syndromes in many regards with the exception that the pulmonary artery pressure is not elevated. The following vasoactive drugs may be of benefit in the treatment of right heart syndromes. The administration of intravenous fluids may not necessarily be beneficial and may actually be detrimental in patients with acute right heart syndromes. A fluid challenge should generally be given to test its effect, but if fluid does not improve perfusion, it should not continue to be given.

DOBUTAMINE

The drug best studied in human right heart shock (both in massive pulmonary embolism and right ventricular infarction) is DBT, which can improve RV function without worsening ischemia. The effects of dobutamine are described above.

NOREPINEPHRINE

Animal models suggest that norepinephrine (by raising coronary pressure but not pulmonary artery resistance) is also a good choice. Norepinephrine (NE) is one of the most powerful adrenergic vasoconstrictors because of its effect on α receptors and lack of effect on β_2 receptors. It may also have a moderate effect on β_1 receptors and thus may increase cardiac output at low doses. Coronary and cerebral blood flow may be spared because of a difference in the distribution of α receptors in these areas. Interestingly, recent studies have suggested that NE may improve end-organ perfusion in patients with septic shock (see below). Tissue ischemia may be present, especially when high doses are used for prolonged periods. If local extravasation occurs, local tissue necrosis may be prevented by local infiltration with phentolamine, an adrenergic blocker.

NITRIC OXIDE

Nitric oxide (NO) given by the inhaled route is a pulmonary vasodilator with minimal systemic effects. Its vasodilatory actions are mediated through cGMP, as described above. NO has been shown to benefit some patients with acute right heart syndrome by decreasing pulmonary artery pressures and improving RV and subsequently LV function. Inhaled NO is superior to intravenous prostacyclin owing to its lack of deleterious systemic effects. Side effects include methemoglobinemia and nitrogen dioxide accumulation. A subset of patients receiving NO have manifested life-threatening deterioration in hemodynamics upon the withdrawal of NO.

Low-Dose Dopamine for Renal Augmentation/Protection

Low-dose DA (2 to 3 μg/kg per min) is commonly used in hypotensive patients with oliguria and renal dysfunction. However, there are very few data to support this approach.

Low-dose DA infusion may temporarily increase the urine output but may not improve creatinine clearance. For example, Olson and colleagues studied 16 septic, nonoliguric patients. As compared with placebo, low-dose DA raised urine output modestly but failed to enhance creatinine clearance. Other studies show that even this effect is short-lived. Clinical studies have failed to show either augmentation of renal function in shock states or renal protection in perioperative states.

Septic Shock

This diagnosis produces the greatest uncertainty and controversy regarding the use of vasoactive drugs. The concept of pathologic supply dependence (PSD) spawned a school of thought that sought to maximize oxygen delivery, usually through vasoactive drug infusions. With the recognition that mathematical coupling through shared variables probably accounts for the observed PSD in human sepsis, controversy exists as to the benefit of maximizing oxygen delivery. Further, most trials of maximizing oxygen delivery have failed to demonstrate a benefit, and some have shown a detriment.

Several studies over the past decade have shown that different vasoactive drugs titrated to identical systemic effect (as judged by blood pressure or cardiac output) may have different effects on renal (urine output), gastric (tonometric P_{CO_2}; indocyanine green), and hepatic perfusion. For example, in one study of human sepsis, DBT reduced the lactate concentration, augmented gut mucosal blood flow (laser Doppler flowmetry), and lowered the gastric-arterial P_{CO_2} gradient (tonometry), while DA raised lactate, lowered gut flow, and increased the gastric-arterial P_{CO_2} gradient.

Similarly, the combination of NE and DBT was superior to epinephrine (EPI) in two studies when judged by splanchnic perfusion. NE was found to be superior to DA in maintaining or enhancing splanchnic perfusion. These studies and several others suggest that DA and epinephrine are ineffective in maintaining splanchnic perfusion. In light of these data, a reasonable approach in a septic patient in whom fluids fail to restore adequate perfusion (e.g., mean BP

<70 mmHg, oliguria, acidosis) is to infuse DBT beginning at 5 μg/kg per min (and increased to 10 to 20 μg/kg per min if needed) and then to add NE beginning at 0.1 μg/kg per min.

There have been small trials of the use of vasopressin (at one-tenth the dose used in variceal hemorrhage) and angiotensin in patients with sepsis suggesting that these drugs might be both beneficial and effective in raising blood pressure. In one such study, vasopressin levels were found to be strikingly low, suggesting a deficiency of vasopressin release in sepsis.

Anaphylactic Shock

Anaphylactic shock is the result of the effect of histamine and other mediators of anaphylaxis on the cardiopulmonary system. The mainstay of therapy includes intravenous fluids and epinephrine.

EPINEPHRINE

Epinephrine is an endogenous catecholamine with both α and β effects, although mainly α effects are observed at higher doses. In general, epinephrine is the drug of choice in anaphylactic shock, where it causes vasoconstriction and bronchodilation to counteract the commonly seen vasodilation and bronchospasm associated with this disorder. Although it may also be used as a vasoconstrictor in patients with refractory hypotension, epinephrine tends to shunt blood away from vital organs and is therefore not an ideal drug to use in other types of shock. Epinephrine is also the drug of choice during cardiac arrests.

For a more detailed discussion, see Chaps. 19, 20, 21, and 25 in *Principles of Critical Care*, 2d ed.

Chapter 6

MINIMIZING COMPLICATIONS OF CRITICAL CARE

SHANNON S. CARSON

Complications resulting from invasive monitoring and life-support measures are common occurrences in critically ill patients, accounting for substantial morbidity and mortality. The challenge for the intensive care unit (ICU) team during their daily management of the patient is to anticipate and prevent as many of these mishaps as possible. A discussion of common complications by organ system is presented in this chapter. Further discussion of many of these problems can be found in appropriate chapters elsewhere in the text.

Neurologic Complications

ICU PSYCHOSIS

Abnormalities in behavior, perception, or cognition occur frequently in adults managed in the ICU. These problems often manifest in an intermittent fashion and during the night. Close communication with nursing and ancillary staff and especially the patient's family is essential to detect and characterize the behaviors. A number of potential etiologies can be responsible for these disturbances, therefore a systematic evaluation as to the underlying cause is warranted in each case. An approach is outlined in Table 6-1. The evaluation begins with a careful neurologic exam looking for evidence of a structural central nervous system (CNS) lesion. An early assessment to rule out CNS infection, including lumbar puncture, is important, followed by a search for possible metabolic disturbances, especially hypoglycemia, hypoxemia, electrolyte abnormalities, and hepatic dysfunction. The polypharmacy of ICU medicine is frequently the culprit,

TABLE 6-1   Evaluation of the Critically Ill Patient
with Abnormal Behavior

Perform neurologic examination to exclude a focal abnormality
   suggesting structural injury
Seek evidence of CNS infection
Exclude metabolic disturbances
Consider withdrawal state
Consider prior psychiatric disorder
Review medication history to exclude drug side effects
Consider "ICU psychosis"

---

so a careful review of all medications should occur, with a
focus on dosages and intervals relative to the patient's age,
renal function, and hepatic function. Withdrawal from substances such as alcohol, cocaine, and prescription benzodiazepines should be considered, as should any prior history
of psychiatric illness.

Once all of the above etiologies have been carefully ruled
out, and only then, one can consider the possibility of ICU
psychosis as a diagnosis of exclusion. This clinical entity is
usually observed after 5 to 7 days of admission to the ICU
(earlier in elderly patients) and manifests as disorientation or
hallucination, most often at night. The patient can usually be
managed effectively with quiet assurance and attention, but
soft physical restraints or sedation with a short-acting benzodiazepine may occasionally be warranted if the patient is
posing a clear danger to himself or herself by reaching for the
endotracheal tube, arterial lines, or pulmonary artery catheter
or thrashing in the presence of unstable traumatic injuries.
Prevention of ICU psychosis is maintained by preservation of
sleep/wake cycles through appropriate lighting and daytime
scheduling of procedures, frequent orientation of the patient
as to time and activities, and addressing emotional stress by
regular bedside presence of the family as well as counseling
by clergy and social work.

STUPOR AND COMA

Extreme depression of consciousness requires the same diagnostic approach as outlined in Table 6-1. Depending on the
neurologic exam, one should have a low threshold for diag-

nostic imaging in the form of computed tomography (CT) or magnetic resonance imaging (MRI) of the head. A lumbar puncture is indicated provided there are adequate platelets ($>20,000/mm^3$) and no evidence of disseminated intravascular coagulation (DIC) or elevations of intracranial pressure. Large accumulations of sedatives and muscle relaxants are common causes of prolonged depression of consciousness, as are accumulations of lidocaine and sodium nitroprusside. Regular review of continued need and dosing of these agents usually prevents this complication. Status epilepticus may present without tonic-clonic activity and should be ruled out with an electroencephalogram (EEG), especially in the setting of an examination that varies over time in a patient with a history of seizures. Only after the evaluation outlined above can depressed consciousness be attributed to underlying illnesses such as sepsis or other metabolic causes of encephalopathy.

Pulmonary Complications

VENTILATOR-INDUCED LUNG INJURY

Barotrauma, defined as the abnormal presence of extraalveolar air in patients receiving mechanical ventilation, takes several forms, as outlined in Table 6-2. It develops from rupture of an overdistended alveolus leading to introduction of air into the perivascular adventitia, which may track along perivascular sheaths into the mediastinum, peritoneum, and pleural space. The presence of air in these locations can lead to severe respiratory and hemodynamic compromise; therefore prevention and early detection of these processes is essential.

TABLE 6-2   Forms of Barotrauma

Pulmonary interstitial emphysema (PIE)
Lung and subpleural air cysts
Pneumomediastinum
Pneumopericardium
Subcutaneous emphysema
Pneumothorax
Pneumoperitoneum

Prevention of barotrauma begins with assessment and minimization of alveolar pressures. Alveolar pressures can be measured indirectly by assessment of proximal airway pressures as illustrated in Fig. 6-1. These measurements assume that (1) the PEEP or $PEEP_i$ level reflects the least alveolar volume during the respiratory cycle; (2) the Pplat reflects the

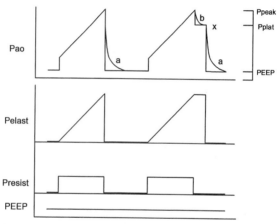

FIGURE 6-1   An idealized demonstration of the components of the pressure at the airway opening (Pao) during positive-pressure ventilation. The peak airway pressure (Ppeak) reflects several individual contributions, as shown together in the top panel and individually in the bottom three panels. The end-expiratory pressure (PEEP) is the pressure at the onset of inspiration. Pressure then rises abruptly as airflow across the resistance of the artificial and native airways is established. This resistant pressure (Presist) is shown in the second panel from the bottom and can be estimated at the bedside by the difference between the Ppeak and Pplat pressures (*b on the top panel*). After the initial abrupt rise in pressure, Pao rises linearly, at a slope determined by the compliance of the respiratory system and to an end-inspiratory point determined by the volume delivered. The elastic pressure (Pelast) is shown in the second panel from the top and is represented as distance *a* on the top panel, or the Pplat–PEEP pressures.

maximal alveolar volume at end-inspiration, although lung and chest wall compliances should be considered when relating Pplat to alveolar volume; and (3) Ppeak may be much greater than Pplat when airway resistance is high and thus, under these conditions, would poorly reflect alveolar volume and risk of barotrauma.

Measures to decrease alveolar inflation include maintaining PEEP at <15 cmH$_2$O and Pplat at <35 cmH$_2$O. Low tidal volume ventilation, permissive hypercapnea, and pressure-controlled ventilation may be necessary to stay within these parameters.

One should consider the presence of a pneumothorax in the setting of agitation, progressive hypoxemia, hypotension, or cardiovascular collapse in a ventilated patient. The presence of crepitations anywhere in the upper body is indicative of subcutaneous emphysema. One of the earliest signs of barotrauma can be detected radiographically by the presence of pulmonary interstitial emphysema (PIE) on the chest radiograph. This manifests as small parenchymal cysts, linear streaks of air radiating toward the hilus, perivascular halos, intraseptal air collection, pneumatoceles, or large subpleural air collections. PIE often precedes more overt manifestations of barotrauma, such as tension pneumothorax. Pneumothoraces in the critically ill supine patients are not often demonstrated radiographically in an apicolateral location but rather tend to present as anteromediastinal, subpulmonic, or posteromedial pleural air collections. Anteromedial pneumothorax presents as a linear air density adjacent to the mediastinum or increased sharpness of the mediastinal border outlined by intrapleural air. Subpulmonic pneumothorax can be recognized by hyperlucency of the upper abdominal quadrants and visualization of the anterior costophrenic sulcus. A tension pneumothorax is suggested by marked collapse of the lung with contralateral shift of the heart and mediastinum or inversion of the diaphragm.

PIE and pneumomediastinum are considered benign, but they should alert the clinician to the possibility of worse forms of barotrauma, and efforts to decrease alveolar distension should begin in earnest. Pneumothorax and tension pneumothorax should be managed by tube thoracostomy. Pneumoperitoneum related to barotrauma is usually accompanied by other signs of barotrauma, described above. If other signs are not present, a surgical evaluation for possible abdominal emergency is indicated.

PULMONARY FIBROSIS

In some patients with adult pulmonary distress syndrome (ARDS), a chronic fibrotic phase of lung injury can develop, usually by 2 weeks into their course. Prevention of this process may depend upon limiting exposure to toxic levels of oxygen and positive-pressure ventilation. The risk of barotrauma can be minimized by using low V_T (6 to 7 mL/kg). Early in the course of ARDS, the clinician should titrate PEEP to achieve 90% saturation of arterial hemoglobin with an $F_{IO_2} \leq 0.6$. Adequate saturation of arterial hemoglobin can be facilitated by maintaining a hematocrit >35% and using vasoactive drugs to increase cardiac output for increased oxygen delivery and by decreasing oxygen consumption with sedation, muscle relaxation, management of hyperthermia, and nutritional modification. If the chronic fibrotic phase of ARDS develops, the stiff, noncompliant lungs produce alveolar pressures that approach pulmonary vascular pressures and perfusion of ventilated alveoli becomes compromised with a resulting increase in dead space. Therefore, hypovolemia will need to be avoided and the patient may benefit from lower PEEP and V_T at this stage.

PREVENTION OF AIRWAY COMPLICATIONS

Translaryngeal intubation is associated with laryngeal edema, ulceration, and hemorrhage in most patients. Clinically, this can lead to hoarseness or tracheal stenosis after extubation. An uncommon but potentially serious consequence is stridor and severe upper airway obstruction immediately after extubation, requiring reintubation or, rarely, emergent tracheostomy. Tracheostomy can be associated with tracheal stensosis (most commonly at the stoma site) as well as tracheoesophageal fistula or tracheoinnominate fistula. Massive hemorrhage associated with tracheoinnominate fistula is managed with hyperinflation of the cuff or a newly placed endotracheal tube.

Prevention of these airway complications begins with attention to daily management of the airway, as outlined in

TABLE 6-3   Daily Management of the Airway

Ensure adequately sized tube with normal patency
Minimize cuff pressure by minimal leak or measured pressure
   <25 mmHg
Minimize cuff movement and tube flexion or torsion
Confirm position by inspection, auscultation, palpation, and
   radiologic imaging
Assess duration of intubation

Table 6-3. A properly sized tube, with a cuff that is not over-inflated, properly positioned 3 to 7 cm above the carina is required. An endotracheal tube should not remain in place more than 7 to 14 days unless reversal of the underlying illness and extubation seems likely within several days.

Occlusion of the endotracheal tube or tracheostomy tube occurs occasionally, sometimes rather suddenly. This would be heralded by a distressed patient with high airway pressures and inability to deliver adequate V_T. Management begins with bagging the patient with 100% O_2. If bagging is difficult, a suction catheter or bronchoscope should be passed to ensure patency. If occlusion is present at the level of the teeth, a bite block should be placed or the patient should receive a dose of a short-acting muscle relaxant. Most tube obstructions are caused by concretized secretions and mucous plugs requiring replacement of the tube. Small tubes, airway bleeding, excessive secretions, and inadequate humidification of inspired gas predispose to tube occlusions.

ARTERIAL HEMOGLOBIN DESATURATION OR HYPOVENTILATION

Arterial hemoglobin desaturation can be the first sign of a number of complications of critical illness. The evaluation begins with bedside assessment of the patient and review of the ventilator and true F_{I_O}, followed by chest radiograph, arterial blood gas, and mixed venous oxygen saturation if available. Evaluation of these data within the context of the clinical presentation will usually distinguish between the potential causes of hypoxemia outlined in Table 6-4.

TABLE 6-4   Causes of Worsening Hypoxemia
in the Critically Ill Patient

---

1. Artifact
2. Alterations in $F_{I_{O_2}}$
3. Hypoventilation $(A - a)_{O_2}$ unchanged
   a. Diminished patient effort (fatigue, depressed drive)
   b. Ventilator malfunction or inadvertent change in settings
   c. Gas leak
   d. Alterations in physiologic dead space
      Hypovolemia
      PEEPi
      Increased alveolar pressures in restrictive lung disease
4. $\dot{V}/\dot{Q}$ mismatch
   a. Airway
      Bronchospasm
      Secretions
      Mucous plugging
      Endotracheal tube suctioning
   b. Vasculature
      Use of vasoactive drugs (inhaled or intravenous)
      Pulmonary embolus
5. Shunt
   a. Atelectasis
   b. Pulmonary edema
   c. Pulmonary hemorrhage
   d. Positional change in nonhomogeneous disease
   e. Lobar collapse (acutely)
   f. Pneumonia
   g. Cardiac shunt
6. Mixed venous hypoxemia
   Low O_2 delivery due to reduced flow, hematocrit, saturation or
      increased $\dot{V}_{O_2} \rightarrow$ low mixed venous saturation $\rightarrow$ arterial
      hypoxemia in shunt or lung disease with large numbers of
      low $\dot{V}/\dot{Q}$ units

Atelectasis and lobar collapse are potential causes of hypoxemia that deserve mention because of their frequent occurrence and often preventable nature. Three-point turning, early mobilization to a chair, incentive spirometry, and upright positioning should be applied to patients at the earliest possible time. Patients requiring mechanical ventilation benefit from PEEP and sighs rather than high V_T, which can predispose to barotrauma. Reexpansion of a collapsed lobe can be accomplished by transiently increasing tidal volumes (maintaining peak airway pressures <50 cmH$_2$O) accompanied by chest physical therapy and vigorous suctioning. Bronchoscopy may be required if these measures fail.

CARDIOVASCULAR COMPLICATIONS

Positive-pressure ventilation can lead to significant elevation of right atrial pressures and compromised venous return. Significant decreases in cardiac output and hypoperfusion of vital organs are more likely to occur in patients with severe airway obstruction and high PEEP$_i$ and in patients whose autonomic adaptive responses are compromised by sedation, muscle relaxation, or hypovolemia. In these circumstances, a patient should be removed from the ventilator to allow lung deflation and slowly bagged until heart rate and blood pressure improve. Hypovolemia should then be corrected and more appropriate ventilator settings should be chosen to allow a longer expiratory phase and minimization of PEEP$_i$. As discussed above, patients with noncompliant lungs, such as those in the proliferative phase of ARDS, may have alveolar pressures that approach pulmonary vascular pressures and are subject to compromised perfusion of those lung units. This will result in increased dead space, evidenced by a rising P$_{CO_2}$ that does not respond to increases in PEEP or minute ventilation. Volume replacement or vasoactive drug support may be necessary in this instance if the patient does not respond to decreases in V_T rate, or PEEP.

PULMONARY EMBOLUS

The incidence of pulmonary emboli (PE) in the ICU is difficult to determine, but it is thought to be 8 to 27% based upon autopsy studies. The incidence of deep venous thrombosis (DVT) in the lower extremity, the most common source of PE, is as high as 30% in some reports. PE must be considered in any patient presenting acutely with hypoxemia, dyspnea, elevated right atrial or pulmonary artery pressures, or hypotension. Clinical signs and symptoms are very nonspecific for PE, and lung scanning is often complicated by existing lung disease. Therefore the clinician must rely on noninvasive leg studies, echocardiography, helical CT scanning, and pulmonary angiography for assistance in making the diagnosis.

Prevention centers on prevention of DVT with the use of heparin, 5000 units given subcutaneously every 8 to 12 hours. Intermittent pneumatic compression devices (IPC) or warfarin is indicated if the patient has heparin-induced thrombocytopenia, and IPC devices are warranted if there are absolute contraindications to anticoagulation, such as active bleeding or neurosurgery. Some authors recommend placement of an inferior vena cava filter for prophylaxis of PE in patients at very high risk, such as immobilized trauma patients, but this may not become standard practice until removable devices become more available.

COMPLICATIONS ASSOCIATED WITH
PULMONARY ARTERY CATHETERS

Complications associated with pulmonary artery catheters include arrhythmias, vascular injury, air embolism, pneumothorax, hemothorax, infusion of substances into the pleural space, right ventricular puncture, pulmonary vascular rupture, pulmonary embolus, and infection. A recent nonrandomized study suggests that pulmonary artery (PA) catheters may be associated with increased mortality. Although PA catheters will remain in use until more definitive studies recommend otherwise, careful attention should be given to prevention of the numerous potential complications mentioned. Prevention of complications begins with a clear discussion of whether the information gained from placement and continued presence of the catheter is necessary for patient management and whether that information can be gained by less invasive means such as echocardiography. Also, it is clear that significant errors occur in the interpretation of data from PA catheters, with important consequences for patient management. Adequate training and competency assessment in data interpretation for all personnel cannot be emphasized enough.

Arrhythmias occur commonly during placement of the catheter. Premature ventricular complexes usually resolve with forward advancement of the catheter. The risk for sustained ventricular tachycardia is increased in patients with acidosis (pH <7.20), recent myocardial infarction (MI), and hypoxemia, especially in the setting of prolonged catheterization. These patients may benefit from prophylactic lidocaine. Patients with MI and left bundle branch block should have a transvenous pacemaker during catheter placement to manage potential complete heart block. Pulmonary artery rupture is a rare complication with high mortality. Presence of a false pulmonary artery aneurysm is suggested radiographically by a mass or nodule near the tip of the catheter. These complications are prevented by avoidance of permanent catheter wedging and balloon hyperinflation. One should anticipate distal catheter migration and monitor for this occurrence by assessment of the waveforms and location on the chest radiograph. The incidence of clinically important pulmonary emboli attributable to fibrin sheath thrombus or mural thrombus associated with PA catheters is unclear, so prophylaxis with anticoagulation is not common practice. Heparin-bonded catheters have been shown to decrease the incidence of fibrin sheaths, but only for 1 to 2 days. The presence of these catheters should be remembered if heparin-induced thrombocytopenia is noted. Once again, the most effective way to prevent thrombi is to minimize the length of time that the catheter remains in place.

ISCHEMIA AND ARRHYTHMIAS

Most critically ill adults are at risk for myocardial ischemia, but their presentation may be atypical. In addition to typical chest pain, ischemia should be expected in any patient with sudden pulmonary edema or elevations in pulmonary capillary wedge pressure or unexplained agitation or dyspnea with abnormalities in heart rate. Patients with known risk factors should receive a daily 12-lead electrocardiogram (ECG) to monitor for asymptomatic changes.

Likewise, critically ill adults are uniformly at risk for cardiac arrhythmias, making continuous ECG monitoring routine for all ICU admissions. Patients at highest risk for ventricular arrhythmias are those with coronary artery disease and patients undergoing central-line or PA catheter placement.

Risks are heightened by the presence of hypoxemia; acidosis; electrolyte abnormalities including hypokalemia, hyperkalemia, hypocalcemia, and hypomagnesemia; and catecholamine infusions. Levels of drugs such as theophylline, digoxin, or other antiarrhythmic agents known to cause rhythm disturbances should be followed closely. Patients with severe lung disease or pulmonary hypertension are subject to the occurrence of multifocal atrial tachycardia, which often responds to verapamil or adenosine.

Gastrointestinal Complications

An important complication of critical illness with a high level of morbidity and mortality is gastrointestinal hemorrhage in patients without primary gastrointestinal disease. The etiology of this complication relates to hypoperfusion of gastric mucosa that compromises protective mechanisms and results in ulceration. Patients at highest risk for clinically significant gastrointestinal bleeding are those requiring mechanical ventilation or those with underlying coagulopathies. Some additional risk factors include major trauma, shock of any type, sepsis, and renal failure. The clinician should identify high-risk patients early and initiate an appropriate prophylactic regimen, although the benefit of prophylactic regimens for overall mortality remains unproven.

Prophylactic regimens that have been proven effective include H_2 blockers, antacids, enteral feedings, and possibly proton-pump inhibitors. In a recent randomized, controlled trial, H_2 blockers were shown to be more effective in prevention of clinically significant bleeding than sucralfate, but sucralfate was associated with a trend toward lower incidence of pneumonia. The increased risk for pneumonia with H_2 blockers stems from increased gastric pH, facilitating colonization of the stomach by enteric organisms that may be aspirated (see below). Enteric feeding has also been shown to be an effective prophylaxis for gastrointestinal bleeding in ventilated patients, but this also predisposes to gastric colonization and pneumonia. Whichever method is chosen, effectiveness of prophylaxis should be monitored in high-risk patients by regular assessment of gastric aspirate pH.

Altered gastrointestinal motility is another common problem in critically ill patients. Decreased motility and ileus are frequently observed in patients receiving mechanical ventilation. Narcotic agents and hypoperfusion are important contributors, as are electrolyte abnormalities such as hypocalcemia. Motility agents such as metoclopramide and cisapride may be helpful, but the clinician must monitor for adverse effects of these agents. Serious arrhythmias have been attributed to interactions of cisapride with erythromycin, clarithromycin, or antifungal agents such as fluconazole, itraconazole, or ketoconazole. Correction of diarrhea begins with attention to causes including *Clostridium difficile* colitis, antacids, or rapid advancement of enteral feedings containing a high fraction of lipids. The patient care team should avoid responding to diarrhea with the use of rectal tubes, as these devices have been associated with significant morbidity, including erosion of bowel mucosa and bowel perforation.

Nutritional Complications

One of the most preventable nutritional complications in the ICU is malnutrition. The ICU team frequently becomes focused on dramatic and rapidly changing hemodynamic issues or diagnostic interventions, and nutrition becomes an afterthought several days into the ICU course. Unfortunately, protein catabolism occurs very early in the face of inadequate nutrition, and this will have adverse effects on respiratory muscle strength, ventilatory drive, immune function, and gut permeability. All critically ill patients should have some form of nutrition in place within 24 hours of ICU admission. Enteral nutrition is preferred because of proven benefits in the preservation of bowel mucosal function and prevention of gastrointestinal bleeding. If gut motility is profoundly compromised such that a patient's caloric needs cannot be met by enteral feeding, parenteral nutrition should be initiated.

Conversely, excessive calorie administration can lead to an increased respiratory quotient and a high ventilatory burden. This is especially problematic for patients with COPD or respiratory muscle weakness. This problem can be identified by indirect calorimetry, and it can be corrected by following nutritional formulas and nitrogen excretion and by providing a higher percentage of calories in the form of lipid.

Complications of nutritional support are more common with parenteral modalities and include hyperlipidemia, hyperglycemia, electrolyte abnormalities, cholestasis, and infection from venous access devices or contaminated products. Electrolytes, glucose, and triglyceride levels should be measured at least every 3 to 5 days in critically ill patients. Diabetic patients need very close monitoring of glucose levels. Glycemic control can be facilitated by inclusion of insulin in the formulas. New infectious symptoms warrant assessment for line infection and cholecystitis. For unclear reasons, some patients who require prolonged parenteral nutrition are at risk for severe hepatic dysfunction, including triaditis, fatty liver, and severe cholestasis. Avoidance of formulas with high quantities of protein and carbohydrates may be preventive. Some 10 to 30% of nonprotein calories should be supplied as lipid.

Complications associated with enteral feeding include aspiration; mishaps associated with placement of nasogastric tubes, such as pneumothorax and empyema; gastric colonization with enteric organisms; and diarrhea. Patients should remain at least 30 degrees upright to help prevent aspiration. The significance of high gastric residuals during enteral feeding remains controversial. When high residuals are associated with abdominal distension and hypoactive or high-pitched bowel sounds, an abdominal x-ray should be obtained. If signs of obstruction or ileus are present, the feedings should be held. Otherwise, the rate should be modified and gastrointestinal motility agents may be considered. Proper nasogastric tube placement must be confirmed by (1) listening in the epigastric region while instilling 20 mL of air; (2) aspiration of bilious fluid; and (3) ensuring phonation in patients who are not endotracheally intubated. Adequate placement of wire-guided Dubhoff-type tubes should be confirmed by x-ray, especially in the neurologically impaired patient. Tubes should be secured well, and continued appropriate placement should be monitored by the methods outlined. Many nasogastric tubes have a proximal port that is visible on x-ray. It is important that this port be beyond the gastroesophageal junction to ensure that feedings are not instilled into the esophagus.

Infectious Complications

Nosocomial infections in the ICU are a major source of morbidity, and the problem is intensified by the evolution of multidrug-resistant organisms, such as vancomycin-resistant enterococcus. Onset of infectious signs and symptoms should provoke a systematic evaluation that searches for the more common ICU-associated infections—including pneumonia, line-related sepsis, and urinary tract infection—but also less obvious sources such as meningitis, sinusitis (especially common in patients with nasogastric and nasotracheal tubes), empyema, endocarditis, abdominal or perirectal abscess, acalculous cholecystitis, peritonitis, and arthritis. While fever and leukocytosis are often present, other signs of infection or sepsis in the critically ill patient may include hypothermia, leukopenia, hypotension, tachycardia, mental status changes, and increased ventilatory requirements.

NOSOCOMIAL PNEUMONIA

Nosocomial pneumonia occurs in approximately 20% of patients receiving mechanical ventilation and accounts for delays in liberation from the ventilator and a prolonged ICU stay. The impact of ventilator-associated pneumonia on mortality in patients with complex and severe illness is unclear. Gram-negative bacilli account for the majority of these pneumonias. It is felt that these infections result from colonization of the oropharynx and stomach, followed by the tracheobronchial tree, by organisms that are able to capitalize on impaired host defenses. Increased availability of bacterial receptor sites and elevated gastric pH due to antacids or H_2 blockade are important mechanisms promoting colonization. Diagnosis of ventilator-associated pneumonia is complicated in that usual clinical criteria are very nonspecific. The diagnosis may be facilitated by quantitative culture of protected specimen brush (PSB) or bronchoalveolar lavage (BAL) samples that yield $>10^3$ CFU/mL for PSB and $>10^4$ CFU/mL for BAL.

Prevention of nosocomial pneumonia relies on adequate nutrition, avoidance of obtundation, upright positioning, pulmonary toilet, and proper endotracheal tube placement. Other measures under investigation include oral and gut decontamination, rotating beds, and endotracheal tubes that provide continuous suctioning above the cuff.

Hematologic Complications

Thrombocytopenia is a common occurrence in the ICU, with multiple etiologies. Medications are often the cause, especially antibiotics and H_2 blockers. The presence of heparin-induced platelet antibodies can be confirmed with serologic studies. When a decline in the platelet count is observed, a careful review of medication lists is important, even in the presence of illnesses that predispose to underproduction or sequestration of platelets. Folate deficiency is another preventable cause that should be considered. Unexplained neutropenia also requires a review of medication lists.

Slight decreases in the hematocrit are often observed in the critically ill patient and can be attributed to phlebotomy or other benign causes, but decreases of more than 2 to 3% require explanation. The gastrointestinal tract is a common site of hemorrhage (see above). Other important but much less obvious sites include the thigh and retroperitoneum, where spontaneous or iatrogenic hemorrhage may occur. CT scanning of these areas is indicated when blood loss unrelated to hemolysis or other obvious hemorrhage is noted.

Renal Complications

Acute renal failure in the critically ill patient is usually due to prerenal causes such as shock or hypovolemia or nephrotoxicity related to medications. Any change in urine output or blood urea nitrogen or creatinine levels should prompt a thorough evaluation of hemodynamics, volume status, and recent medications, especially nonsteroidal anti-inflammatory drugs (NSAIDs), angiotensin converting enzyme (ACE) inhibitors, aminoglycosides, amphotericin, or contrast dye. Obstructive uropathy is less common, but early consideration of this possibility and evaluation with ultrasound is important, since the management is substantially different. Foley catheter obstruction should be considered in the setting of hematuria with clots in the bladder. Prevention of acute renal failure depends on maintaining adequate renal perfusion, with the help of volume and inotropic agents when appropriate. The role of low-dose dopamine to enhance renal perfusion remains unclear. When procedures requiring contrast dye are required, additional hydration before and during the procedure may be protective.

Endocrinologic Complications

Glucose intolerance is extremely common in critically ill patients, especially in the setting of sepsis or multisystem organ failure. Maintenance of blood sugars below 150 to 200 mg/dL in the previously nondiabetic patient would be difficult and may not be beneficial. Adrenal insufficiency can be caused by shock, hemorrhage, infections, or medications such as ketoconazole or rifampin. More commonly, however, adrenal insufficiency is related to previous or current corticosteroid administration. Stress doses of corticosteroids should be administered to critically ill patients who were previously receiving corticosteroids. Adrenal insufficiency should be suspected in a patient presenting with persistent hemodynamic instability of unexplained etiology, and stress doses of dexamethasone should be administered while an adrenocorticotropin hormone (ACTH) stimulation test is performed.

Pharmacologic Complications

Pharmacologic complications are minimized by careful daily review of a patient's medication lists, with a focus on proper dosing, safe and appropriate routes of administration, important drug interactions, and whether each drug is still necessary in the patient's care. Participation in rounds by pharmacy staff can be helpful in managing these issues.

For a more detailed discussion, see Chap. 15 in *Principles of Critical Care*, 2d ed.

Chapter 7

NUTRITION IN THE INTENSIVE CARE UNIT

WILLIAM M. SANDERS

The need to provide nutrition early in the course of critical illness is well accepted, even though it has been difficult to prove that feeding has a positive effect on short-term outcome. Studies of nutrition in critical illness are faced with a number of inherent limitations. First, it is difficult to justify ethically not feeding patients in randomized, controlled comparisons. Moreover, the heterogeneity of illness in the intensive care unit makes comparisons between groups of patients difficult. Nonetheless, there is support for the notion that feeding, particularly by the enteral route, will improve wound healing, enhance immune function, and reduce infectious complications.

The long-term benefits of feeding are easier to identify. Without nutrition, a patient will starve and eventually die. During starvation, the metabolic needs of the central nervous system (CNS) are generally preserved, often at the expense of other tissues. The brain's requirement of 90 g of glucose per day is initially generated from the breakdown of glycogen stores in muscle and liver as well as hepatic gluconeogenesis, a process that converts amino acids from muscle proteins and glycerol from lipolysis to glucose. However, glycogen stores are depleted in 4 to 5 days, and eventually 50% of the brain's energy requirements are met by the oxidation of ketone bodies. The balance of glucose is generated from the catabolism of proteins and fat. Other organs can meet their metabolic needs through the metabolism of fat stores. During starvation, fat stores are normally exhausted within 60 days. However, the hypermetabolic state of critical illness can lead to protein-calorie malnutrition in a much shorter period.

Most organs suffer a decrease in nitrogen content as proteins are metabolized. CNS proteins are preserved, and the requirement of 75 g of protein per day is generated primarily from the breakdown of muscle. Protein metabolism generates nitrogen, which is excreted in the urine as urea nitrogen. Therefore, nitrogen losses in the urine can be considered equivalent to nitrogen balance. Normals excrete approximately 4 g per day, whereas fasting normals excrete approximately twice as much. Patients with severe burns can be highly catabolic and may lose up to 27 g per day of nitrogen. This is equivalent to 170 g of protein or 1 kg of body cell mass. At this rate of loss, a burned patient can become severely malnourished in less than 3 weeks.

Calculation of Metabolic Needs

CALORIC REQUIREMENTS

Complications of over- or underfeeding can be prevented by accurately determining a patient's metabolic needs. For some patients in the ICU, a rough estimate of metabolic requirements is adequate. In general, most patients can be fed adequately with 36 kcal/kg per day, or about 2500 kcal/day for a 70-kg person. Protein administration should be at least 0.6 g/kg per day. Many patients with more complex illness require more precise estimation of their nutritional requirements to prevent over- or underfeeding.

Empiric Formulas for Calculating Metabolic Demand

Empiric formulas have long been used to estimate the basal energy expenditure (BEE). The best known is the Harris-Benedict equation. In general, BEE is calculated from the patient's height in centimeters (H), weight in kilograms (W), and age in years (A):

For men: $EE = 66.5 + 13.7W + 5.00H - 6.78A$
For women: $EE = 66.5 + 9.56W + 1.85H - 4.68A$

This formula allows a more precise estimate of BEE; however, significant error in the estimate can arise from difficulties in measuring the patient's height and weight. The estimate can be multiplied by factors that take into account the patient's activity and severity of injury:

Activity:	On a ventilator	0.85
	Unconscious	1.00
	Awake in bed	1.10
	Sitting in a chair	1.20
	Walking in ward	1.30
Stress:	Minor surgery	1.20
	Trauma	1.30
	Sepsis	1.60
	Severe burns	2.10

For patients with fever, an additional 10% per degree over 37°C can be added to the energy expenditure.

Indirect Calorimetry

Indirect calorimetry is probably the most precise and convenient method to determine the energy requirements of critically ill patients and should be used when there is doubt about a patient's metabolic demands. A metabolic cart measures the minute volume and the exhaled concentration of oxygen and carbon dioxide. Oxygen consumption ($\dot{V}_{O_2}$) and carbon dioxide production ($\dot{V}_{CO_2}$) are then calculated. Sometimes urine urea nitrogen losses are measured and included in the calculation of caloric requirement. Energy expenditure is then determined by the following formulas:

$$EE \text{ (kcal)} = 3.6 \times \dot{V}_{O_2} + 1.4 \times \dot{V}_{CO_2}$$
$$- 1.2 \times \text{(nitrogen metabolism)}$$

or

$$EE \text{ (kcal)} = 3.6 \times \dot{V}_{O_2} + 1.4 \times \dot{V}_{CO_2} - 21.5$$

In most patients, the EE can be calculated to within 2% using a metabolic cart and an estimate of 21.5 kcal in protein metabolism, so quantification of urine nitrogen may not be necessary.

The Fick Principle

When a Swan-Ganz pulmonary artery catheter is in place, $\dot{V}_{O_2}$ can be measured by a modified Fick principle using measurements of cardiac output (Qt) and the difference of oxygen content in the arterial and mixed-venous blood:

$$\dot{V}_{O_2} \text{ (mL/min)} = \dot{Q}_T \text{ (mL/min)}$$
$$\times \frac{Ca_{O_2} \text{ (mL/dL)} - C\bar{v}_{O_2} \text{ (mL/dL)}}{100}$$

Assuming a diet with a normal balance of carbohydrate, protein, and fat 4.8 kcal will be liberated for each liter of oxygen consumed. Therefore:

$$EE \text{ (kcal)} = \dot{V}_{O_2} \text{ (mL/min)}/1000 \times 4.8 \text{ (kcal/L)}$$
$$\times 1440 \text{ (min/day)}$$

or

$$EE \text{ (kcal)} = \dot{V}_{O_2} \times 7.0$$

Measuring oxygen consumption by either method is subject to sampling error, because the patient's present level of activity and state of injury or infection will affect the oxygen consumption. Ideally, the average or steady-state oxygen consumption should be measured to calculate the patient's daily caloric requirement.

PROTEIN REQUIREMENTS

Critically ill patients metabolize protein in favor of carbohydrate or fat to a greater extent than healthy patients. The goal in providing protein is to try to limit the catabolism of constitutive proteins to glucose; however, providing greater than 14 g/day of nitrogen has been shown to be of little additional benefit, and may incur further complications of overfeeding. In general, the amount of protein can be estimated in relation to the patient's total caloric requirement. For most patients a calorie-to-nitrogen ratio of 150:1 will provide the appropriate amount of protein. Therefore, a patient who requires 2000 kcal/day should receive 13 g/day of nitrogen.

If protein losses are unusually large, protein catabolism may be estimated by measuring the nitrogen excreted in the urine. The goal is to administer enough protein to achieve positive nitrogen balance, with the realization that this may not be possible until the underlying illness resolves. Since 1 g of urine urea nitrogen is produced for each 6.25 g of protein and approximately 4 g of nitrogen is lost each day from stool and through the skin, the necessary protein or amino acid to administer can be calculated with the following formula:

Nitrogen balance = (grams of amino acid/6.25)
$$- \text{(24-h urine urea nitrogen in grams)} - 4 \text{ g}$$

Gastrointestinal hemorrhage can confound this calculation, because protein is lost in the stool in the form of blood and is virtually impossible to measure. Proteinuria can also confound this calculation, but this protein loss can be measured in the 24-h collection and included in the calculation.

FAT REQUIREMENTS

Calories that cannot be provided in the form of carbohydrate can be given as fat. There is a maximum amount of glucose that critically ill patients can metabolize—approximately 24 kcal/day. Providing carbohydrate calories above this does not result in greater glucose oxidation or protein synthesis. Fat provides a greater concentration of calories per gram (9 kcal/g), and can be infused in a smaller volume when administered with total parenteral nutrition (TPN). The usual formulations are 10 or 20% lipid derived from soybean oil. Absence of fat in the diet can lead to a fatty acid–deficiency syndrome.

Benefits and Risks of Enteral Feeding

Whenever possible, feeding should be attempted by an enteral route because it is less expensive, easier, and may allow for better delivery of nutrients. Enteral feeding may provide further benefits including reduced incidence of stress-related hemorrhagic gastritis and improved host immune response. In particular, enteral feeding may promote the gut mucosal barrier and may prevent the translocation of bacteria and endotoxins.

Nasogastric tubes are convenient for short-term enteral feeding. Standard Salem sump tubes can be placed into the stomach easily. Thin tubes with weighted ends (Dobhoff) have the advantage that they are smaller and therefore more comfortable for the patient. Moreover, they can sometimes be passed into the duodenum endoscopically or by peristalsis, and, by feeding into the duodenum, the risk of aspiration may be less. Placement of the tube within the stomach can be verified by injecting air through the tube and auscultating the abdomen. With any feeding tube, it is advisable to obtain radiographic confirmation that the tube tip is below the level of the diaphragms and beyond the gastroesophageal junction. This is particularly important with small-bore Dobhoff tubes, which can inadvertently be passed into the patient's airway.

Enteral feeding does carry some risk in critically ill patients. Massive aspiration can cause respiratory failure. Smaller aspiration events can lead to aspiration pneumonitis and pneumonia. Small-bore feeding tubes are thought to present less aspiration risk, but this has not been borne out in investigation. The supine position has been shown to significantly increase the risk of aspiration, so all patients receiving enteral feedings should have the head of their beds elevated to greater than 30 degrees. Aspiration can be detected by measurement of glucose in tracheal secretions or more sensitively by detecting the presence of methylene blue added to the feeding.

Nasogastric tubes are also associated with an increased incidence of sinusitis. When long-term feeding is required, percutaneous endoscopic gastrostomy or surgically placed gastrostomy may be preferred, particularly for patient comfort. Complications of these tubes include bleeding, infection, and erosion at the site of insertion by pressure necrosis or leakage of gastric acid. Occasionally the tubes can be dislodged into the peritoneum, resulting in peritonitis. When tubes fall out or are removed, they should be replaced promptly by experienced personnel and their position verified.

Ileus and gastroparesis are common in critical illness because of the hypercholinergic state, the hemodynamic effects of positive-pressure ventilation, the use of narcotic analgesics and paralytic agents, and immobility. Decreased gastric motility can increase the risk of aspiration and lead to failure to provide adequate nutrition. Metoclopramide and cisapride can often enhance gastrointestinal motility enough to overcome these problems.

Metabolic complications—including hyperglycemia, hypophosphatemia, and other electrolyte imbalances—can result from feeding. Monitoring of serum glucose and electrolyte composition on a regular basis can detect these complications. Sometimes an excess of calories can cause hypercapnea.

As soon as a patient loses the ability to eat due to critical illness, delivering nutrition by other means should be considered. If the patient is expected to eat in 2 to 3 days, intravenous fluid and glucose infusion alone may be adequate. If enteral feeding is possible, a tube should be placed and feedings started at full strength at one-third to one-half the goal rate (usually about 30 mL/h). The rate should then be systematically increased to reach the goal rate. Gastric contents can be periodically aspirated through the feeding tube to measure the gastric residual. A residual greater than 120 mL might indicate that the patient is not tolerating the feed, and very large residuals (200 to 300 mL) might increase the risk of aspiration.

If a patient continues to have large residuals, agents such as metoclopramide or cisapride can be used to enhance gastrointestinal motility. Moreover, pharmacologic agents such as narcotic analgesics should be minimized or removed.

Enteral feeding can sometimes cause diarrhea, either because the gut mucosa is abnormal or the feedings are hyperosmolar and draw fluid into the intestinal lumen. This can be treated by reducing the osmolarity of the feeding or by using a formula with added fiber. After infection is ruled out as a cause of the diarrhea, agents that decrease motility, such as loperamide, can be used.

Benefits and Risks of Parenteral Feeding

If nutrition cannot be delivered by the enteral route, hyperalimentation may be considered. This can be given through a peripheral vein (peripheral parenteral nutrition, or PPN) or through a central vein. PPN has the advantage that risks of central venous access are avoided; however, less concentrated formulas must be used to prevent irritation and sclerosis of the peripheral vein. Therefore, it may not be possible to deliver adequate calories with PPN.

Total parenteral nutrition (TPN) can be administered through a central vein and provides a patient with a complete complement of calories, as the concentration of glucose solutions can be much higher. Most hospitals supply a number of standard TPN solutions. The concentrations of glucose, amino acids, and electrolytes can be adjusted daily. Vitamins and essential trace elements are also added. Addition of insulin in the TPN solution can aid in the control of hyperglycemia.

Line-related complications are the major concern when nutrition is delivered through a central vein. These include bleeding, pneumothorax, local infection, thrombosis, and line-related bacteremia. There is also evidence that TPN may be associated with a decrease in host immune function, including inhibition of macrophage function, atrophy in gut-associated lymphoid tissue, depression in the CD4:CD8 ratio, and suppression of gut IgA. These changes are difficult to attribute solely to TPN and may be due to the absence of enteral feeding. Metabolic complications of TPN administration include hyperglycemia, hyperlipidemia, and liver dysfunction. Therefore, electrolytes, glucose, and liver function tests should be monitored routinely. Many complications of TPN administration can be avoided when dedicated nutrition support teams are utilized to formulate TPN solutions and monitor their use.

Special Considerations

RENAL FAILURE

Patients with renal failure are at risk for malnutrition due to protein losses in the urine and subsequent catabolism of constitutive proteins. In acute renal failure, appropriate nutritional support may improve nutritional status enough to promote healing of the damaged kidney. When large protein losses are suspected, as in the nephrotic syndrome, the urine protein and urea nitrogen should be measured in order to promote positive nitrogen balance.

HEPATIC FAILURE

The deranged metabolism of protein by the liver in hepatic failure leads to the generation of excess ammonia and other toxic metabolites that are thought to cause hepatic encephalopathy. The branched-chain amino acids (leucine, isoleucine, and valine) can be metabolized even when there is virtually no liver function left. Therefore, special diets for patients have been formulated using branched-chain amino acids. These formulas may lessen the degree of hepatic encephalopathy but have not been proven to improve outcome.

RESPIRATORY FAILURE

The beneficial effects of providing optimal nutrition in acute respiratory failure are well accepted. The goal is to improve patient strength without adding to the load of the respiratory system. Overfeeding with nonprotein calories can induce lipogenesis, which in turn generates excess carbon dioxide. Measurement of caloric needs with a metabolic cart may help to prevent this overfeeding. Diets that provide a greater percentage of calories as fat rather than carbohydrate can also decrease the generation of carbon dioxide while providing the same number of calories.

For a more detailed discussion, see Chaps. 16 and 78 in *Principles of Critical Care*, 2d ed.

Chapter 8

SYSTEMIC INFLAMMATORY RESPONSE SYNDROME

DELBERT DORSCHEID

The difference between the terms *systemic inflammatory response syndrome* (SIRS), *multiple organ dysfunction syndrome* (MODS), and *multiple organ system failure* (MOSF) resides in specific criteria defining each condition. Functionally they represent similar end-organ physiologic derangements arising during critical illness.

MOSF is the dysfunction of at least two organ systems for more than 24 h. Tables 8-1 and 8-2 summarize the defining criteria of and risks for this syndrome. MOSF is a major therapeutic challenge, occurring in up to 15 percent of patients admitted to the intensive care unit (ICU), and this number may increase as our ability to maintain the severely ill with advances in monitoring, imaging, antibiotics, and single-organ support extends. Many critical illnesses—most notably sepsis, trauma, severe inflammatory disorders, burns, and hypoperfused states—precipitate MOSF. It appears that these inciting events impair host defenses and cause inappropriate host regulation of acute immune and inflammatory responses (Fig. 8-1). Previously, MOSF was defined with subjective criteria of variable single-organ dysfunctions. This has been markedly improved with the standardization of APACHE II (see Chap. 17).

SIRS is a similar condition, defined as including one or more of the following: body temperature >38°C or <36°C; HR >90 beats per minute; respiratory status with a rate >20 respirations per minute or Pa_{CO_2} <32 mmHg; WBC >12,000/μL or <4000 μL or >10 percent of band neutrophils. It should be noted that at least 15 percent of people meeting these criteria are not infected.

TABLE 8-1   Modified Apache II Criteria for Organ System Failure[a]

Cardiovascular failure (presence of one or more of the following):
   Heart rate ≤ 54/min
   Mean arterial blood pressure ≤ 49 mmHg (systolic blood pressure ≤ 60 mmHg)
   Occurrence of ventricular tachycardia and/or ventricular fibrillation
   Serum pH ≤ 7.24 with a Pa_{CO_2} of ≤ 40 mmHg

Respiratory failure (presence of one or more of the following):
   Respiratory rate ≤ 5/min or >49/min
   $Pa_{CO_2} \geq 50$ mmHg
   $(A-a)_{O_2} \geq 350$ mmHg $(A-a)_{O_2} = 713$ $F_{I_{O_2}} - Pa_{CO_2} - Pa_{O_2}$
   Dependent on ventilator or CPAP on the 2nd day of OSF (i.e., not applicable for the initial 24 h of OSF)

Renal failure (presence of one or more of the following)[b]:
   Urine output ≤ 479 mL/24 h or ≤ 159 mL/8 h
   Serum BUN ≥ 100 μg/100 mL (>36 μmol/L)
   Serum creatinine ≥ 3.5 μg/100 mL (>310 μmol/L)

Hematologic failure (presence of one or more of the following):
   WBC ≤ 1000 μL
   Platelets $\leq 20,000$ μL
   Hematocrit $\leq 20\%$

Neurologic failure
   Glasgow Coma Scale score ≤ 6 (in absence of sedation)
   Glasgow Coma Scale score: Sum of best eye opening, best verbal, and best motor responses

Scoring of responses as follows (points):

Eye	Open: spontaneously (4); to verbal command (3); to pain (2); no response (1)
Motor	Obeys verbal command (6); response to painful stimuli—localized pain (5); flexion-withdrawal (4); decorticate rigidity (3); decerebrate rigidity (2); no response (1); movement without any control (4)
Verbal	Oriented and converses (5); disoriented and converses (4); inappropriate words (3); incomprehensible sounds (2); no response (1) If intubated, use clinical judgment for verbal responses as follows: patient generally unresponsive (1); patient's ability to converse in question (3), patient appears able to converse (5)

(Continued)

TABLE 8-1 (*Continued*)

Hepatic failure (presence of both of the following):
  Serum bilirubin >6 mg %
  Prothrombin time >4 s over control (in the absence of systemic
    anticoagulation)

ABBREVIATIONS: WBC, white blood count; BUN, blood urea nitrogen; Pa_{CO_2}, arterial partial pressure of carbon dioxide; $(A-a)_{O_2}$, alveolar-arterial difference in oxygen tension; FI_{O_2}, fraction of inspired oxygen; Pa_{O_2}, arterial partial pressure of oxygen; CPAP, continuous positive airway pressure.
[a]If the patient had one or more of the following during a 24-h period (regardless of other values), organ system failure (OSF) existed on that day.
[b]Excluding patients on chronic dialysis prior to hospital admission.
SOURCE: Modified from Knaus WA, Wagner D: Multiple systems organ failure: Epidemiology and prognosis. *Crit Care Clin* 5:221, 1989, with permission.

MODS is another entity defined by a scoring system assessing the extent of organ dysfunction (Table 8-3), for use in sepsis trials. A thorough understanding of the pathogenesis of MOSF may facilitate the development of effective prevention or treatment. Although these classification systems are useful to determine prognosis, they do not detail the role of

TABLE 8-2   Clinical Risk Factors for the Development and/or Lethal Progression of MOSF

Severity of disease (e.g., APACHE II, APACHE III score[a])
Severe trauma (injury severity score >25)
Age >65 years (>55 years in trauma patients)
Sepsis or infection at ICU admission
Systemic sepsis
  Bacteremic
  Nonbacteremic
  Nonbacterial
Arterial hypotension 24 h after ICU admission
Deficit in O_2 delivery/uptake after resuscitation from shock—
  persistently elevated serial blood lactate values
Focus of devitalized/injured tissue
Major operations
Aortic cross-clamp time >1.5 h during cardiopulmonary bypass
Preexisting liver dysfunction
Chronic alcohol abuse

[a]APACHE II score >20; APACHE III score >30

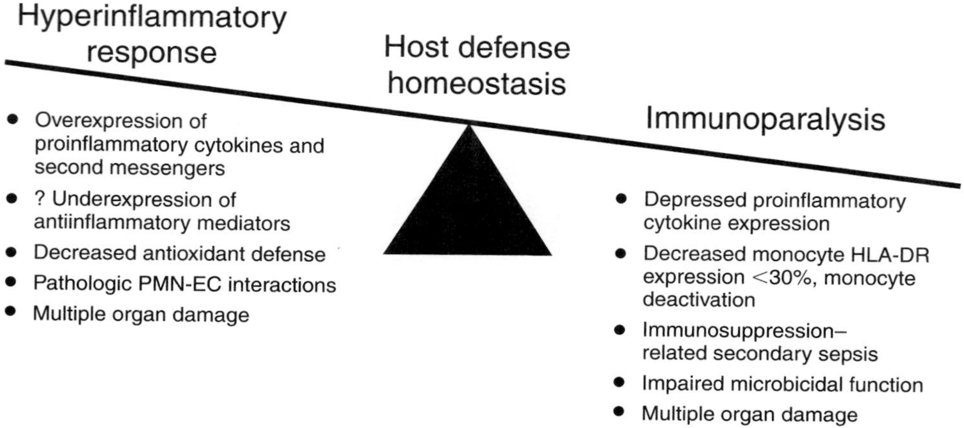

Hyperinflammatory response

- Overexpression of proinflammatory cytokines and second messengers
- ? Underexpression of antiinflammatory mediators
- Decreased antioxidant defense
- Pathologic PMN-EC interactions
- Multiple organ damage

Host defense homeostasis

Immunoparalysis

- Depressed proinflammatory cytokine expression
- Decreased monocyte HLA-DR expression <30%, monocyte deactivation
- Immunosuppression– related secondary sepsis
- Impaired microbicidal function
- Multiple organ damage

FIGURE 8-1 Bimodal immunologic risk periods for MOSF in relation to host defense homeostasis. Both hyperinflammatory responses from early overexpression of cytokines and cytokine-induced second-messenger systems, and delayed immunosuppression from trauma, burns, programmed cell death (apoptosis), and reduced immunostimulatory cytokine production with secondary sepsis share similar SIRS-related clinical features.

TABLE 8-3 The Sepsis-Related Organ Failure (SOFA) Score

SOFA Score	1	2	3	4
Respiration				
$Pa_{CO_2}/F_{I_{O_2}}$, mmHg	<400	<300	<200 with ventilatory support	<100
Coagulation				
Platelets $\times 10^3/\mu L$	<150	<100	<50	<20
Liver				
Bilirubin, mg/dL	1.2–1.9	2.0–5.9	6.0–11.9	>12.0
(μmol/L)	(20–32)	(33–101)	(102–204)	(>204)
Cardiovascular				
Hypotension	MAP <70 mmHg	Dopamine ≤5 or dobutamine (any dose)	Dopamine >5 or epinephrine 0.1 or norepinephrine ≤0.1	Dopamine >15 or epinephrine >0.1 or norepinephrine ≤0.1
Central nervous system				
Glasgow Coma Scale score	13–14	10–12	6–9	<6
Renal				
Creatinine, mg/dL	1.2–1.9	2.0–3.4	3.5–4.9	>5.0
(μmol/L) or urine	(110–170)	(171–299)	(300–440)	(>440)
output			or <500 mL/day	or <200 mL/day

[a]Adrenergic agents administered for at least 1 h (doses given are in μg/kg per minute).

89

specific, single-organ dysfunction and how the individual dysfunctions may interact.

Common Organ Failures

PULMONARY

The lung is the most common organ to fail in MOSF; the acute respiratory distress syndrome (ARDS) is the most typical lesion. Sepsis, aspiration, trauma, and pneumonia contribute to the inflammatory events underlying its pathogenesis. Mortality from ARDS alone exceeds 50 percent in some series. In addition, ARDS may itself lead to MOSF, with high mortality seemingly unrelated to the initial pulmonary dysfunction.

RENAL

Acute renal failure secondary to acute tubular necrosis (ATN) is the most common renal lesion in MOSF. ATN usually follows an episode of shock, but has been noted in the absence of well-defined episodes of hypoperfusion. The complex hemodynamic alterations that typify sepsis, in which renal blood flow is often preserved but metabolic demand is increased, may explain this phenomenon. The frequent superimposition of nephrotoxic drugs may also contribute. Acute renal failure related to sepsis still has a 40 to 60 percent mortality rate that has not changed in over 30 years. Improved survival has been noted with new dialytic therapy (continuous venovenous hemodialysis, for example) but is largely limited to patients with diabetes-related renal failure, nonseptic postoperative complications, or contrast nephropathy.

OTHER

Encephalopathy, hypermetabolism, hyperglycemia, acidosis, cardiac depression, disseminated intravascular coagulation (DIC), thrombocytopenia, leukopenia, stress ulceration, cholestasis, and liver synthetic failure also occur in MOSF, although less commonly than ARDS and ATN.

MODELS FOR MOSF

Tabulating and summing the multiple organ systems failures has been exemplified by the APACHE II score. However, this "summative model," based on the presumed equivalence of

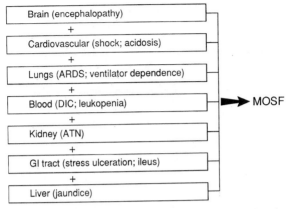

FIGURE 8-2 Summative model of organ system interactions in MOSF. Organs are assumed to have equivalent pathogenetic importance in the clinical expression of MOSF, the outcome of which depends on the numerical sum of organ-specific failures. MOSF, multiple organ system failure; ARDS, acute respiratory distress syndrome; DIC, disseminated intravascular coagulation; ATN, acute tubular necrosis.

organs (Fig. 8-2), is inadequate to explain the fundamental dysregulation of inflammation that amplifies organ failure. An alternative "relational" model emphasizes derangement of organs with immunoregulatory function, especially the liver and gastrointestinal tract (Fig. 8-3).

Pathogenesis

The most common etiology for MOSF is shock, typically septic shock. Yet many other diseases—including pancreatitis, thermal injury, trauma, connective tissue disease, and hepatic failure—can lead to MOSF. Less than 50 percent of trauma patients who die of MOSF have documented bacterial sepsis. Each of these processes may activate host inflammatory defenses, which are intended to be protective but instead become self-perpetuating, leading to tissue injury. Tissue damage itself incites more inflammation, propagating the hemodynamic and end-organ manifestations of MOSF. If

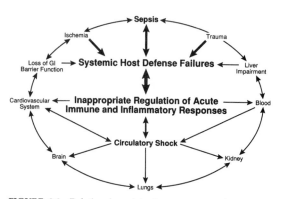

FIGURE 8-3 Relational model of organ system interactions in MOSF. Preexisting or acquired impairment of organs with immunoregulatory functions (e.g., liver, GI tract, lungs) amplify fundamental alterations in systemic host defense induced by severe sepsis, oxidant stress associated with ischemia-reperfusion and hypoxia-reoxygenation injuries, or trauma to cause remote organ dysfunction. Inappropriate host regulation of acute immune and inflammatory responses by genetic factors (e.g., allelic polymorphism at TNF- and IL-1 loci), pathologic signaling within a complex cytokine network, and cross-talk among cytokine and noncytokine second-messenger pathways result in overexpression of proinflammatory mediators. These processes synergize to produce circulatory shock, pansystemic endothelial injury, and organ dysfunction. Alternatively, subsequent development of a relative cytokine deficiency state predisposes to immunosuppression, secondary nosocomial infection, and MOSF by compromising antimicrobial defense. Bidirectional arrows depict interdependent effects.

homeostasis cannot be maintained, inflammation leads to a final common pathway of humorally mediated end-organ failure. This is the presumed mechanism whereby a large variety of different insults can activate the same set of defenses and eventuate in a form of self-perpetuating inflammation with organ damage. Even when the initial precipitant is successfully treated, the subsequent humoral cascade may be self-sustaining and continue the autoactivation of intravascular inflammation. This may explain why some patients deteriorate despite successful treatment of the inciting disease (Fig. 8-4).

THE ROLE OF THE GUT-LIVER AXIS

A widely accepted model for MOSF suggests that the gut may play a pivotal role as the "engine" of the system failure. Integrity of the gut mucosal barrier normally limits the translocation of bacteria and entry of bacterial products (such as endotoxin) into the portal circulation. Shock, infection, pancreatitis, trauma, and burns are believed to increase gut permeability by upregulation in local metabolism. An increased gut oxygen demand ($\dot{V}_{O_2}$) and/or a limit in the supply ($\dot{Q}_{O_2}$), possibly through inadequate oxygen delivery or derangements in the metabolism of glutamine, may lead to gut ischemia. The villi, which usually limit the translocation of bacteria and endotoxin, fail, leading to portal endotoxemia (Figs. 8-5 and 8-6). Liver Kupffer cells readily clear the endotoxin, which results in release of tumor necrosis factor and other cytokines in the initiation of the "protective" humoral cascade. This release of mediators then in turn may cause a further increase in $\dot{V}_{O_2}$ with risk for potentiating local hypoxia. Parenteral nutrition and disruption of the indigenous bowel flora may further compromise the gut mucosal barrier. When the capacity of the liver to clear endotoxin is exceeded, the hepatopulmonary axis and lung macrophages act as the second line of defense. This process may possibly explain the frequency of ARDS in MOSF, as endotoxin is a known experimental precipitant of ARDS. Preexisting hepatic dysfunction would be expected to accelerate the development of MOSF—a hypothesis that may explain the particularly poor outcome of critically ill patients with liver disease.

Prognosis

Table 8-4 summarizes data of Knaus and colleagues, who examined the prognosis of patients with MOSF. Prognosis clearly relates to the number and duration of organ failures. Although pooled data regarding prognosis cannot be applied to an individual patient with confidence and precision, this information may be used as a rough guideline to determine the appropriateness of continued treatment for cure or if therapy and support should be withdrawn. Generally, if three or more organ systems have failed for more than 3 days, the

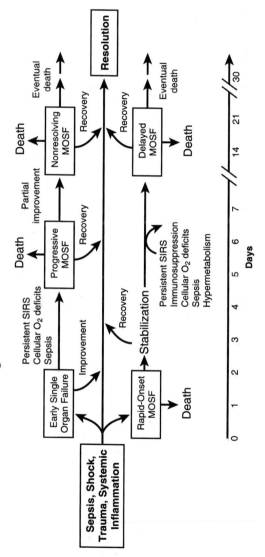

Progression vs Resolution of MOSF

◀ **FIGURE 8-4   Progression** *vs.* **clinical resolution of MOSF demonstrating diverse temporal sequences of onset and outcome. Rapid-onset single organ failure or early MOSF results from hyperinflammatory host responses within 3 days of such "single-hit" insults as acute sepsis, shock, trauma, or systemic inflammation (e.g., pancreatitis). By contrast, progressive or delayed MOSF reflects cumulative reductions in organ functional reserve because of underlying disease plus ongoing inflammation, immunosuppression, reductions in the cellular O_2 supply, secondary sepsis, and other multiple-hit processes. SIRS, systemic inflammatory response syndrome.** *(Modified from Civetta JM, Taylor RW, Kirby RR (eds): Critical Care, 3d ed. Philadelphia, Lippincott-Raven, 1997, p 343, with permission).*

patient is extremely unlikely to live, and withdrawal of therapy may be indicated if no improvement is noted in the patient's condition. This general observation has been made by multiple other investigators.

Treatment

A thorough understanding of the pathogenesis of MOSF may facilitate the development of effective prevention or treatment. Table 8-5 presents potential interventions to improve morbidity and mortality in MOSF. None are of proven efficacy in reducing morbidity or mortality, but they suggest avenues for further research. The recognition of endotoxemia dictated the study of antiendotoxin antibodies. As this therapy did not provide survival benefit to patients with sepsis, it is not likely these antibodies have a role in the larger universe of patients with SIRS/MOSF.

Steroids have on a number of occasions been investigated in the treatment of both ARDS and sepsis syndrome. Large prospective studies have not shown any benefit in these instances; many of these patients met criteria for MOSF. Thus it is not likely that the anti-inflammatory effects of corticosteroids will be useful in countering the unchecked inflammation of MOSF/SIRS.

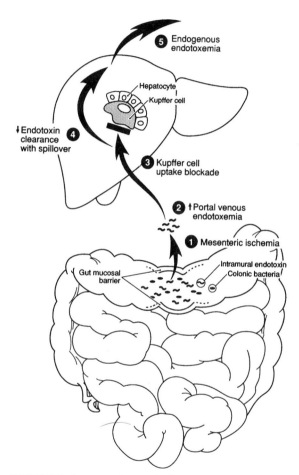

FIGURE 8-5 Sequence of events in the gut-liver axis involved in endogenous endotoxemia.

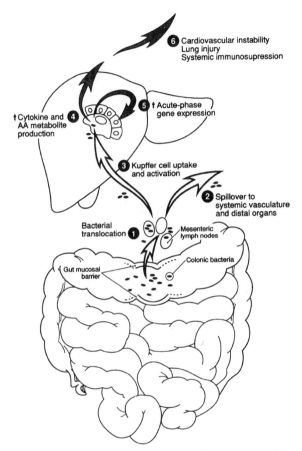

FIGURE 8-6   Sequence of events in the gut-liver axis involved in bacterial translocation.

TABLE 8-4 Mortality Statistics in a Large Cohort of Patients with MOSF.

Number of Organ System Failures	Day of Failure						
	1st	2nd	3rd	4th	5th	6th	7th
1	440/2297 19% / 37% 488/1323	294/1291 23% / 41% 347/842	248/1036 24% / 46% 309/672	221/846 26% / 47% 264/561	198/729 27% / 48% 235/491	170/615 28% / 50% 222/441	145/542 27% / 51% 179/353
2	313/718 44% / 64% 267/419	262/561 47% / 73% 221/302	219/415 53% / 71% 153/214	185/350 53% / 73% 139/191	160/311 51% / 72% 128/178	146/270 54% / 80% 111/138	126/217 58% / 83% 87/105
≥3	404/491 82%	302/322 94%	208/223 93%	152/159 95%	127/131 97%	103/105 98%	103/105 98%

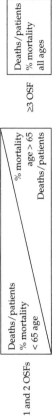

1 and 2 OSFs —
Deaths/patients
% mortality <65 age
% mortality age >65
Deaths/patients

≥3 OSF —
Deaths/patients
% mortality all ages

(Knaus et.al., Critical Care Clinics, 1989) (Reprinted with permission from Knaus W: Multiple Systems Organ Failure: Epidemiology and Prognosis, in Pinsky MR, Matuschak GM: Critical Care Clinics, Saunders WB, Philadelphia, 1989.)

TABLE 8-5   Mechanism-Oriented Prophylactic
and Therapeutic Options for Sepsis-Induced MOSF

Reduction in frequency/duration of deficits in systemic O_2 delivery
    by timely resuscitation and maintenance of intravascular blood
    volume

Therapeutic goals for O_2 delivery based on values from survivors

Source control of infection
    Antibiotics
    Drainage of purulent collections

Meticulous management of intravascular lines

Prevention of nosocomial pneumonia

Prevention of mesenteric/hepatic ischemia

Selective mesenteric dopaminergic receptor stimulation (e.g.,
    dopamine 1-3 μg/kg per minute)

Amelioration of oxidant stress by inhibition of xanthine oxidase-
    mediated generation of O_2 radicals

Allopurinol, sulfhydryl donors (e.g., N-acetylcysteine), other agents

Extracorporeal blood filtration to dampen malignant intravascular
    inflammation

Plasma exchange

Specific absorption (e.g., polymyxin B for endotoxin) or removal if
    inflammatory cytokines

Antiendotoxin approaches

Recombinant BPI

Anti-LBP antibodies

TFN-α/IL-1 antagonism
    Monoclonal antibodies or antibody fragments
    Chimeric soluble receptor fusion proteins
    Receptor antagonists (e.g., IL-1ra)
    Organ-specific transfection with antisense oligonucleotides
    Inhibitors of nuclear gene transcription/signal transduction

Administration of anti-inflammatory cytokines/CSFs:
    IL-10
    G-CSF

Stimulation with inflammatory cytokines to correct secondary
    immunosuppression
    Gamma interferon
    TNF-α
    Anti-IL-10 antibodies

NO inhibition
    Selective iNOS inhibitors
    Methylene blue

(Cont.)

TABLE 8-5 Mechanism-Oriented Prophylactic and Therapeutic Options for Sepsis-Induced MOSF *(Cont.)*

Modulation of coagulation cascade components
   Anti-tissue factor antibodies
   Administration of recombinant protein C, antithrombin III, of
      TFPI
Pharmacologic modulation of intracellular cyclic AMP in
   inflammatory cells
   Pentoxifylline
Pharmacologic modulation of cytokine gene expression
   or tissue effects
   Corticosteroids
   PAF synthesis inhibitors or PAF receptor blockade
   Cyclooxygenase pathway inhibition
   Lipoxygenase pathway inhibition or leukotriene
   receptor blockade

Study of other cytokines and their receptors, specifically interleukin-1 and tumor necrosis factor, have also led to clinical trials of biologic blockade of these systems, which did not confer benefit to patients with sepsis syndrome. Finally, there is early evidence from human trials of benefit when parenteral nutrition is supplemented with glutamine (thought by some to be an essential factor for maintaining gut mucosal integrity).

Given the current limitations in our understanding of MOSF, prevention is essential. Early resuscitation from shock to avoid tissue ischemia and end-organ failure is paramount. Organ-specific supportive therapy such as mechanical ventilation, renal dialysis, and nutritional support are indicated while reversible precipitants of MOSF are treated.

For a more detailed discussion, see Chap. 17 in *Principles of Critical Care,* 2d ed.

Chapter 9

PAIN CONTROL, SEDATION, AND USE OF MUSCLE RELAXANTS

MICHAEL O'CONNOR

Most critical care practitioners would agree that the ideal patient would be comfortable, cooperative, and accepting of care yet lucid. This state can be obtained in rare patients through the use of a regional anesthetic technique, such as a continuous epidural infusion. Unfortunately, many critically ill patients are not candidates for this technique, as it is relatively contraindicated in infected or coagulopathic patients. Consequently, opiates, benzodiazpines, propofol, and major tranquilizers such as haldol are frequently used to sedate critically ill patients. All of these classes of agents depress mentation in a dose-dependent fashion. A variety of tools are used to assess the level of sedation in critically ill patients, including the Glasgow Coma Scale and the Ramsey Scale (Table 9-1).

Most critically ill patients are sedated to control what we refer to as *distress behavior (agitation)*, which is usually nonverbal behavior in intubated patients suggesting distress (Table 9-2). Desire to control undesirable hypertension and tachycardia, rest the fatigued patient, and decrease oxygen

TABLE 9-1   Ramsey Scale

1—Patient anxious, agitated, or restless
2—Patient cooperative, oriented, and tranquil
3—Patient responds to commands only
4—Brisk response to glabellar tap or loud auditory stimulus
5—Sluggish response to glabellar tap or loud auditory stimulus
6—No response to glabellar tap or loud auditory stimulus

TABLE 9-2   Indications for Sedation

For distress behavior ("bucking" the ventilator, combativeness, behavior signaling discomfort)

To control unacceptable hemodynamics (delerium tremens, etc.)

To rest the fatigued patient (severe asthma or emphysema)

To decrease oxygen consumption in acute hypoxemic respiratory failure

---

consumption all also motivate practitioners to use sedation. Hypertension and tachycardia are frequently a consequence of pain and anxiety in the critically ill and are manifestations of a broader biological response commonly referred to as the *stress response*. It occurs as a consequence of psychological and physical stress to the organism and is associated with a complex cascade of changes that can last several days, including increased cortisol levels, increased catecholamine levels, increased ADH levels, hyperglycemia, and a variety of other neurologic, endocrine, and autocrine responses. Also associated with the stress response is a hypercoagulable state, which is obviously potentially beneficial in some circumstances and potentially very problematic in others. The stress response is potentially adaptive in the settings of hypovolemic and septic shock but is probably significantly detrimental in the setting of ischemic cardiac disease or other vasculopathy. Controlling pain can significantly reduce the magnitude of the stress response and the changes in patient physiology associated with it. Attempts to control the stress response associated with pain using agents other than analgesics are certain to fail and allow the stress response to continue unabated. When a patient manifests hypertension and tachycardia, his or her caregivers should consider using analgesics and anxiolytics as therapy as much as vasoactive drugs. Indeed, therapy with sedatives instead of vasoactive drugs is desirable in patients with ischemic heart disease, as vasoactive drugs treat only one limb of the stress response, whereas sedative agents treat all components of it. Control of the stress response in critically ill patients with ischemic heart disease improves their outcome.

TABLE 9-3   Underlying Causes of Agitation/
Distress Behavior

Pain
Dyspnea
Anxiety
Disorientation
Delirium (substance withdrawal)
Encephalopathy (renal/hepatic)
Psychosis
Others (e.g., nausea)

Distress behavior has a huge range of manifestations but a relatively small number of causes (Table 9-3). Pain or discomfort is the most common cause of distress behavior in critically ill patients. Mechanical ventilation is intrinsically uncomfortable and anxiety-producing, and the appliances associated with it—endotracheal and gastric tubes—can be very uncomfortable. Pain and discomfort are frequently underestimated as causes of agitation in critically ill patients, with the result that huge quantities of benzodiazepines are used where small quantities of opiates would suffice. Dyspnea is a frequently underestimated cause of distress behavior or agitation, because most patients with severe lung disease end up intubated and mechanically ventilated. Hence it is most severe in patients who lack ability to communicate verbally. Anxiety is a feature present in less critically ill patients. As patients become more ill, they tend to have diminished mentation and insight into their circumstances. Anxiety is a major feature in patients with acute-on-chronic respiratory failure, such as asthma or emphysema. Disorientation, encephalopathy, delirium, and psychosis can all cause patients to manifest the same kinds of behavior as pain, dyspnea, and anxiety and should therefore be included in any list of causes of distress behavior; they should be considered or investigated as possible causes in appropriate patients. Disorientation should be regarded as an almost unavoidable consequence of admission to the intensive care unit (ICU). It afflicts the elderly and debilitated very quickly, usually within days, but will ultimately afflict almost any patient who remains resident

TABLE 9-4   Strategies for Maintaining Orientation
in Critically Ill Patients

Repeatedly orient the patient as to the day of the week, time of day
  (morning, afternoon, evening, night) and place

Open window curtains during daylight hours

Turn down the lights and keep noise to a minimum during the
  night

Repeatedly apprise patients of their condition and interventions
  being performed on their behalf

Encourage all bedside caregivers to introduce themselves every time
  they interact with a patient

Encourage visits from family and friends; ask them to bring in
  objects which might help orient the patient (pictures, etc.)

Inquire as to favorite television or radio shows watched by the
  patient and provide them to the patient if possible

---

in the ICU long enough. Strategies to maintain orientation in
critically ill patients are included in Table 9-4.

Bedside caregivers should assess patients in distress and
estimate the contributions of pain, dyspnea, and anxiety to
their distress, and select sedative agents as appropriate (Table
9-5). Almost all classes of sedative agents depress consciousness in a dose-dependent fashion; hence all can be used to
depress mentation. By selecting appropriate agents, caregivers can achieve patient comfort with minimal depression
of mentation, lower doses of drugs, and fewer side effects.
The use of benzodiazepines to treat pain will not succeed and

TABLE 9-5   Properties of Commonly Used Sedative Agents

Class	Analgesia	Anxiolysis	Suppress Dyspnea	Amnesia
Opiates	+ + + +	+ +	+ + + +	0
Benzodiazepines	0	+ + + +	0	+ +
Propofol	+	+ + +	?	+ +
Haloperidol	+	+ + + +	0	0
Paralytics	0	0	0	0

will lead to the infusion of large doses of drug. On the other hand, benzodiazepines and propofol, especially when used in doses associated with unconsciousness, are likely to be associated with amnesia, whereas opiates are not. Major tranquilizers, such as haloperidol, are frequently used as sedatives in the ICU, but in much larger doses than have been used in other domains; hence our understanding of their actions in this application is limited. Paralytic agents have no effect on the CNS and hence have none of the properties sought in sedative agents.

The mainstay of most sedation regimens in the ICU should be opiates. Opiates will treat the discomfort and pain almost universally present in critically ill patients and suppress the dyspnea that is commonly present in mechanically ventilated patients; they are also far more efficacious in treating anxiety than is commonly believed. Anxiolytic agents such as benzodiazepines, haloperidol, and propofol should be administered as supplements to the opiate regimen. Since the pain and dyspnea that critically ill patients suffer from do not fluctuate significantly during a day, it is reasonable to use longer-acting opiate agents. Shorter-acting opiates are superficially attractive for this purpose but have a variety of limitations, including more rapid development of tolerance, greater expense, and larger infused volumes. Morphine, methadone, and hydromorphone are all appropriate for use in the ICU. Patient-controlled analgesia (PCA) requires patient self-assessment and ability to self-medicate, which is frequently not possible in critically ill patients. PCA is certainly a very viable and effective modality to control patient pain, but its use is likely to be limited to less sick patients and patients whose discharge from the ICU is imminent. Although we do not encourage their widespread use, meperidine and fentanyl are also commonly used in the ICU. The use of large doses of meperidine over time can be complicated by the accumulation of an active metabolite, normeperidine, which can lower the seizure threshold and precipitate seizures. Fentanyl is shorter acting than necessary in most ICU patients, and as a rule patients rapidly develop a tolerance to it. Bolus doses of fentanyl are very appropriate for analgesia for bedside procedures performed in the ICU, such as dressing changes, chest tube insertion, etc. Because opiates decrease gut motility in a dose-dependent fashion, strong consideration should be given to prescribing medications to maintain gut motility whenever opiates are used in the ICU. Stool softeners such as ducosate, bowel irritants such as bisacodyl, and osmotic agents such as lactulose are all appropriate choices.

Among the large numbers of benzodiazepines available to present-day practitioners, lorazepam, midazolam, and diazepam are by far the most commonly used in the ICU. All can be used safely and effectively for sedation in the ICU. Diazepam has active metabolites, including oxazepam, that can accumulate in critically ill patients. It is not clear whether this is a real or hypothetical concern, but its use in recent years has diminished in favor of midazolam and lorazepam. Midazolam is attractive because it is relatively short-acting, is not associated with pain upon injection (a consequence of its water-solubility), and can be administered via continuous infusion. Experience with midazolam suggests that the drug or an active metabolite may accumulate, that tolerance to the drug may occur rapidly, and that the cost and infused volumes associated with continuous infusions may be far greater than many appreciate. Lorazepam is consequently the benzodiazepine of choice in many ICUs. Although it is associated with some pain upon injection, clinical experience suggests that it is less costly and perhaps even more titratable than midazolam (surprising, since it is a longer-acting agent).

Propofol infusions enjoy growing popularity because of the ease of titrating sedation with this agent. Infusions can be turned down or off, and abdominal and neurologic exams may be performed on otherwise very deeply sedated patients. The timing of liberation from ventilation and extubation can also usually be well controlled with propofol infusions. Concerns about the consequences of the obligatory infused volume of fat emulsion continue to trouble many. For this reason, infusions should be limited to a dose of no higher than 60 μg/kg per min in most settings. Finally, haloperidol, when given in large doses, can be used to achieve long-lasting sedation. Haloperidol is especially effective in patients who are otherwise tolerant to the effects of opiates and benzodiazepines, such as oncology patients and intravenous drug abusers. Drawbacks to haloperidol include a host of side effects, such as extrapyramidal symptoms and neuroleptic malignant syndrome. Because the risk of extrapyramidal side effects is substantial at the doses of haloperidol used in the ICU, practitioners should seriously consider using empiric prophylactic treatment for them. Table 9-6 lists the more commonly used agents, some relevant clinical pharmacokinetics and dynamics, and dose ranges for bolus doses and continuous infusion in the ICU. The onset of action of these agents may be enhanced by a hyperdynamic circulation and delayed by a depressed circulation. Similarly, the duration of effect can be prolonged in patients with hepatic and renal dysfunction. Bolus doses in the lower range are more appropriate for hypotensive, elderly, and frail patients. Bolus doses in the higher range are more appropriate for healthier patients with significant circulatory reserve (i.e., an intubated, young, healthy asthmatic patient). Infusions should generally be started at the lower end of the range and titrated upward as needed.

The role of paralytic agents in the ICU has changed dramatically over the past 10 years. In the past, they were almost automatically incorporated into any sedation regimen in intubated, mechanically ventilated patients. Concerns about their potential to cause the polyneuropathy of critical illness and their expense have resulted in a significant decline in their use in critical care. Whereas most mechanically ventilated patients were paralyzed 10 years ago, only 3 to 5% are now. The use of paralytic agents is now reserved for patients who cannot be adequately sedated because they are being ventilated with very uncomfortable modes of mechanical ventilation, such as jet ventilation, pressure-control ventilation, inverse ratio ventilation, and high PEEP. Table 9-7 lists the accepted indications for paralysis in the ICU.

Although a large number of paralytic agents are available for use today, most ICU practitioners need only know how to use one or two of these. The choice of which paralytic agent to use is usually determined by the drug's route of elimination. Renally excreted drugs such as pancuronium, are undesirable in patients with renal failure or evolving multisystem organ dysfunction. Pancuronium will accumulate in patients with renal failure, and a few doses can produce neuromuscular blockade lasting for days. Paralytic agents that depend upon the liver for their elimination, such as vecuro-

TABLE 9-6 Comparison of Sedative Agents and Their Effects

Agent	Onset of Action, min	Single-Dose Duration	Risk of Prolonged Effect	Equipotent Dose, mg	Suggested Dosing Bolus	Infusion
Morphine	5–10	4 h	++	10	1–5 mg	1–20 mg/h
Methadone	30–60	6–24 h	+	10	5–20 mg	NA
Hydromorphone	5–10	4–6 h	+	1.5	0.5–1.0 mg	0.5–2.0 mg/h
Fentanyl	2–5	0.5–1 h	++	0.1	25–100 μg	1–10 μg/kg/h
Midazolam	1–5	0.5–2 h	+++	3	0.5–5 mg	0.01–0.3 mg/kg/h
Lorazepam	15–20	6–10 h	++	1	0.5–4 mg	0.01–0.1 mg/kg/h
Diazepam	2–5	30–60 min	++++	5	5–10 mg	
Propofol	1–5	2–8 min	0		NA	1–60 μg/kg/min
Haloperidol	2–5	2–24 h	+		2.5–20 mg	

TABLE 9-7   Indications for the Use of
Paralytic Agents in the ICU

To facilitate mechanical ventilation, typically with unusual modes,
    such as high frequency ventilation, inverse ratio ventilation, or
    very high PEEP
For Endotracheal intubation and other bedside procedures (the use
    of paralytics in this setting should be restricted to experts trained
    in their use)
To treat tetanus refractory to medical therapy
To treat poisoning (strychnine, methaqualone)
To treat hypothermia/shivering
To treat status epilepticus associated with inability to ventilate the
    patient (very rare)

---

nium and rocuronium, can cause similar problems in patients
with hepatic insufficiency. Atracurium and cisatracurium are
eliminated by their spontaneous degradation in the blood, a
process referred to as Hofmann elimination, and are thus
quite safe to give to patients with renal or hepatic insufficiency. Table 9-8 lists pertinent pharmacokinetic and phar-
macodynamic information for paralytic agents commonly
used in the ICU.

Pancuronium is the paralytic agent of choice for patients
with normal renal function. Atracurium and cisatracurium
should be used in patients with impaired renal function, impaired hepatic function, or substantial risk of developing multisystem organ failure. Rocuronium and vecuronium should
only rarely be used in the ICU. Succinylcholine in the ICU
should be restricted to airway management and administered
by individuals who are trained experts.

It is imperative that all paralytic agents be carefully monitored in the ICU. In most settings, this entails the use of a
neuromuscular stimulator and the train-of-four mode by personnel trained to use these devices. The neuromuscular stimulator is a device used to deliver electrical impulses to peripheral nerves (usually the ulnar nerve) and assess the level
of muscular response. Normal muscular contraction is consistent with normal muscle function; the absence of muscular contraction is consistent with deep neuromuscular block-

TABLE 9-8 Dosage and Administration of Paralytic Agents

Agent	Intubating Dose, mg/kg	Duration of Intubating Dose, min	Infusion Rate	Elimination
Pancuronium	0.10	60–120	0.025 mg/kg/h	70% renal 30% biliary
Cisatracurium	0.20	25–50	1–10 µg/kg/min	Hofmann
Rocuronium	0.6–1.2	50–80	10–20 µg/kg/min	Biliary
Vecuronium	0.10	30–45	0.07 mg/kg/h	20% renal 40% biliary
Atracurium	0.50	30–45	0.25 mg/kg/h	Hofmann
Succinylcholine	1	2–7	NA	Pseudocholinesterase

ade with paralytic agents. It is also desirable to stop or turn down the infusion of paralytic agents on a daily basis to assess patients and their ability to recover from the agent that has been administered.

For a more detailed discussion, see Chap. 10 in *Principles of Critical Care,* 2d ed.

Chapter 10

OVERVIEW OF RESPIRATORY FAILURE

MICHAEL WALDMAN

The function of the respiratory system is to provide oxygen to the tissues and to eliminate carbon dioxide that is produced as a waste product of tissue metabolism. These two functions of the lung are frequently independent of each other. Therefore, respiratory failure can be defined as the failure to provide adequate oxygen delivery to the tissues and/or the failure to adequately eliminate carbon dioxide. There are four classes of respiratory failure, all of which lead to arterial hypoxemia, arterial hypercarbia, or both.

Causes of Inadequate Oxygen Delivery

Before discussing the types of respiratory failure it is useful to review the physiology that leads to hypoxia or hypercarbia. Oxygen delivery is dependent on arterial oxygen content, hemoglobin concentration, cardiac output, and the tissue metabolism of oxygen. While the focus here is on arterial hypoxemia, it is important to recognize that critically ill patients frequently have anemia, diminished cardiac output, and increased tissue metabolism from fevers or increased work of breathing. Addressing these issues can be as important to preventing anaerobic metabolism as correcting alveolar hypoxia.

Arterial hypoxia is usually caused by alveolar hypoventilation, ventilation/perfusion ($\dot{V}/\dot{Q}$) mismatch, shunt, or diminished mixed venous oxygenation. Alveolar hypoventilation produces mild hypoxemia when the required oxygen uptake is greater than the partial pressure of oxygen in the alveolus. The partial pressure of oxygen is diminished as arterial carbon dioxide increases. However, small increments in inspired oxygen fraction will correct the hypoxemia ($P_{A_{O_2}} = P_{I_{O_2}} - Pa_{CO_2}/R$). Causes of alveolar hypoventilation are discussed later in the chapter.

$\dot{V}/\dot{Q}$ mismatch describes the situation where some lung units have increased ventilation relative to perfusion (high $\dot{V}A/\dot{Q}$ units) and other lung units have decreased ventilation relative to perfusion (low $\dot{V}A/\dot{Q}$ units). This can occur in obstructive lung disease, where the high $\dot{V}A/\dot{Q}$ units lead to increased dead space and increased arterial carbon dioxide, and the low $\dot{V}A/\dot{Q}$ units lead to hypoxemia. Modest increments in inspired oxygen fraction will correct the hypoxemia (see Fig. 10-1).

In shunt, some lung units are perfused but not ventilated, as there is a lung-filling process (e.g., pulmonary edema, pneumonia, pulmonary hemorrhage). The blood leaving these lung units has oxygen and carbon dioxide content equal to that of the mixed venous content. The arterial oxygen content is independent of the inspired fraction of oxygen, as there is no gas exchange in the flooded lung units (see Fig. 10-1).

Decreased mixed venous oxygenation usually has little influence on arterial oxygenation, as the functional reserve of the lungs is normally able to fully oxygenate the venous blood as it passes, no matter how deoxygenated it may be. However, if the mixed venous saturation decreases due to diminished cardiac output in a patient with shunt or $\dot{V}/\dot{Q}$ mismatch, it will significantly worsen the arterial hypoxemia.

Correction of arterial hypoxemia is accomplished by optimizing oxygen delivery in the individual patient. In patients with hypoventilation and/or $\dot{V}/\dot{Q}$ mismatch, this is readily accomplished with supplemental oxygen for the reasons given above. In patients with acute hypoxemic respiratory failure (AHRF) arising from intrapulmonary shunt, the goals of therapy are somewhat different because of the lack of an adequate response to oxygen alone. In patients with AHRF, reasonable goals are to have the minimal positive end-expiratory pressure (PEEP) to obtain 90% oxygen saturation of an adequate circulating hemoglobin concentration on a nontoxic $F_{I_{O_2}}$, with the lowest pulmonary vascular pressures compatible with an adequate cardiac output. In addition, efforts should be made to limit tissue metabolism of oxygen by decreasing the work of breathing with mechanical ventilation and sedation and cooling the febrile patient if necessary (see Chap. 15).

Causes of Hypercapnea

The clearance of carbon dioxide is dependent upon minute ventilation, dead-space fraction, and carbon dioxide production from the tissues. To maintain adequate minute ventilation, a patient must have both sufficient respiratory drive to breathe and sufficient respiratory muscle strength to overcome the respiratory load to expand the lungs.

Arterial carbon dioxide content is dependent upon metabolic CO_2 production (V_{CO_2}), dead-space volume (V_D), and the minute ventilation (MV) as described in the relation $P_{CO_2} = k \times V_{CO_2}/\{MV \times [1-(V_D/V_T)]\}$, where V_T is the tidal volume. Therefore, hypercarbia can occur when metabolic production of carbon dioxide increases in the presence of the inability to increase alveolar ventilation, decreased minute ventilation, or the dead-space fraction increases in the presence of the inability to increase minute ventilation.

Most disease states having an effect on the neurohormonal inputs in the brainstem result in augmented central respiratory drive. Most commonly, decreased central respiratory drive results from the use of drugs (narcotics, alcohol, sedatives, anesthetics). Some toxins, central nervous system (CNS) injuries, and severe hypothyroidism may also cause diminished central respiratory drive. However, with the exception of drugs and toxins, failure of central respiratory drive is rarely the sole etiology of respiratory failure.

Before discussing respiratory muscle strength and respiratory load, it is useful to review respiratory mechanics. A pressure must be generated by the respiratory muscles to expand the chest wall and lungs against their elastance and generate an inspiratory flow past the airway resistance. Therefore, the respiratory muscles are working against the lungs, the chest wall, and the airway resistance. When a patient is mechanically ventilated, the airway pressures as measured by the ventilator may offer insight into the etiology of respiratory failure. In airway obstruction, the peak inspiratory pressure to overcome the airway resistance is often as elevated as 60 cmH$_2$O. However, during an inspiratory pause with no flow across the airways, the pressure measured is that of the elastic recoil of the lungs and the chest wall. In the case of

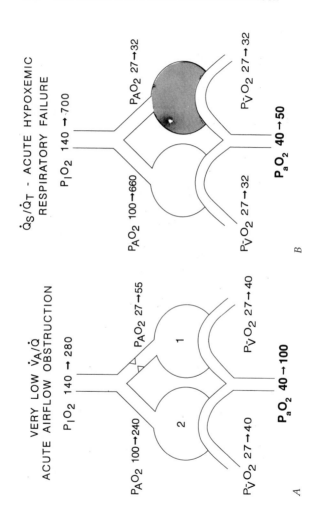

◀ FIGURE 10-1   Schematic illustration showing the effects of oxygen therapy on arterial P_{O_2} (Pa_{O_2}) in two conditions: (A) acute airflow obstruction and (B) airspace flooding with acute hypoxemic respiratory failure (AHRF). Each panel depicts a two-compartment lung in which each airspace is perfused by half the mixed venous blood with a P_{O_2} ($P\bar{v}_{O_2}$) of 27 mmHg while breathing room air, which has a fractional concentration of oxygen in the inspired gas ($F_{I_{O_2}}$) of 0.21. Acute airflow obstruction causes severe hypoxemia that is relatively easily corrected by breathing supplementary oxygen, but hypoxemia in AHRF is much more refractory to oxygen administration and so requires adjunctive therapies. A. Because the airspace distal to the obstruction is so poorly ventilated, all its inspired oxygen is absorbed and alveolar P_{O_2} values (PA_{O_2}) approach mixed venous P_{O_2} values (27 mmHg). By contrast, because alveolar P_{O_2} in the well-ventilated alveolus is considerably higher (100 mmHg), its effluent blood becomes fully saturated (S_{O_2} = 100%); when this blood mixes with an equal amount of effluent blood from the obstructed unit (S_{O_2} = 50%), the resulting arterial blood (Sa_{O_2} = 75%) has a very low P_{O_2} (40 mmHg). Raising $F_{I_{O_2}}$ to 0.4 (P_{O_2} = 280 mmHg) increases both the amount of oxygen ventilating the obstructed unit and the alveolar P_{O_2} (55 mmHg). Accordingly, effluent blood from the obstructed airspace (S_{O_2} = 90%) mixes with fully saturated blood from the well-ventilated alveolus, which also contains more dissolved oxygen, causing arterial S_{O_2} to approach 100% and arterial P_{O_2} to approach 100 mmHg. Note that this increased arterial oxygen transport is associated with increased mixed venous P_{O_2} (27 to 40 mmHg). B. During room air breathing, the oxygen exchange is as described in A because half the mixed venous blood traverses the flooded airspace from which no oxygen can be absorbed; accordingly, arterial P_{O_2} is 40 mmHg and mixed venous P_{O_2} is 27 mmHg. Raising $F_{I_{O_2}}$ to 1.0 increases the dissolved oxygen content in the fully saturated blood exiting the well-ventilated alveolus by about 2 mL/dL (because alveolar P_{O_2} increases from 100 to 660 mmHg), but oxygen is still not absorbed from the flooded airspace. Accordingly, arterial P_{O_2} increases slightly (40 to 50 mmHg), and the increased O_2 delivery allows mixed venous P_{O_2} to increase slightly (27 to 32 mmHg).

airway obstruction, the lungs and chest wall are normal, so the elastic pressure is 10 cmH$_2$O. The large gradient between the two pressures is indicative of a high airway resistance. In a patient with pulmonary edema, the peak inspiratory pressure to inflate the lungs may again be 60 cmH$_2$O. However, in this patient the elastic pressure will be elevated to 50 cmH$_2$O, as the tidal volume is overdistending the small

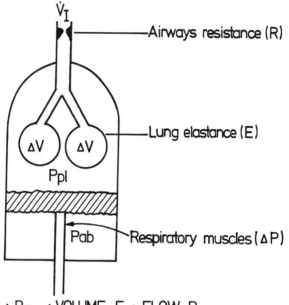

$$\Delta P = \Delta VOLUME \cdot E + FLOW \cdot R$$

A

FIGURE 10-2 *A.* Schematic depicts the mechanical characteristics of the respiratory system. Inspiratory flow ($\dot{V}_I$) is delivered through an airway with resistance (R) to a two-compartment lung model, the units of which have elastance (E) and are distended by the delivered volume (V). During positive-pressure ventilation, lung distention raises the pressure between the lungs and chest wall (Ppl) to increase the volume of the chest wall, in part by pushing the diaphragm downward (see piston at the floor of the thorax) to raise the abdominal pressure (Pab); during a spontaneous breath, the respiratory muscles (P) pull the piston down to lower Ppl and inspire V across R. In either case, ΔP = the elastic pressure (Pel = V × E) plus the resistive pressure (Pr = $\dot{V}_I$ × R).

number of aerated alveoli. The normal gradient between the peak and elastic pressures indicates that the cause of the elevated pressure is either from the lungs, the chest wall, or the abdominal cavity (see Fig. 10-2).

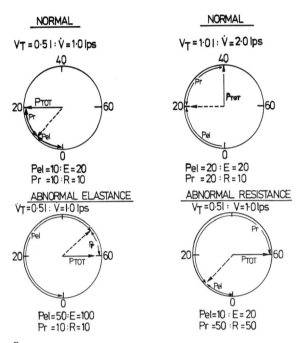

B

FIGURE 10-2 (*Continued*)   *B*. Schematic of the pressure dial on a mechanical ventilator illustrating the measurement of respiratory elastic pressure (Pel) and resistive pressures (Pr) and a calculation of E and R. The upper panels illustrate normal respiratory mechanics for a normal tidal volume and flow rate (*left*) and for a large tidal volume and flow rate (*right*). The lower panels illustrate abnormal elastance (*left*) and abnormal resistance (*right*). For discussion, see text.

In normal patients the maximal negative inspiratory force exceeds 100 cmH$_2$O, whereas the work of spontaneous breathing is 10 cmH$_2$O or less, providing considerable respiratory muscle reserve. As long as the work of spontaneous breathing is less than one-third of the maximal inspiratory force, respiratory failure should not occur. However, many conditions may impinge on this reserve. The main groups of disorders that cause respiratory muscle weakness are neuromuscular diseases (amyotrophic lateral sclerosis, muscular dystrophies, myasthenia gravis), toxic or metabolic neuromuscular dysfunction (electrolyte abnormalities, sepsis, malnutrition, drugs), circulatory insufficiency, respiratory muscle fatigue (acute on chronic respiratory failure), and

TABLE 10-1 Liberation of the Patient from Mechanical Ventilation

Correctable Factors Decreasing Respiratory Muscle Load	Correctable Factors Increasing Respiratory Muscle Strength
Type I: AHRF	Type VI: Shock
Reduce edema production	Hypoperfusion
Enhance edema clearance	Hypotension
Treat pneumonia	Anemia
Drain pleural effusions	Hypoxia
Stabilize chest wall	Sepsis
Least PEEP	Fever
Minimize dead space	Acidosis
	Electrolytes (K^+, Ca^{2+}, Mg^{2+}, PO_4^{2-})
Type II: Airflow obstruction	Protein-calorie nutrition
Hypoxemia—give O_2	Aminophylline
Reverse sedation	
Bronchodilation	Common confounding conditions
Clear bronchial secretions	Neuromuscular disease
Treat bronchial infection	Muscle-relaxing drugs
Pneumothorax—chest tube	Coma, sedation
Fractured ribs—nerve block	Cerebrovascular accident
Decrease intrinsic PEEP	Subclinical status epilepticus
Allow HCO_3 accumulation	Hypothyroidism
Reduce CO_2 production	Phrenic nerve paralysis
Type III: Perioperative RF	Respiratory muscle fatigue
Posturize and pummel	
Ventilate 45 degrees upright	Respiratory muscle exercise program
Treat incisional/abdominal pain	Tone
Drain ascites	Power
Reexpand atelectasis early	Coordination
Stop smoking 6 weeks preop	Animation
Avoid overhydration	

respiratory muscle atrophy (chronically mechanically ventilated patients).

Increased mechanical load may be from increased resistance (obstructive pulmonary diseases), increased lung elastance (airspace filling, pulmonary fibrosis), increased chest wall elastance (obesity, bandages, scar), or increased abdominal wall elastance (ascites, postoperative state). Any of these conditions will lead to respiratory muscle fatigue if the pressure to expand the lungs increases to a level that cannot be sustained by the neuromuscular system (see Table 10-1).

Any condition that necessitates increased minute ventilation may cause an increased respiratory load that may produce respiratory failure if there is not sufficient respiratory muscle reserve. These situations include the causes of hypercarbia (mismatch, increased dead space), hypoxia (shunt), and metabolic acidosis (renal failure, lactic acidosis), which all trigger compensatory hyperventilation.

Clinical Classification of Respiratory Failure

The utility of classifying respiratory failure is that the different types tend to have distinct presentations, clinical settings, and, therefore, specific treatments (see Table 10-2).

Type I, or acute hypoxemic respiratory failure (AHRF), is a failure of oxygenation due to airspace flooding. This produces a shunt lesion that is refractory to supplemental oxygen. The patients typically have a hyperventilation response, which produces a low arterial carbon dioxide until late in the course of respiratory failure. The treatment is to optimize oxygen delivery, as discussed above.

Type II, or hypoventilatory respiratory failure, is the primary failure of alveolar ventilation, leading to hypercarbia. Hypoxemia in these cases corrects easily with supplemental oxygen. Hypoventilation may be due to inadequate central respiratory drive, decreased respiratory muscle strength, increased respiratory load, increased dead space fraction, or increased metabolic production of carbon dioxide.

TABLE 10-2 Mechanistic Approach to Respiratory Failure

	Type I, Acute Hypoxemic	Type II, Ventilatory	Type III, Perioperative	Type IV, Shock
Mechanism	$\dot{Q}s/\dot{Q}T$	$\dot{V}_A$	Atelectasis	Hypoperfusion
Etiology	Airspace flooding	1. CNS drive 2. N-M coupling 3. Work/dead-space	1. FRC 2. CV	1. Cardiogenic 2. Hypovolemic 3. Septic
Clinical Description	Pulmonary edema Cardiogenic ARDS Pneumonia Lung hemorrhage	1. Overdose/CNS injury 2. Myasthenia gravis, polyradiculitis/ALS, botulism/curare 3. Asthma/COPD, pulmonary fibrosis, kyphoscoliosis	1. Supine/obese, ascites/peritonitis, upper abdominal incision, anesthesia 2. Age/smoking, fluid overload, bronchospasm, airway secretions	1. Myocardial infarct, pulmonary hypertension 2. Hemorrhage, dehydration, tamponade 3. Endotoxemia, bacteremia

Type III, or perioperative respiratory failure, is seen in patients who have their functional residual capacity (FRC) reduced below the increased closing volumes, leading to progressive collapse of dependent lung units. The resultant atelectasis may cause hypoxemia, hypercarbia, or both. Factors that predispose postoperative patients to atelectasis are the supine position, anesthesia, splinting from incisional pain, obesity, ascites, and diminished cough. The closing volume increases with age, fluid overload, bronchospasm, interbronchial secretions, and cigarette smoking within 6 months of surgery. Treatment should focus on preventing atelectasis. These measures include frequent turning, chest physiotherapy (including pummeling, chest vibration, endotracheal suctioning, and positioning the patient 30 to 45 degrees upright), CPAP or PEEP to return the end-expired lung volume over the closing volume, sighs dialed into the ventilator, and attention to postoperative pain.

Type IV, or hypoperfusion respiratory failure, results from the circulation's inability to provide sufficient oxygen delivery to the respiratory muscles. This is most frequently due to cardiogenic, hypovolemic, or septic shock. Mechanical ventilation is usually required to decrease the work of breathing and the metabolic demands of the tissues. Patients with hypovolemic shock can usually be resuscitated without mechanical ventilation. If hypovolemia is present, mechanical ventilation is particularly contraindicated, since increased intrathoracic pressure secondary to positive-pressure ventilation can reduce venous return and hence cardiac output further. Care should be taken to ensure that the patient is not working to breathe against the ventilator. Adjusting the ventilator to meet the patient's desired minute ventilation and sedation may be required. Usually, once the hypoperfusion state is corrected, spontaneous breathing can be resumed.

In the ICU, patients frequently have multiple factors contributing to respiratory failure. Attention to all the contributing factors of respiratory failure will result in a more rapid return of spontaneous respiration so that the patient can be liberated from mechanical ventilation.

For a more detailed discussion, see Chaps. 30 through 36 and 39 in *Principles of Critical Care*, 2d ed.

Chapter 11

AIRWAY MANAGEMENT AND TRACHEOSTOMY

MICHAEL O'CONNOR

Intensivists are currently armed with an increasingly diverse array of technology to manage patients with respiratory failure. One of the most important decisions they make is whether to attempt a course of noninvasive ventilation or proceed directly to more invasive airway management and mechanical ventilation. As a rule, noninvasive ventilation should be initiated in a more closely monitored setting, such as a stepdown unit or intensive care unit (ICU) and *not* on the ward. The decision as to whom to intubate and whom to ventilate noninvasively is determined by a multitude of factors, including institutional resources, the presumed cause of the patient's respiratory failure, and the logistics of providing care. Only rarely are these decisions clear-cut and can, in retrospect, appear unreasonable as patients do better or worse than expected. Table 11-1 summarizes the commonly accepted indications for a trial of noninvasive ventilation in the acute-care setting. Table 11-2 presents a list of contraindications to noninvasive ventilation. These contraindications are not absolute and must be weighed in combination with other factors in the care of individual patients. Table 11-3 presents a summary of the indications for endotracheal intubation.

Once the decision to intubate the trachea has been made, there are several routes available to accomplish this goal. The most commonly chosen is translaryngeal orotracheal

TABLE 11-1   Indications for Noninvasive Ventilation

Acute cardiogenic pulmonary edema from a readily reversible cause
Acute on chronic respiratory failure (COPD exacerbation)
Neuromuscular disease?

TABLE 11-2   Contraindications to Noninvasive Ventilation

Shock
Hypotension
Requirement for cardioversion (or defibrillation)
Procedures requiring prolonged supine positioning such as intraaortic
   balloon pump placement, cardiac catheterization, or surgery
Nonresolving ischemia
LV failure refractory to medical therapy
Full stomach
Diminished mental status associated with impaired airway reflexes

TABLE 11-3   Indications for Endotracheal Intubation

Airway support
   Diminished mental status/decreased ability to maintain airway
      and clear secretions (e.g., new quadriplegia, hepatic
      encephalopathy)
   Compromised airway anatomy (e.g., edema)
   Diminished airway reflexes, full stomach, and fluctuating
      consciousness
   Requirement for sedation in circumstances where airway control
      may not be easy to establish (e.g., computed tomography,
      magnetic resonance imaging)
   Pharyngeal instability (e.g., facial fractures)
Pulmonary disease
   Acute hypoxemic respiratory failure
   Hypoventilation (including central nervous system causes and
      weakness)
   Lung disease with a work of breathing which exceeds the
      patient's ability to breath (e.g., severe obstruction or restriction
      of any cause)
Circulatory disorders
   Cardiopulmonary arrest
   Refractory or unresuscitated shock
   Sepsis
Other
   Elevated intracranial pressure requiring hyperventilation
   Transportation of a patient at risk for deterioration
   Severe metabolic acidosis

intubation. The advantages of the transoral route include familiarity for most practitioners, minimal risk of trauma associated with the procedure, and the ability to accommodate relatively large endotracheal tubes without difficulty. Disadvantages of this route include patient biting on the tube, difficult oral care, difficulty securing the tube in the setting of copious oral secretions or weeping skin edema, and dental damage during placement. Nasotracheal intubation has several advantages, including the ability to be accomplished blindly, minimal or no need for sedation, placement with the patient sitting upright in bed, and a very stable endotracheal tube. Disadvantages of nasotracheal intubation include trauma to nasal structures during insertion, requirement for a slightly smaller tube than might be inserted transorally, and risk of sinusitis associated with prolonged intubation. Tracheostomy can be performed instead of either of these approaches and is discussed in greater detail further on.

Tables 11-4 and 11-5 list the medical and anatomic issues that need to be considered prior to making any plan for airway management in a critically ill patient.

Of all considerations mentioned above, it is the risks associated with aspiration and elevated intracranial pressure that are most often underestimated by those with little experience in airway management. Unless it is specifically contraindicated, the Sellick maneuver—pressure on the cricoid cartilage anteriorly to occlude the esophagus posteriorly—should be performed during all airway management in the ICU where aspiration is considered even a remote risk. If a patient has a full stomach and cannot be intubated awake with topical anesthesia or minimal sedation, most practitioners elect to perform a rapid sequence induction of a brief intravenous general anesthetic to facilitate intubation.

In patients with elevated intracranial pressure, it is imperative that the airway manager be acutely aware of the tradeoffs to be made to limit the elevation of intracranial pressure. In patients with favorable airways, most practitioners will elect to perform a rapid sequence induction as outlined in Table 11-6. If there is significant concern about anatomy and the ability to obtain an airway in a timely fashion, serious consideration should be given to performing an awake tracheostomy. If this is not practical, careful topical

TABLE 11-4   Medical Evaluation for Intubation

Neurologic
  Elevated intracranial pressure
  Presence of intracranial bleed, arteriovenous malformation,
    or aneurysm
  Cervical spine disease
Cardiovascular
  Ischemia, hypovolemia, history of myocardial infarction, congestive
    heart failure, dysrhythmias
  Drug allergies
Pulmonary
  Severity of hypoxemia, obstruction
Aspiration risk
  "Nothing by mouth"
  Morbid obesity
  Impaired gastric emptying/gastroparesis
  Pregnancy
Coagulation
  Thrombocytopenia, anticoagulant therapy, coagulopathy
  Recent or anticipated therapy with thrombolytics
Contraindications to succinylcholine
  History of burns, crush injuries, spinal cord injuries, malignant
    hyperthermia

---

anesthesia followed by careful awake or fiberoptic laryngoscopy should be considered as the most desirable method to secure the airway.

The list of basic equipment required to manipulate the airway has grown over time, reflecting the higher standards to which practitioners are being held in this activity. A list of basic equipment as well as a more complete list of desirable equipment for more elective circumstances is given in Table 11-7.

Pharmacologic Aids

The goals of pharmacologic preparation of the patient include creating conditions that allow for safe and effective laryngoscopy; providing relief from the discomfort and hemodynamic consequences associated with laryngoscopy, airway manipulation, and endotracheal intubation; and decreasing

TABLE 11-5   Anatomic Evaluation for Intubation

Obesity
Pregnancy
Short neck
Large tongue
Poor mouth opening/temporomandibular joint dysfunction
Small mandible
Limited flexion at the base of the neck or extension at the base of
    the skull
Cervical instability
Dentures
Loose teeth
Tumor (adenoma, carcinoma, abscess)
Large epiglottis
Copious secretions or blood
Trauma
History of prior intubations
Mallampati classification (a measure of ability to visualize the
    retropharynx with normal mouth opening)

TABLE 11-6   Algorithm for Intubation in the Presence of
Elevated Intracranial Pressure (and a Clinically Favorable
Airway)

 1. *d*-Tubocurarine 3 mg or vecuronium/pancuronium 1 mg
 2. Preoxygenation/hyperventilation for 3 min
 3. Cricoid pressure
 4. Midazolam 0.03 mg/kg
 5. Fentanyl 1–2 μg/kg
 6. Lidocaine 100 mg
 7. Thiopental 3–5 mg/kg or propofol 2 mg/kg
 8. Succinylcholine 1.5 mg/kg or rocuronium 1.0 mg/kg
 9. Hyperventilate for 45 s with ambu bag/mask following
    succinylcholine, 90 s following rocuronium
10. Laryngoscopy/intubation
11. Confirm intubation with auscultation/capnography
12. Elevate head of bed and hyperventilate

TABLE 11-7   Equipment List for Intubation

Cardiac arrest
   Two laryngoscopes with functioning lights
   Macintosh 3 and 4 and Miller 3 blades
   Small, medium, and large face masks
   Suction with Yankauer tip
   ETTs, cuffs checked, 6.5, 7.0, 7.5, 8.0, and 8.5 mm
   Malleable metal stylet
   10-mL syringe for inflation of ETT cuff
   Tape
   Oxygen supply
   Ambu bag or other circuit to ventilate patient
   Stethoscope
   Gloves and eye protection
Urgent and elective intubation
   Functioning IV line
   Monitors:
      Pulse oximeter
      Blood pressure
      Electrocardiograph
      Exhaled CO_2 monitor (e.g., capnograph)
   Resuscitation cart
   Drugs
      Atropine
      IV lidocaine
      Ephedrine
      Epinephrine
      Glycopyrrolate
      Succinylcholine
      Rocuronium
      Topical anesthetics (lidocaine jelly, benzocaine spray)
   Magill forceps
   Size 7, 8, 9, and 10 oral airways
   Nasal trumpets, 28, 30, 32, and 34Fr
   Full variety of endotracheal tubes (including 7.0 and 8.0 mm
     endotrol tubes)
   Laryngeal mask airways
   Fiberoptic bronchoscope
   Cricothyroidotomy kit
   Jet ventilator

the hormonal, endocrinologic, and neurologic consequences of the procedure. The spectrum of pharmacologic preparation ranges from topical anesthesia at one end to intravenous anesthesia on the other. Most airway manipulation in the ICU can be accomplished by an experienced operator with topical anesthesia alone. Intravenous general anesthesia is indicated in the setting of elevated intracranial pressure and straightforward airway anatomy. There are many institutions where an intravenous general anesthetic is administered at the time of airway manipulation, but this practice should be strongly discouraged. Patients who require urgent intubation may benefit from pharmacologic preparation. Many operators routinely administer 0.2 mg glycopyrrolate IV to dry the mouth so as to facilitate direct laryngoscopy. The oropharynx can be anesthetized topically with either 4% lidocaine spray or benzocaine spray, followed by approximately 4 mL of 2% lidocaine jelly on an oral airway of appropriate size for that patient. The oral airway can be used to direct the topical anesthetic at the vocal cords of the patient as well. Care should be taken to avoid giving high doses (>6 mg/kg) of lidocaine for topical anesthesia, as lidocaine is readily absorbed by the mucosa of the pharynx. Some practitioners routinely perform transtracheal and superior laryngeal nerve blocks to facilitate airway manipulation, but these procedures are not universally necessary. Topical/local anesthesia schemes that avoid anesthetizing the trachea have several advantages in the ICU setting: they allow patients to retain some ability to protect themselves from aspiration and also allow confirmation of endotracheal intubation when patients cough in response to introduction of the endotracheal tube into the trachea.

The use of intravenous agents to facilitate endotracheal intubation in the ICU is fraught with hazard. The degree of hypovolemia, myocardial dysfunction, and shock in these patients is difficult or impossible to ascertain prior to manipulating the airway in an urgent situation. Doses of intravenous agents that are well tolerated or even subtherapeutic in healthy patients can precipitate respiratory arrest or circulatory collapse in the critically ill, converting a serious situation into a desperate one. 100 mg of lidocaine IV is frequently sufficient to induce general anesthesia in patients with shock. Intravenous agents such as midazolam, fentanyl, thiopental, etomidate, propofol, and ketamine should be used only by experienced practitioners who can guess at what the appropriate dose may be. When indicated, these agents may be cautiously titrated to an acceptable level of sedation (which will be accompanied by a corresponding decrease in both hemodynamics and minute ventilation, with the attendant worsening of hypoxemia and hypercarbia) or to very deliberately induce a (hopefully) short general anesthetic.

The Role of Paralytic Agents in ICU Airway Management

The use of paralytic agents to facilitate airway management in the ICU remains controversial. When anesthesiologists are confronted with patients who have airway anatomy that causes concern or whom it may not be possible to oxygenate or ventilate with a bag and mask, they tend to opt for awake intubation strategies, as outlined in this chapter. The use of paralytic agents—including succinylcholine, vecuronium, mivacurium, rocuronium, and cisatracurium—should be restricted to those who are experienced in managing the airway with an Ambu bag and mask and who are thoroughly versed in all the techniques used to manage the difficult airway. The reason for this is that once these agents are administered, it is imperative that a definitive airway be obtained within minutes. Attempts at ventilating most patients with respiratory failure with an Ambu bag and mask are very difficult and usually futile, as the underlying decreased compliance of the lung or increased airway resistance makes it difficult or impossible to maintain adequate minute ventilation, given the mechanical disadvantage and lack of seal associated with mask ventilation. The impulse of inexperienced operators to attempt to use these intravenous agents to compensate for lack of confidence and skill should be strongly discouraged.

Complications

There are a large number of complications of endotracheal intubation in the ICU, of which hypotension, hypertension, arrhythmias/cardiac arrest, aspiration, trauma, and tube mis-placement in either the right mainstem bronchus or esophagus are the most common (Table 11-8). Hypotension typically occurs in the setting of prior existing hemodynamic instability and can have a variety of causes, including diminished venous return associated with the institution of positive-pressure ventilation, intrinsic PEEP from vigorous ventilation subsequent to tracheal intubation, and myocardial ischemia in

TABLE 11-8   Complications of Intubation

Immediate
   Right mainstem intubation
   Esophageal intubation
   Gastric aspiration
   Dental injury, tooth aspiration
   Tracheal or esophageal tear
   Hypertension/tachycardia
   Myocardial ischemia
   Elevated intracranial pressure
   Hypotension
   Arrhythmias
      Ventricular premature beats
      Ventricular tachycardia
      Ventricular fibrillation
      Bradycardia (especially in the young)
   Bronchospasm
   Vocal cord trauma
   Dislocation of arytenoid cartilage
   Epistaxis
   Avulsed turbinate
   Pain
Delayed
   Serous or purulent otitis
   Sinusitis
   Necrosis of lip or nose
   Dental damage from biting
   Tracheal mucosal injury
   Tracheomalacia
   Tracheoinnominate fistula
   Laryngeal stricture
      Vocal cord synechiae
      Posterior cricoarytenoid edema
      Tracheal stenosis

patients ssusceptible to it. Hypertension occurs more commonly in patients with uncomplicated respiratory failure and a stable circulation, such as those with asthma or neuromuscular disease. Bradyarrhythmias predominate in children and young adults, whereas supraventricular tachyarrhythmias and ventricular dysrrhythmias predominate in older patients. Approximately 3 percent of patients will succumb to cardiac arrest around the time they are intubated. Although this is an expected event in some, it is unexpected in many and may be less likely to occur if minimal sedation is used and practitioners are poised to resuscitate the patient around the time of intubation. Right mainstem intubation is more frequently done by inexperienced practitioners and may occur more often in women and short patients. It can be difficult to detect clinically, especially in patients with severe airway obstruction. Esophageal intubation can similarly be difficult to detect in these patients. If the patient has a spontaneous circulation, capnography can be used to confirm endotracheal intubation expeditiously. Capnography is of no use in confirming endotracheal intubation in patients with cardiac arrest. Repeat laryngoscopy can be helpful if there is doubt about endotracheal tube position. It is imperative to recognize esophageal intubation in the critically ill patient in a timely fashion, as most of these patients will otherwise desaturate very quickly to dangerous levels of hypoxemia.

Tracheostomy

The role of tracheostomy has evolved considerably over the past 15 years and will continue to evolve with critical care medicine. The most uncontroversial indication for tracheostomy is evolving upper airway obstruction. Tracheostomy is also widely accepted as preferable to transglottic intubation for long-term mechanical ventilation. Tracheostomy is also indicated when a patient is unable to clear airway secretions, and will not become able to do so in the foreseeable future. Finally, tracheostomy is frequently used to facilitate liberation from mechanical ventilation.

Tracheostomy in the face of evolving upper airway obstruction is a lifesaving procedure. It has several benefits in

TABLE 11-9   Complications of Tracheostomy

Early
  Hemorrhage
    Subcutaneous vessels
    Anterior neck veins
    Thyroid vessels
    Thyroid gland
    Coagulopathy
  Malpositioning/dislodgement
  Pneumothorax/pneumomediastinum
Late
  Hemorrhage
    Tracheoinnominate fistula
  Pneumonia
  Tracheoesophageal fistula
  Tracheomalacia/stenosis

---

patients who will require long-term mechanical ventilation, allowing much easier and safer access to the mouth, which in turn allows oral hygiene to be easily maintained. It is substantially more comfortable than translaryngeal intubation. When combined with specially designed tracheostomy tubes, it allows for speech and even normal eating. Finally, it allows easy discontinuation and reinstitution of mechanical ventilation. There was a time when patients underwent tracheostomy after only very brief periods of translaryngeal intubation and mechanical ventilation. As more inert materials have come to be used in the manufacture of endotracheal tubes and the tubes have become softer, the complications associated with translaryngeal intubation have declined. The threshold for performing tracheostomy has therefore changed; tracheostomy is usually reserved for patients who may take weeks or months to be liberated from the mechanical ventilator or who may require relatively frequent reinstitution of mechanical ventilation. Females and patients with diabetes mellitus, purulent pneumonia, rheumatoid arthritis, ankylosing spondylitis, and a history of keloid formation are at increased risk for the complications of translaryngeal intubation and may benefit from earlier tracheostomy.

TABLE 11-10   Some Practical Bedside Rules of Thumb

1. Save the brain.
2. Spare the circulation.
3. A spontaneously breathing patient has at least one vital sign; an apneic patient may soon have none.
4. Mask ventilation is better than esophageal intubation.
5. The worst time for a patient to aspirate is when it is time for intubation.
6. If you do not give any IV anesthetics, the CODE cannot be blamed on you.
7. A patient who does not mind a tube needs one.
8. The patient who asks for a tube needs one.
9. The best procedure for a patient may be the one that you know how to do best.

Tracheostomy has the great benefit of substantially reducing the anatomic dead space, resulting in substantially greater alveolar minute ventilation for any given minute ventilation. This effect is unimportant in patients with normal muscle strength and normal lung/chest wall mechanics, but it may be of critical importance in patients whose strength is very closely matched to their requirement for minute ventilation. The wide bore and short length of tracheostomy tubes is also of benefit in these circumstances.

For a more detailed discussion, see Chap. 11 in *Principles of Critical Care*, 2d ed.

Chapter 12

MONITORING OF THE RESPIRATORY SYSTEM

SANGEETA BHORADE

Monitoring Gas Exchange

The most important function of the lungs is the uptake of oxygen from air into arterial blood and the disposal of carbon dioxide from the mixed venous blood to the environment. Failure of the respiratory system to perform this function may result in arterial hypoxemia and/or hypercarbia. Several monitoring systems—including arterial blood gas analysis, blood oximetry (both transmission and reflectance oximetry) and capnography—are available to clinically assess the adequacy of the respiratory system in oxygen and carbon dioxide exchange.

ARTERIAL BLOOD GAS ANALYSIS

Arterial blood gas (ABG) analysis is fundamental to the management of the critically ill patient. Importantly, one must remember that in increasing or decreasing the level of supplemental oxygen delivered to the patient, one should wait approximately 15 minutes prior to obtaining an ABG to allow for equilibration of arterial oxygenation. Likewise, in decreasing the ventilation delivered to a patient, one should take into account the 16-minute half-time (t_2^1) for carbon dioxide (CO_2) accumulation due to the dependence on metabolic generation of CO_2. However, during hyperventilation, arterial CO_2 concentrations respond relatively quickly ($t_2^1 > 3$ minutes).

BLOOD OXIMETRY

The advent of oximetry has made possible a quick, inexpensive method for the on-line assessment of arterial and mixed venous oxygen saturation on a continuous basis. Recent studies describing the benefit of oximetry in settings such as the operating room and the emergency department suggest that this monitoring tool probably has had a significant impact in the management of critically ill patients as well.

TRANSMISSION OXIMETRY (ARTERIAL PULSE OXIMETRY)

Pulse oximetry uses the absorptive properties of oxygenated and deoxygenated hemoglobin to determine the oxygen saturation of arterial blood (Sp_{O_2}). Light of two specific wavelengths in the red (660 nm) and infrared (940 nm) range is reflected or absorbed in proportion to oxygen saturation; the differences in absorption between wavelengths permits determination of Sp_{O_2}. With recent developments in the pulse oximeter, output stabilization requires less than 1 minute. After stabilization is obtained, less than 10 seconds is required before a change in the arterial oxygen saturation is reflected in the Sp_{O_2}. Response time to step changes in saturation is slightly slower for finger than for ear probes.

Pulse oximeters are highly accurate (within 1% to 4%) for oxygen saturations greater than 70%. However, this accuracy decreases at lower oxygen saturations, with pulse oximeters overestimating the true value at lower saturations. In addition, oximeters tend to provide falsely low values of Sp_{O_2} in the setting of hypoperfusion, deep pigmentation, intravenous dyes (including methylene blue), and green, black, or blue nail polish. Pulse oximeters tend to overestimate Sp_{O_2} in the presence of high levels of methemoglobin or carboxyhemoglobin. In such patients, accurate measurements of oxygenation should be obtained via co-oximeter and ABG samples.

REFLECTANCE OXIMETRY (MIXED VENOUS OXIMETRY)

Fiberoptic pulmonary artery (PA) catheters use reflectance oximetry to determine the mixed venous oxygen saturation ($S\bar{v}_{O_2}$) in the pulmonary artery blood. The accuracy of $S\bar{v}_{O_2}$ determination is less than that for Sp_{O_2}, and, in general, $S\bar{v}_{O_2}$ obtained in this manner should be correlated with mixed venous blood gas samples to ensure accurate values.

Blood samples drawn from the distal port of the PA catheter may provide intermittent samples to determine the adequacy of oxygen delivery. To obtain accurate values, the catheter tip must be positioned in the proximal pulmonary artery. In addition, catheter dead space (approximately 3 to 5 mL) must be cleared and the sample should be drawn over 20 seconds to avoid contamination with oxygenated pulmonary capillary blood. The clinical application and utility of the $S\bar{v}_{O_2}$ is addressed further on.

CAPNOMETRY AND CAPNOGRAPHY

Capnometry is the measurement of exhaled CO_2, while capnography is the graphic waveform display of CO_2. After anatomic dead space has been cleared, the end-exhalation CO_2 ($P_{ET_{CO_2}}$) tension generally tracks the mean alveolar CO_2 concentration. Clinical applications of capnography include estimation of the partial pressure of CO_2 in arterial blood (Pa_{CO_2}), estimation of CO_2 excretion, and dead-space calculation. In patients with parenchymal or obstructive airway disease, caution must be used with these devices, as estimation of Pa_{CO_2} by $P_{ET_{CO_2}}$ is fraught with inaccuracies.

COLORIMETRIC CAPNOMETRY

Colorimetric capnometry is a technique that uses a portable, disposable device to monitor the presence of CO_2 in the exhaled gas. This device is useful for distinguishing tracheal intubation from esophageal intubation. This instrument is designed for short-term analysis and caution must be exercised in its use, as this device may be affected by circuit humidification and may deteriorate with prolonged use. In addition, significant quantitative analysis cannot be determined by this technique.

INFRARED AND MASS SPECTROSCOPY CAPNOMETRY

These capnometers provide a quantitative measure of exhaled CO_2. In general, mass spectrometers are more expensive and are used less often than infrared capnometers. These analyzers may be placed in the mainstream or sidestream of the ventilator tubing of intubated patients. Advantages and disadvantages are associated with both methods of placement, and the decision to use one method over the other is based on personal preference and availability in the specific institution.

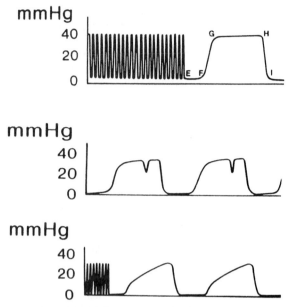

FIGURE 12-1   Tidal capnography. *Top*. The expiratory phase of normal capnogram consists of a base-line (dead space) segment, a segment in which dead space and tidal gas are mixed (FG), a segment during which gas is primarily from the alveolar compartment (GH), and an inspiratory segment (HI). *Middle*. Capnogram of patient recovering from neuromuscular paralysis. The notch in the plateau indicates the patient's attempt to inspire. *Bottom*. Deformed capnographic tracing of patient with airflow obstruction. Note that in this latter instance, end-tidal CO_2 gas tensions will vary with breathing frequency. (Adapted from Stock MC: Noninvasive carbon dioxide monitoring. Crit Care Clin 4(3):511, 1988, with permission.)

The normal capnogram, the graphic waveform display of exhaled CO_2 concentration, is composed of a baseline, an ascending portion, a plateau, and a descending portion (Fig. 12-1). It is important to examine the entire tracing rather than depending upon the digital readout for the end-tidal value, as several variations in the waveform may result in erroneous digital readouts. $P_{ET_{CO_2}}$ normally underestimates Pa_{CO_2} by 1 to 3 mmHg because of alveolar dead space that dilutes CO_2

from well-perfused alveoli. Although the correlation between PET_{CO_2} and Pa_{CO_2} is excellent for patients with normal lungs breathing at low frequencies, the difference widens when $\dot{V}/\dot{Q}$ mismatch increases. The shape of the waveform may provide information regarding the discrepancy between PET_{CO_2} and Pa_{CO_2}. Common conditions that may increase the Pa_{CO_2}–PET_{CO_2} gradient include any disorder that increases either the physiologic and/or anatomic dead space, such as obstructive lung disease, pulmonary embolism, hyperinflation, low cardiac output, ventilator disconnection, and hyperventilation. The Pa_{CO_2}–PET_{CO_2} can be useful to diagnose air embolus when acute increases in the gradient are noted in patients at risk. This gradient may also be useful in identifying the optimal PEEP level, as the arterial to end-tidal CO_2 difference should be minimal when perfused alveoli are maximally recruited.

Monitoring the Efficiency of O_2 Exchange

Although the partial pressure of O_2 in arterial blood (Pa_{O_2}) is a simple, rapid measure of oxygenation by itself, it is an inadequate estimate of the efficiency of gas exchange. Several other indices have been developed for a more accurate estimation of the efficiency of gas exchange; these account for the fraction of inspired oxygen being delivered (see below).

ALVEOLAR-ARTERIAL OXYGEN TENSION DIFFERENCE

The alveolar-arterial oxygen tension difference $[P(A − a)_{O_2}]$ is obtained by subtracting the Pa_{O_2} from the PA_{O_2}, where $PA_{O_2} = (PB − P_{H_2O}) FI_{O_2} − P_{CO_2})/R$ [PA_{O_2} = partial pressure of alveolar oxygen, PB = the barometric pressure in millimeters of mercury, P_{H_2O} = partial pressure of H_2O in millimeters of mercury, FI_{O_2} = fraction of inspired oxygen, and R = respiratory quotient (typically = 0.8)]. At sea level with the patient breathing room air, where $FI_{O_2} = 0.21$, $PB = 760$ mmHg, $P_{H_2O} = 47$ mmHg, and R = 0.8, this equation can be simplified to $PA_{O_2} = 147 − 1.25 (P_{CO_2}) − Pa_{O_2}$.

The $P(A − a)_{O_2}$ difference provides an estimation of the efficiency of gas exchange and can identify hypoventilation as the sole cause of hypoxemia (the gradient will be normal). Normally, this gradient is less than 10 mmHg in young, healthy persons breathing room air. However, both increasing $F_{I_{O_2}}$ requirements and increasing age affect this difference and limit its usefulness in monitoring the efficiency of gas exchange.

VENOUS ADMIXTURE AND SHUNT

Venous admixture ($\dot{Q}s/\dot{Q}T$) represents pulmonary blood flow that is shunted through poorly ventilated and well-perfused alveoli [ventilation/perfusion ($\dot{V}/\dot{Q}$) ratio approaching zero]. Venous admixture causes hypoxemia when venous blood with low oxygen content combines with well-oxygenated blood from nonshunted blood flow. In the steady state, $\dot{Q}s/\dot{Q}T = (C_{C_{O_2}} - Ca_{O_2})/(C_{C_{O_2}} - C\bar{v}_{O_2})$, where $C_{C_{O_2}}$ = oxygen content in pulmonary capillary blood, Ca_{O_2} = oxygen content in arterial blood, and $C\bar{v}_{O_2}$ = oxygen content in mixed venous blood. Since low $\dot{V}/\dot{Q}$ units may cause hypoxemia and low Ca_{O_2}, leading to overestimation of shunt, true shunt is best estimated on a $F_{I_{O_2}} > 0.6$.

THE $Pa_{O_2}/F_{I_{O_2}}$(P/F) RATIO

The P/F ratio is an easy and convenient way to measure oxygen exchange that attempts to adjust for fluctuating $F_{I_{O_2}}$. Although useful when the primary cause for hypoxemia is $\dot{V}/\dot{Q}$ mismatch, this ratio fluctuates with the level of $F_{I_{O_2}}$ when shunt is a major cause of hypoxemia.

THE Pa_{O_2}/Pa_{O_2} RATIO

This ratio of arterial to alveolar oxygen tension is a useful bedside index and is relatively unaffected by changing values of $F_{I_{O_2}}$. However, it loses reliability with increasing shunt.

Monitoring the Efficiency of CO_2 Exchange

Pa_{CO_2} alone is insufficient to determine the efficiency of gas exchange of the lung and must be interpreted in conjunction with minute ventilation. Pa_{CO_2} may rise when diminished respiratory drive or marked neuromuscular weakness impairs total ventilation and CO_2 excretion, even in the presence of normal lung function. Increased CO_2 production ($\dot{V}_{CO_2}$) may accentuate this tendency and must be taken into account in assessing the etiology of hypercarbia.

MEASURING CO_2 PRODUCTION

The rate of CO_2 excretion, an estimate of metabolic CO_2 production ($\dot{V}_{CO_2}$), is the product of the expired fraction of CO_2 ($F_{E_{CO_2}}$) and the total volume of all gas (minute ventilation) expelled over the assessed interval. Accurate estimation of CO_2 excretion requires collection over an adequate time and a sample that is adequately mixed and analyzed. CO_2 excretion may also be estimated as the product of minute ventilation and the mean expired CO_2 partial pressure from a capnograph divided by barometric pressure. In addition, metabolic carts may also measure $\dot{V}_{CO_2}$ directly. Regardless of technique, accurate $\dot{V}_{CO_2}$ measurement depends on the stability of the patient during the period of gas collection not only with regard to $\dot{V}_{CO_2}$ but also in terms of acid-base homeostasis, perfusion, and ventilation.

THE RATIO OF DEAD SPACE TO TIDAL VOLUME (V_D/V_T)

Dead-space (V_D) ventilation is characterized by ventilation that does not participate in gas exchange with blood. The physiologic dead space is the sum of the anatomic and alveolar components of dead space. The ratio of dead space to tidal volume (V_D/V_T) ratio reflects the ability of the lung to transfer CO_2 from the pulmonary vasculature to the alveoli. The fraction of wasted ventilation can be estimated from the following equation: $V_D/V_T = (Pa_{CO_2} - PE_{CO_2})/Pa_{CO_2}$ where Pa_{CO_2} is the partial pressure of CO_2 in the arterial blood and the PE_{CO_2} is the partial pressure of CO_2 in expired gas. In general, in normal subjects, V_D/V_T is between 0.15 and 0.35.

Monitoring Oxygen Delivery ($\dot{Q}_{O_2}$) and Oxygen Consumption ($\dot{V}_{O_2}$)

Total body oxygen delivery ($\dot{Q}_{O_2}$) is the product of total oxygen content of arterial blood (Ca_{O_2}) and the rate of delivery of blood to body tissues ($\dot{Q}_T$). The Ca_{O_2} is dependent on hemoglobin and oxygen saturation. The following equation describes this relationship: $\dot{Q}_{O_2} = (\dot{Q}_T \times Ca_{O_2}) = \dot{Q}_T[(1.39 \times [Hgb] \times Sa_{O_2}) + (0.003 \times Pa_{O_2})]$, where $[Hgb]$ is the blood hemoglobin level in mg/dL and Sa_{O_2} is the oxygen saturation of arterial blood.

$\dot{V}_{O_2}$ is difficult to measure accurately at the bedside. Total body oxygen uptake ($\dot{V}_{O_2}$) is the difference between the arterial oxygen delivery and the oxygen returning in the mixed venous blood. Two primary methods are used to determine $\dot{V}_{O_2}$: (1) direct analysis of the inspired and expired gases and (2) Fick's method, which is the calculation of the $\dot{V}_{O_2}$ from the cardiac output ($\dot{Q}_T$) and the difference in oxygen content between the arterial and mixed venous blood ($Ca_{O_2} - C\bar{v}_{O_2}$).

Both of these methods are fraught with problems that may lead to inaccuracy of $\dot{V}_{O_2}$ determination; therefore they should be used with caution. The metabolic cart and indirect calorimetry are used to determine $\dot{V}_{O_2}$ by subtracting the expired from the inspired volume of oxygen. Expired oxygen concentration is determined by the fraction of mixed expired oxygen concentration and the expired minute volume, and the inspired concentration is determined by the $F_{I_{O_2}}$ and the inspired minute volume. The presence of high $F_{I_{O_2}}$ requirement, air leaks, and high airway pressures lead to inaccurate measurements. The Fick equation may be rearranged to determine the $\dot{V}_{O_2}$ in the following manner: $\dot{V}_{O_2} = \dot{Q}_T (Ca_{O_2} - C\bar{v}_{O_2})$. This method may also be associated with problems due to errors in measurement of any one of the variables used in determining $\dot{V}_{O_2}$. In addition, neither method is accurate when the patient is not in a metabolic steady state.

Monitoring Lung and Chest Wall Mechanics

Gas flows to and from alveoli are driven by differences in pressure. When a mechanical ventilator performs the entire inflation work of breathing, the difference between airway and atmospheric pressures can be accounted for in two ways: (1) to drive gas between the airway opening and the alveolus and (2) to expand the alveoli against the combined elastic recoil of the lung and chest wall.

ESOPHAGEAL PRESSURE (Pes)
MEASUREMENT

Esophageal pressure (Pes) measurements provide a significant aid in the assessment of intrathoracic pressures. By enabling the clinician to indirectly measure pleural pressures (Ppl), the Pes measurement enables one to partition respiratory system compliance and resistance into pulmonary and chest wall components. Changes in the Pes (ΔPes) can be used to measure end-expiratory wedge pressure, to calculate lung compliance and airway resistance during spontaneous breathing, and to separate total elastic recoil of the respiratory system into its lung and chest wall components. In addition, in research settings, the ΔPes can be used to calculate the work of breathing or the product of developed pressure and the duration of inspiratory effort (the pressure-time product).

The Pes is measured with a thin plastic balloon (approximately 10 cm long) affixed to a multiperforated catheter stent and positioned in the lower or middle third of the esophagus. The balloon is typically filled with 0.2 to 0.5 mL of air in order to transmit changes in intrathoracic pressures accurately during spontaneous cycles. While the accuracy of Pes measurements in reflecting true Ppl may vary due to position of the patient, the ΔPes correlates extremely well with ΔPpl.

To position the esophageal balloon properly, it must first be passed into the stomach, where positive-pressure deflections during forceful inspiratory efforts are transduced and displayed. The catheter is then withdrawn until negative deflections appear, reflecting Ppl and indicating that the uppermost portion of the balloon is in the esophagus. The catheter is withdrawn further until the entire balloon is within the esophagus. Confirmation of appropriate positioning is obtained by observing nearly equivalent deflections of airway and esophageal pressures.

STATIC PRESSURE-VOLUME
RELATIONSHIPS

The transpulmonary pressure (PTP) is defined as the alveolar pressure (PA) minus the pleural pressure Ppl and reflects the pressure required to expand the lung by a certain volume. Lung compliance (CL) is defined by the change in volume

(ΔV) elicited by a change in the transpulmonary pressure ΔPtp: $C_L = \Delta V/\Delta Ptp$. Chest wall compliance is determined by the change in pleural pressure required to expand the chest wall by ΔV: ($C_{CW} = \Delta V/\Delta Ppl$), and the compliance of the total respiratory system is a combination of the lung and chest wall compliance: $\Delta V/\Delta P_A$ (Fig. 12-2).

Caution must be exercised in attempting to use the respiratory system compliance as an indicator of tissue elastance. Respiratory system compliance is linear only over the central portion and becomes flatter at both high and low volumes owing to alterations in the lung and chest wall compliance at these volumes, respectively. In addition, C_{RS} may also be altered at lower lung volumes in a mechanically ventilated patient with pulmonary edema if substantial alveolar recruitment occurs during tidal inflation.

CALCULATING COMPLIANCE AND RESISTANCE OF THE RESPIRATORY SYSTEM

Airway pressure (Paw) overcomes the frictional and elastic forces characterized by resistance and compliance of the respiratory system. Thus, the airway opening pressure is the sum of the respiratory system compliance, the expiratory resistance, and the level of total positive end-expiratory pressure (PEEP) (applied PEEP + intrinsic PEEP).

When an inspiratory pause is temporarily inserted at end-inspiration, the end-inspiratory pressure (Pst) (static, plateau, or pause pressure) can be determined. Pst is the end-inspiratory inflation pressure required to overcome the elastic forces of tidal inflation (Fig. 12-3). Pst may be elevated in any condition that decreases the compliance of the respiratory system, including any alveolar filling process, auto-PEEP, chest wall deformity, and any condition that increases pleural pressure. An estimate of the static Cst may be calculated by the following equation: $C_{st} = V_T/(Pplat - PEEP_T)$, where V_T is the delivered tidal volume.

The peak dynamic pressure or Ppk is the total pressure required at a given flow rate to drive gas into the alveoli and expand the lung and chest wall by a set tidal volume. Thus, at a constant inflation volume, Ppk is a function of the flow resistance in the airways and the elastic recoil of the lungs

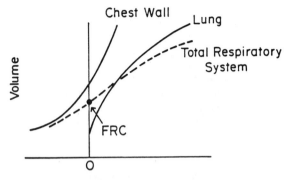

Transmural Pressure

FIGURE 12-2   Static pressure-volume relationships of the lung, re-
laxed chest wall, and total respiratory system. Transmural pressures
of the lung, chest wall, and total respiratory system are (Palv-Ppl),
(Ppl), and (Palv), respectively. Functional residual capacity (FRC) defines the equilibrium volume at which the opposing recoil forces of
lung and chest wall are balanced. (Adapted from Marini JJ: *Respiratory Medicine for the Houseofficer,* 2nd ed. Baltimore, Williams
Wilkins, 1987, p 4, with permission.)

and the chest wall. The difference between Ppk and Pst, the
pressure gradient that is driving flow, is determined by the
resistance of the airways and the endotracheal tube. Elevated
Ppk pressures without a significant rise in Pst are typically
suggestive of airflow obstruction—that is, mechanical obstruction of the airways or the endotracheal tube.

Dynamic hyperinflation and auto-PEEP occur when insufficient time has elapsed between inflation cycles to allow
for complete expiration of the tidal volume. Thus, alveolar
pressure remains continuously positive during both inspiration and expiration. Auto-PEEP may occur in any situation in
which there is a high demand for ventilation, even in patients
without severe airflow obstruction. At the bedside, auto-PEEP
is suspected when significant flow persists to the very end of
exhalation. Auto-PEEP may be quantified by occluding the
expiratory port of the ventilator at the end of exhalation (Fig.
12-4). For accuracy, occlusion must occur just prior to the next
ventilator-delivered breath and persist for 0.5 second or
longer.

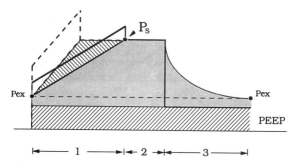

FIGURE 12-3 Schematic of the airway pressure-time profile during passive ventilation at two rates of constant flow (heavy solid and dashed lines). An end-inspirator pause (segment 2) is interposed between inflation (segment 1) and deflation (segment 3). Airway pressure is outlined in a heavy solid line and alveolar pressure in a fine solid line enclosing shaded and crosshatched areas. Under these constant flow conditions, the length of the inspiratory period reflects the V_I, and the slope of the airway pressure tracing $[(PS - Pex)/V_T]$ indicates the elastance of the respiratory system. (Note that Pex > PEEP in this instance, the difference being auto-PEEP.)

Monitoring Breathing Pattern

The breathing pattern provides valuable information that is often underutilized in the clinical setting. In normals, as minute ventilation increases, RR and V_T increase to a plateau V_T, after which RR increases further to meet the ventilation requirement. This elevated RR is a sign of ventilatory muscle decompensation. Tobin and Yang evaluated the ratio of RR/V_T in the mechanically ventilated patients and found that a rapid, shallow breathing index $(RR/V_T) > 100$ breaths per minute per liter suggests impending muscle fatigue in patients being weaned from the ventilator.

As the ventilatory muscles fatigue, the fraction of inspiratory time (T_I) to total cycle length (T_{tot}) changes. This ratio (T_I/T_{tot}) increases from approximately 0.35 to 0.5, and this longer T_I may tax the respiratory muscles because of the increased workload.

Monitoring Strength and Muscle Reserve

The ability of the mechanically ventilated individual to sustain independent breathing is depending upon workload as well as muscle strength and reserve.

MAXIMAL INSPIRATORY PRESSURE (MIP)

The maneuver to obtain this pressure must be performed in an alert, cooperative patient. The patient is asked to exhale to between residual volume (RV) and functional residual capacity (FRC) to optimize the mechanical advantage of the inspiratory muscles. The patient is then asked to inspire forcefully against a closed valve. The MIP generally exceeds 100 cmH$_2$O in normal, spontaneously breathing subjects,

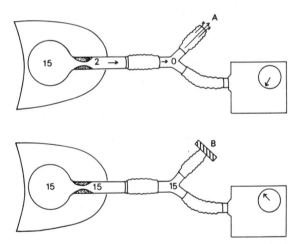

FIGURE 12-4   The auto-PEEP effect and its measurement by the end-expiratory port occlusion maneuver. Just before the next ventilator inflation cycle, alveolar pressure remains markedly positive (15 cmH$_2$O) as flow continues through critically narrowed airways. The ventilator manometer approximates auto-PEEP only when pressures equilibrate following occlusion of the expiratory port at end exhalation. (Adapted from Collee GG, Lynch KE, Hill RD, Zapol WM: Bedside measurement of pulmonary capillary pressure in patients with acute respiratory failure. *Anesthesiology* 66:614, 1987 with permission.)

whereas the work of spontaneous breathing is $<10\,\text{cmH}_2\text{O}$. Patients with acute respiratory failure require a MIP $>30\,\text{cmH}_2\text{O}$ in order to be liberated from the ventilator.

VITAL CAPACITY

Another measure of respiratory muscle strength in mechanically ventilated patients is the vital capacity (VC). In general, when the VC is at least three times the V_T necessary to maintain eucapnia and a normal pH, respiratory muscle fatigue is unlikely. In the supine position, the VC may fall by 20% in normal individuals and only slightly more in patients with unilateral diaphragmatic dysfunction. When a change in position elicits a decrease of $>30\%$ in VC, bilateral diaphragmatic dysfunction should be considered, especially if paradoxical abdominal motion or orthopnea is observed.

Monitoring Liberation of the Mechanically Ventilated Patient

Evaluation of the patient's ability to resume spontaneous ventilation includes measurements of the MIP, VC, RR, V_T, and V_E; observation of respiratory motion during a period of spontaneous breathing; and communication with the patient. Factors that increase CO_2 production, dead space, or metabolic acidosis may increase the ventilation requirements and thus increase respiratory muscle fatigue. In addition, attention to the correctable factors of each patient's underlying disease in conjunction with increasing respiratory muscle strength is an effective approach to the liberation of these patients. General guidelines of acceptable parameters to discontinue mechanical ventilation include (1) MIP $>30\,\text{cmH}_2\text{O}$, (2) VC $>$ three times the V_T, (3) $V_T > 5\,\text{mL/kg}$, (4) RR <30 breaths per minute, (5) $V_E < 10\,\text{L/min}$, and (6) RR/$V_T < 100$ breaths per minute per liter. Once again, it must be emphasized that determining whether a patient should be taken off the ventilator should not be based on a set of parameters alone but on the overall condition of the patient.

For a more detailed discussion, see Chap. 13 in *Principles of Critical Care*, 2d ed.

Chapter 13

MECHANICAL VENTILATORS

G. SCOTT BUDINGER

The first part of this chapter is designed as a rapid reference for the modes of mechanical ventilation and the standard settings on most ventilators. Choice of ventilator settings is then discussed, followed by alternative modes of mechanical ventilation.

Types of Mechanical Ventilators

It is important for the intensivist to realize that there are substantial differences in the software protocols used in different ventilators and to become familiar with the ventilator most frequently used in his or her institution. For example, a decelerating inspiratory flow pattern nearly doubles the inspiratory time on a Puritan-Bennet 7200 ventilator, whereas the same setting does not change the inspiratory time with a Hamilton-Veolar ventilator. When it is necessary to use more than one type of ventilator, more complicated patients should be placed on the more commonly used ventilator. If possible, monitoring devices to graphically monitor pressure and volume tracings should be used with difficult patients.

Common Modes of Mechanical Ventilation

The vast majority of patients in the intensive care unit (ICU) are managed using one of four modes of mechanical ventilation. Broadly, these modes are either volume-preset or pressure-preset. In the volume-preset modes (synchronized intermittent mechanical ventilation and assist control ventilation), the clinician sets the rate and tidal volume and the ventilator delivers whatever pressure is required to achieve that tidal volume. In the pressure-preset modes (pressure support ventilation and pressure control ventilation), the clinician sets a maximal inspiratory pressure and the ventilator delivers whatever tidal volume is generated by that pressure.

Both pressure- and volume-preset ventilation can provide full ventilatory support or allow for substantial patient exercise. Volume-preset modes are commonly used, are familiar to most physicians, and allow for easy measurement of respiratory mechanics. However, they can lead to significant elevations in ventilator pressures in response to decreased respiratory compliance or increased airways resistance. Pressure-preset modes limit airway and alveolar pressures, which may be beneficial in patients with acute lung injury. However, changes in respiratory system resistance or compliance can lead to substantial decrements in minute ventilation.

VOLUME-PRESET MODES

In *synchronized intermittent mandatory ventilation* (SIMV) (Fig. 13-1), the clinician sets the respiratory rate and tidal volume and the ventilator delivers exactly that number of tidal volumes every minute. The ventilator attempts to synchronize these mandatory breaths with the patient's triggering efforts. Spontaneous efforts between ventilator-delivered breaths are unassisted and tend to be smaller and shorter. As the set rate is progressively decreased, the patient must increase the work of breathing to maintain the same minute ventilation.

In *assist control or controlled mandatory ventilation* (AC or CMV) (Fig. 13-2), the clinician sets the tidal volume and a *minimum* respiratory rate. The ventilator then delivers the set tidal volume each time a breath is triggered by the patient. If the patient's spontaneous rate is less than the ventilator's set rate or if the patient is paralyzed, the ventilator delivers tidal volumes at the minimum backup rate (identical to SIMV). Increases in the patient's spontaneous respiratory rate increase the minute ventilation delivered by the ventilator. AC is often used when the goal of therapy is to minimize the patient's work of breathing. However, in obstructed patients increases in minute ventilation associated with tachypnea can increase PEEPi.

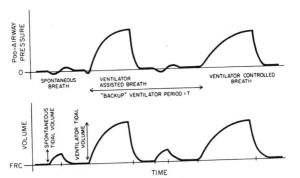

FIGURE 13-1 Airway pressure (Pao) and tidal volume versus time profiles for *assist-control ventilation*. Inspiratory effort by the patient is detected by the machine as a drop in airway pressure below a specific threshold. When this occurs, a full positive pressure tidal volume is delivered in synchrony with the patient's effort. If the patient fails to initiate a breath during the user-specified "backup" period, a positive pressure breath is delivered by the machine.

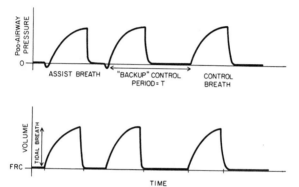

FIGURE 13-2   Airway pressure and tidal volume versus time profiles for *synchronized intermittent mandatory ventilation*. The ventilator "waits" a preset time for the patient to initiate a breath, detected as a decrease in airway pressure below a preset trigger value,
similar to assist control ventilation. Full tidal volume positive pressure breaths are then delivered in synchrony with the patient's effort. If no attempt is made to initiate a breath during the backup period, a positive pressure breath is delivered by the machine. Between
full tidal breaths, the inspiratory valve to the patient is open, allowing for spontaneous breathing.

PRESSURE-PRESET MODES

In *pressure support ventilation* (PSV) (Fig. 13-3), the clinician sets
only the inspiratory pressure above PEEP. The ventilator then
delivers this pressure whenever the patient triggers a breath.
Inspiration is terminated (i.e., the airway pressure is again reduced to PEEP) when a threshold decrease in the inspiratory
flow rate is reached. Some investigators believe that this mode
of ventilation allows for titration of patient effort during liberation from mechanical ventilation. Disadvantages include the
lack of a backup respiratory rate in the event of apnea and potential decreases in minute ventilation in the event of changes
in respiratory system resistance or compliance. As with AC,
high spontaneous respiratory rates can lead to the development of intrinsic PEEP. Often, PSV will be used with SIMV set
at a low rate to provide a backup in the event of apnea.

In *pressure control ventilation* (PCV) (Fig. 13-4), the clinician
sets the inspiratory pressure above PEEP, the rate, and the inspiratory time. In some ventilators the I:E ratio is set to determine the inspiratory time, while in others inspiratory time
is set directly. The ventilator then delivers whatever flow rate
and volume are required to maintain the set inspiratory pressure for the set inspiratory time. The major advantage of this
mode is that alveolar pressure can never exceed the set inspiratory pressure. This mode of ventilation is increasingly
used in patients with the acute respiratory distress syndrome
(ARDS) as it both prevents high alveolar pressures and allows for inverse ratio ventilation (IRV) (see below). Disadvantages include the potential for marked hypoventilation in
the setting of increased airway resistance or decreased respiratory system compliance and the development of PEEPi with
use of prolonged inspiratory times.

Continuous positive airway pressure (CPAP) is not actually
a mode of ventilatory support. Rather, it is a setting on the
ventilator that allows for spontaneous breathing trials while
the ventilator's monitoring functions are in place. The presence of CPAP may also slightly increase FRC in normal patients and decrease the work of breathing in obstructed patients with intrinsic PEEP.

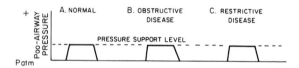

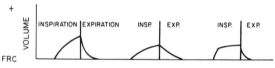

FIGURE 13-3 This figure demonstrates how differences in lung impedance influence tidal volume profiles during pressure support ventilation. Example A depicts airway pressure and tidal volume in a patient with normal airway resistance and lung compliance. Examples B and C depict how airway obstruction and decreased lung compliance affect tidal volume delivered when the airway pressure profile remains the same.

Other Ventilator Settings

F_{IO_2} AND PEEP

The use of oxygen therapy and PEEP in hypoxemic patients is discussed in Chap. 15. These parameters almost exclusively affect arterial oxygenation. The sole exception is the patient with severe airflow obstruction and intrinsic PEEP where the application of PEEP may decrease the work of breathing and improve gas exchange.

INSPIRATORY FLOW RATE

Most intensivists begin mechanical ventilation with an inspiratory flow rate of 60 L/min. This is comfortable for most patients and usually provides adequate expiratory times. Inspiratory flow rates may be increased in patients with air hunger to improve patient ventilator synchrony or in patients with substantial levels of intrinsic PEEP and acceptable peak

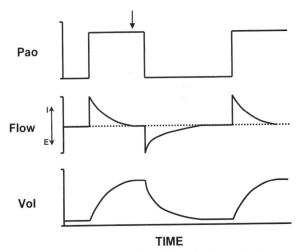

TIME

FIGURE 13-4   Pressure-control ventilation of a therapeutically paralyzed patient. In this patient, the airway pressure equilibrates with alveolar pressure before the ventilator's inspiratory phase is terminated, so flow ceases.

airway pressures to increase expiratory time. However, *inspiratory flow rates should be reduced only after careful consideration*. All too often, inspiratory flow rates are reduced in response to high peak pressures. In obstructed patients, this will decrease peak pressure at the expense of elevated work of breathing and PEEPi, while in ARDS patients it will decrease the contribution of airway resistance to the peak pressure without altering the plateau pressure Pplat. In all patients, it is important to include the inspiratory flow rate when measuring airway resistance = (Ppk − Pplat)/inspiratory flow rate.

INSPIRATORY WAVEFORMS

In volume-preset ventilation, virtually all ventilators include a "square" inspiratory waveform, where the inspiratory flow rate rises as quickly as possible to the set level at the beginning of inspiration and remains constant until the breath is terminated. This pattern usually provides adequate expiratory times and allows measurement of airway resistance. Many ventilators have optional settings, such as decelerating flow waveforms or sine-wave patterns. These settings may be useful in certain clinical settings (for example, a decelerating waveform pattern during AC in a Puritan Bennet 7200 ventilator produces a tracheal pressure waveform nearly indistinguishable from PCV). However, the effect of most alterations in the inspiratory flow pattern is to reduce the average inspiratory flow rate, resulting in the potential complications listed above.

SENSITIVITY

This refers to the negative pressure the patient must generate in the ventilator circuit to initiate a breath. It is usually set at −2 cmH$_2$O but may be lowered (e.g., −1 or −0.5) in very weak patients. "Flow-by" is an alternative mode of triggering the ventilator where reductions in a continuous flow of gas through the circuit rather than a threshold decrease in pressure initiate the breath. Flow-by has been shown to decrease the work of breathing in some patients during pressure-preset ventilation. Historically, increases in sensitivity were used to exercise patients on the ventilator, but this practice has fallen out of favor.

HIGH-PRESSURE LIMIT

Generally this limit (typically 60 to 80 cmH$_2$O) is set by the respiratory therapist. However, if the high-pressure limit is exceeded during volume-preset ventilation, the tidal volume will be cut off. This can lead to substantial hypoventilation even though the patient is connected to the ventilator and the ventilator is cycling. Marked elevations of peak pressures require emergent evaluation (Chap. 12).

Initial Ventilator Settings

No firm guidelines for initial ventilator settings are applicable to all patients. Table 13-1 gives some clinical scenarios with suggested initial settings.

MODE

In general, the choice of ventilator mode should be made based on (1) comfort and familiarity of the physician, (2) achieving optimal patient-ventilator synchrony, (3) etiology of respiratory failure [e.g., ARDS versus chronic obstructive pulmonary disease (COPD) exacerbation], and (4) anticipated duration of illness (e.g., continued need for full support, movement toward liberation, possibility for central apnea etc.)

As a starting point, assist control ventilation is often chosen to provide full ventilatory support in the setting of hypoxemic respiratory failure, hypoventilatory respiratory failure due to central nervous system or neuromuscular disease, postoperative respiratory failure, and shock. IMV ventilation combined with sedation is often used to limit minute ventilation in patients with severe airflow obstruction and dynamic hyperinflation, but this requires deep sedation or therapeutic paralysis. Pressure support, CPAP, or T-piece trials are frequently used during liberation from mechanical ventilation (Chap. 22). Pressure control ventilation is considered in patients with ARDS to prevent the development of alveolar overdistention.

RATE, VOLUME, AND PRESSURE

When starting volume-preset ventilation, a tidal volume of about 7 mL/kg achieves adequate minute ventilation at acceptable respiratory rates and ventilator pressures in most

TABLE 13-1 Some Clinical Scenarios with Suggested Initial Settings

Clinical Scenario	Mode	Rate (bpm)	Tidal Volume or Pressure	Flow (L/min)/Pattern	Principle of Therapy
Severe airflow obstruction	IMV	10	500 mL	60 or higher/square	Minimizing minute ventilation and maximizing expiratory time to limit the development of PEEPi while tolerating some respiratory acidosis
ARDS	PCV or AC	20	$PIP = 35$ cmH_2O V_T titrated to $P_{peak} < 35$	N/A 60/square or decelerating	Use PEEP to prevent end-expiratory atelectasis and low tidal volumes to prevent lung injury from alveolar overdistension while tolerating respiratory acidosis
Postoperative	AC or IMV	10–15	7–10 mL/kg or larger	60/square	Ensure adequate minute ventilation in the setting of decreased drive and prevent atelectasis
Shock with normal lungs	AC	20	7–10 mL/kg	60 or higher/square	Perform as much as possible of the work of breathing in the setting of high minute ventilatory requirements
Weaning	PSV	N/A	Adjust to $f < 30$ and decrease progressively[a]	60 or higher	Gradually decrease support from the ventilator allowing the patient to assume more of the work of breathing

ABBREVIATIONS: ARDS, acute respiratory distress syndrome; IMV, intermittent mandatory ventilation; PCV, pressure control ventilation; AC, assist control; PSV, pressure support ventilation; I:E, ratio of inspiratory to expiratory time; PIP, peak inspiratory pressure; V_T, tidal volume; f, respiratory rate; PEEP, positive end-expiratory pressure; PEEPi, intrinsic PEEP patients. Tidal volume can be increased as needed to improve patient-ventilator synchrony or to prevent atelectasis while monitoring lung mechanics, while it may be decreased in patients with dynamic hyperinflation or very stiff lungs.

Initial pressure support levels should be chosen to achieve adequate tidal volumes with a respiratory rate $(f) < 30$. When used during liberation from mechanical ventilation, pressure support levels should be decreased 2 to 4 cmH_2O once or twice daily as long as f remains < 30.

In beginning pressure control ventilation in ARDS, a rate of 20 with a pressure of 35 cmH_2O and I:E of 1:3 are reasonable starting points. PEEP and F_{IO_2} should be titrated to gas exchange or perhaps the pressure-volume curve of the lung (Chap. 15). Prolonging the inspiratory time may improve oxygenation (see IRV, below), but care must be taken to monitor the development of PEEPi.

OTHER SETTINGS AND MONITORING

The inspiratory flow rate and waveform should be specified with all ventilator orders. All patients should be evaluated within minutes of initiation of changes in mechanical ventilation. History, physical examination, and measurement of lung mechanics should be used to titrate ventilator settings to the patient's comfort and treatment goals. Virtually all patients require sedation; however, sedation can often be minimized by adjusting the ventilator settings to improve patient comfort.

Alternative Modes of Mechanical Ventilation

PROPORTIONAL ASSIST VENTILATION (PAV)

In this mode, flow, volume, and pressure are all determined by patient effort. Strong respiratory efforts by the patient result in higher flows, larger tidal volumes, and potentially higher pressures. Physicians set the flow gain and volume gain of the system. This mode of ventilation provides patients' comfort even while they are receiving substantial levels of ventilatory support, and it may reduce the need for sedation.

Preliminary data suggest that alveolar pressures do not increase to levels associated with alveolar overdistention.

AIRWAY PRESSURE RELEASE VENTILATION

In this mode, airway pressures are maintained at moderate to high levels (15 to 20 cmH$_2$O) throughout most of the respiratory cycle, with brief periods of deflation. The prolonged elevation of airway pressures enhances alveolar recruitment and the brief deflation allows for adequate gas exchange without alveolar collapse. In addition, spontaneous unsupported breaths are permitted, potentially decreasing the need for sedation.

INVERSE RATIO VENTILATION

This is not really a mode of mechanical ventilation but involves reversal of the normal I:E ratio (2: or 3:1) to a level less than 1:1 during any mode of mechanical ventilation, with the goal of improving oxygenation. During volume-preset ventilation, this can be achieved by decreasing the inspiratory flow rate or adding an end-inspiratory pause. In PVC, the inspiratory time can be adjusted directly. IRV typically requires paralysis. PEEPi often develops with IRV and must be monitored. The mechanism of improvement in oxygenation with IRV remains controversial.

TRACHEAL GAS INSUFFLATION (TGI)

This is an adjunct to mechanical ventilation in which oxygen-enriched gas is insufflated into the trachea. The goal is to ventilate the anatomic dead space during expiration and so reduce the Pa$_{CO_2}$ at any given level of inspiratory minute ventilation. The extra flow associated with TGI can lead to the development of high airway pressures and dynamic hyperinflation. Special devices to time TGI to expiration have been developed. In general, TGI should be attempted only by experienced physicians, with careful monitoring of airway pressures and respiratory mechanics.

For a more detailed discussion, see Chap. 32 in *Principles of Critical Care,* 2d ed.

Chapter 14

NONINVASIVE VENTILATION

MICHAEL WALDMAN

Noninvasive positive-pressure ventilation (NIPPV) has been developed in response to questions regarding the invasiveness of endotracheal intubation, which has many complications and risks, including laryngospasm, tracheal trauma, nosocomial pneumonia, and prolonged weaning secondary to sedative medications. The main goal of NIPPV when applied to patients with acute respiratory failure is to provide respiratory assistance while reducing complications by decreasing the need for invasive mechanical ventilation. NIPPV also provides an alternative treatment to patients refusing endotracheal intubation or in patients with poor underlying status.

Physiologic Effects

NIPPV frequently results in improvement of arterial oxygenation in patients with hypoxemic respiratory failure. The exact mechanism behind the improvement is unclear, but it is likely due to either increased inspired oxygen fraction or improved functional residual capacity as a result of the positive end-expiratory pressure. Improvement in oxygenation in patients with hypoventilatory respiratory failure is also seen with the use of NIPPV. It is unclear whether this effect is due to increased inspired oxygen fraction or a result of improvement in alveolar ventilation.

The initiation of NIPPV has been shown to lessen the work of breathing both in stable patients and in those with acute respiratory failure. The combination of PEEP and pressure support has been shown to decrease diaphragmatic efforts in patients with chronic obstructive pulmonary disease more efficiently than either method alone. After initiation of NIPPV, the respiratory rate decreases and minute ventilation increases, usually leading to improvement in the sense of dyspnea.

Features of NIPPV

In most cases NIPPV is intended as an intermittent means of respiratory support. It is rarely successful in patients requiring prolonged or permanent ventilatory support. As patients are awake and nonsedated while using NIPPV, they must have a sufficient central drive to breathe. The success of NIPPV is dependent on preventing leaks in the system. The presence of a leak can lead to increased patient discomfort, dyssynchrony between the patient and the ventilator, and loss of the ability to maintain positive end-expiratory pressure.

Mode of Ventilation

Several modes of ventilation have been proposed with NIPPV, including assist-control, pressure-support, and assist-pressure-control ventilation. All modes have benefits and limitations. Volume-targeted modes are more prone to develop leaks and to provoke skin necrosis, gastric distention, and lack of tolerance. It has been suggested that pressure-support modes are better tolerated, but if a leak is present, the cycling from inspiration to exhalation will not be detected. Setting an inspiratory time limit, as in assist-pressure-control ventilation, may solve this problem.

The initial bedside management is critical to the success of NIPPV (Table 14-1). The physician must determine the best patient-ventilator interface (nasal mask, full face mask, or mouthpiece as bridge to face mask). Time is required to educate the patient and elicit full cooperation. Typical initial ventilator settings are pressure-support of 8 cmH_2O and PEEP 2 cmH_2O with a plan to advance these settings as needed to 10 to 15 cmH_2O and PEEP 5 cmH_2O (equivalent to an inspiratory pressure of 15 to 20 cmH_2O and expiratory pressure of 5 cmH_2O). Relief of dyspnea should be obvious, often within the first 10 minutes. Pulse oximetry and arterial blood gases should be followed closely during the first 1 to 2 hours of treatment.

TABLE 14-1   The Technique of NIPPV

Select patients likely to benefit from NIPPV (see Table 14-2).

Exclude patients who are hemodynamically unstable, unable to
protect the airway, or who are in respiratory arrest.

Explain the procedure to the patient and encourage cooperation.

Monitor the patient continuously with pulse oximetry.

Choose a well-fitting nasal or full face mask.

Before fixing the mask tightly, apply it gently to the patient's face by
hand—with the ventilator connected—so the patient can feel the
relief of dyspnea.

Initiate NIPPV using pressure-support ventilation, beginning with
5 cmH$_2$O pressure-support and 2 cmH$_2$O CPAP.

Gradually increase the levels of pressure-support to 10 cmH$_2$O and
CPAP to 5 cmH$_2$O until the patient's respiratory rate falls and the
patient appears more comfortable.

Be prepared to intubate the patient if there is no apparent beneficial
response.

Sedatives or anxiolytics will occasionally allow successful NIPPV,
but these drugs may increase the risk of aspiration, ventilatory
failure, and respiratory arrest.

The level of pressure-support can be raised to 25 cmH$_2$O but this is
usually not necessary and risks pressure necrosis of the facial skin
and gastric distention.

Analyze arterial blood-gas levels after 1 hour.

Indications

Successful outcomes can be expected in patients with acute
ventilatory failure with no other organ dysfunction, without
central nervous system disorders, and with no urgent need
for endotracheal intubation (respiratory arrest or the inability to protect the airway). The group that most clearly benefits from NIPPV contains patients with hypercapnic ventilatory failure (Table 14-2) based on improvement in arterial pH,
symptoms of breathlessness, and need for endotracheal intubation. In fact, NIPPV is the current standard for ventilation
of patients with acute-on-chronic respiratory failure from
COPD who are hemodynamically stable and can maintain
their airways. Other groups of patients who clearly benefit
from NIPPV are those with postoperative respiratory failure
and those with acute cardiogenic pulmonary edema—probably also patients with status asthmaticus. The benefits of

TABLE 14-2 Indications for Noninvasive Ventilation and Expected Efficacy

Disease	Specific Cause	Efficacy	Mode of Ventilation
Acute hypercapnic respiratory failure			
COPD	No specific cause	Proven	PSV, ACV, PSV + PEEP
COPD	Specific cause such as pneumonia, cardiac failure	Unproven and higher likelihood for failure	PSV, ACV, PSV + PEEP
Chronic restrictive disease		Likely	PSV, ACV, PSV + PEEP
Postextubation respiratory failure	Reversible upper airway obstruction, or inability to clear secretions, or post surgical	Likely	PSV, ACV, PSV + PEEP
Cardiogenic pulmonary edema (hypercapnic forms)	Absence of cardiogenic shock	Proven	CPAP or PSV + PEEP or ACV + PEEP
Coma	Central nervous system disorders	Contraindicated except when secondary to reversible hypercapnia	

Acute hypoxemic respiratory failure		
Acute Respiratory Distress Syndrome	Unlikely or contra-indicated in case of multisystem organ dysfunction	CPAP or PSV + PEEP
Pneumocystis carinii	Unproven but possible benefit	CPAP or PSV + PEEP or ACV + PEEP
Infectious pneumonia	Unproven or unlikely to benefit	
Other		
Patients who are not candidates for endotracheal intubation		
Refuse endotracheal intubation	Likely	PSV or ACV
Elderly		

ABBREVIATIONS: PSV, pressure-support ventilation; ACV, assist-control ventilation; PEEP, positive end-expiratory pressure; CPAP, continuous positive airway pressure.

NIPPV in patients with acute hypoxic respiratory failure are less clear. NIPPV may be a useful tool in liberating patients from the ventilator. Early data have shown significant benefits in outcomes from deliberate early extubation with a switch to NIPPV. Patients with hemodynamic instability should not receive NIPPV.

Complications

Complications seen with NIPPV include skin pressure lesions, facial pain, dry nose, eye irritation, discomfort, poor sleep, mask leakage, and gastric distention. Occasionally these complications are significant enough to necessitate withdrawal of the technique. The most common reasons for failure of NIPPV are difficulties with proper mask fit and inability to maintain adequate gas exchange. Skin necrosis and gastric distention can usually be avoided by limiting peak mask pressure to 20 to 25 cmH$_2$O. Nosocomial pneumonia, thromboembolic disease, and gastrointestinal disorders are also seen, but with an incidence less than that with invasive mechanical ventilation.

For a more detailed discussion, see Chap. 31 in *Principles of Critical Care*, 2d ed.

Chapter 15

ACUTE HYPOXEMIC RESPIRATORY FAILURE

SANGEETA BHORADE

Acute hypoxemic respiratory failure (AHRF) or type 1 respiratory failure is the result of alveolar filling and/or alveolar collapse and is characterized by hypoxemia that is minimally responsive to oxygen therapy. AHRF results in decreased lung compliance and increased work of breathing; ultimately, it may lead to respiratory arrest. Diffuse lung lesions are either high-pressure (hydrostatic, cardiogenic) or low-pressure [high permeability, pulmonary capillary leak syndrome, adult respiratory distress syndrome (ARDS)] pulmonary edema. Focal lesions are often caused by lobar pneumonia or lung contusion. A list of causes of AHRF is presented in Table 15-1.

Diffuse AHRF

Liquid flux in the lung is determined by the integrity of the pulmonary vasculature and by the driving hydrostatic pressure. Accordingly, elevated hydrostatic pressure due to heart failure, volume overload, or any increase in volume in the central pulmonary circulation can result in high-pressure pulmonary edema. On the other hand, any lung injury that decreases the integrity of the pulmonary vasculature and the oncotic pressure gradient between the intravascular and interstitial spaces can result in low-pressure pulmonary edema (Fig. 15-1).

HIGH-PRESSURE OR CARDIOGENIC PULMONARY EDEMA (CPE)

CPE typically occurs in the setting of increased left ventricular end-diastolic pressure from either myocardial ischemia/infarct or congestive heart failure. CPE may also occur with

TABLE 15-1   Causes of Acute Hypoxemic
Respiratory Failure

Diffuse lung lesions
  Cardiogenic (hydrostatic) edema
    Left ventricular failure
    Acute ischemia
    Mitral regurgitation
    Mitral stenosis
    Ball-valve thrombus
    Volume overload, particularly with
      coexisting renal and cardiac disease
  Permeability (low-pressure) edema (ARDS)
    Most common
      Sepsis and sepsis syndrome
      Acid aspiration
      Multiple transfusions for hypovolemic shock
    Less common
      Near drowning
      Pancreatitis
      Air or fat embolism
      Cardiopulmonary bypass
      Pneumonia
      Drug reaction or overdose
      Leukoagglutination
      Inhalation injury
      Infusion of biologics (e.g., IL-2)
  Edema of unclear or mixed etiology
    Reexpansion
    Neurogenic, postictal
    Tocolysis-associated
    High-altitude
  Alveolar hemorrhage
    Collagen-vascular diseases
    Thrombocytopenia
    Bone marrow transplantation
    Infection in immunocompromised patients
  Focal lung lesions
  Lobar pneumonia
  Lung contusion
  Lobar atelectasis (acutely)

---

any obstruction of the mitral valve or volume overload in the
setting of renal and cardiac failure. In addition, patients in
the Trendelenburg position or those who receive vasoactive

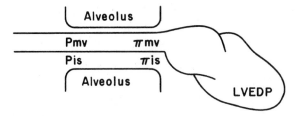

$$\text{Edema Flow} = \left[\,(Pmv-Pis) - (\pi mv - \pi is)\,\sigma\,\right] Kf$$

FIGURE 15-1 The Starling equation for edema flow in the lungs. Hydrostatic edema most typically occurs in conditions in which the pulmonary microvascular pressure (Pmv) is high because of elevations in LVEDP secondary to cardiac dysfunction.

medications, both of which shift intravascular volume from the peripheral circulation to the more central circulation, are at risk for CPE.

LOW-PRESSURE PULMONARY EDEMA OR ARDS

ARDS occurs directly as a result of lung injury (e.g., aspiration, inhalation, or infectious agents) or indirectly by systemic processes (e.g., sepsis, shock with large-volume blood product resuscitation). It is helpful to separate the various phases of lung injury associated with ARDS in order to understand the pathophysiology of this entity and, subsequently, the management of patients in the different phases of ARDS (Fig. 15-2).

The early phase of ARDS, also termed the *exudative phase,* usually occurs within the first 7 days of lung injury. It is characterized by the influx of proteinaceous fluid, with minimal evidence of cellular injury by light microscopy. The proliferative phase of ARDS generally occurs approximately 7 to 10 days following the initial pulmonary insult. This phase is characterized by hyaline membrane formation, increased numbers of inflammatory cells, progressive fibrosis with increased dead-space fraction, high minute ventilation requirements, and decreased responsiveness to PEEP.

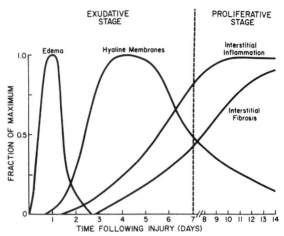

FIGURE 15-2   A schematic representation showing the time course of evolution of the adult respiratory distress syndrome (ARDS). During the early or exudative phase, the lesion is characterized by a pulmonary capillary leak with edema and then, shortly thereafter, hyaline membrane formation. Within as short a period of time as 7 to 10 days, a proliferative phase may appear with marked interstitial inflammation, fibrosis, and disordered healing (see text for discussion). (*Reproduced with permission from Katzenstein AA, Askin FB: Surgical Pathology of Non-Neoplastic Lung Diseases. Philadelphia, Saunders, 1982.*)

Because of the difference between these two phases, their management differs. Therapeutic measures to reduce lung water are likely to be most effective during the exudative phase of ARDS. On the other hand, increased circulating volume may be beneficial during the proliferative phase of ARDS, when increased dead space is often present.

The etiology of some forms of pulmonary edema is still unclear. For example, neurogenic pulmonary edema, reexpansion pulmonary edema, and pulmonary edema induced by tocolysis are thought to be the result of both increased hydrostatic pressure and pulmonary capillary leak.

Focal AHRF

Either lobar pneumonia or lung contusion may cause focal AHRF. In patients with lobar pneumonia, loss of hypoxic vasoconstriction contributes to the shunt and worsening hypoxemia. In patients with lung contusion, lung regions adjacent to the contusion may be hypoventilated. Thus in contusion, unlike lobar pneumonia, much of the hypoxemia is due to low ventilation perfusion $(\dot{V}/\dot{Q})$ ratios, which may be corrected by oxygen therapy. Contusions are often associated with direct injury to the pulmonary microcirculation and hemorrhage, which occur within minutes to hours of injury. Caution must be taken when using positive-pressure ventilation or PEEP in patients with focal injury, as these modes may worsen the lung injury. Thus, when PEEP is applied, frequent determinations of benefit should be made. Other measures include positioning the patient with the unaffected lung in the dependent position, which may improve ventilation and perfusion matching.

Clinical Presentation

The clinical presentation of the different etiologies of AHRF is very similar. Physical examination usually reveals tachypnea (respiratory rate > 30) and dyspnea; lung exam reveals diffuse crackles in pulmonary edema or focal findings over an area of consolidation in patients with lobar infiltrates. CPE may be associated with wheezing. Often patients who are dehydrated at presentation may be extremely dyspneic, with minimal findings on chest radiographs or physical examination. Once hydrated, these patients often develop significant findings. Arterial blood gas (ABG) usually reveals significant hypoxemia with oxygen saturation (Sa_{O_2}) < 85%. If the oxygenation can be corrected easily with supplemental oxygen therapy, a significant shunt is unlikely to be present and other causes for dyspnea should be considered. On rare occasions, if the chest radiograph (CXR) is completely clear and the ABG reveals significant hypoxemia that does not respond to oxygen therapy, an alternative explanation of right-to-left shunt should be considered, including intracardiac shunt or arteriovenous malformation.

Determining the Etiology of Pulmonary Edema

CLINICAL SETTING

The clinical setting of pulmonary edema is usually the most helpful factor in determining its etiology. If a patient has evidence of cardiac dysfunction by history, physical exam, electrocardiogram (ECG), or other laboratory studies, cardiogenic edema should lead the list of differential diagnoses. The volume status of each patient should always be assessed as either the primary etiology or complicating factor in pulmonary edema. ARDS typically arises in several clinical contexts (see Table 15-1).

CHEST RADIOGRAPH (CXR)

Unfortunately, although CXR is an easily available clinical diagnostic test, its accuracy in distinguishing high-pressure from low-pressure pulmonary edema is low. Criteria that support high-pressure pulmonary edema include increased heart size, increased width of the vascular pedicle, vascular redistribution toward upper lobes, septal lines, and a perihilar "batwing" distribution of the edema. The lack of these findings along with patchy peripheral infiltrates is suggestive of ARDS.

EDEMA FLUID ANALYSIS

Measurement of protein in edema fluid suctioned from the endotracheal tube may provide information useful in distinguishing high-pressure pulmonary edema from ARDS. The ratio of protein content of edema fluid (E) to protein content in plasma (P) in ARDS is 70 to 90%, while the E/P ratio in

CPE is less than 50%. This analysis should be performed early in the course of AHRF, since active clearance of water from pulmonary edema by alveolar cells may cause the E/P ratio to increase as patients recover. Interestingly, failure to concentrate alveolar protein suggests persistent capillary leak and poorer prognosis.

ECHOCARDIOGRAPHY

Echocardiography is a useful noninvasive method of detecting ventricular or valvular abnormalities, including left ventricular dilatation, regional or global wall motion abnormalities, and mitral regurgitation supporting an etiology for CPE. However, one should remember that a normal echocardiogram does not universally rule out a cardiac etiology for pulmonary edema, as prior ventricular or valvular disease may intermittently improve with therapy.

INVASIVE HEMODYNAMIC MONITORING

Recently, controversy surrounding the benefits versus the risks of the right heart catheter has escalated. Concerns regarding complications of insertion and placement of the catheter as well as misinterpretation of data obtained from the catheter have added to the controversy surrounding its use. Thus, it is important to formulate specific questions regarding ventricular function, adequacy of volume resuscitation, degree of intrapulmonary shunt, and adequacy of oxygen delivery prior to placement of the catheter. In mechanically ventilated patients with normal lung function and normal serum oncotic pressure, CPE is typically associated with a pulmonary capillary wedge pressure (Ppw) ≤ 25 to 35 mmHg. Patients with ARDS typically have Ppw of 0 to 18 mmHg.

Defining and Scoring ARDS

ARDS has been defined and stratified according to the criteria presented in Table 15-2. Acute lung injury is a less severe form of this syndrome, characterized by the same criteria except that the Pa_{O_2}/F_{IO_2} is < 300. The Lung Injury Score (LIS),

TABLE 15-2   Criteria for Diagnosis of ARDS

Clinical presentation
  Tachypnea and dyspnea
  Crackles on auscultation
Clinical setting
  Direct lung insult (e.g., aspiration) or
    systemic process with potential for
    lung injury (e.g., sepsis)
Radiologic appearance
  Three- or four-quadrant alveolar flooding
Lung mechanics
  Diminished compliance (<40 mL/cmH$_2$O)
Gas exchange
  Severe hypoxemia refractory to oxygen
    therapy (Pa$_{O_2}$/F$_{I_{O_2}}$ < 200)
Normal pulmonary vascular pressures
  Pulmonary capillary wedge pressure <18 mmHg

---

a scoring system developed in 1988 by Murray and Matthay, is a widely accepted method of determining the severity of lung diseases in order to compare patients across different settings (Table 15-3).

Treatment of AHRF

While supportive therapy for AHRF is initiated, a search for and treatment of the underlying cause of AHRF is of utmost importance. If the underlying disease is not addressed, increasing complications and irreversible organ failure will inevitably occur. Initial therapy includes supplemental oxygen therapy in the highest concentration available. It is well to remember that the maximal F$_{I_{O_2}}$ attainable with high-flow masks and rebreathing devices is 0.6 to 0.7 under most clinical conditions.

MANAGING CARDIOGENIC PULMONARY EDEMA

The management of CPE requires management of left ventricular systolic and diastolic dysfunction. In general, hypox-

TABLE 15-3 Scoring System for ARDS

Chest roentgenogram score	
No alveolar consolidation	0
1-quadrant consolidation	1
2-quadrant consolidation	2
3-quadrant consolidation	3
4-quadrant consolidation	4
Hypoxemia score	
$Pa_{O_2}/F_{I_{O_2}} \geq 300$	0
$Pa_{O_2}/F_{I_{O_2}}$ 225–299	1
$Pa_{O_2}/F_{I_{O_2}}$ 175–224	2
$Pa_{O_2}/F_{I_{O_2}}$ 100–174	3
$Pa_{O_2}/F_{I_{O_2}} \leq 100$	4
Compliance (when ventilated) (mL/cmH_2O)	
≥ 80	0
60–79	1
40–59	2
20–39	3
≤ 19	4
PEEP required (when ventilated) (cmH_2O)	
≤ 5	0
6–8	1
9–11	2
12–14	3
≥ 15	4
Final value is obtained by dividing the aggregate sum by the number of components used	
Score:	
No injury	0
Mild to moderate injury	0.1–2.5
Severe injury (ARDS)	>2.5

SOURCE: Modified and reproduced with permission from Murray JF, Matthay MA, Luce J, et al: An expanded definition of the adult respiratory distress syndrome. *Am J Respir Crit Care Med* 138:720, 1988.

emia associated with CPE responds quickly to appropriate pharmacologic therapy, and mechanical ventilatory support is often not required if therapy is instituted in a timely fashion. Nonetheless, patients with CPE often have hypoxemia that is severe and, like other forms of AHRF, minimally responsive to oxygen therapy.

The goals of therapy are threefold: (1) to reduce myocardial ischemia, (2) to decrease the elevated filling pressures that are often responsible for CPE, and (3) to maintain perfusion to end organs. In order to accomplish these goals, one must focus on titrating therapy to optimize preload, decrease afterload, and increase contractility.

Therapy should begin with oxygen by nasal cannula or mask titrated against oximetry or ABG measurements. Preload may be optimized in several ways. Positioning of the patient in an upright position, even after intubation, is preferable if arterial blood pressure allows. Preload is reduced with a combination of nitrates, diuretics, and morphine. Nitroglycerin (10 to 30 μg/min IV) and furosemide (20 to 40 mg) both increase venodilation and pooling of blood in the periphery. Furosemide may also reduce intrapulmonary shunt directly. The initial dose of furosemide may be doubled if the desired response is not elicited. Alternatively, bumetanide (1 to 2 mg IV) or furosemide and metolazone (2.5 to 10 mg PO) may be administered. Morphine sulfate reduces anxiety and excessive sympathetic tone; 2 to 4 mg IV of morphine sulfate may be repeated every 5 to 10 minutes and titrated to patient comfort, mental status, and blood pressure. If renal function is compromised and hemodialysis is delayed, preload may be reduced by rotating tourniquets or phlebotomy. Longer-term diuresis in patients with acceptable renal function may be enhanced by administration of dopamine (1 to 4 μg/kg per minute). Afterload reduction includes morphine to decrease sympathetic output. For persistent elevations of blood pressure, angiotensin converting enzyme (ACE) inhibitors or sodium nitroprusside may be instituted until blood pressure is reduced to the desired level. Dobutamine is the preferred inotrope in CPE, since it also causes afterload reduction. It should be administered at a dose of 5 to 15 μg/kg per minute and titrated to cardiac output and clinical parameters of perfusion. Tachyphylaxis may occur, and the dose may need to be increased to yield the same effect over several days.

Positive-pressure ventilation applied by mask reduces the work of breathing as well as ventricular afterload without the risks associated with endotracheal intubation. There is a growing literature suggesting that noninvasive ventilation in selected patients with CPE is associated with improved out-

TABLE 15-4   Contraindications to Noninvasive Ventilation

Hemodynamic instability
Left ventricular failure refractory to medical support
Difficult airway anatomy/poor mask fit
Full stomach (pregnancy, morbid obesity, diabetic
  gastroparesis)
Decreased mentation/airway reflexes
Complex dysrhythmias requiring cardioversion
Need for intraaortic balloon pump, angiography, or
  surgery

---

come. Contraindications to noninvasive ventilation are commonly encountered in patients with CPE and should motivate early elective intubation and mechanical ventilation (Table 15-4). Patients with mask ventilation must be monitored continuously by experienced staff, since the mask must be tight-fitting to provide continuous positive pressure, and loss of a seal can have immediate adverse effects on arterial hemoglobin saturation. Gastric dilatation with vomiting may also have disastrous consequences.

Mechanical ventilation has beneficial cardiovascular effects, which include decreasing the work of breathing, decreasing oxygen consumption, decreasing the perfusion requirements of the respiratory muscles, and reducing the afterload on a dysfunctional left ventricle. Volume control modes including assist-control (A/C) and synchronized intermittent mandatory ventilation (SIMV) may be used. Initial ventilator settings should include an $F_{I_{O_2}}$ of 1.0, tidal volume (TV) of 6 to 8 mL/kg, and a respiratory rate (RR) of 25 breaths per minute. PEEP may then be titrated against arterial saturation to permit a reduction in the $F_{I_{O_2}}$ to 0.6 or less. As the patient improves, spontaneous breathing modes, including pressure support (PS) and continuous positive airway pressure (CPAP), may be instituted.

MANAGING ARDS

Emphasis must be placed on aggressive diagnosis and treatment of the underlying condition. *Because ARDS is a syndrome, recognizing its existence is not equivalent to diagnosing the patient's underlying problem.* Having made this important point, focus will be on the supportive management of these patients, which sustains the patient while parallel diagnostic and therapeutic interventions are made for the underlying disease(s) that caused the acute lung injury.

CIRCULATORY STRATEGIES

The circulatory management of these patients remains a therapeutic dilemma. Previously, strategies involving maximizing oxygen delivery to peripheral tissues by augmenting cardiac output were felt to be beneficial in ARDS. However, recent studies have not confirmed a benefit, presumably owing to the fact that the proposed oxygen extraction deficit may not be clinically relevant. In addition, maximizing oxygen delivery may escalate requirements for mechanical ventilation, oxygen, and PEEP, which may be associated with increased complications. As a result, we favor a strategy that would reduce preload without decreasing cardiac output early in the course of ARDS.

This strategy requires careful titration of the volume status at times. On the one hand, intravascular volume reduction may reduce pulmonary edema, ultimately reducing the duration of mechanical ventilation and improving outcome. However, if this approach is taken to the other extreme, hypoperfusion and other organ failure may occur. Thus, the clinician must focus on end-organ function, including mental status, urine output and concentration, and any evidence of inadequate peripheral tissue perfusion while also reducing the pulmonary capillary wedge pressure to the lowest level compatible with an adequate cardiac output and oxygen delivery.

Measures to optimize the circulatory status should follow the above guidelines. All excess intravenous fluids should be limited and intravenous drips with medications should be maximally concentrated. In patients with systolic dysfunction, dobutamine may be used to maintain perfusion at a reduced preload. If preload is reduced excessively, red blood cell transfusion, as opposed to crystalloid, should be administered.

The task of interpreting right heart catheter data during mechanical ventilation with high levels of PEEP may be challenging. If alveolar pressure is greater than left atrial pressure at the site of measurement (West zone 1 or 2 conditions), then the pulmonary capillary wedge pressure (Ppw) reflects alveolar pressure as opposed to left ventricular end-diastolic pressure. Even in zone 3 lung conditions, PEEP may increase pericardial pressure, making the Ppw an inaccurate reflection of transmural filling pressure of the left ventricle. However, it must be remembered that these data simply contribute to all trended measurements that guide the clinician in seeking the lowest pulmonary wedge pressure consistent with an adequate cardiac output.

VENTILATOR STRATEGIES

Over the past decade, a body of knowledge has accrued regarding appropriate ventilation strategies in patients with ARDS. Results of these studies suggest that lung injury in ARDS is often inhomogeneous; thus, the tidal volume is delivered to a functionally reduced population of alveoli or "small lung," with the potential for overdistention and lung injury.

The lung pressure–volume (PV) relationship in ARDS has a sigmoidal shape, with a lower inflection point (LIP) and an upper inflection point (UIP); it exhibits hysteresis when the inflation and deflation limbs are compared (Fig. 15-3). The LIP has been taken to reflect a two-compartment structure, with some alveoli that exhibit relatively normal compliance and others that require higher transpulmonary pressure to inflate. The UIP has been taken to reflect the point where a pressure increase will result in less volume change, presumably because some alveoli are maximally stretched. These mechanical properties of the lung have been use to guide innovative ventilator strategies: (1) limiting the end-inspiratory lung volume to avoid alveolar overdistention and (2) applying sufficient PEEP to prevent end-expiratory derecruitment. Principles that guide ventilatory management of ARDS are: (1) avoid alveolar overdistention; (2) maintain $F_{I_{O_2}} < 0.6$; (3) use sufficient PEEP to prevent derecruitment; (4) remember that the mode of ventilation is less important; and (5) tolerate hypercapnia, if necessary, to limit alveolar overdistention.

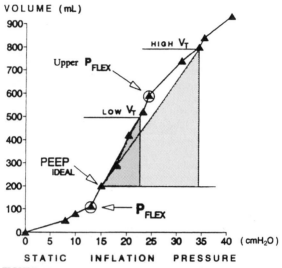

FIGURE 15-3 An inspiratory static pressure-volume curve of the respiratory system obtained from one of the patients entered in a recent study of open-lung ventilation in ARDS. Note that at an inflation pressure between 10 and 15 cmH$_2$O, a lower inflection point is noted, designated P$_{FLEX}$. This describes a lung inflation point below which alveolar closure is hypothesized to occur, and selecting a PEEP level below this point causes alveolar recruitment-derecruitment with each respiratory cycle. It is speculated that such inflation-deflation with its associated shear forces can cause lung injury. Thus a PEEP level above this lower inflection point is shown as "Ideal PEEP." As volume increases along the inflation curve, note that a second or upper inflection point, designated *upper* P$_{FLEX}$, is encountered. This upper inflection point is believed to reflect a point at which overdistention of alveolar units occurs, risking volutrauma. Utilization of high tidal volumes, as shown, can result in lung inflation exceeding this inflection point and risking alveolar overdistention and injury. The goal of open-lung ventilation is to maintain inflation-deflation between the two inflection points during the entire respiratory cycle. (Reproduced and adapted with permission from Amato MBP, Barbas CSV, Medeiros DM, et al: Beneficial effects of the "open lung approach" with low distending pressures in acute respiratory distress syndrome: A prospective randomized study on mechanical ventilation. *Am J Respir Crit Care Med* 152:1835, 1995.

On presentation, the patient should receive oxygen provided by high-low or rebreather mask, although these devices rarely achieve a tracheal F_{IO_2} much above 0.6. If a patient responds dramatically to oxygen therapy, he or she probably has a large component of $\dot{V}/\dot{Q}$ mismatch and a small component of shunt disease. When Pa_{O_2} improves only slightly, indicating a large shunt, oxygen delivery may still rise substantially because of the steep nature of the hemoglobin saturation relationship at low Pa_{O_2}. The role of noninvasive positive-pressure ventilation (NIPPV) has not been established in ARDS.

Intubation should be performed early and electively when it is clear that mechanical ventilation will be required. The initial ventilator settings include an F_{IO_2} of 1.0, RR of 20 to 30 breaths per minute, and TV of 6 to 8 mL/kg when using assist-control (AC) or synchronized intermittent mandatory ventilation (SIMV). Most authorities recommend using tidal volumes that maintain the plateau pressures (Pplat) below 30 to 35 cm, which typically correspond to the UIP on the PV curve in ARDS. When pressure-control ventilation (PCV) is being used, the inspiratory pressure should be 30 to 35 cmH_2O. By restricting this inspiratory pressure (Pinsp) level, the TV delivered to the patient may be limited. Such a decrease in TV may result in an elevated P_{CO_2}, termed *permissive hypercapnia* (described below). One of the first goals of ventilator management is to reduce the F_{IO_2} to less than 0.6 to minimize further lung injury. PEEP is used to recruit alveoli by expanding collapsed units and translocating fluid from flooded units to the interstitial space. In this way, respiratory system compliance increases and gas exchange is improved.

Since the approach to PEEP in patients with ARDS is evolving, intensivists must currently manage patients without the benefit of definitive clinical studies. We provide guidelines for both "least PEEP" and "open-lung strategies."

LEAST-PEEP APPROACH

With this approach PEEP is increased in increments of 5 cmH_2O, with pulse oximetry to monitor the oxygen saturation (Sa_{O_2}). If hypotension occurs secondary to decreased venous return, PEEP may be temporarily reduced and intravenous fluids and vasoactive medications administered to increase the cardiac output. After the Sa_{O_2} rises to 90%, the $F_{I_{O_2}}$ should be reduced to 0.6 if possible. The least PEEP required to maintain $(Sa_{O_2}) > 90\%$ on an $F_{I_{O_2}} \leq 0.6$ is used. The Sa_{O_2} should be confirmed by ABG analysis.

OPEN-LUNG APPROACH

This approach is based on the LIP of the PV curve, as described in recent clinical trials. The PV curve is constructed by increasing the tidal volume from 100 to 1000 mL and documenting the pressure after an inspiratory pause (on zero PEEP). The PEEP is then set 2 cmH_2O higher than the LIP. If the patient will not be able to tolerate zero PEEP for 30 minutes (the time it takes to construct the PV curve), the PV curve may be determined with a PEEP of 10 to 15 cmH_2O. PEEP is then adjusted upward until the LIP is eliminated. Since it may be impractical to determine PV curves on a daily basis, the PEEP may be based on values that exceed the LIP in other studies, approximately 17 cmH_2O. As oxygenation improves, the PEEP and $F_{I_{O_2}}$ are adjusted downward.

PERMISSIVE HYPERCAPNIA

Over the past decade, the benefit of ventilating patients with smaller tidal volumes to prevent alveolar overdistention and thus avoid ventilator-induced injury appears to outweigh maintaining normocarbia. The resulting respiratory acidosis has many physiologic effects that may serve as contraindications to permissive hypercapnia. While the manner and degree in which permissive hypercapnic ventilation should be conducted have not been well defined, a common approach is to allow the P_{CO_2} to rise gradually (10 mmHg/h) in order to allow time for cellular compensation. The role of sodium bicarbonate administration has not been validated in this clinical scenario and has theoretical adverse effects.

In patients with refractory hypoxemia, ancillary strategies—including increasing oxygen-carrying capacity by blood transfusion or augmentation of cardiac output with vasoactive agents, specifically dobutamine—should be considered. In addition, reduction of oxygen consumption via sedation, paralysis, and cooling may improve Sa_{O_2}.

SALVAGE THERAPIES FOR ARDS

The following therapies are currently regarded as salvage therapies in patients who do not improve or continue to deteriorate with the previously mentioned measures. These therapies may be proven to be more effective in the future.

Prone Position

Several studies have shown that patients with ARDS exhibit improved oxygenation with prone positioning. Hypotheses to explain the improvement in oxygenation include (1) increased FRC, (2) change in regional diaphragm motion, (3) redistribution of perfusion, and (4) better clearance of secretions. Prone positioning, if desired, should be performed early in the course of ARDS, and special attention should focus on preventing pressure ulcers on the nose, face, and ears. In addition, special care is needed to prevent pressure on the eye, which may lead to retinal ischemia.

Tracheal Gas Insufflation (TGI)

TGI is an adjunctive technique that introduces fresh gas near the carina through a modified endotracheal tube. This added flow washes CO_2-rich gas out of the trachea, thus reducing anatomic dead space as well as P_{CO_2} during permissive hypercapnia. Potential risks include tracheal erosion, oxygen toxicity related to the unknown $F_{I_{O_2}}$, and increases in auto-PEEP.

High-Frequency Ventilation (HFV)

HFV typically employs tidal volumes of 1 to 5 ml/kg with respiratory rates of 60 to 300 breaths per minute. Gas exchange is poorly understood under these conditions but is thought to occur as much through augmented axial diffusion as through bulk flow. However, HFV has not been shown to be superior to conventional modes of ventilation. Until future studies comparing this mode of ventilation with current standard approaches are conducted, this technique is best viewed as salvage therapy.

Inverse Ratio Ventilation (IRV)

IRV entails the use of prolonged inspiratory times (I:E ratio > 1). IRV is thought to improve gas exchange by alveolar recruitment at lower airway pressures and more optimal distribution of ventilation. An important caution when using this mode is that both auto-PEEP and higher mean alveolar pressure may reduce cardiac output.

ECMO and IVOX

The use of extracorporeal gas exchange (ECMO) to adequately oxygenate and ventilate the blood while allowing the lung to rest has not been supported by clinical outcome studies in patients with AHRF. IVOX is an intravenous oxygenator consisting of a very small membrane gas exchanger that is inserted into the inferior vena cava. Currently, these technologies are not being used in adults.

Perflubron

Perflubron is a perfluorocarbon that is instilled into the trachea and improves oxygenation by recruiting dependent alveoli by a hydraulic column. This approach is known as *partial liquid lung ventilation*. A practical problem is that perflubron is radiodense, making the lungs appear white, so that it is impossible to use chest radiographs for diagnostic and monitoring purposes. This therapy remains under investigation and is not available outside of clinical trials.

Pharmacotherapy

The development of pharmacotherapy for ARDS involves improving gas exchange by reducing intrapulmonary shunt and limiting acute lung injury.

Nitric oxide (NO) is hypothesized to be the primary endogenous mediator of vascular smooth muscle relaxation. Inhaled NO is a selective pulmonary vasodilator that preferentially dilates blood vessels of well-ventilated alveoli, reducing shunt. Pulmonary vascular resistance may also be lowered due to the vasodilating effects of NO. While there is a large literature documenting these beneficial physiologic effects of NO, outcome studies have not demonstrated long-term benefit in adults. Currently, NO is not an FDA-approved drug and may not be given outside the realm of research protocols.

Surfactant levels are decreased in patients with ARDS. However in a recent large prospective study of surfactant, no benefit was associated with therapy. At this point, surfactant therapy for ARDS remains experimental.

Corticosteroids in the early phase of ARDS have not been shown to improve outcome, gas exchange, or lung mechanics. The only acute lung lesion that does benefit from steroid therapy is acute eosinophilic pneumonia. The role of corticosteroids in the later phases of ARDS has yet to be defined. Several anecdotal reports suggest that there may be some benefit to corticosteroids use in the proliferative phase of ARDS.

Monitoring ARDS

Some patients may recover rapidly from ARDS, within 2 to 3 days, presumably secondary to resolution of the predisposing cause and appropriate cardiovascular interventions. However, a subset of patients may progress over the first week to disordered healing and severe lung fibrosis. Nutritional support is crucial and should be instituted early in the course of ARDS. If the patient has not improved substantially after 10 to 14 days of mechanical ventilation, tracheostomy should be considered. Most studies indicate that approximately one-fourth of long-term ARDS survivors show no impairment at one year, one-fourth show moderate impairment, roughly half show only mild impairment, and a very small fraction show severe impairment.

For a more detailed discussion, see Chap. 33 in *Principles of Critical Care*, 2d ed.

Chapter 16

VENTILATOR-INDUCED LUNG INJURY

JOHN KRESS

The goals of mechanical ventilation (adequate tissue oxygenation and ventilation) have been traditionally met using tidal volumes in the range of 10 to 15 mL/kg, with variable levels of positive end-expiratory pressure (PEEP) and F_{IO_2}. There is now a large body of evidence that mechanical ventilation, particularly in the setting of lung disease, contributes to lung injury. "Normal" blood gases may come at the cost of ventilator-induced lung injury (VILI). Newer ventilation strategies have been developed in an attempt to reduce peak airway pressures and avoid overdistention and resultant VILI (Table 16-1).

Acute Respiratory Distress Syndrome

In ARDS, plain chest radiographs are frequently misleading, in that they suggest that the lung damage is uniformly distributed, whereas CT scans of the chest show heterogeneous regions of airspace disease neighbored by normal lung. Dependent lung regions show progressively more areas of decreased aeration and compressed alveoli. ARDS is also characterized by a decrease in lung compliance due to a loss of alveolar units. Therefore, in ARDS, there are alveoli with normal compliance next to fluid-filled alveoli with markedly decreased compliance. This functional dropout of alveoli has led to the notion that smaller tidal volumes—like those used in pediatric patients ("baby lungs")—may be appropriate for these patients. Traditional tidal volumes (10 to 15 mL/kg) are inappropriate and result in overdistention of lung units with relatively normal compliance, which may in itself lead to lung injury identical to that seen in ARDS.

189

TABLE 16-1 Goals of Mechanical Ventilation Modified
to Reduce the Risk of Ventilator-Induced Lung Injury

Oxygenation
  Maintain saturation > 90%
  Ensure adequate oxygen delivery
Avoid overdistention
  Plateau lung inflation < upper inflection point
  Limit plateau pressure to < 30–35 cmH$_2$O?
  Limit tidal volumes to 6–8 mL/kg?
Recruit alveoli
  Pressure preset ventilation waveform?
Keep alveoli patent
  End-expiratory volume > LIP
  Titrate end-expiratory volume to best lung compliance
  Keep PEEP above LIP (often ~15 cmH$_2$O)
Ventilation
  Permissive hypercapnia

Ventilator-Induced Lung Injury

MACROSCOPIC INJURY

Recent work has expanded our understanding of the scope
of VILI, which may be broadly classified into macroscopic
and microscopic injury (Table 16-2). Macroscopic injury consists of what has been classically described as barotrauma
(pneumothorax, pneumomediastinum, pneumoperitoneum,
and subcutaneous emphysema), leading to the presence of
extraalveolar air. During positive-pressure ventilation, alveolar rupture at the border of the alveolar base and bronchovascular sheath occurs. Air then dissects along the vascular sheaths toward the mediastinum, hilum, and
mediastinal soft tissues, with subsequent rupture of the mediastinal parietal pleura—a pneumothorax.

Macroscopic barotrauma correlates with a variety of factors. Retrospective studies have found peak airway pressure, level of PEEP, tidal volume, and minute ventilation to
correlate with the development of barotrauma, though a
subsequent prospective study found only the presence of
ARDS to be associated with the development of baro-

TABLE 16-2   The Scope of Ventilator-Induced Lung Injury

Ventilator-Induced Lung Injury
  Macroscopic
    Pneumothorax
    Pneumomediastinum
    Pneumopericardium
    Pneumoperitoneum
    Subcutaneous emphysema
    Parenchymal emphysema
    Cystic lung spaces
  Microscopic
    Lung edema
    Damage to alveolar-capillary barrier
    Surfactant dysfunction
    Hyaline membranes
    Histologic features of ARDS
    Cytokine release
    Fibrosis?

---

trauma. Patients with severe lung disease often require higher levels of PEEP to maintain oxygenation, so underlying lung disease, rather than PEEP per se, likely begets barotrauma. Gas trapping has also been associated with barotrauma.

MICROSCOPIC INJURY

Mechanical ventilation, even at modest airway pressures, is capable of producing functional impairment of the lung—with loss of integrity of the alveolar-capillary barrier, surfactant dysfunction, and parenchymal damage—that mimics the histologic appearance of ARDS.

With progressive lung inflation, a *decrease* in interstitial pressure and dilation of extra-alveolar vessels occurs. The net effect is an increase in the hydrostatic gradient for fluid to move from the capillaries into the interstitial space. Ventilation with high lung volumes may also cause a reduction in the integrity of the alveolar-capillary barrier, increasing its protein permeability. There appears to be a cumulative effect of mechanical ventilation with an increase in exposure to high airway pressures, resulting in progressive and eventually sustained lung injury.

High airway pressures themselves are not likely responsible for lung injury. Recently the emphasis has shifted away from pressure-induced injury (*baro*trauma) to lung overdistention (*volu*trauma). Peak inspiratory pressure (PIP) is a marker for the *degree* of lung inflation as opposed to the *cause* of lung injury per se. Transpulmonary pressure (alveolar pressure–pleural pressure) is a better indicator of the degree of lung inflation/overdistention. In addition to elastance, PIP incorporates a dynamic component—the drop in flow across the endotracheal tube and conducting airways. *Plateau* pressure (at end-inspiration after airway occlusion) more closely reflects alveolar pressure. Normally, transpulmonary pressures of 20 to 25 cmH$_2$O lead to full inspiration to TLC. Ventilation of patients with ARDS often leads to transpulmonary pressures > 20 to 25 cmH$_2$O. As a rule, plateau pressures > 30–35 cmH$_2$O overdistend normal alveoli in patients with ARDS and may propagate lung injury. The gradient between peak and plateau pressures in usually small (< 10 cmH$_2$O) in ARDS (but not always, so it should be measured). Heterogeneous lung injury with regional differences in lung compliance may lead to regional differences in lung inflation, making a "safe" plateau airway pressure difficult to identify.

Any ventilator mode strategy that adheres to the principles outlined above is acceptable. Pressure-control mode is particularly attractive because it assures an upper pressure limit. Also, the PIP is reached quickly and maintained throughout the rest of the inspiratory cycle, which may result in better alveolar recruitment and improved gas exchange and compliance. Other, more complex modes (volume-regulated pressure control, pressure-release ventilation) have been recommended by investigators, but currently there is no evidence to support the use of one specific mode of ventilation over another.

Pressure-Volume Curve in ARDS

The static pressure-volume (P-V) relationship of the lung in ARDS provides a conceptualization of changes that occur during ARDS and has helped develop strategies of mechanical ventilation to reduce lung injury (Fig. 16-1). The P-V curve in ARDS typically shows two points where the slope of the curve changes. The lower inflection point (LIP) corresponds to the transition from collapsed alveoli at low lung volumes to reexpanded ("recruited") alveoli. After the LIP, the slope of the P-V curve is relatively constant until a flattened portion of the curve is reached—the upper inflection point (UIP). Here, lung inflation approaches total lung capacity (TLC); continued inflation beyond this point risks overdistention of alveoli and lung injury.

There are several techniques for measuring static P-V curves in ARDS. One method is to gradually increase the tidal volume in 50- or 100-mL increments using constant flow and observing the plateau airway pressure generated. One can then graphically plot these points (Fig. 16-1). An abrupt increase in plateau airway pressure indicates that the upper inflection point has been reached and, to avoid barotrauma, no further measurements should be done. As previously mentioned, patients with ARDS have a decrease in aerated lung, and the upper inflection point often occurs at a lower tidal volume than in normal lungs.

At volumes and pressures below the LIP, partially aerated lung units may collapse at the end of a tidal breath, only to be reopened during the subsequent breath. Such cyclical opening and closing of alveoli may propagate lung injury. It is known to disrupt surfactant and is speculated to disrupt epithelial structures and contribute to failure of the alveolar-capillary barrier. Keeping PEEP slightly above the LIP may keep alveoli patent during the entire respiratory cycle, and this strategy has been shown to improve outcomes in patients with ARDS. In addition to a purely mechanical splint, PEEP may keep alveoli patent by preserving surfactant function (which has been observed to be functionally altered in ARDS), thereby reducing surface tension and the tendency of alveoli to close. If one chooses to set PEEP above the LIP, high levels (~15 cmH$_2$O) are often needed. One must simultaneously decrease tidal volumes (~6 to 8 mL/kg, sometimes lower), as PEEP is increased to keep ventilation along the steep portion of the P-V curve *below the UIP* where alveolar overdistention

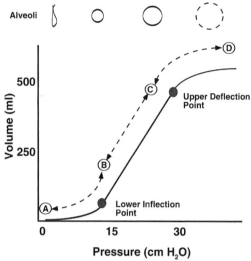

FIGURE 16-1   The sigmoidal shape of the pressure-volume curve of the respiratory system in a patient with ARDS. The relative state of inflation of alveoli is provided in the upper portion of the figure. At airway pressures above the upper inflection point C (30 cmH$_2$O), the curve flattens as the limits of lung compliance are reached and there is progressive overdistention of alveoli. Airway pressures below the lower inflection point B are also associated with lower compliance and result in alveolar collapse. A typical ventilation strategy using 15 cmH$_2$O PEEP and PIP of 40 cmH$_2$O (points B to D) would lead to repetitive inflation above the upper inflection point and potentially disrupt alveoli and the alveolar-capillary barrier (see text). A strategy that attempts to reduce lung distention by reducing PIP (points A to C) would still lead to repetitive opening and closure of alveoli (also associated with lung injury). An optimal ventilation strategy should consider both the lower inflection and upper inflection points of the pressure-volume cure (points B to C). Note also that for the same driving pressure (points A to B, B to C, C to D), a change in pressure from points B to C is associated with the largest change in lung volume. Thus an optimal ventilation strategy should aim for volume excursions along the steepest portion of the pressure-volume curve (maximal compliance).

TABLE 16-3   Goals of PEEP

Maximize oxygen delivery
  Optimize PEEP to cardiac output
  Increase oxygen content by reducing venous
    admixture
Maximize respiratory compliance
  Recruit alveoli
  Prevent derecruitment of alveoli
Minimize ventilator lung injury
  Maintain end-expiratory lung volume above lower inflection point

---

and barotrauma may occur (Table 16-3). Ventilation strategies discussed above may not pertain to patients with abnormalities in chest wall–abdominal compliance (e.g. burns, ascites), which confound P-V curve measurements. Under these circumstances, high airway pressures may not be reflective of alveolar overdistention but rather of chest wall stiffness.

TABLE 16-4   The Potential Consequences of Hypercapnea

Cardiovascular
  Decreased ventricular contractility
  Increased heart rate
  Decreased afterload
  Increased or no change in stroke volume/cardiac output
  Decreased responsiveness to catecholamines?
Pulmonary
  Increased pulmonary vascular resistance
  Bronchodilation
Decreased affinity of hemoglobin for oxygen
Central nervous system
  Increased cerebral blood flow
  Increased intracranial pressure
  Agitation
  Reduced level of consciousness
Renal
  Decreased renal blood flow
  Decreased filtration rate

PERMISSIVE HYPERCAPNIA

Strategies outlined above frequently lead to use of very small tidal volumes, with resulting hypercapnia—so called permissive hypercapnia. This does not represent a method of mechanical ventilation per se; rather it is the consequence of a strategy that limits lung volume excursions in an attempt to minimize alveolar overdistention and hence VILI. The physiologic consequences of hypercapnia and respiratory acidosis are summarized in Table 16-4.. The degree of acceptable respiratory acidosis is not clear, though most clinicians will accept a pH down to ~7.15. Studies of permissive hypercapnia in patients with ARDS have not observed clinically important side effects from an elevation of Pa_{CO_2}. At present, the only absolute contraindication is increased intracranial pressure.

For a more detailed discussion, see Chaps. 12 and 33 in *Principles of Critical Care*, 2d ed.

Chapter 17

ACUTE-ON-CHRONIC RESPIRATORY FAILURE

BRIAN GEHLBACH

Patients with chronic obstructive pulmonary disease (COPD) may deteriorate acutely following even minor insults. The acute deterioration of these patients is termed *acute-on-chronic respiratory failure* (ACRF).

Pathophysiology

Patients with COPD develop ventilatory failure from inspiratory muscle fatigue when respiratory system load exceeds neuromuscular competence. The work of breathing of patients with chronic stable disease may be up to five times that of normal persons. Balanced against this increased load is a disadvantaged neuromuscular apparatus. Insults in the form of either increased load or decreased strength may result in ACRF.

INCREASED LOAD

Both *resistive* and *elastic* loads contribute to the increased work of breathing in patients with stable COPD (Figs. 17-1 and 17-2). Resistive work is increased by airway inflammation, mucus, and bronchospasm. Elastic work is increased primarily by dynamic hyperinflation. Airway obstruction and decreased elastic recoil prolong expiration, so that the lung is not emptied before the ensuing inspiration. Consequently, alveolar pressure remains positive with respect to the mouth at end-expiration. This positive elastic recoil pressure, called intrinsic positive end-expiratory pressure (PEEPi), must be overcome by the inspiratory muscles before flow (the next breath) occurs. Further increments in load may overcome neuromuscular competence and provoke ventilatory failure.

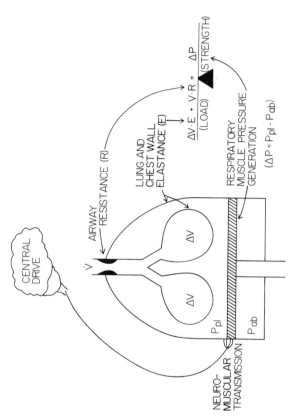

FIGURE 17-1   A drawing of the key elements of the respiratory system. The drive to breathe derives from CNS regulators of respiratory pattern. Neural afferents are the path for signals causing respiratory muscle contraction. Diaphragm contraction generates a pleural pressure (Ppl) and is opposed by any increased abdominal pressure (Pab). The Ppl generated must overcome the resistive (R) and elastic (E) forces acting on the respiratory system in producing a given minute ventilation (Ve). *(From Schmidt GA, Hall JB: Acute on chronic respiratory failure: Assessment and management of patients with COPD in the emergent setting. JAMA 261:3444, 1989.)*

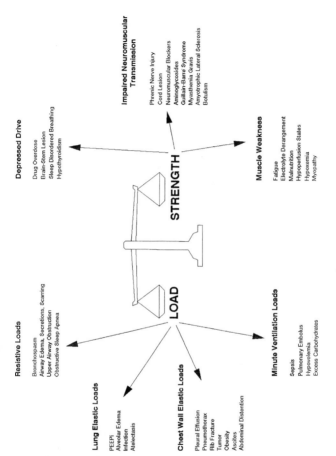

FIGURE 17-2   The balance between the load on the respiratory system and the strength of the system determines progression to and resolution of ACRF.

DECREASED NEUROMUSCULAR COMPETENCE

Dynamic hyperinflation places the inspiratory muscles in a mechanically disadvantageous position for force generation. Further decrements in strength may stem from protein-calorie malnutrition associated with COPD or from steroid myopathy. Additional causes of diminished neuromuscular competence are numerous and are shown in Fig. 17-2.

Treatment of ACRF

PHASE 1: BEFORE INTUBATION

The physician treating the patient with ACRF should forestall mechanical ventilation when this is possible yet recognize when progressive respiratory failure makes it inevitable. This discrimination requires an understanding of each patient's strength-load relationship and the reason(s) for the patient's decompensation. This may be achieved by asking three simple questions: (1) What is the patient's premorbid condition (i.e., how much reserve does he or she have)? (2) What caused the deterioration (increased load/decreased strength)? (3) Are these insults reversible, and how quickly? Contrast the middle-aged patient with stable, well-compensated COPD and congestive heart failure (CHF) who deteriorates acutely following volume overload with the elderly, malnourished one with an FEV_1 of 800 mL and multilobar pneumonia. The former patient has an identifiable precipitant with a rapidly effective treatment and is unlikely to require mechanical ventilation. The latter patient begins with more severe disease and less strength, suffering from a precipitant likely to respond less rapidly to therapy. Mechanical ventilation in this situation is a virtual certainty and should not be delayed while the patient continues to fatigue.

Oxygen should be given to all patients with COPD and hypoxemia. Many physicians still believe that patients with COPD rely on hypoxic drive to breathe and that administration of oxygen is liable to precipitate ventilatory failure. This is a myth. Several well-designed studies have convincingly shown that patients with ACRF nearly maintain alveolar ventilation despite treatment with 100% oxygen. A rise in P_{CO_2} does occur in these patients, but primarily as a consequence of $\dot{V}/\dot{Q}$ mismatch rather than hypoventilation. The risks of oxygen administration are small compared with those of untreated hypoxemia. The goal of oxygen therapy is to raise the hemoglobin saturation to 90% or greater. Since hypoxemia from COPD is generally caused by $\dot{V}/\dot{Q}$ mismatch, adequate saturation usually is achieved through the use of a nasal cannula or 35% face mask.

Bronchospasm may be treated by the administration of inhaled β agonists and anticholinergics (Table 17-1). Ipratropium bromide is the agent of choice for chronic stable COPD, and is as effective as β agonists in the treatment of acute exacerbations. β_2-selective agonists such as albuterol should be given in combination unless contraindicated (e.g., excessive tachycardia). Bronchodilators may be given by nebulization or, in the cooperative patient, by MDI.

Corticosteroids have been shown to improve spirometric values of patients with ACRF within the first day of administration. Beyond this, the role of steroids is uncertain. We administer methylprednisolone 0.5 mg/kg every 6 hours to patients with ACRF and reevaluate their role after several days.

Antibiotics have been administered to patients with ACRF with conflicting results. Since bronchitis is a common precipitant of ACRF, we administer an inexpensive broad-spectrum antibiotic (e.g., trimethoprim-sulfamethoxasole, ampicillin, etc.) to all patients with ACRF not explained by another cause.

Aminophylline and theophylline are mild bronchodilators in patients with COPD. Beneficial effects on the diaphragm—increased inotropy and resistance to fatigue—have also been observed in experimental settings. Also, addition of theophylline to a regimen of inhaled β agonists and ipratropium has been shown to be beneficial in patients with stable COPD. Nonetheless, the role of these agents in the treatment of ACRF is uncertain given the absence of benefit in controlled trials and the potential for arrhythmias. Aminophylline should be used in patients with a history of prior benefit or as a second-line agent when other therapies have failed. A loading dose of 5 mg/kg infused over 30 minutes is followed by a continuous infusion of 0.5 mg/kg per hour. Patients already on theophylline should have therapy guided by serum levels.

Noninvasive positive-pressure ventilation (NIPPV) is now preferred over invasive mechanical ventilation for selected patients with ACRF (see Chap. 14). A tight-fitting mask

TABLE 17-1　Bronchodilator Therapy in ACRF

β Agonists
  Albuterol or metaproterenol by MDI (three to six puffs every
  30–60 min)
  or
  Albuterol or metaproterenol by nebulizer (0.5 mL albuterol or
  0.3 mL metaproterenol in 2.5 mL normal saline solution every 2 h)
Ipratropium
  Three to ten puffs every 2–6 h by MDI
  Consider high doses (400 μg every 2–6 h) in intubated patients
Aminophylline
  Loading dose is 5 mg/kg
  Maintenance dose is approximately 0.5 mg/kg per hour
  Must be titrated against serum levels
Corticosteroids
  Methylprednisolone, 0.5–1 mg/kg every 6 h
  Assess ongoing need after 72 h

---

allows for variable amounts of inspiratory and expiratory pressure to be applied, either by a conventional ICU ventilator or a portable unit designed for this purpose. This therapy may unload the respiratory muscles (via inspiratory support) and overcome the effects of PEEPi (via expiratory support) without subjecting the patient to the potential complications of endotracheal intubation and mechanical ventilation (sinusitis, ventilator-associated pneumonia, tracheal stenosis, etc.). Also, readiness for spontaneous breathing may be more easily assessed, since failure does not require reintubation. Complications of NIPPV are infrequent; skin necrosis may occur at pressures greater than 20 cmH$_2$O and gastric distention and aspiration are possible. Endotracheal intubation and mechanical ventilation are preferred when one or more of the following is present: (1) shock or frequent arrhythmias; (2) severely decreased mental status, evolving airway edema, or another threat to airway patency; (3) preexisting gastric distention, ileus, or obstruction; or (4) craniofacial trauma.

When a patient is said not to tolerate NIPPV, the physician's approach may be to blame. Strapping a mask onto an already distressed and dyspneic patient and applying 10 to 15 cmH$_2$O pressure may only serve to *increase* patient discomfort. A better approach is to begin with low pressures (e.g., inspiratory positive pressure of 5 cmH$_2$O and expiratory positive pressure of 2.5 cmH$_2$O) and offer the mask to the patient, helping him or her to place it. The patient is then encouraged to take several breaths before the mask is removed. The mask is reoffered several times in this way, with simple verbal instruction. This allows patients to discover for themselves how the mask will aid breathing. The mask is then secured in place, with careful attention to the elimination of air leaks. The inspiratory and expiratory pressures are titrated upward in increments of 2.5 cmH$_2$O until a goal of 15/5 is reached or the patient appears more comfortable. (It is important to be aware of the difference in terminology between the settings on a NIPPV machine and those on a mechanical ventilator. NIPPV settings of 5 cmH$_2$O positive expiratory pressure and 15 cmH$_2$O positive inspiratory pressure are equivalent to 5 cmH$_2$O PEEP with 10 cmH$_2$O pressure-support on a ventilator.) Success of NIPPV is often apparent within 10 minutes of application and may be gauged by improvement in dyspnea and a decline in respiratory rate.

PHASE 2: FOLLOWING INTUBATION

The decision to intubate is a clinical one and requires a physician at the bedside. Predictors of frank ventilatory failure are listed in Table 17-2 and include persistent tachypnea despite NIPPV, mental status deterioration, and subjective exhaustion.

Two common problems occur immediately following intubation—life-threatening alkalemia and hypotension. Both occur as a consequence of excessive ventilation and thus are usually avoidable. Patients with ACRF usually have minute ventilations of 10 L/min or less, with tidal volumes of approximately 300 mL. It is common for patients to be ventilated in excess of this immediately following intubation. At the same time that ventilation is increased, production of CO$_2$ by respiratory muscles declines, often by as much as 20%. The resulting fall in P$_{CO_2}$ is often coupled with a preexisting compensatory metabolic alkalosis. A serum pH > 7.7 may result. Excessive ventilation also leads to dynamic hyperinflation with auto-PEEP. Venous return is impaired, and hypotension

TABLE 17-2   Assessment of the Need
for Intubation in ACRF

---

1. This judgment must be made by the physician at the bedside.
2. Predictors of frank respiratory failure:
   Respiratory rates which remain > 36/min despite NIPPV
   Worsening tachycardia
   Continued use of all accessory muscles
   Mental status deterioration
   Patient's subjective sense of exhaustion
3. Arterial blood-gas studies are of limited use in making this judgment, usually merely confirming clinical assessment.
4. Concomitant hemodynamic instability or inability to protect the airway mandate intubation.

---

may result. This process may be reversed by disconnecting the patient from the ventilator for 30 seconds and then resuming ventilation while efforts to reduce PEEPi as well as restore intravascular volume ensue.

Initial ventilator settings on assist-control mode should consist of tidal volumes of 5 to 7 mL/kg with respiratory rates of 20 to 24/min. PEEPi must be overcome by the patient before flow results and a breath is delivered. The resulting inspiratory load to the patient cannot be circumvented by lowering the triggering sensitivity. If PEEPi exists, external PEEP should be applied in a nearly equal amount (about 75% of the PEEPi value if this is known) to counterbalance this pressure and eliminate this inspiratory load. The occasional patient will respond to the application of external PEEP with additional hyperinflation, increasing the risk of hypotension and barotrauma.

The goal following intubation for respiratory failure is to restore a favorable strength-load relationship. Restoring strength may occur only through rest. Most patients are exhausted at the time of intubation and will require very little or no sedation as they sleep the following day. Between 48 and 72 hours are required for full recovery of respiratory muscle strength; attempts to restore spontaneous breathing before such time has elapsed are frequently counterproductive unless a clearly identifiable precipitant has been eliminated.

Causes of increased load should be identified and treated. Pulmonary embolism, congestive heart failure, infection, and bronchospasm are examples of common precipitants of ACRF. Similarly, contributors to decreased neuromuscular competence should be reviewed daily and addressed. Malnutrition is common in patients with COPD and should not be overlooked. Nutrition should be supported early; however, excessive refeeding should be avoided, as increased carbon dioxide production may unnecessarily load the respiratory system. This may be avoided in part by supplying 50% or more of the calories in the form of lipids to minimize the respiratory quotient.

Once the respiratory muscles have been rested adequately, a daily exercise program should begin. This may be achieved through any method that increases the demand on the patient—reducing the backup rate on intermittent mandatory ventilation (IMV), lowering the triggering sensitivity on assist-control, decreasing pressure support, or performing T-piece sprints. Decreasing the IMV rate seems least useful in speeding liberation from the ventilator (see Chap. 22). The patient should never be exercised to exhaustion and rest at night should be ensured.

All patients undergoing mechanical ventilation for ACRF should receive subcutaneous heparin for thromboembolism prophylaxis and antacids or sucralfate for prevention of gastrointestinal hemorrhage. Many physicians choose sucralfate over acid suppression therapies with the goal of reducing the risk of ventilator-associated pneumonia (VAP), although the evidence for this is controversial.

PHASE 3: LIBERATION FROM THE VENTILATOR

Successful liberation from the ventilator requires that strength exceed load. Once the contributors to increased load and/or decreased strength are identified and reversed, the ventilator is no longer necessary. The details of ventilator management are largely irrelevant once this stage is reached. Recent trials have confirmed this by demonstrating the superiority of frequent T-piece trials over other methods of diminishing ventilator support in leading to spontaneous breathing. This is probably because no other method so clearly conveys readiness for spontaneous breathing.

Determination of a patient's readiness for spontaneous breathing may be aided through the analysis of respiratory variables that attempt to quantify various components of strength and load. These variables (negative inspiratory force, peak pressure, static pressure, minute ventilation, PEEPi, and frequency:tidal volume ratio) should be assessed daily and are useful objective measures of therapeutic interventions. For example, if ventilatory failure was precipitated by the minute volume load associated with sepsis, a return of this variable to normal should predict successful liberation as long as no additional insults have occurred.

The transition to spontaneous breathing is likely to be smoother if ventilator settings that mimic the patient's own pattern of respiration are chosen [i.e., tidal volume (TV) 7 mL/kg with assist/control (AC) 18]. The patient with a more precarious strength-load relationship may be extubated to NIPPV, allowing a more gradual resumption of spontaneous breathing.

For a more detailed discussion, see Chap. 34 in *Principles of Critical Care*, 2d ed.

Chapter 18
STATUS ASTHMATICUS
THOMAS CORBRIDGE

Status asthmaticus (SA) is defined as asthma that is either sudden and severe at exacerbation onset or that is progressive over hours to days despite standard pharmacotherapy. Enhanced pharmacotherapy restores most of these patients, without complication, to a state of unlabored breathing. A small subset of patients fail enhanced pharmacotherapy and are intubated in hospital. Fortunately for these patients, the prognosis is quite good if lung hyperinflation is assessed and minimized as a part of the ventilation protocol—in stark contrast is the poor prognosis of patients who arrest out of hospital and present with anoxic brain injury.

The presence of SA speaks to failure of outpatient management, particularly in the subgroup of patients that depend on crisis-oriented management. These patients often reside in inner cities, have lower incomes, and are less knowledgeable about asthma. In an attempt to interrupt crisis-oriented care and decrease future risk of SA, the patient's outpatient regimen should be reviewed and optimized while he or she is in the acute care setting.

Pathophysiology of Acute Airflow Obstruction

Sudden asphyxic asthma is characterized by smooth muscle–mediated bronchospasm with airway submucosal neutrophilia (in contrast to the airway wall eosinophilia of chronic asthma) and fewer secretions. Triggers include medications (e.g., aspirin or β-blocker ingestion), allergens, ingestion of foods containing sulfites, and inhalation of illicit drugs (especially "crack" cocaine and heroin). Slowly progressive disease—which is triggered by a variety of infectious, allergic, and nonspecific irritant exposures—is characterized by bronchospasm, extensive airway wall inflammation, and mucous plugging. It is not surprising that patients who treat this disease with β agonists alone fail for lack of accelerated antiinflammatory therapy.

Expiratory airflow obstruction predisposes to incomplete emptying of alveolar gas and positive end-expiratory alveolar pressure (auto-PEEP). Inspiratory work of breathing is increased by airway narrowing, auto-PEEP (a pressure that must be overcome to establish inspiratory flow), and decreased static lung compliance due to lung hyperinflation. At the same time, diaphragmatic force generation is decreased by the mechanically disadvantageous position of the diaphragm in the hyperinflated chest and by adverse effects of hypoperfusion and respiratory acidosis. When the load is too great for the strength, ventilatory failure occurs.

Maldistribution of alveolar ventilation relative to perfusion produces low $\dot{V}/\dot{Q}$ units and hypoxemia. The degree of hypoxemia correlates with the severity of airway obstruction. However, hypoxemia (which is influenced more by peripheral airway obstruction) may occur sooner and/or resolve more slowly than airflow rates that predominantly reflect large airway function. Acute respiratory alkalosis often accompanies hypoxemia in early or mild disease. As the severity of airflow obstruction increases, Pa_{CO_2} increases because of inadequate minute ventilation and an increase in the ratio of dead space to tidal volume (V_D/V_T).

Circulatory effects of SA result from labored breathing in the setting of airway obstruction. During forced expiration, positive intrathoracic pressure decreases blood return to the right ventricle. Blood flow to the right ventricle increases as intrathoracic pressure falls during vigorous inspiration. Right ventricular filling shifts the intraventricular septum leftward and impedes left ventricular (LV) filling. Negative inspiratory pleural pressure also directly impairs LV emptying by increasing LV afterload. The net effect of these cyclic respiratory events is to accentuate the normal inspiratory fall in stroke volume and systolic blood pressure, a phenomenon termed *pulsus paradoxus* (PP).

Clinical Presentation and Differential Diagnosis

Features of severe SA include tachypnea, monosyllabic speech, tachycardia, hyperinflation, accessory muscle use, PP, upright posture, altered mental status, and diaphoresis. Wheeze is an unreliable marker of disease severity because the chest is silent in cases of extremely low airflow. Accessory muscle use and PP indicate severe airflow obstruction, but severe disease can occur in their absence.

The differential diagnosis of SA includes exacerbation of chronic obstructive pulmonary disease (COPD), upper airway obstruction, aspiration with or without foreign body, endotracheal or endobronchial stenosis, congestive heart failure with "cardiac asthma," and, rarely, pulmonary embolism. In most cases, the history and physical examination help to distinguish these disorders.

Assessment of Severity, Initial Testing, and Disposition

Physician estimates of airflow are inaccurate, giving credence to serial determinations of peak expiratory flow rate (PEFR). In severely dyspneic patients, however, we defer PEFR measurement because it rarely alters initial management and may worsen bronchospasm. In severe SA, PEFR is below 30 to 50% predicted or the patient's personal best (usually corresponding to a PEFR less than 120 L/min). Failure of therapy to improve PEFR after 30 minutes predicts a more severe course and need for hospitalization.

When PEFR is less than 120 L/min and there is an inadequate response to initial therapy, an arterial blood gas is useful. Early SA is characterized by mild hypoxemia and respiratory alkalosis. Hypercapnia indicates severe disease, but the absence of hypercapnia does not exclude impending respiratory failure. Hypercapnia alone is not an indication for intubation, because many hypercapneic patients respond adequately to drug therapy. Serial blood gases are not needed because most patients can be followed by close examination with attention to posture, speech, accessory muscle use, diaphoresis, and qualitative estimates of air movement and by serial peak flows. Patients who deteriorate by these measures should be considered for intubation irrespective of Pa_{CO_2}.

Metabolic acidosis with a normal anion gap occurs when patients waste serum bicarbonate in response to respiratory alkalosis. Metabolic acidosis with an elevated anion gap generally reflects excess lactate. Lactic acidosis is more common in men, in severely obstructed patients, and when parenteral β agonists are prescribed.

Chest radiographs are indicated in intubated patients and when there are lateralizing signs or concern regarding barotrauma. Unselected chest radiography rarely alters therapy.

Risk factors for fatal or near-fatal SA should be considered prior to patient disposition (Table 18-1). In general, patients who demonstrate a good response to initial therapy in the emergency department may be discharged home with close follow-up. These patients should demonstrate significant improvements in dyspnea and airflow and have a PEFR of $\geq 80\%$ predicted or personal best. Observation for 30 min

TABLE 18-1   Risk Factors for Fatal or Near Fatal SA

Late arrival for care
Sleep deprivation
Abnormal mental status
Frequent emergency department visits
Frequent hospitalization
Intensive care unit admission
Prior intubation
Hypercapnia
Barotrauma
Psychiatric illness
Medical noncompliance
Illicit drug abuse
Low socioeconomic status
Use of more than two canisters per month of inhaled β agonist
Difficulty perceiving airflow obstruction
Comorbidities such as coronary artery disease
Sensitivity to *Alternaria* species

after the last dose of β agonist helps ensure stability. Before discharge, patients should receive written medication instructions and a written plan of action. Most patients should be discharged on oral corticosteroids at a fixed dose (e.g., 40 mg daily) with instructions for close follow-up. Fixed-dose regimens are easier to understand and minimize the risk of premature taper. We initiate or accelerate inhaled corticosteroids depending on the situation in the emergency department.

Patients in severe exacerbation (PEFR < 50% predicted or personal best) who demonstrate a poor response to initial therapy (e.g., less than 10% increase in PEFR) or any patient who deteriorates despite therapy should be admitted to an intensive care unit. Intensive care unit admission is also indicated for patients in respiratory arrest, an altered mental status, and/or cardiac toxicity.

An incomplete response to treatment is defined as the persistence of symptoms and a PEFR between 50 and 80% predicted. Patients in this group require ongoing treatment either in the emergency room or in hospital. Admission is recommended when the home environment is of concern or directly observed therapy is needed in noncompliant patients.

Pharmacologic Therapy

OXYGEN

Low-flow oxygen should be prescribed to maintain arterial oxygen saturation > 90% (> 95% in pregnant women and in patients with coronary artery disease). Supplemental oxygen improves oxygen delivery to the respiratory muscles, reverses hypoxic pulmonary vasoconstriction, protects against β-agonist-induced pulmonary vasodilation and $\dot{V}/\dot{Q}$ mismatch, and may result in some airway bronchodilation.

β AGONISTS

Inhaled β-agonists are indicated for the immediate relief of bronchospasm. They should be prescribed in a repetitive or continuous manner until there is a convincing clinical

TABLE 18-2   Pharmacotherapy of Status Asthmaticus

Albuterol: 2.5 mg in 2.5 mL normal saline by nebulization every
   15–20 minutes or 4–6 puffs by MDI with spacer every 10–20 min;
   for intubated patients, titrate to physiologic effect and side effects.
Epinephrine: 0.3 mL of a 1:1000 solution subcutaneously every
   20 min × 3. Terbutaline is favored in pregnant patients when
   parenteral therapy is indicated. Use with caution in patients over
   age 40 and in patients with coronary artery disease.
Corticosteroids: Methylprednisolone 60 mg IV every 6 hours or
   prednisone 40 mg PO every 6 hours
Anticholinergics: Ipratropium bromide 0.5 mg by nebulization every
   1–4 h combined with albuterol concentrate or 4–10 puffs by MDI
   with spacer every 20 minutes.
Theophylline: 5 mg/kg IV over 30 min loading dose in patients not
   on theophylline followed by 0.4 mg/kg/h IV maintenance dose.
   Check serum level within 6 hours of loading dose. Watch for drug
   interactions and disease states that alter clearance.
Magnesium sulfate: 2 g IV over 20 minutes, repeat in 20 minutes
   (total dose 4 g unless hypomagnesemic).
Heliox: 80:20 or 70:30 helium:oxygen mix by tight-fitting,
   nonrebreathing face mask. Higher helium concentrations are
   needed for maximal effect.

---

response or side effects limit further administration (Table 18-2). Recent heavy use of β agonists should not preclude high-dose administration unless serious side effects are identified. Albuterol is slightly preferred over metaproterenol because of its greater β_2 selectivity. Long-acting β agonists are not indicated in the initial treatment of SA because of their slow onset of action.

Inhaled β agonists may be delivered equally well by a metered dose inhaler (MDI) with spacer or by a hand-held nebulizer. Anywhere from 4 to 12 puffs of albuterol by MDI with spacer achieves the same degree of bronchodilation as one nebulized treatment, even in severely obstructed patients. MDIs with spacers are cheaper and faster; hand-held nebulizers require fewer instructions, less supervision, and less coordination.

Subcutaneous epinephrine is no better than inhaled albuterol in the initial management of SA unless patients are unable to comply with inhaled therapy (e.g., in the arrest or impending arrest situation). Patients not responding adequately to inhaled therapy, however, may benefit from sub-cutaneous epinephrine. Parenteral therapy is relatively contraindicated in patients with cardiac disease and in those above age 40. Epinephrine should not be used in pregnant asthmatics because of its vasoconstrictive action on the utero-placental circulation. Intravenous infusions of β agonists should be avoided because they are more toxic and less efficacious than inhaled drug.

CORTICOSTEROIDS

Systemic corticosteroids by mouth or vein should be started quickly to treat airway wall inflammation and to upregulate β receptors. Oral administration should be avoided in the setting of dyspepsia or impending respiratory failure. The recommended dose of methylprednisolone is 60 mg IV every 6 hours; lower doses are less effective and higher doses have not been shown to be more so. Still, many clinicians prefer higher initial doses (e.g., 125 mg methylprednisolone IV q 6h) in steroid-dependent patients and in the setting of impending respiratory failure.

Improving patients can receive prednisone in doses ranging from 60 to 80 mg daily (in single or divided doses). This dose should be continued until the PEFR returns to baseline, after which prednisone may be stopped or tapered at various rates depending on durability of the clinical response, duration of high-dose therapy, and whether oral corticosteroids have been used as maintenance therapy. Inhaled steroids should be continued or restarted during oral corticosteroid taper.

IPRATROPIUM BROMIDE

Limited date support the use of ipratropium bromide in SA. This drug produces less bronchodilation at peak effect than β agonists and achieves a more variable clinical response. Despite its "second line" status in SA, ipratropium bromide is widely used because of its favorable side-effects profile. It can be administered by MDI with spacer (4 to 10 puffs every 20 minutes) or by nebulizer (0.5 mg per unit-dose vial every 1 to 4 hours combined with albuterol concentrate).

THEOPHYLLINE

Theophylline does not add to maximal doses of β agonists in the first few hours of treatment but does increase the incidence of tremor, nausea, anxiety, and tachyarrhythmias. However, emergency department use of theophylline may decrease risk of hospitalization—even in the absence of improved airflow, raising the possibility that theophylline acts in ways distinct from bronchodilation (e.g., through anti-inflammatory properties or effects on respiratory muscle function). Furthermore, negative short-term studies do not rule out a delayed benefit from the early use of theophylline. Our approach is to use theophylline when there is a poor response to β agonists and corticosteroids. The loading dose of theophylline is 5 mg/kg (6 mg/kg aminophylline) by peripheral vein over 30 minutes followed by a continuous infusion of 0.4 mg/kg per hour (0.5 mg/kg per hour aminophylline). In patients taking theophylline, serum levels should be checked before additional theophylline is given. If the level is therapeutic, a continuous infusion may be started or the oral preparation may be continued. Serum levels should be checked within 6 hours of intravenous loading to avoid toxic levels and guide further dosing. We aim for levels between 8 and 12 μg/mL to avoid toxicity. Attention should be paid to the multiple factors that increase serum levels.

MAGNESIUM SULFATE

Prospective trials have failed to confirm the efficacy of magnesium sulfate in SA except in the subgroup of patients presenting with a $FEV_1 < 25\%$ of predicted. Additional data are needed before magnesium sulfate can be recommended for routine use in severe SA. Side effects from the usual dose of 2 g IV over 20 minutes are trivial.

HELIOX

Heliox is a gas consisting of 20% oxygen and 80% helium (30:70% mixtures are also available) that has a greater kinematic viscosity (the ratio of gas viscosity to gas density) than air. This property decreases the driving pressure required for gas flow, particularly in the setting of upper airway obstruction. In SA, limited data demonstrate that heliox delivered by a tight-fitting, nonrebreathing face mask improves airway resistance and decreases work of breathing, thereby possibly "buying time" for concurrent pharmacologic therapy to take hold. Heliox reduces airway resistance in intubated patients but is rarely necessary during mechanical ventilation and requires substantial institutional expertise for safe use.

ANTIBIOTICS

Prospective evaluation of asthmatics admitted to hospital has not demonstrated a benefit from routine antibiotic use. Sputum that looks purulent typically contains an abundance of eosinophils and not polymorphonuclear leukocytes. Antibiotics should be reserved for patients with concurrent sinusitis or when mycoplasmal or chlamydial infection is suspected.

Mechanical Ventilation

Limited observational data suggest noninvasive positive-pressure ventilation (NPPV) is useful in patients with SA who are not in need of immediate intubation. NPPV appears to improve gas exchange and decrease dyspnea, heart rate, and respiratory rate by decreasing inspiratory work of breathing. Recommended settings are $0 \, cmH_2O$ CPAP and $10 \, cmH_2O$ pressure support, with subsequent titration of CPAP to 3 to $5 \, cmH_2O$ and pressure support as necessary to achieve an exhaled tidal volume of $7 \, mL/kg$ and a respiratory rate $< 25/min$.

Intubation is indicated for patients who are apneic, somnolent, or in impending respiratory failure. Progressive hypercapnia and exhaustion also indicate the need for intubation. Oral intubation is preferred because it allows for a larger endotracheal tube—important to decrease airway resistance and remove excess mucus. Nasal intubation mandates a smaller tube and increases the risk of sinusitis.

Sedation can be achieved with either a benzodiazepine or propofol combined with an opioid in low dose (Table 18-3). When sedation alone is unable to achieve patient-ventilator

TABLE 18-3   Sedatives in Status Asthmaticus

Agent	Dose	Cautions
	Peri-intubation period	
Midazolam	1 mg IV slow push	Hypotension
	Repeat every 2–3 min	Respiratory
	as needed	depression
Propofol	60–80 mg/min IV initial	Respiratory
	infusion up to 2.0 mg/kg	depression
	Sedation for Protracted Mechanical Ventilation	
Lorazepam	1–5 mg/h IV continuous	Drug
	infusion or IV bolus prn	accumulation
Propofol	1–5 mg/kg/h IV	Seizures
		Hyperlipidemia
Morphine Sulfate	1–5 mg/h IV continous	Ileus
	infusion; avoid bolus	

synchrony, neuromuscular blockade with *cis*-atracurium or vecuronium should be considered. The use of a nerve stimulator or intermittent interruption of a continuous infusion avoids drug accumulation. In all cases, paralytic agents should be restricted to aggressively sedated patients and discontinued as soon as possible to decrease the risk of acute paralytic-steroid-induced myopathy.

During mechanical ventilation, expiratory time (T_E) must be prolonged to allow for adequate gas emptying. High respiratory rates shorten T_E and may result in life-threatening lung hyperinflation, with hemodynamic sequelae of hypotension and tachycardia. When this occurs, the lung may be acutely deflated by a trial of hypoventilation (2 to 3 breaths per minute). If hemodynamic stability is not quickly restored, tension pneumothorax should be considered. A respiratory rate between 11 and 14 breaths per minute with a tidal volume between 7 and 8 mL/kg is unlikely to result in life-threatening hyperinflation (assuming an adequate inspiratory flow rate) (see Fig. 18-1 and Table 18-4). The degree of lung hyperinflation may be assessed by quantifying the total volume of gas exhaled from full inflation or, more practically, by measuring end-inspiratory plateau pressure (Pplat), or auto-PEEP. Pplat is an estimate of the average end-inspiratory alveolar pressure, determined by stopping flow at end-inspiration. During this maneuver, airway opening pressure falls from peak to plateau as inspiratory resistive pressure falls to zero. Extensive experience, but limited data, suggest that complications of lung hyperinflation are rare when Pplat is $< 30\ cmH_2O$. Auto-PEEP is the lowest average alveolar pressure achieved during the respiratory cycle. During an end-expiratory hold maneuver, equilibration of airway opening pressure with alveolar pressure generally occurs, permitting measurement of auto-PEEP. The presence of expiratory gas flow at the beginning of inspiration also demonstrates the presence of auto-PEEP. In general, auto-PEEP $< 15\ cmH_2O$ is safe; however, low levels of auto-PEEP have been reported in severely hyperinflated patients, suggesting the presence of noncommunicating gas. Low levels of ventilator-applied PEEP (e.g., $5\ cmH_2O$) decrease inspiratory work of breathing in patients triggering the ventilator without adding to lung inflation.

This low minute ventilation strategy often results in hypercapnia. Fortunately, hypercapnia is well tolerated as long as Pa_{CO_2} does not exceed 90 mmHg and acute changes are avoided. Ensuing acidemia is similarly well tolerated, raising the unanswered question as to whether buffer therapy is required in severely acidemic patients. Permissive hypercapnia should be avoided in patients with raised intracranial pressure (as might occur in the setting of an arrest with anoxic brain injury) and in those with severe myocardial dysfunction.

High inspiratory flow rates with a square inspiratory flow waveform are associated with a high inspiratory resistive and peak pressure (Ppk). Recent data, however, do not show a relationship between Ppk and complications of mechanical ventilation. The reason may be that Ppk does not predict alveolar pressure or the degree of lung hyperinflation. We currently accept high peak pressures for the greater good of reducing lung inflation.

Bronchodilators can be administered effectively to intubated patients using either a MDI with spacer or a nebulizer. Higher drug dosages are required and should be titrated upward until a convincing bronchodilator response is seen by a fall in the peak-to-pause airway pressure gradient or side

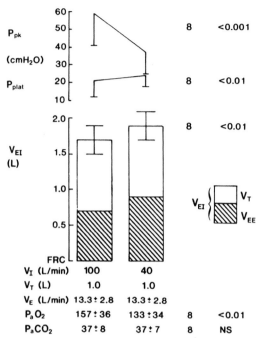

FIGURE 18-1   Effects of ventilator settings on airway pressures and lung volumes during normocapneic ventilation of eight paralyzed asthmatic patients. V_{EE}=lung volume at end-expiration; V_{EI}=lung volume at end-inspiration; Ppk=peak airway pressure; Pplat=end-inspiratory plateau pressure; V_E=minute ventilation; V_I=inspiratory flow. **A.** As inspiratory flow is decreased from 100 L/min to 40 L/min at the same V_E, Ppk falls, but hyperinflation increases due to dynamic gas trapping. **B.** Dynamic hyperinflation is reduced by low respiratory rates and high tidal volumes (as long as V_E is decreased), but high tidal volumes result in high Pplat. (Reproduced with permission from Tuxen DV, Lane S: The effects of ventilatory pattern on hyperinflation, airway pressures, and circulation in mechanical ventilation of patients with severe air-flow obstruction. *Am Rev Respir Dis* 136:872, 1987.

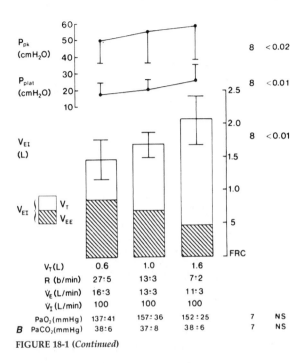

FIGURE 18-1 (Continued)

effects occur. If a nebulizer is used, it should be placed close to the ventilator. In-line humidifiers should be stopped and inspiratory flow should be temporarily reduced to 40 L/min to minimize turbulence. The MDI is effective only if combined

TABLE 18-4   Initial Ventilator Settings in SA

F_{IO_2}	1.0
Vt	7–8 mL/kg
RR	11–14/min
PEEP	0–5 cmH$_2$O
Vi	80 L/min
Wave form	Square
Mode	SIMV

with a spacer placed on the inspiratory limb of the ventilator. Patient-ventilator synchrony is crucial to optimize drug delivery.

Patients with labile asthma may respond to therapy within hours. Others require prolonged pharmacotherapy before there is a convincing fall in airway pressure. Once this occurs and Pa_{CO_2} normalizes, sedatives should be held in anticipation of extubation. If pneumonia, central nervous system injury, or muscle weakness have not complicated the patient's course, we favor a quick return to spontaneous breathing and extubation to prevent complications of mechanical ventilation. After extubation, close observation in the ICU is recommended for an additional 12 to 24 hours, during which the focus can switch to safe transfer to the medical ward and outpatient management.

For a more detailed discussion, see Chap. 35 in *Principles of Critical Care,* 2d ed.

Chapter 19

NEUROMUSCULAR DISEASES LEADING TO RESPIRATORY FAILURE

IKEADI MAURICE NDUKWU

MANAGEMENT IN THE INTENSIVE CARE UNIT (ICU)

The general management of patients with neuromuscular disease may be divided into five overlapping areas: diagnosis and treatment of the specific neuromuscular disease, diagnosis of precipitating factors prompting admission, evaluation of the need for respiratory support, provision of such support on an acute basis, and consideration of chronic support when required.

Precipitating Factors

The identification of precipitating factors is essential, because they may be more amenable to therapy than the neuromuscular disease itself. Upper airway obstruction and aspiration should be suspected in patients with bulbar involvement. Pulmonary hypertension and right-sided heart failure should be anticipated in chronically hypoxemic patients, including those whose muscle weakness is compounded by kyphoscoliosis.

Evaluation of the Need for Respiratory Support

The finding of severe hypoxemia, hypercapnia, and acidemia on arterial blood gas analysis is perhaps the most compelling indication for such support; but by the time blood gas abnormalities occur, respiratory failure is already profound. Respiratory failure is suggested by a rapid, shallow breathing pattern and by the presence of abdominal paradox. Patients with neuromuscular disease should be observed during sleep for signs of upper rib cage paradox and upper airway obstruction. Respiratory muscle dysfunction may be documented by having a patient exhale forcefully or cough.

Determination of maximum inspiratory and expiratory pressures (PI_{max} and PE_{max}) is the most sensitive way to quantitate respiratory muscle weakness. These pressures should be measured while the patient is breathing with maximum effort against mouthpiece systems that are occluded at residual volume (RV) and total lung capacity (TLC), respectively. The PE_{max} averages approximately 100 cmH$_2$O in normal adults, whereas a pressure of less than 40 cmH$_2$O precludes effective coughing (Table 19-1).

Vital capacity (VC) may be measured by spirometry, and RV and TLC by pulmonary function testing. The VC averages approximately 50 mL/kg in normal adults; impaired secretion clearance occurs at a VC of less than 30 mL/kg, and ventilatory failure occurs at a VC of around 10 mL/kg (Table 19-1).

TABLE 19-1   Respiratory Compromise
due to Neuromuscular Diseases Causing Weakness

Finding	Compromise
Maximum pressures	
Maximum expiratory pressure < 40 cmH$_2$O	Inability to cough and clear secretions
Maximum inspiratory pressure < −20 cmH$_2$O	Inability to ventilate adequately
Vital capacity	
< 30 mL/kg	Inability to cough adequately
< 20 mL/kg	Inability to sigh or prevent atelectasis
< 10 mL/kg	Inability to ventilate adequately
Bulbar weakness or paralysis	Inability to protect airway and avoid aspiration
Arterial blood gases	
Hypercapnia	Inability to ventilate adequately
Hypoxemia	Inability to oxygenate adequately

Providing Respiratory Support

Noninvasive mechanical ventilation or mechanical ventilation delivered via an endotracheal tube or tracheostomy is usually needed if lung volumes and muscle strength have declined to the levels indicated in Table 19-1 and is necessary if hypercapnia is acute and severe. Tracheostomy is indicated for any patient who requires intubation for more than a few weeks. Atelectasis can be prevented or treated with frequent sighs or moderate to high tidal volumes.

Patients with neuromuscular disorders require scrupulous nursing care to avoid nerve compression (especially involving the ulnar and peroneal nerves) and bedsores. They should be turned frequently and may benefit from insulating pads or kinetic beds. Foot boards and wrist splints should be provided; physical therapy may prevent disuse (but not denervation) atrophy and improve patient morale. Nutrition should be provided by the enteral route whenever possible and oral feedings may be used for tracheostomized patients who can swallow. Nasointestinal feedings are desirable for patients who cannot swallow but are likely to regain neuromuscular function, whereas feeding jejunostomies may be more appropriate for those who are permanently weak or paralyzed. Low-dose subcutaneous heparin or pneumatic leg compression devices are indicated to prevent deep venous thrombosis and pulmonary embolism.

Patients receiving mechanical respiratory assistance on an acute basis also require emotional support. These patients frequently regress psychologically—sometimes because of central nervous system involvement by their disease but more commonly because of their complete dependence on the people caring for them.

Consideration of Chronic Support

Some patients who accept chronic support and whose phrenic nuclei are damaged but whose nerves and hemidiaphragms are intact may be candidates for electrophrenic ventilation, in which the nerves are repetitively stimulated in the lower neck or upper thorax. Others who maintain near-normal arterial blood gas measurements only while awake may be ventilated during sleep with rocking beds, chest cuirasses, and other intermittent negative-pressure devices or by intermittent positive pressure delivered through the mouth or nose or via a tracheostomy. Most patients with severe chronic neuromuscular disease must receive negative- or positive-pressure ventilation around the clock. Chronic home ventilation of this sort is effective, although it requires attendant care and is expensive. It is ethically permissible to withhold or withdraw life support from these patients if they or their surrogates so desire.

Disorders of Upper Motor Neurons

Neuromuscular dysfunction can involve any or all of the components of normal neuromuscular function (Table 19-2). Damage to the upper motor neurons extending from the motor cortex to synapse with lower motor neurons in the brainstem or spinal cord characteristically causes unilateral weakness. Lesions above the corticospinal tract decussation in the medulla produce contralateral weakness or paralysis, whereas those below the medulla produce ipsilateral weakness below the level of involvement if only one side of the spinal cord is damaged; most spinal cord lesions cause bilateral weakness because of the close proximity of the tracts.

Hemiplegia is the contralateral upper and lower extremities weakness caused by cerebral infarction involving the motor cortex. Hemiplegia may be associated with sensory changes if the infarction involves the neighboring sensory cortex, decreased chest wall motion on the side of extremity weakness, and elevated hemidiaphragm on the affected side. Therefore there is reduced activity during voluntary inspirations in both the parasternal intercostal muscles and the hemidiaphragm on electromyography (EMG), leading to limited regional lung ventilation and causing hypoxemia, especially when the patient lies in a lateral position.

Quadriplegia may result from acute cervical spinal cord trauma, spinal artery infarction, or cord compression by tumor. Severe damage at or above cord segments C3 to C5 involves the phrenic nerves and causes partial or complete bilateral hemidiaphragmatic paralysis. Sternocleidomastoid, scalene, and trapezoid activity persists in high spinal cord injuries, but contraction of these muscles causes an increase primarily in the anteroposterior dimensions of the upper rib cage and pulls the hemidiaphragms toward the head. Abdominal paradox (Pab), in which the abdominal wall is sucked in by the negative abdominal pressure as the hemidiaphragms ascend, is a sign of hemidiaphragmatic dysfunction in patients who inspire only with their accessory muscles. The ventilatory consequences of high cervical quadriplegia include inability to generate an adequate tidal volume, leading to hypercapnia, and low arterial oxygenation. The hypoxemia results from both hypoventilation and microatelectasis.

Lower cervical spinal cord lesions spare the phrenic nerves, but the intercostal muscle activity necessary to stabilize the rib cage, so that the hemidiaphragms can function properly, is lost. Hemidiaphragmatic contraction therefore results in paradoxical inward motion of the upper and middle rib cage during inspiration, until the chest wall stiffens due to spasticity or fibrosis of muscles. VC and total lung TLC are reduced and are worse in the upright position. The combination of expiratory and inspiratory weakness prevents these patients from coughing and clearing secretions, putting them at an increased risk for respiratory tract infection.

Disorders of Lower Motor Neurons

Lower motor neuron dysfunction is characterized by weakness, loss of deep tendon reflexes, and denervation atrophy of muscles whose motor neurons are destroyed. Diseases of the anterior horn cells also cause fasciculations, in which irritability of the motor neurons leads to sporadic discharges of the muscle fibers under their control. Motor nerve root lesions resulting from herniated disks cause a myotonic distribution of weakness; because these lesions are not selective for anterior roots, they are usually accompanied by pain and sensory loss.

POLIOMYELITIS

Poliomyelitis is an acute febrile illness that may produce signs of meningeal irritation and flaccid paralysis. The disease is caused by a ribonucleic acid virus that spreads from person

TABLE 19-2 Disorders of Neuromuscular Function

Level	Examples	Clinical Characteristics	Cerebrospinal Fluid	Nerve Conduction	Electromyography
Upper motor neurons	Hemiplegia Quadriplegia	Weakness Spasticity Hyperreflexia Many have sensory and autonomic changes	Normal	Normal	Normal
Lower motor neurons	Paralytic poliomyelitis Amyotrophic lateral sclerosis	Weakness Atrophy Flaccidity Hyporeflexia Fasciculations Bulbar involvement No sensory changes	Little or no inflammation	Normal	Denervation potentials
Peripheral neurons	Guillian-Barré syndrome Diphtheria Critical illness polyneuropathy	Weakness Flaccidity Hyporeflexia Bulbar involvement Sensory and autonomic changes	Increased protein	Reduced	Denervation potentials late in course

| Myoneural junction | Myasthenia gravis
Botulism
Eaton-Lambert syndrome
Organophosphate poisoning
Tick paralysis | Fluctuating weakness
Fatigability
Normal reflexes
Bulbar involvement (esp. eyes)
No sensory changes
May have autonomic changes
May respond to cholinergic agents | Normal | Normal | Changes in muscle action potential during repetitive stimulation |
| Muscles | Muscular dystrophies
Polymyositis
Trichinosis
Endocrinologic disease | Weakness
Normal reflexes
No sensory or autonomic changes
May have pain | Normal | Normal | Small motor units |

to person via fecal-oral transmission and infects motor neurons in the spinal cord and brainstem. Paralysis may develop within hours of acute infection or may take an indolent course. Muscle weakness is usually asymmetrical, may be widely distributed, and tends to involve the lower extremities and lower trunk. Patients with upper cord and brainstem lesions usually lose diaphragmatic function. Bulbar poliomyelitis may also cause paralysis of the muscles involved in swallowing and speech. Weakness of the laryngeal muscles may precipitate upper airway obstruction, and aspiration may occur if the gag reflex is lost. Therapy is supportive. The prognosis is excellent except in the elderly and those with the bulbar form of the disease. Most recover some or all motor function except in areas of total paralysis.

AMYOTROPHIC LATERAL SCLEROSIS

Amyotrophic lateral sclerosis (ALS) is the most common lower motor neuron disorder in industrialized countries. The etiology is unknown. Patients may present with progressive muscle weakness and wasting that often involves the distal muscles initially. Although the extraocular muscles are spared in ALS, bulbar involvement may lead to impairment of the gag reflex, lingual atrophy and fasciculations, and laryngeal dysfunction. The coexistence of upper and lower motor signs should strongly suggest the diagnosis. No specific therapy is available for ALS, and more than 50% of patients die from complications such as aspiration and pneumonia within 3 years of diagnosis. Severe hypercapnia and hypoxemia can be corrected only by mechanical ventilatory support.

Disorders of Peripheral Nerves

Damage to the peripheral nervous system results in a variable combination of muscle weakness, sensory change, autonomic dysfunction, and reflex loss.

GUILLAIN-BARRÉ SYNDROME

Guillain-Barré syndrome (GBS; acute postinfectious polyneuropathy) is characterized by a widespread, patchy, inflammatory demyelination of the peripheral and autonomic nervous systems that is thought to result from a hypersensitivity reaction. The predisposing factors include antecedent upper respiratory infection or gastrointestinal illness within 1 month of onset, surgery, pregnancy, malignancy, and acute seroconversion to the human immunodeficiency virus. Characteristic features include progressive, usually symmetrical weakness that often includes facial and bulbar paresis and external ophthalmoplegia. This is accompanied by areflexia; mild sensory changes, such as distal paresthesias; and autonomic abnormalities, such as tachycardia, arrhythmias, and postural hypotension.

While not all patients with GBS develop respiratory failure, all should have vital capacity (VC) and respiratory muscle strength measured daily. Patients with decreasing respiratory reserve should be moved to the intensive care unit (ICU) before hypercapnea supervenes. Patients should be intubated and ventilated electively when signs of respiratory distress are present and before the Pa_{CO_2} rises or VC falls below 10 mL/kg. Plasmapheresis reduces hospital stay and the time spent on the ventilator if it is given to patients who do not improve or who worsen within the first 7 days. Corticosteroids are of no proven value in treating GBS. Recovery usually begins within 2 to 4 weeks after progression ceases. Although most patients eventually recover complete motor function, approximately 15% remain significantly handicapped by weakness.

CRITICAL ILLNESS POLYNEUROPATHY

Critical illness polyneuropathy is defined as a predominantly motor axonal polyneuropathy whose features are flaccid quadriparesis, respiratory muscle weakness, hyporeflexia, muscle atrophy, and distal sensory disturbances. It most often occurs in patients with sepsis and multiple organ failure who are difficult to wean from prolonged mechanical ventilation. The EMG shows predominantly axonopathic features of fibrillations and sharp positive waves on concentric needle studies as well as diminished amplitudes of muscle or nerve action potentials after stimulation. Histologic studies reveal primary axonal degeneration of motor and sensory fibers. Patients with critical illness polyneuropathy have a high mortality in the ICU relating to their underlying disorders. Over 50% of patients who survive show complete recovery, but some remain weak for years. Conduction slowing on repeat EMG studies suggest a particularly poor prognosis. No treatment exists for this condition other than supportive care.

Disorders of the Myoneural Junction

Disorders of the muoneural junction are caused by abnormalities of acetylcholine release or reception. They are characterized by fluctuating weakness and fatigability that is particularly striking in the extraocular muscles, the eyelid levators, and other muscles of the head and neck, but is not associated with sensory loss, altered reflexes, profound muscle atrophy, or the EMG findings of upper or lower motor neuron disease. The EMG reveals changes in muscle action potential during repetitive stimulation that can often be altered by drugs affecting ACh activity.

MYASTHENIA GRAVIS

Myasthenia gravis results from circulating antibodies directed against ACh receptors in the myoneural junction. Cell-mediated immunity, involving sensitized lymphocytes and the thymus gland, is also involved. The result is that potential interactions between ACh and receptor molecules are reduced, causing weakness and fatigability superficially resembling those seen in poisoning by botulinum toxin.

The most common presenting symptom is weakness of the eye muscles, manifest by diplopia or ptosis. Dysarthria and dysphagia are also common, as is proximal weakness of the upper and lower extremities. Myasthenia gravis may be precipitated or exacerbated by infection, surgical stress, or the administration of an aminoglycoside, neuromuscular blocking agents, or cholinergic agents. Myasthenia can be diagnosed on clinical grounds, and by giving short-acting acetylcholinesterase-inhibiting agents that increase the interaction between ACh and its receptors. Transiently increased strength should be achieved within seconds following the intravenous injection of edrophonium (Tensilon). Antibodies to the ACh receptor can also be detected in 90% of patients with unequivocal generalized myasthenia gravis. A rapid decline in muscle action potentials on repetitive stimulation is seen on the EMG.

Myasthenia is treated on a chronic basis with relatively long-acting anticholinesterase agents, such as pyridostigmine (Mestinon), at a dosage that improves muscle weakness with a minimum of cholinergic side effects. Plasmapheresis, which presumably removes antireceptor antibodies, may improve motor function for longer periods. Thymectomy leads to complete remission or substantial improvement in about 85% of patients. Corticosteroids and other immunosuppressive agents are routinely given to patients with generalized disease. Approximately 10% of patients with generalized disease will require mechanical ventilation.

BOTULISM

Botulism is caused by a sporulating, gram-positive anaerobic bacterium, *Clostridium botulinum.* Ubiquitous in nature, this organism produces potent neurotoxins, designated A through G, that bind irreversibly to the presynaptic terminal and inhibit ACh release. Botulism occurs in three forms: food-borne botulism, in which preformed toxin is ingested in nonacidic home-canned or factory-canned vegetables or meat; infant botulism, in which the organism and its spores are ingested in honey, other foods, or from the environment; and wound botulism, in which *C. botulinum* and its spores contaminate traumatic or surgical wounds.

Neuromuscular symptoms follow exposure to *C. botulinum* neutotoxin within 2 to 24 hours. The bulbar musculature is affected first, with resultant diplopia and dysphagia. Ptosis, extraocular muscle weakness, and diminution of the gag reflex are also common. Because the neurotoxin also involves the autonomic nervous system, gastrointestinal symptoms such as nausea, vomiting, and ileus may also occur, and the pupils may be dilated. Mentation remains normal, and there is no fever. Severe respiratory muscle involvement is paralleled by decreases in VC and TLC and an increase in RV, reflected in hypercapnia, hypoxemia, and the need for mechanical ventilation.

Diagnosis is confirmed by the detection of the neurotoxin in serum, stool, or contaminated food. Botulism can be distinguished from myasthenia gravis through EMG, which shows small evoked muscle action potentials that increase in amplitude after repetitive stimulation.

Botulism therapy involves elimination of unabsorbed neurotoxin from the gut by means of enemas and gastric lavage; administration of trivalent antitoxin (against neurotoxins A, B, and E) to neutralize circulating neurotoxin in the serum; administration of high-dose penicillin (3 million units intravenously every 4 hours) to kill *C. botulinum* organisms, and surgical debridment of offending wounds. Only about one-third of patients with botulism have respiratory failure severe enough to require mechanical ventilation, although aspiration is common.

Disorders of Muscles

Myopathies may be genetic (e.g., the various muscular dystrophies), inflammatory (e.g., polymyositis), metabolic (e.g., glycogen storage diseases, such as acid maltase deficiency), or endocrinologic (e.g., hypo- and hyperthyroidism). Myopathic processes commonly involve the shoulder and pelvic girdles in a symmetrical fashion. Sensory loss does not occur with the myopathies, reflex changes are minimal, muscle wasting is uncommon, and pseudohypertrophy may occur early in the course of certain dystrophies. Pain may be prominent, as may an increase in the serum concentration of creatine phosphokinase (CPK) and other muscle enzymes. Nerve conduction studies are normal. A predominance of small motor units is seen on EMG.

POSTPARALYTIC MYOPATHY

Recent years have seen the increasing recognition of a syndrome of muscle weakness following mechanical ventilation, usually for status asthmaticus. The clinical presentation varies from mild weakness to severe flaccid paralysis requiring continued mechanical ventilation. The pathogenesis of postparalytic myopathy is unknown. There is a clear association with the use of neuromuscular blocking drugs and corticosteroids. Early on it was speculated that the steroidal nucleus of vecuronium and pancuronium was important in combining with high-dose corticosteroids to produce myopathy, but it is now recognized that atracurium (a nonsteroidal paralytic agent) does not prevent or reduce the incidence of the syndrome. The likelihood of suffering this complication is related to the duration of paralysis. Many units have reduced the use of paralytic agents in light of the frequent occurrence of post-paralytic myopathy. When paralytic agents are given, it is advisable to use a nerve stimulator to ensure that the minimum dose necessary for paralysis is not exceeded; however, this approach has not been shown to reduce the incidence of the syndrome. There is no known treatment.

MUSCULAR DYSTROPHIES

Muscular dystrophies have three characteristics: hereditary transmission, progressive weakness, and biopsy evidence of muscle degeneration without evidence of stored material or structural abnormality. The Duchenne type is the best known and is associated with an X-chromosomal deficiency of the protein dystrophin, which produces progressive proximal weakness starting in childhood. This is paralleled by expiratory muscle weakness that limits cough and later by inspiratory weakness that reduces RV and TLC.

Eventually patients become unable to walk and develop muscle contractures and kyphoscoliosis. These thoracic cage abnormalities then combine with respiratory muscle weakness to cause severe respiratory failure. Respiratory tract infections become progressively more frequent, and most patients die in the third decade.

Duchenne dystrophy is transmitted as a sex-linked recessive trait, but in one-third of cases, spontaneous mutations arise. There is no specific treatment beyond the possible use of corticosteroids, which increase muscle strength but do not reduce wheelchair requirements. The question of whether to provide chronic ventilatory support for patients with advanced illness raises great ethical difficulties, although non-invasive intermittent positive-pressure ventilation has been shown to stabilize pulmonary function and prolong the lives of patients with Duchenne dystrophy.

For a more detailed discussion, see Chaps. 30 and 36 in *Principles of Critical Care*, 2d ed.

Chapter 20

MASSIVE HEMOPTYSIS AND DIFFUSE ALVEOLAR HEMORRHAGE

SEAN FORSYTHE

Massive Hemoptysis

Massive hemoptysis has varying definitions but is usually considered to be the expectoration of > 600 mL of blood in a 48-hour period. It is a medical emergency and if untreated has a high mortality. The causes of massive hemoptysis are listed in Table 20-1.

PATHOPHYSIOLOGY

It is unusual for the pulmonary circulation to be the cause of massive hemoptysis, as it is a low-pressure system and involved only with airways below the level of the terminal bronchiole. The bronchial circulation, on the other hand, is a high-pressure system associated with the entire length of the bronchial tree and is a much more common cause of hemoptysis. It is also a much more variable system with plexiform anastamoses and a propensity to hypertrophy and collateralize with nonbronchial systemic vessels in chronic inflammatory disease. This becomes problematic when attempting to embolize bleeding vessels.

MANAGEMENT

Initial management of massive hemoptysis should focus on deciding if the airway needs securing to prevent asphyxiation or aspiration, resuscitating the circulating volume, ensuring adequate oxygenation, and treating the underlying cause. Intensive care unit monitoring, dependent positioning of the bleeding lung, correction of any coagulopathy and early

TABLE 20-1   Causes of Massive Hemoptysis

Infectious
  Bronchitis
  Bronchiectasis
  Necrotizing pneumonia
  Mycetoma
  Lung abscess
  Mycobacterial infection
    Active infection
    Rupture of Rasmussen's aneurysm
    Broncholithiasis
    Bronchiectasis
    Scar carcinoma
Tumors
  Carcinoma
  Bronchial adenoma
Cardiovascular
  Mitral stenosis
  Congenital heart disease
Arteriovenous malformations
  Osler-Weber-Rendu
Trauma
Broncholithiasis
Sarcoidosis
  Endobronchial granulomas
  Complications of sarcoid cavities
Coagulopathy
  Disseminated intravascular coagulation
  Thrombotic thrombocytopenic purpura
  Thrombocytopenia
Drug- and toxin-induced
Iatrogenic
  Pulmonary artery catheter–induced rupture
  Bronchoscopy complication

---

involvement of a pulmonary physician, thoracic surgeon, and interventional radiologists should then take place. Localization of the bleeding with bronchoscopy may help guide further therapeutic interventions. Topical interventions during bronchoscopy, including iced saline lavage, epinephrine, or balloon tamponade, are of questionable efficacy and should not delay more definitive therapy. Computed tomography

(CT) scanning adds little to the acute evaluation and should be reserved for the evaluation of stable patients with submassive hemoptysis. Traditionally it has been felt that every patient should be considered for surgery immediately, but arteriography and embolization have become more popular because of their relatively noninvasive nature and preservation of lung function. Embolization may not be an option for every patient because of variable bronchial circulation. Surgery should be considered in massive uncontrollable bleeding, bleeding that has failed embolization, or when embolization is not possible. Once the patient has stabilized, surgery should also be considered as definitive therapy for certain underlying causes, such as mycetomas or carcinomas.

Diffuse Alveolar Hemorrhage (Alveolar Hemorrhage Syndromes)

Diffuse alveolar hemorrhage is caused by a group of idiopathic or autoimmune diseases (Table 20-2). The bleeding arises from the pulmonary circulation (small capillaries, arterioles, and venules) at the alveolar level. It typically presents with symptoms of cough, shortness of breath, and

TABLE 20-2   Causes of Diffuse Alveolar Hemorrhage

Anti – basement membrane antibody disease (Goodpasture's syndrome)
Wegener's granulomatosis
Essential mixed cryoglobulinemia
Systemic lupus erythematosus (SLE)
Polyarteritis
Allergic granulomatosis (Churg-Strauss syndrome)
Henoch-Schönlein purpura
Behçet's disease
Lymphomatoid granulomatosis
Hypersensitivity angiitis
Other collagen vascular diseases (mixed connective tissue disease, systemic sclerosis, rheumatoid arthritis)
Isolated pulmonary capillaritis
Idiopathic pulmonary hemosiderosis

hemoptysis. The hemoptysis may be the major feature or may not present at all initially. The chest radiograph typically shows a diffuse or patchy alveolar infiltrate. Chest CT confirms the airspace-filling process and in chronic processes can show interstitial infiltrates as well. Laboratories show an iron-deficiency anemia and hypoxemia.

The diagnosis of diffuse alveolar hemorrhage may be difficult and is often missed initially. The pulmonary manifestations of these diseases are very similar, and one must often rely on the extrapulmonary manifestations to help make the diagnosis (sinus disease, renal disease, and/or dermatologic disease). An aggressive workup and early institution of therapy are important to prevent progression of the lung disease and manifestation of extrapulmonary complications.

Management should consist of stabilizing the patient and searching for the underlying disease process. The exact evaluation should be guided by the history and physical but should typically consist of screening laboratory values, a sedimentation rate, a urinalysis, and a serologic workup (ANA, ANCA, and anti–glomerular basement membrane antibodies). Diagnosis is made with the help of serologic results and tissue pathology (either lung or kidney, depending on the sites of involvement). Specific therapy depends on the underlying cause but usually consists of steroids and immunosuppressive drugs. An aggressive workup and early institution of therapy are important to prevent progression of the lung disease and manifestation of extrapulmonary complications. This means that it may be necessary to start immunosuppressive therapy empirically pending full evaluation (which may take several days or longer), when the presentation strongly suggests an underlying treatable vasculitis.

For a more detailed discussion, see Chaps. 33 and 97 in *Principles of Critical Care*, 2d ed.

Chapter 21

PLEURAL DISEASES AND CHEST TUBES

SCOTT BUDINGER

Pneumothorax

ETIOLOGY AND PATHOGENESIS

Pneumothorax, or air in the pleural space, remains a common complication of mechanical ventilation. While pneumothoraces may result from direct injury to the pleura (e.g., during central venous catheterization), more often they begin with rupture of overdistended alveoli. Air then dissects into the pulmonary interstitium and from there to the pleural space, mediastinum, subcutaneous tissues, or peritoneum.

While pneumothoraces result from excess alveolar volume, this cannot be measured directly. Therefore, we rely on measurements of alveolar pressure in assessing the risk of barotrauma in ventilated patients. Pressure estimates of lung volume are inexact, as they vary with lung and chest wall compliance and cannot account for the large heterogeneity of compliance in diseased lungs. That being the case, the best pressure estimates of alveolar volume are the level of PEEP (extrinsic or intrinsic), which reflects end-expiratory alveolar volume, and the plateau pressure, which reflects end-inspiratory alveolar volume.

It is important to remember that many pneumothoraces result from the underlying disease process rather than high ventilator pressures. This is especially true in adult respiratory distress syndrome (ARDS), which has been documented to be an independent risk factor for the development of barotrauma in multiple studies among patients in intensive care units (ICUs). Other lung diseases associated with an increased incidence of barotrauma include interstitial fibrosis, necrotizing infections, and preexisting blebs. In addition, multiple procedures including central venous catheterization, transbronchial biopsy, and thoracentesis carry a significant risk of pneumothorax.

The most feared complication of pneumothoraces is the development of a "tension pneumothorax." This occurs when more air enters the pleural space during inspiration than leaves on expiration, resulting in a continuous rise is pleural pressure. As the pressure in the pleural space approaches right atrial pressure, cardiac filling is impaired, resulting in circulatory collapse. Tension pneumothoraces seldom develop in spontaneously breathing patients, as air ceases to enter the pleural space once inspiratory pleural pressure exceeds atmospheric pressure. However, during mechanical ventilation, up to 50% of unrecognized pneumothoraces will evolve into tension pneumothoraces.

DIAGNOSIS

Diagnosis of pneumothorax in mechanically ventilated patients can be difficult. The patient may be agitated or tachypneic, and tachycardia is common. The blood pressure may be elevated initially but falls within the development of tension physiology. Decreased breath sounds, hyperresonance to percussion ipsilateral to the pneumothorax, and shift of the trachea contralateral to the pneumothorax may be subtle or masked by other pathology. Plateau pressures will be elevated compared with baseline, although the change may be small prior to the development of tension physiology (Table 21-1).

Chest radiography is an important tool in diagnosing pneumothorax. However, a substantial fraction of pneumothoraces in supine patients will not result in the typical

TABLE 21-1   Clinical Signs of Pneumothorax

Ipsilateral decreased breath sounds
Ipsilateral hyperresonance to percussion
Contralateral mediastinal shift
Tachycardia
Hypotension (late)
Increased plateau pressure

TABLE 21-2   Radiologic Signs of Pneumothorax

Finding	Type of Pneumothorax
Apicolateral pleural line	Apicolateral
Linear air density adjacent to the mediastinum	Anteromedial
Increased sharpness of mediastinal border	Anteromedial
Caudal displacement of the costophrenic angle (deep sulcus sign)	Anterolateral
Hyperlucency of the upper abdominal quadrants	Subpulmonic
Visualization of the anterior costophrenic sulcus	Subpulmonic
Ipsilateral increased volume	All
Contralateral shift of the mediastinum	Tension
Ipsilateral flattening of the hemidiaphragm	Tension

apicolateral line seen in upright patients. Instead, pneumothoraces may loculate in the anteromedial recess, producing a "deep sulcus sign," or in the subpulmonic recess, leading to hyperlucency of the upper abdominal quadrants (Table 21-2). In addition, many ICU patients have prominent skin folds, which may mimic pneumothorax (Table 21-3). If doubt exists, serial radiographs, cross-table lateral films, or even chest CT may be helpful in establishing the diagnosis.

MANAGEMENT

Management of pneumothoraces in mechanically ventilated patients requires tube thoracostomy drainage due to the high rate of development of tension physiology (see below). In

TABLE 21-3   Differentiation of Pneumothorax from Skin Fold

Pneumothorax	Skin Fold
Pleural line (black/white line/black)[a]	Edge (one shade of gray to another[a])
Stays inside thorax	Continues outside thorax
Limited by anatomic boundaries (lobes/fissures)	Violates anatomic boundaries
No lung markings past line	Lung markings past edge

[a]Most reliable.

cases of suspected tension pneumothorax with circulatory compromise, empiric tube thoracostomy is warranted even prior to chest radiography. Prophylactic tubes should not be placed in patients with evidence of extrapulmonary air without a pneumothorax (pulmonary interstitial emphysema, pneumomediastinum, subcutaneous emphysema, pneumoperitoneum). However, increased surveillance in these patients is warranted. Preventive strategies that limit ventilator pressures and are compatible with acceptable gas exchange are appropriate in all patients.

Pleural Effusions

GENERAL CONSIDERATIONS

Pleural effusions may be seen in up to 60% of ICU patients. The vast majority of these effusions are small, easily attributable to a known disorder, and require no specific therapy. In addition, thoracentesis is associated with increased risk in critically ill patients, especially those receiving positive-pressure ventilation. Therefore, the majority of effusions in the ICU need not be investigated.

In general, effusions should be tapped when there is a suspicion of pleural space infection (e.g., parapneumonic effusion, unexplained sepsis), an increase in the size of the effusion despite empiric therapy, loculation in the effusion, or a possibility of pleural fluid analysis establishing a specific diagnosis of a systemic illness. Small effusions in the setting of atelectasis, known congestive heart failure (CHF) or cirrhosis, or postoperatively need not be tapped (Table 21-4). CT and perhaps ultrasound increase the sensitivity over chest radiography of detecting small effusions but do not decrease the risk of complications of thoracentesis. Therefore, their routine use is not recommended.

DIAGNOSIS

All pleural fluid should be sent for determination of LDH, total protein, glucose, cell count, and microbiologic studies, and, if empyema is a possibility, pH (under anaerobic collection technique). When appropriate, other studies such as cytology, triglycerides (suspected chylous effusions), cholesterol, and

TABLE 21-4 Causes of Pleural Effusions in the ICU

Generally Should Be Tapped	Generally Should Not Be Tapped
Infection adjacent to the pleura	Congestive heart failure
Pneumonia	Malignancy (when the diagnosis is known)
Upper abdominal sepsis	Atelectasis
Suspected mediastinal sepsis	Massive fluid resuscitation
High-grade systemic sepsis	Hepatic hydrothorax
Endocarditis	Line complication
Life-threatening line sepsis	Hypoalbuminemia
Suspected malignancy	Peritoneal dialysis
Vasculitis	Pulmonary embolism
Pancreatitis	Uremia
Drug-induced	Postoperative
	Postesophageal sclerotherapy

amylase can be performed. An exudative effusion is defined by Light et al. as pleural fluid with one or more of the following: (1) fluid protein/serum protein > 0.5, (2) fluid LDH/serum LDH > 0.6, or fluid LDH greater than two-thirds of the normal value. Transudative effusions meet none of the above criteria. These criteria are useful, as transudates are caused by a relatively small group of disorders including CHF, pericardial disease, nephrotic syndrome, cirrhosis, pulmonary embolism (also associated with exudates), and myxedema and by peritoneal dialysis (Table 21-5).

MANAGEMENT

Management of pleural effusions is usually aimed at treatment of the underlying disease. However, some effusions require drainage (Table 21-6):

Complicated Parapneumonic Effusions/Empyema

The presence of pus or microorganisms in the pleural space (empyema) requires immediate drainage with tube thoracostomy. If this does not adequately drain the effusion, radiologically guided catheter draining with or without concomitant administration of streptokinase or urokinase into the pleural space is an appropriate next step. Thoracoscopic or open surgical decortication should probably be reserved for patients who fail the above therapies. Even in the absence of frank pus or a positive Gram stain on initial thoracentesis, some parapneumonic effusions rapidly develop into loculated empyemas. Effusions with a high likelihood of becoming empyemas are termed *complicated parapneumonic effusions* and should be drained. While some controversy over the definition persists, most authors agree that nonmalignant effusions with a pH < 7.10, glucose < 40, or an LDH > 1000 should be drained immediately. Free-flowing effusions with pH > 7.30, glucose > 60, and LDH < 100 can be treated with antibiotic therapy alone. Effusion with a pH between 7.10 and 7.30 and LDH < 1000 should be resampled in 12 to 24 hours. A falling pH, or development of empyema should prompt immediate drainage.

TABLE 22-5 Selected Causes of Pleural Effusions

Cause of Pleural Effusion	Lateralization	Pleural Chemistries	Treatment
CHF	Bilateral	T	Treat CHF
Cirrhosis	Right	T	Decrease ascites
Nephrotic syndrome	None	T	Increase protein/exclude pulmonary embolus
Pulmonary embolus	None	T or E, may be bloody	Anticoagulation
Uncomplicated parapneumonic effusion	None	E, pH ≥ 7.30, LDH < 1000, glucose > 40	Antibiotics
Complicated parapneumonic effusion	None	E, pH ≤ 7.10, LDH > 1000, glucose < 40	Tube thoracostomy
Empyema	None	E, Frank pus or (+) Gram stain/culture	Tube thoracostomy
Pancreatitis	Left	E, ↑ amylase	Treat pancreatitis
Esophageal perforation (iatrogenic or spontaneous)	Left (spontaneous only)	E, ↑ amylase, pH < 7.10	Emergent mediastinal exploration
Chylothorax (trauma or malignancy)	None	E, triglycerides > 110 or chylomicrons present	Nutrition, surgery if traumatic
Hemothorax	None	E, pleural HCT/serum HCT > 50%	Observation or tube thoracostomy

ABBREVIATIONS: T, transudate; E, exudate; HCT, hematocrit; CHF, congestive heart failure.

245

TABLE 21-6   Indications for Tube Thoracostomy

Complicated parapneumonic effusion/empyema
Pneumothorax in mechanically ventilated patients
Pneumothorax with respiratory compromise in any patient
Traumatic hemothorax
Rapidly reaccumulating effusions with symptoms

Mechanically Important Effusions

Pleural effusions have rarely been reported to impair venous return and to compromise systemic perfusion; when this occurs, however, it requires prompt drainage. More commonly, the small increase in chest wall volume and decrease in functional residual capacity (FRC) associated with moderate-sized effusions may impede liberation from mechanical ventilation in marginal patients. Such effusions can usually be managed with one-time or intermittent thoracentesis.

Trauma

Most trauma patients with pleural effusions (usually hemothorax) or hemopneumothoraces should undergo large-bore tube thoracostomy. The presence of 2 L of blood after initial tube placement or drainage of > 100 mL blood per hour should prompt consideration of surgical exploration.

Chest Tube Placement and Management

PLACEMENT

Chest tubes are placed in the fourth or fifth intercostal space anterior to the midaxillary line or at the second intercostal space in the midclavicular line (usually only for pneumothorax) (Figure 21-1). In general, larger tubes are preferred. Simple pneumothoraces can be treated with small-bore tubes attached to a Heimlich valve in selected patients; however, they are often inadequate to achieve complete drainage in mechanically ventilated patients.

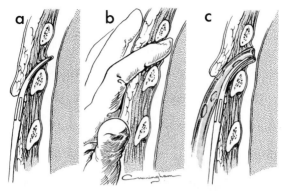

FIGURE 21-1   Technique of chest tube insertion. The incision is made 2 cm below the chose interspace, and the clamp (*a*) followed by the finger (*b*) is inserted into the pleural space above the upper border of the rib. The tube is inserted and directed with the Kelly clamp (*c*). The tube is then gently directed posteriorly and toward the open space.

MANAGEMENT

Once placed, the chest tube should be connected to a three-chamber chest drainage collection system (Figure 21-2). Commercially available systems contain all three chambers in a sealed apparatus. Pleural fluid and air from the patient flow into chamber 1. This is attached in series to chamber 2, which contains a column of water with an underwater seal. When pleural pressure (and therefore chamber 1 pressure) becomes negative relative to the atmosphere, this "water seal" prevents backflow of air into the pleural space. Chamber 2 is connected in series to chamber 3, which contains another column of fluid, open to the atmosphere, to which suction is applied. The height of the column of fluid in chamber 3 (not the wall suction pressure) determines the amount of suction applied to the system. Wall suction should be adjusted to provide a slow stream of bubbles in chamber 3. Excessive wall suction can lead to accelerated evaporation of water in chamber 3, effectively decreasing the applied suction.

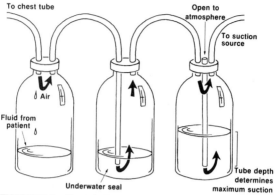

FIGURE 21-2 Chest drainage collection systems. The underwater seal is provided before exposure to the atmosphere or to suction.

Daily chest x-rays should be checked in all patients with chest tubes. In addition, the drainage system should be inspected initially and at least daily thereafter. The quantity and gross appearance of the fluid should be noted. The suction system should be inspected for bubbles in the water-seal chamber. The presence of bubbles indicates entry of air into the system from a bronchopleural fistula in the patient, a leak around the tube at the insertion site, or a leak in the connecting tubing or the collecting system.

REMOVAL

Chest tubes placed for pneumothoraces are removed when the air leak has resolved, the risk factor for the development of the pneumothorax has improved, and no pneumothorax has accumulated after 24 h without suction (water seal). Chest tubes placed for pleural effusions or empyema are generally removed when the inciting event has resolved and fluid drainage is minimal.

For a more detailed discussion, see Chap. 98 in *Principles of Critical Care*, 2d ed.

Chapter 22 _____

LIBERATION FROM MECHANICAL VENTILATION

JOHN McCONVILLE

Overview

The determination of who can be liberated from mechanical ventilation is not an exact science. There is no predictive factor or integrated formula that can unfailingly predict who is ready to breathe spontaneously and who still requires mechanical ventilation. However, even before the clinician determines whether a patient is able to resume spontaneous breathing, it is important to remember why the patient required mechanical ventilation in the first place. There are four different types of respiratory failure that require intubation and mechanical ventilation: (1) type I or hypoxemic respiratory failure, (2) type II or ventilatory failure, (3) type III respiratory failure that is a combination of hypoxemic and ventilatory failure occurring in the perioperative period, and (4) type IV or shock related respiratory failure. In all of these instances, the respiratory system is unable to oxygenate and/or ventilate adequately; thus mechanical ventilation is started in an effort to provide adequate gas exchange while giving a "rest" to the respiratory muscles. After the patient is intubated, it is the clinician's task to diagnose and treat the underlying cause of respiratory failure. *Once the underlying cause of respiratory failure is treated, most patients are able to resume spontaneous respiration immediately.* This chapter helps to identify those patients who are appropriate candidates for liberation from mechanical ventilation and describes an approach to patients who initially fail liberation from mechanical ventilation.

Physiologic Effects of Mechanical Ventilation

Positive-pressure ventilation (PPV) is the most common mode of mechanical ventilation in the intensive care unit (ICU). Because this mode of ventilation provides a fixed volume or pressure to the respiratory system, the cardiopulmonary circuit operates slightly differently than it does during spontaneous respiration. Normally, inspiration creates a negative intrathoracic pressure, which increases venous blood return to the right side of the heart. During positive-pressure ventilation, however, the pressure generated by the ventilator is partially transmitted to the lungs and heart. Thus, the intrathoracic pressure, which is negative during spontaneous respiration, becomes positive during mechanical ventilation. This results in two important physiologic changes: (1) venous blood return to the right atrium decreases during PPV and (2) positive-pressure ventilation reduces left ventricular afterload. These alterations in cardiopulmonary function are important to consider when one is deciding whether a particular patient can be liberated from mechanical ventilation.

Positive end-expiratory pressure (PEEP) is another component of PPV that is important to consider in deciding who can be liberated from mechanical ventilation. PEEP is utilized to prevent alveolar collapse during the terminal portions of expiration. The utilization of PEEP in patients with hypoxic respiratory failure is a common method of improving oxygenation. During the conversion from positive-pressure ventilation to spontaneous respiration, some patients may develop alveolar collapse/atelectasis and worsening oxygenation when no PEEP is supplied by the ventilator.

Determining Who Can Be Liberated

Occasionally, it is quite obvious that some patients are able to resume spontaneous respiration. For example, an otherwise healthy individual undergoing an operation to repair a torn anterior cruciate ligament is typically able to breathe spontaneously as soon as the anesthetic wears off. In this situation, as soon as the patient is able to follow commands and cooperate, he or she can assume the work of breathing and then quickly be extubated. This example brings out a subtle yet important distinction. Liberation from mechanical ventilation is *not* the same as extubation. Liberation from mechanical ventilation implies that the patient is able to perform all the work of spontaneous respiration without any assistance from the ventilator. Extubation, on the other hand, refers to pulling the endotracheal tube out of the airway. There are plenty of situations where the patient is liberated from mechanical respiration yet is unable to be extubated—a cirrhosis patient with grade 4 encephalopathy, for example.

Because complications are associated with endotracheal intubation and mechanical ventilation (Table 22-1), it is important for clinicians to ask themselves every day whether or not the intubated patient can be liberated from mechanical

TABLE 22-1   Complications Associated with Endotracheal Intubation and Mechanical Ventilation

Complications Related to the Endotracheal Tube

Endotracheal tube malfunction—mucous plug, cuff leak
Endotracheal tube malposition
Self-extubation
Nasal or oral necrosis
Pneumonia
Laryngeal edema
Tracheal erosion
Sinusitis

Complications Related to the Ventilator

Alveolar hypoventilation/hyperventilation
Atelectasis
Hypotension
Pneumothorax
Diffuse alveolar damage

Effects on Other Organ Systems

Gastrointestinal hypomotility
Pneumoperitoneum
Stress gastropathy and gastrointestinal hemorrhage
Arrhythmias
Salt and water retention
Malnutrition

ventilation. As stated above, the clinician's first task is to treat the underlying cause of respiratory failure. For example, the patient who is intubated for type I respiratory failure secondary to pulmonary edema arising from cardiac ischemia should receive treatment for the underlying coronary artery disease prior to being extubated. Only after the underlying ischemia has been treated with medications and/or angioplasty/stenting can liberation from mechanical ventilation be considered. Once the underlying coronary artery disease is treated, there are several additional factors to be considered. To consider a patient for a trial of spontaneous breathing, oxygenation must be adequate (Pa_{CO_2} greater than 60 mmHg) on a concentration of oxygen less than or equal to 50% that can be increased as needed at nominal levels of PEEP (less than or equal to 5 cmH_2O). The patient should be hemodynamically stable and, preferably, not excessively tachycardic. In addition, excessive respiratory muscle loads, such as severe bronchospasm, should be reversed before considering a patient for liberation from mechanical ventilation, since excessive loads are likely to precipitate failure. However, even if a patient is hemodynamically stable, with excellent oxygenation on minimal amounts of supplemental oxygen, the clinician often wants additional proof that the patient will be able to succeed at a trial of spontaneous breathing.

Weaning parameters are objective criteria used to assess the readiness of patients to sustain spontaneous ventilation and maintain oxygenation. Unfortunately, the term *weaning* implies a slow process of separating the patient from the ventilator. *In actuality, most patients are able to breathe spontaneously as soon as the underlying cause or causes of respiratory failure are treated.* Nevertheless, some assessment of the patient's ability to breathe spontaneously should be made prior to a trial of spontaneous respiration. Since oxygenation is easily measured by pulse oximetry, most weaning parameters focus on respiratory muscle strength of respiratory muscle load.

The capacity of the respiratory muscles to perform work against mechanical and metabolic loads depends upon intact neuromuscular function—from the medullary control center, to the spinal cord, the phrenic nerves, and the respiratory muscles. Weaning parameters can measure neuromuscular function at several of these levels. The maximal inspiratory pressure, airway occlusion pressure, vital capacity, and maximum voluntary ventilation are all measures of the respiratory muscles' ability to do work. There has been much investigation of these weaning parameters and their ability to predict who can and cannot succeed at a trial of spontaneous respiration. For example, a mechanically ventilated patient who is able to generate a maximal inspiratory pressure (MIP) of 25 mmH$_2$O is predicted to succeed if given the opportunity to breathe spontaneously. Thus, a clinician, trying to decide whether or not a particular patient can be liberated from the ventilator, might check the patient's MIP. If the MIP is greater than 25 cmH$_2$O, the clinician would be more confident that the patient would tolerate a trial of spontaneous respiration. Unfortunately, none of the measures of neuromuscular function are entirely accurate in predicting who can and cannot breath spontaneously. This is because normal neuromuscular function can be associated with a failed attempt at spontaneous respiration if it is coupled with an excessive load (a large pleural effusion, for example). A similar argument holds true for those weaning parameters that attempt to quantify respiratory muscle load. Minute volume, respiratory compliance, and airway resistance are all measures of respiratory muscle load that have been validated in studies as being able to predict who can succeed at a trial of spontaneous respiration. Unfortunately, like the weaning parameters that assess neuromuscular strength, the weaning parameters that assess respiratory muscle load are not perfect prognosticators. Thus, a patient may have a normal airway resistance and still not be able to breathe without assistance of the ventilator.

While no measured variable is perfect, one index has now been studied in a large number of patients and appears to have a predictive utility superior to that of other commonly used parameters. The rate-volume ratio (RVR) measures the respiratory rate:tidal volume ratio (breaths per minute per liter) during a 1-min T-piece trial, and 105 is the threshold value that best predicts weaning outcome. Patients who have an RVR of less than 105 breaths per minute per liter have a much greater chance of succeeding at spontaneous respiration. Several studies have demonstrated excellent sensitivity and specificity of the RVR. In one particular study, the predictive value was even better when the RVR was remeasured after 30 min of spontaneous breathing. Nevertheless, the RVR is not a perfect predictor of who will succeed. The principal defect in this index appears to be false-positive results (patients with RVR less than 105 breaths per minute per liter who fail). Accordingly, an RVR of less than 105 breaths per minute per liter does not necessarily ensure successful liberation from mechanical ventilation but should prompt a spontaneous breathing trial of 30 to 120 min to further assess patient readiness.

Liberation

Before the patient's ability to breathe spontaneously is assessed, sedatives and narcotics should be discontinued for several hours. This reduces the likelihood of iatrogenic hypoventilation. Patients should be awake and able to cooperate while sitting up at greater than a 30 degree angle. In addition, tube feeds should be turned off to allow enough time for the stomach to empty, in case a trial of spontaneous respiration leads to extubation.

Which mode on the ventilator is used to assess the patient's ability to breathe spontaneously is a question of style. One common method is to place the patient on a T piece and to watch for signs of failure (see below). A nurse or physician should remain at the bedside. If the patient has an RVR of less than 105 breaths per minute per liter without developing excessive tachypnea, tachycardia, hypertension, significant distress, or mental status changes, then he or she should be carefully watched for 30 to 120 min on a T-piece trial. If the patient tolerates a trial of spontaneous respiration, then he or she can be considered for extubation.

Some data suggests that breathing through an endotracheal tube on a T piece is more work than spontaneous respiration. This is thought to be the result of the resistance to airflow caused by the endotracheal tube. Therefore, some clinicians suggest that a pressure support of 5 to 8 cmH_2O or a continuous positive airway pressure (CPAP) of 5 to 8 cmH_2O can be used instead of a T piece to assess the patient's ability to breathe spontaneously. This limited amount of positive pressure is felt to be enough assistance to overcome the added resistance of the endotracheal tube but not enough additional positive pressure to significantly reduce the work of respiration. Utilizing CPAP or pressure support as means of assessing a patient's ability to breathe spontaneously has recently been validated in clinical trials. Thus, a T-piece trial or a trial of CPAP or pressure support of 5 to 8 cmH_2O can be utilized to assess a patient's ability to breathe spontaneously.

The Patient Who Fails

The clinical signs demonstrated by a patient who is failing a trial of spontaneous respiration include tachypnea, tachycardia, hypertension, mental status changes, and subjective distress. These signs result from (1) decrements in gas exchange, (2) cardiovascular events and (3) noncardiopulmonary events. Hypercapnia and hypoxia are the measured values that suggest a decrement in gas exchange. Hypercapnia is often the result of rapid shallow breathing during a spontaneous breathing trial. Acute hypercapnia during a liberation trial frequently results from an imbalance between respiratory pump capacity and respiratory load. The three components of respiratory load are resistance, elastance, and minute ventilation. Figure 22-1 shows some of the causes of increased respiratory load and illustrates how this load must be counterbalanced by neuromuscular competence. Table 22-2 explains how respiratory load can be reduced and respiratory strength improved in patients who initially fail extubation.

Patients with preexisting coronary artery disease often develop ischemia during the transition from mechanical ventilation to spontaneous respiration. As stated earlier, this transition is associated with increased venous return and increased afterload. In a patient with limited cardiopulmonary reserve, increases in the venous return and afterload can result in an increased myocardial oxygen demand that is unable to be met by the diseased coronary arteries. Often, the result is myocardial ischemia. This can contribute to the signs of failure seen during an unsuccessful trial of spontaneous respiration.

The ventilator and its circuitry can contribute to weaning failure by two mechanisms: (1) by increasing respiratory loads during a spontaneous breathing trial enough to fatigue the respiratory muscles and (2) by imposing significant respiratory muscle work during "rest" periods. The resistance of the endotracheal tube increases with time, and this increase can occasionally be of sufficient magnitude to impede weaning.

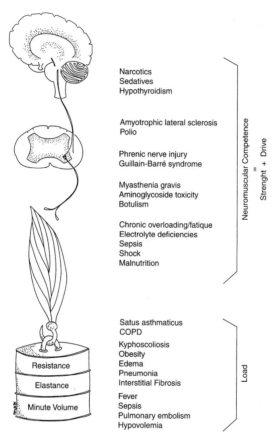

FIGURE 22-1   The neuromuscular circuit. This diagram summarizes the components of neuromuscular competence (strength) and respiratory muscle load and illustrates processes that can affect the strength-load balance leading to ventilatory failure. *(From Manthous CA, Siegel M: Ventilatory failure, in Matthay et al (eds): Pulmonary and Critical Care Yearbook, vol 3. St. Louis, Mosby, 1996, chap. 2, with permission.)*

TABLE 22-2 Reversible Factors Contributing to Ventilatory Failure—Daily Correction of Reversible Contributors to Ventilatory Failure Expedites Patient Recovery

Reduce Respiratory Load	Improve Respiratory Strength
Resistance	Replace K^+, Mg^{2+}, PO_4^{2-} to normal
Inhaled bronchodilators	Treat sepsis
Corticosteroids	Nutritional support without
Removal of excess airway secretions	overfeeding (aim to achieve a normal prealbumin)
Treatment of upper airway obstructions	Consider stopping aminoglycosides
	Rule out:
	Neurologic disease/ occult seizures
Elastance	Hypothyroidism
Treat pneumonia	Oversedation
Treat pulmonary edema	Critical illness myopathy/ polyneuropathy
Reduce dynamic hyperinflation	
Drain large pleural effusions	
Evacuate pneumothoraces	
Treat ileus	
Minute volume	
Detect intrinsic PEEP	
Bronchodilators	
Antipyretics	
Treat sepsis	
Therapy for pulmonary embolism	
Maintain least PEEP possible	
Correct metabolic acidoses	
Resuscitate shock	
Prevent hypovolemia	
Avoid overfeeding	

In addition, the ventilator circuit provides increased dead space and in some modes (for older ventilators) can require excessive work to trigger a "sticky" demand valve. In this manner, the ventilator circuit can load and covertly fatigue the respiratory muscles when patients are presumed to be "resting" as well as when they are weaning. Patient-ventilator synchrony during "rest" periods reduces the likelihood that the ventilator is contributing to weaning failure.

Liberating Strategies after a Failed Attempt

Many intensivists have reasoned that by gradually reducing ventilatory support, the respiratory muscles exercise at sub-fatiguing loads, leading to gradual improvement of function. However, there are no studies proving that respiratory muscle training through the use of decremental ventilatory support hastens the recovery of unassisted breathing. Two recent studies have assessed the role of "weaning" strategies in expediting liberation from mechanical ventilation. These studies randomized patients to one of several weaning strategies: daily T-piece trials of increasing duration, intermittent mandatory ventilation (SIMV) with a gradual reduction in the rate, or pressure support (PSV) with a gradual reduction in pressure. One of these studies supported the use of pressure support after failed liberation and another supported T-piece trials of increasing duration. However, there are many different "weaning trials" that come to many different conclusions. Ultimately, there is no consensus as to the best "exercise mode" of ventilation for patients who have previously failed attempts at spontaneous respiration. However, several important conclusions can be drawn from these studies. First, and most important, the majority of patients can be successfully extubated on the first day that physicians recognize readiness after a brief (30- to 120-min) trial of breathing through a T piece. *Weaning is not necessary for most patients.* Second, both of the recent studies suggest that those patients who have failed an initial T-piece trial will have a longer duration of mechanical ventilation if the SIMV mode is utilized. However, if one considers all the results of these studies together, choices of ventilator mode do not appear to have a major impact in speeding that recovery to unassisted breathing.

Extubation

Once a patient is able to breathe without assistance from the ventilator, the clinician has to decide whether the patient can be extubated. Before the endotracheal tube is removed, it is important to consider whether the patient will be able to maintain an adequate airway without the endotracheal tube in place. Even if a patient is able to breathe without assistance from the ventilator, the patient's mental status, airway protective mechanisms, ability to cough, and amount of secretions must be assessed prior to extubation. While in place, the endotracheal tube provides an avenue for positive pressure ventilation and a means to have secretions removed by suctioning. Once the endotracheal tube is removed, the patient must be able to maintain a patent upper airway, clear secretions, and cough. The determination of whether a patient can be extubated is somewhat subjective and is one reason why patients can fail extubation even if they are able to breathe spontaneously. However, there are some clinical scenarios in which the clinician should be suspicious of the patient's ability to maintain an adequate airway. Recognition of these situations may prevent some extubation failures. For example, laryngeal edema, vocal cord damage, and tracheal stricture are all complications of a prolonged intubation that may make it difficult for a patient to tolerate extubation. In addition, patients intubated for stridor or those with a cancerous upper airway lesion may have difficulty upon extubation because of an upper airway that is critically narrowed. Poor mental status is another situation that can require continued intubation despite the ability to breathe unassisted. Patients with poor mental status, such as severe hepatic encephalopathy, are unable to clear secretions and cough appropriately. However, when the cause of impaired airway protection is thought to be reversible, treating and attempting a trial of extubation at a later time is reasonable. Finally, if a recently extubated patient develops some breathing difficulty in the postextubation period, noninvasive face-mask positive-pressure ventilation may prevent the need for reintubation.

A Practical Approach

The most important step in limiting the time a patient spends on the ventilator is for the clinician to ask: Can the patient be liberated from the ventilator? This question should be asked every day. One approach to liberation from the ventilator is outlined in Fig. 22-2. If the patient is awake and triggering the ventilator with a Pa_{O_2} greater than 60 mmHg on an inspired oxygen of less than 50% and PEEP less than or equal to 5 mmH$_2$O, the RVR should be assessed. If the RVR is less than 125 breaths per minute per liter, we place the patient on a T piece or pressure support trial (40 to 50% oxygen) of 30 to 120 minutes. If the patient remains comfortable, with oxygen saturation greater than 90%, without tachycardia or hypertension, and the RVR remains less than 125 breaths per minute per liter at 30 min, we will obtain an arterial blood

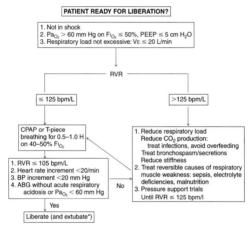

FIGURE 22-2 A simple bedside algorithm for weaning patients with ventilatory (and hypoxemic) failure from mechanical ventilation. "The decision to extubate depends upon the patient's level of consciousness, ability to protect her or his airway (cough, gag reflex), and the amount of endotracheal secretions (see text). This algorithm should be individualized for every patient; when other parameters are favorable, no single unfavorable parameter should prevent a trial of liberation. (RVR = respiratory rate:tidal volume ratio, V_E = minute volume, CPAP = continuous positive airway pressure, BP = blood pressure.) (*Adapted from Manthous CA, Siegel M: Ventilatory failure, in Matthay et al: (eds): Pulmonary and Critical Care Yearbook, vol 3. St. Louis, Mosby, 1996, Chap. 2, with permission.*)

gas and consider a trial of extubation. Patients who still require an artificial airway can continue to breathe as much as they are able off of the ventilator until they are ready for extubation. For patients with RVR greater than 125 breaths per minute per liter or for those who fail on an initial trial of spontaneous breathing, we aggressively assess the pathogenesis of their failure and perform daily trials of either T-piece or pressure support breathing until the patient can tolerate a greater than 30-min trial of unassisted breathing. Since the RVR is an abbreviated T-piece trial, an alternative approach would be to perform one extended T-piece trial each day to recognize the earliest day of readiness for liberation.

For a more detailed discussion, see Chap. 39 in *Principles of Critical Care*, 2d ed.

Chapter 23

SHOCK

IMRE NOTH

Definitions

"Shock" is the hypoperfusion of multiple organ systems. Clinical signs of hypoperfusion include tachycardia, tachypnea, low mean blood pressure, diaphoresis, poorly perfused skin and extremities, altered mental status, and decreased urine output. Hypotension, defined as systolic blood pressure less than 90 mmHg or a mean pressure less than 60 mmHg, often occurs in shock states but is not always present. Indeed, eclampsia and hypertensive crisis are shock states with elevated blood pressures. A decreased pulse pressure (defined as a reduction in the difference between systolic and diastolic pressure) may be a clearer sign of a hypoperfusion state in some patients. It should be noted that cuff blood pressure may markedly underestimate central blood pressure in low-flow states. Lactic acidosis may indicate tissue hypoxia but does not necessarily reflect anaerobic metabolism. Hypoperfusion and resuscitation may initiate a systemic inflammatory response (SIRS), and diseases associated with SIRS also produce shock, creating a complex interaction for the clinician to dissect.

Primary Survey

Morbidity and mortality in shock are directly related to rapidity of diagnosis and treatment of the shock state. Cardiac output (CO) and systemic vascular resistance (SVR) determine overall systemic pressure. Hypotension occurs when CO is inadequate (most commonly with hypovolemic or cardiogenic shock) or when SVR becomes abnormally low (typically with septic shock). Initial patient examination should focus on differentiating between types of shock. The following algorithm aids in prompt delineation of these major categories (Table 23-1).

TABLE 23-1 Rapid Formulation of an Early Working Diagnosis of the Etiology of Shock

Defining Features of Shock

Blood pressure	→
Heart rate	←
Respiratory rate	← →
Mentation	→
Urine output	→
Arterial pH	→

	High-Output Hypotension Septic Shock	Low-Cardiac-Output Cardiogenic and Hypovolemic
Is cardiac output reduced?	No	Yes
Pulse pressure	←	→
Diastolic pressure	←	→
Extremities digits	Warm	Cool
Nailbed return	Rapid	Slow
Heart sounds	Crisp	Muffled
Temperature	↑ or →	← →
White cell count	↑ or →	← →
Site of infection	++	–
	Reduced Pump Function Cardiogenic Shock	Reduced Venous Return Hypovolemic Shock

264

Is the heart too full?	Yes	No
Symptoms clinical context	Angina ECG	Hemorrhage dehydration
Jugular venous pressure	↑ ↓	—
S_3, S_4 gallop rhythm	+++ −	—
Respiratory crepitations	+++ −	—
Chest radiograph	Large heart ↑ upper lobe flow Pulmonary edema	Normal

What Does Not Fit?

Overlapping etiologies (septic cardiogenic, septic hypovolemic, cardiogenic hypovolemic)

Short list of other etiologies:

High output hypotension	*High right atrial pressure hypotension*	*Nonresponsive hypovolemia*
Liver failure	Pulmonary hypertension	Adrenal insufficiency
Severe pancreatitis	(most often pulmonary embolus)	Anaphylaxis
Trauma with significant systemic inflammatory response	Right ventricular infarction	Spinal shock
Thyroid storm	Cardiac tamponade	
Arteriovenous fistula		
Paget's disease		

Get more information

Echocardiography, right heart catheterization

265

1. Is cardiac output reduced or elevated? Septic shock is strongly suggested by high-cardiac-output hypotension, which is most often signaled by a widened pulse pressure with marked diastolic reduction relative to systolic pressure, a strong apical cardiac impulse, warm extremities with brisk nail-bed return, and fever or hypothermia, leukocytosis, or leukopenia. Low CO indicates cardiogenic or hypovolemic shock. A small pulse pressure, reduced apical cardiac impulse, and cool extremities with poor nail-bed return signal low cardiac output.

2. Is the heart too full? Volume overload in the low-CO state may present with elevated jugular venous pressure (JVP), peripheral edema, crepitations on lung auscultation, a large heart with extra heart sounds (S3, S4), and chest pain. The electrocardiogram (ECG) may demonstrate ischemic changes and a chest x-ray may show a large heart with prominent upper-lobe vessels and pulmonary edema. Ischemic heart disease is the most common cause of cardiogenic shock. Hypovolemic shock results from blood loss (indicated by hematemesis, tarry stools, abdominal distention, reduced hematocrit, or trauma), or dehydration (indicated by decreased skin turgor, vomiting, diarrhea, or a negative fluid balance). Distinguishing between hypovolemic and cardiogenic shock is critical to help focus therapy directed at volume resuscitation or vasoactive drugs.

3. What does not fit? When bedside examination yields unclear or conflicting information, the answer is often that hypotension is secondary to more than one cause. A mixed shock picture, such as sepsis complicated by myocardial infarction, must be considered. More information perhaps from a right heart catheter, is then needed to separate out these etiologies. The approach to early management, however, does not change—prompt restitution of an adequate intravascular volume with fluids or blood.

Urgent Initial Resuscitation

The objective is to avoid the sequelae of organ hypoperfusion by rapidly restoring circulation. Therapy is directed at (1) improving oxygen delivery (by raising hemoglobin concentration, cardiac output, or arterial saturation); (2) reducing oxygen consumption; and (3) identifying and treating the precipitants of hypoperfusion. Brief examination of the patient as outlined above can help in formulating a hypothesis concerning the type of shock responsible. During this examination, the ABCs (airway, breathing, and circulation) should also be evaluated. Table 23-2 reviews management of factors aggravating the hypoperfusion state.

IMPROVING OXYGEN DELIVERY

Airway and Breathing

Patients with shock frequently develop depressed mentation and obtundation. Tracheal intubation is indicated for these patients to protect the lungs from aspiration of oropharyngeal or gastric contents (Table 23-3). Acute hypoxemic respiratory failure frequently accompanies shock. Metabolic (lactic) acidosis secondary to shock increases respiratory drive, elevates respiratory muscle oxygen demand, while impairing oxygen delivery. Intubation and mechanical ventilation serve to reduce the work of breathing and hence oxygen demand while allowing increased delivery of inspired oxygen and utilization of positive end-expiratory pressure (PEEP). Note that intubation and positive-pressure ventilation frequently reduce venous return in hypovolemic shock, *so greater volume resuscitation may be needed.* Evidence of respiratory muscle fatigue—such as labored breathing, tachypnea > 40/min, thoracoabdominal paradoxical motion, and accessory muscle use—should prompt early elective intubation.

Circulation

Tension pneumothorax or arrhythmias are causes of shock that are rapidly correctable by tube thoracostomy or electrical cardioversion, respectively, and therefore must be considered as part of the primary survey. The immediate therapeutic approach to hypotension in nearly all forms of shock is aggressive volume resuscitation to decisively assure an adequately filled cardiovascular system. Evaluation should be initiated with volume challenge and assessed with short-term endpoints such as blood pressure, jugular venous pressure,

TABLE 23-2   Urgent Resuscitation of the Patient
with Shock—Managing Factors Aggravating
the Hypoperfusion State

Respiratory therapy
Protect the airway—consider early elective intubation
Prevent excess respiratory work—ventilate with small volumes
Avoid respiratory acidosis—keep Pa_{CO_2} low
Maintain oxygen delivery—$F_{I_{O_2}}$, PEEP, hemoglobin
Infection in presumed septic shock—(see Chap. 25)
Empirical rational antibiosis for all probable etiologies
Exclude allergies to antibiotics
Search, incise, and drain abscesses (consider laparotomy)
Arrhythmias aggravating shock (see Chap. 28)
Bradycardia (rate < 80 min in shock)
   Correct hypoxemia—$F_{I_{O_2}}$ 1.0
   Atropine 0.6 mg, repeat × 2 for effect
   Increase dopamine to 10 μg/kg min
   Add isoproterenol (1–10 μg/min)
   Consider transvenous pacer
Ventricular ectopy, tachycardia
   Lidocaine
   Detect and correct K^+, Ca^{2+}, Mg^{2+}
   Detect and treat myocardial ischemia
Supraventricular tachycardia
   Consider defibrillation early
   Digoxin for rate control of atrial fibrillation
Sinus tachycardia > 140 min
   Detect and treat pain and anxiety
      Midazolam fentanyl drip
      Morphine
   Detect and treat hypovolemia
Metabolic (lactic) acidosis
Characterize to confirm anion gap without osmolal gap
Rule out or treat ketoacidosis, aspirin intoxication
Hyperventilate to keep Pa_{CO_2} 25 mmHg
Calculate bicarbonate deficit and replace half if pH < 7.0
Correct ionized hypocalcemia
Consider early dialysis
Hypothermia
Maintain skin dry and covered with warmed blankets
Warm vascular volume expanders
Aggressive rewarming if temperature < 35°C (95°F)

TABLE 23-3   Indications for Intubation in Shock Patients

Indication	Why
Hypoxemia	High F_{IO_2} is not guaranteed by oxygen masks
	PEEP can be added
Ventilatory failure	Ensure adequate CO_2 removal
(inappropriately high P_{CO_2},	Correct hypoxia due to hypoventilation
signs of ventilatory muscle fatigue)	Prevent sudden respiratory arrest
Vital organ hypoperfusion	Rest ventilatory muscles (and divert cardiac output to hypoperfused vital organs)
Obtundation	Protect and ensure an adequate airway

or pulmonary edema. In cases of obvious hemorrhagic shock, immediate hemostasis is essential, blood must be warmed and filtered, and blood substitutes should be administered in large quantities until blood pressure rises or the heart becomes too full. Ultimately, the lowest left ventricular filling pressure needed to maintain adequate cardiac output and oxygen delivery is sought. If shock is not corrected by adequate circulating volume, inotropic or other vasoactive agents are indicated. Too often vasoactive agents are administered before adequate intravascular volume is assured, thereby compromising subsequent delivery of fluid. All hypotensive patients require an adequate circulating volume, so volume infusion should be pushed until a discernible point of "too much" is reached, as evidenced by clinical examination revealing a heart that is too full; then positive inotropic drugs (dobutamine, etc.) can be effective in increasing cardiac output from the heart with adequate preload. The exceptions to aggressive volume resuscitation are in patients with right heart syndromes or ischemic heart disease, when more modest volume challenges (e.g., 500 mL) are indicated. Nevertheless, many patients with acute myocardial infarction are hypovolemic and improve with judicious fluid resuscitation.

Based on initial assessment, a working diagnosis should direct therapy in an effort to maximize oxygen delivery through improving cardiac output, oxygen saturation, or carrying capacity. Blood transfusions offer both oxygen-carrying capacity and effective intravascular volume replacement and therefore should be utilized to achieve a hematocrit of up to 40. Hemoglobin saturation can be maximized by high concentrations of inspired oxygen and PEEP. Temporary use of 100% inspired oxygen, pending additional resuscitation measures, is advisable. PEEP has the potential either to improve oxygen delivery by reducing shunt in diffuse lung lesions or to worsen it by compromising cardiac output.

REDUCING OXYGEN CONSUMPTION

Mechanical ventilation reduces but does not eliminate the work of breathing. The addition of sedation and paralytic agents to relax muscles will also decrease oxygen demand and improve overall tissue oxygenation. Fever increases oxygen demand by about 10% per degree centigrade above 37°C, and antipyretics should be given early in the acute management of hyperthermic (usually septic) shock. Cooling blankets should be restricted to paralyzed, sedated patients, since they cause shivering, which can increase oxygen consumption.

CATHETERS AND OTHER MEASUREMENTS

For large-volume administration, two peripheral intravenous catheters of gauge 16 or better are required. Large-bore central venous catheterization is useful in assessing central venous pressure (CVP) and administering volume or vasoactive drugs. A urinary bladder catheter should be placed to monitor urine output. A nasogastric or orogastric tube should be placed to decompress the stomach and deliver enteral medications and nutrition. Arterial catheterization may be useful in low-flow states to monitor blood pressure and obtain arterial blood gases (ABGs). Placement of a pulmonary artery catheter allows detailed repeated cardiovascular measurements. CVP, right ventricular pressures, pulmonary artery occlusion pressure, and thermodilution cardiac output; this can be measured as frequently as necessary to identify hemodynamic abnormalities and measure the effect of therapeutic interventions as tests of clinical hypotheses (see Chap. 3 for more details).

CORRECTING CONTRIBUTING CAUSES OF SHOCK

During initial resuscitation, one should consider other definitive therapies such as antibiotics in the septic patient or early consultation for surgical problems. Dysrhythmias should be treated appropriately based on specific etiologies.

Diagnosis and correction of acidemia rely on ventilator therapy to keep Pa_{CO_2} low while confirming the presence and magnitude of anion-gap acidosis without the osmolar gap of exogenous poisons. Concurrent exclusion of ketoacidosis suggests the most common cause of shock-related metabolic acidosis—lactic acidosis. Legitimate uncertainty exists concerning the treatment of lactic acidosis with intravenous NaH_{CO_3}, in part because intracellular acidosis may be made worse, lactic acid production may increase, and treatment-associated ionized hypocalcemia may depress cardiovascular function (see Table 23-2).

Goals of Therapy of Shock

The goal of airway intubation and mechanical ventilation is to correct inadequate oxygenation and ventilation, to rest the respiratory muscles so as to decrease their need for the limited blood flow, and to protect the airway. Initially one must choose a high inspiratory oxygen ($F_{I_{O_2}}$) and a ventilatory mode to do all the work of breathing. Muscle paralysis may improve efficiency of mechanical ventilation and reduce oxygen demands.

The next goal is to minimize risk of therapeutic interventions (reducing toxic $F_{I_{O_2}}$, lowering PEEP, and liberating the patient from mechanical ventilation). This is done by seeking the least $F_{I_{O_2}}$ necessary to maintain an adequate arterial oxygenation, using the least PEEP consistent with an arterial oxygenation of sufficient circulatory hemoglobin on a nontoxic $F_{I_{O_2}}$. Although PEEP can reduce venous return in the patient in shock, PEEP often increases cardiac output in patients with cardiogenic shock and pulmonary edema. Similarly, when septic or hypovolemic shock is complicated by pulmonary vascular leak, these patients often tolerate PEEP to correct hypoxemia without reducing their cardiac output or blood pressure provided that their vascular volume is adequate.

Ventilator liberation should not be pursued until the causes leading to shock and hypoperfusion are identified and treated. Correcting these causes is the most important and first step in eliminating the need for mechanical ventilation and airway.

Goals of cardiovascular management are to maintain cardiac output and oxygen delivery adequate to reverse tissue hypoperfusion while avoiding adverse effects of excessive therapy by seeking the lowest ventricular filling pressures and lowest vasoactive drug infusions required to achieve this goal.

VASOACTIVE DRUGS

Clinical assessment is important in selecting inotropic or vasoactive agents. Table 23-4 outlines volume resuscitation and the actions and dosages of various vasoactive agents. Dopamine increases contractility but also increases venous return by constricting the capacitance veins, even in hypovolemic shock, and may acutely appear beneficial. Continued use may mask inadequate fluid resuscitation and is dangerous. Dobutamine increases ventricular contractility and reduces afterload, which may result in increased cardiac output and oxygen delivery in cardiogenic shock. However, if contractility is already adequate, then dobutamine may only serve to decrease afterload and preload, which, in the hypovolemic patient, may cause dangerous hypotension and hypoperfusion. Dopamine in the range of 0.5 to 5 μg/kg per minute may selectively improve renal and mesenteric blood flow in cardiogenic shock but does not appear beneficial in septic states. These drugs should be given and adjusted based on physiologically relevant endpoints, such as adequacy of perfusion, rather than titrated to arbitrary levels of blood pressure.

Types of Shock

Table 23-5 offers an extensive list of common and less common etiologies of shock. In those cases in which no infection, acute hemorrhagic, or myocardial cause is found, other disease processes should be sought.

DECREASED PUMP FUNCTION — CARDIOGENIC SHOCK

Cardiogenic shock is defined as an inappropriately low cardiac output in the face of a normal or high input or right atrial pressure. Causes resulting in shock may be acute or acute-on-chronic left ventricular failure. Clinical findings include pulmonary crackles in dependent lung regions, presence of a third heart sound, absence of crisp heart sounds, and clinical evidence of ventricular dilation. Pulmonary artery catheter

TABLE 23-4 Urgent Resuscitation of the Patient with Shock; Intravenous Volume and Vasoactive Drug Therapy

Hemorrhagic shock including trauma, ruptured aneurysms	Nonhemorrhagic hypovolemia including septic shock	Cardiogenic shock due to myocardial ischemia
	Volume therapy	
Elevate legs, MAST	Elevate legs	When heart is "too full," blood volume
Access infuse emergency blood	3 L/20 min warmed saline	(rotating tourniquets, phlebotomy,
Group match administer warmed blood components	Group match packed RBCs and plasma re dilutional anemia	nitroglycerin, morphine, diuretics)
>3 L/20 min warmed saline	Continue aggressive volume infusion until blood pressure normal or heart "too full"	If the heart is not "too full" or blood pressure with above interventions, NaCl 250 mL/20 min
Equal volumes of colloid or substitutes (albumin, dextran, hetastarch)	Detect and treat tamponade with pericardiocentesis, thoracostomy, peritoneal drainage, or reduced PEEP	Repeat if blood pressure rises until heart too full
Continue aggressive volume infusion until blood pressure normal		
Consider early surgical hemostasis		

274

Vasoactive drug therapy

Awaiting adequate volume repletion, institute multipurpose agent (*dopamine* or *epinephrine*) and increase dose from 1 toward 10 (μg/kg per minute for dopamine; μg/min for epinephrine) as needed to maintain blood pressure. If higher doses are needed, add norepinephrine (2–20 μg/min) Discontinue these drugs as urgently as volume repletion and hemostasis allow (see second column).	Avoid vasoactive drugs until heart "too full." Except dopamine (2–5 μg/kg per minute) for renal perfusion early. Nitroglycerin and nitroprusside are contraindicated. Vasoconstrictors delay adequate volume resuscitation (see left column). In right heart overload with shock, norepinephrine (2–20 μg/min) may help by maintaining RV perfusion. In septic shock, vasoconstrictor may help when adequate volume replacement provides inadequate perfusion pressure (see text).	*Dobutamine* (5–15 μg/kg per minute) to enhance contractility without excess tachycardia, arrhythmia, or vasoconstriction; higher doses dilate skeletal vascular bed. *Dopamine* (2–5 μg/kg per minute) to preserve renal cortical blood flow; at higher dose (4–12 μg/kg per minute) increases heart rate, contractility, venous tone, and preload, like *epinephrine*. *Nitroglycerin* (25–250 μg/min) for venodilation with minimal arterial dilation except for the coronary circulation. *Sodium nitroprusside* (0.1–5 μg/kg per minute) for arterial dilation to reduce afterload and allow greater ejection from a depressed left ventricle or regurgitant aortic mitral valve.

TABLE 23-5   Causes of and Contributors to Shock

Decreased Pump Function of the Heart—Cardiogenic Shock

Left ventricular failure
  Systolic dysfunction—decreased contractility
    Myocardial infarction
    Ischemia and global hypoxemia
    Cardiomyopathy
    Depressant drugs: β blockers, calcium-channel blockers, antiarrhythmics
    Myocardial contusion
    Respiratory acidosis
    Metabolic derangements: acidosis, hypophosphatemia, hypocalcemia
  Diastolic dysfunction—increased myocardial diastolic stiffness
    Ischemia
    Ventricular hypertrophy
    Restrictive cardiomyopathy
    Consequence of prolonged hypovolemic or septic shock
    Ventricular interdependence
    External compression (see cardiac tamponade, below)
  Greatly increased afterload
    Aortic stenosis
    Hypertrophic cardiomyopathy
    Dynamic outflow tract obstruction
    Coarctation of the aorta
    Malignant hypertension
  Valve and structural abnormality
    Mitral stenosis, endocarditis, mitral aortic regurgitation
    Obstruction due to atrial myxoma or thrombus
    Papillary muscle dysfunction or rupture
    Ruptured septum or free wall
  Arrhythmias
Right ventricular failure
  Decreased contractility
    Right ventricular infarction, ischemia, hypoxia, acidosis
  Greatly increased afterload
    Pulmonary embolism
    Pulmonary vascular disease
    Hypoxic pulmonary vasoconstriction, PEEP, high alveolar pressure
    Acidosis
      ARDS, pulmonary fibrosis, sleep-disordered breathing, chronic obstructive pulmonary disease

(Continued)

TABLE 23-5   *(Cont.)* Causes of and Contributors to Shock

Valve and structural abnormality
   Obstruction due to atrial myxoma, thrombus, endocarditis
Arrhythmias

Decreased Venous Return with Normal Pumping Function—Hypovolemic Shock

Cardiac tamponade (increased right atrial pressure—central
  hypovolemia)
  Pericardial fluid collection
    Blood
    Renal failure
    Pericarditis with effusion
  Constrictive pericarditis
  High intrathoracic pressure
    Tension pneumothorax
    Massive pleural effusion
    Positive-pressure ventilation
  High intraabdominal pressure
    Ascites
    Massive obesity
    Post–extensive intraabdominal surgery
Intravascular hypovolemia (reduced mean systemic pressure)
  Hemorrhage
    Gastrointestinal
    Trauma
    Aortic dissection and other internal sources
  Renal losses
    Diuretics
    Osmotic diuresis
    Diabetes (insipidus, mellitus)
  Gastrointestinal losses
    Vomiting
    Diarrhea
    Gastric suctioning
    Loss via surgical stomas
  Redistribution to extravascular space
    Burns
    Trauma
    Postsurgical
    Sepsis
Decreased venous tone (reduced mean systemic pressure)
  Drugs
    Sedatives

(Continued)

TABLE 23-5   (*Cont.*) Causes of and Contributors to Shock

    Narcotics
    Diuretics
  Anaphylactic shock
  Neurogenic shock
Increased resistance to venous return
  Tumor compression or invasion
  Venous thrombosis with obstruction
  PEEP
  Pregnancy

High-Cardiac-Output Hypotension

Septic shock
Sterile endotoxemia with hepatic failure
Arteriovenous shunts
  Dialysis
  Paget's disease

Other Causes of Shock with Unique Etiologies

Thyroid storm
Myxedema coma
Adrenal insufficiency
Hemoglobin and mitochondrial poisons
  Cyanide
  Carbon monoxide
  Iron intoxication

---

measurement in cardiogenic shock should demonstrate a diminished cardiac index $< 2.2 \text{ L/m}^2$ per minute and a pulmonary artery wedge pressure (PAWP) $> 18 \text{ mmHg}$ (see Chap. 26 for more detail).

Systolic dysfunction represents a decreased ability of the ventricle to achieve a normal stroke volume for a given afterload. Mechanisms by which the patient's heart may compensate for this diminished ability to eject blood include increasing end-diastolic volume to increase stroke volume. Mean systolic pressure may increase via increased fluid retention and increased venous tone. Acute myocardial infarction or ischemia is the most common cause of LV failure leading to shock. Incidence of shock is greater with an anterior myocardial infarction than with inferior or posterior infarctions.

In diastolic dysfunction, increased LV diastolic stiffness contributes to cardiogenic shock, particularly during myocardial ischemia. Cardiac function is depressed, since stroke volume is decreased secondary to decreased end-diastolic volume. Echocardiography can identify a small left ventricular end-diastolic volume (LVEDV), indicating diastolic dysfunction in the patient with low cardiac output and high filling pressure. Treatment is difficult except when the problem is caused by immediately reversible etiologies such as ischemia or tamponade. If conventional therapy aimed at improving systolic function is ineffective, one should consider diastolic dysfunction as the cause of failure to improve function. Attempting to decrease diastolic stiffness with calcium-channel blockers or β-blocker agents can be difficult if not impossible in the face of shock.

Treatment of LV failure with shock frequently requires a pulmonary artery catheter to help optimize filling pressures, increase contractility utilizing inotropes, optimize afterload, and improve the ratio of oxygen supply and demand. In the presence of ischemia, one should consider early thrombolytic therapy and revascularization or surgical correction. Using a temporary intraaortic balloon pump (IABP) as a bridge to surgical therapy is effective and should be implemented early when appropriate. Filling pressures should be optimized to improve cardiac output while avoiding pulmonary edema. Patients with hypovolemia should receive smaller bolus increments than those in septic shock. The objective is to attain an adequate cardiac output and oxygen delivery while maintaining the lowest filling pressure possible for this goal. Decreasing oxygen demands, with pain control as an example, will relieve ischemia and may enhance contractility.

Right ventricular (RV) failure leading to cardiogenic shock may demonstrate elevated right atrial pressure and low cardiac output not otherwise explained by LV failure or cardiac tamponade. The most common causes of RV failure leading to shock are RV infarction and pulmonary embolism resulting in greatly increased RV afterload. Therapy includes fluid infusion and dobutamine. Atrioventricular sequential pacing may dramatically improve CO in cases of resultant bradycardia. Appropriate anticoagulation or fibrinolytic therapy should be performed as necessary (see Chap. 29 for more detail).

ACUTE VALVULAR DYSFUNCTION

The acute failure of an aortic or mitral valve may lead to cardiogenic shock. This most often occurs in the setting of infective endocarditis or as a complication of myocardial infarction. Sudden onset of pulmonary edema with a new murmur should prompt consideration of sudden valvular failure. The initial diagnosis is obtained with bedside echocardiography, followed by left heart catheterization if necessary. Management includes reducing LV afterload using drugs such as nitroprusside. Other anatomic processes associated with hypoperfusion include rupture of the ventricular septum leading to left to right shunting and acute obstruction of the mitral valve by left atrial thrombus or myxoma. Surgical management is typically required to reestablish hemodynamic stability in particularly severe cases. Initiation of inotropic drugs like dobutamine may cause a decrease in cardiac output or blood pressure as a result of a dynamic ventricular outflow tract obstruction, which can be demonstrated by echocardiography. The treatment for this is increasing preload and/or afterload and hence end-systolic volume.

CARDIAC ARRHYTHMIAS

Arrhythmias can aggravate hypoperfusion in shock states. Specific therapy warrants a specific diagnosis of the arrhythmia (see Chap. 28). Pain and drug withdrawal should be included in the differential diagnosis. Bradyarrhythmias contributing to shock may respond acutely to atropine, isopreterenol, and/or pacing. Hypoxia or ischemia should be sought as causes and treated.

CARDIAC TAMPONADE

Patients with tamponade are generally short of breath without pulmonary edema but have signs of elevated filling pressures, including jugular venous distentions, peripheral edema, and hepatojugular reflux. A pulsus paradox is often present and a friction rub may be heard on auscultation of the heart. The cardiac silhouette is often enlarged, sometimes in the classic "water-bottle" configuration. The electrocardiogram (ECG) may reveal low voltage, diffuse ST elevation (when pericarditis is present), or electrical alternans. Echocardiography is the diagnostic test of choice. Effusions can be readily identified and the signs of tamponade including diastolic right atrial and systolic ventricular collapse may be seen. Right heart catheterization can be used to confirm the diagnosis (equalization of pressures during diastole). Urgent relief of the tamponade with pericardiocentesis or a pericardial "window" must be accomplished in the hemodynamically unstable patient. While the patient is awaiting surgical therapy, great care must be taken to avoid hypovolemia. Vasoactive agents should be avoided.

DECREASED VENOUS RETURN—HYPOVOLEMIC SHOCK

Venous return to the right atrium may be inadequate due to decreased intravascular volume (hypovolemic shock); decreased tone of the venous capacitance bed so that mean systemic pressure is low (drugs, neurogenic shock); increased intrathoracic pressure (tension pneumothorax, intrinsic PEEP); and, rarely, increased venous resistance (obstruction of the inferior vena cava).

Hypovolemic shock consists of two categories—hemorrhagic and nonhemorrhagic. Trauma and gastrointestinal bleeding (reviewed in Chap. 59) are the most common causes of hemorrhagic shock. The initial urgent management includes placement of at least two large-bore intravenous catheters with the rapid infusion of warmed blood and crystalloid until circulation has been restored. In trauma, correction of the primary bleeding site is critical and must be undertaken as early as possible. Occult bleeding sites include the abdomen, retroperitoneum, thorax, and thighs. Gastrointestinal bleeding also requires early diagnosis and aggressive management with emergent upper endoscopy to look for sites of bleeding and treat them with electrocoagulation or sclerotherapy as appropriate. Diagnosis of lower gastrointestinal bleeding may require angiography, a radiolabeled bleeding scan, or direct visualization of the bleeding site. Therapies include endoscopic laser cautery, embolization, local infusion of vasoactive agents, sclerotherapy, or surgical extirpation of the bleeding segments.

Nonhemorrhagic etiologies of hypovolemic shock include gastrointestinal causes such as vomiting and diarrhea. Fluid replacement is critical in reestablishing adequate intravascular volume while ascertaining and treating the underlying cause. This may include antibiotics for infectious colitis or antiemetics for drug-induced emesis. Renal losses may occur from diabetes insipidus or excessive diuretic therapy. Other less common etiologies include burns, with excessive third-spacing of intravascular fluids and pancreatitis, which may lead to a change in capillary membrane permeability. Care is supportive in these cases.

HIGH CARDIAC OUTPUT HYPOTENSION—SEPTIC SHOCK

Septic shock causes reduced arterial vascular tone and reactivity, often associated with abnormal distribution of blood flow. Gram-negative bacilli are the cause in approximately two-thirds of cases, but only about one-third of patients develop gram-negative bacteremia. Clinically patients present with large pulse pressure, warm extremities, brisk nail-bed capillary filling, and low diastolic and mean blood pressure. Temperature and white blood cell counts are frequently abnormal. Systolic contractility may also be reduced. Sepsis may, of course exist in addition to cardiogenic or hypovolemic shock. Decreased arterial resistance is almost always observed in septic shock.

Initial therapy consists of fluid to correct the frequent hypovolemia of early septic shock (see Fig. 23-1). Blood transfusions will expand the intravascular space and increase oxygen-carrying capacity and therefore delivery. Early institution of antibiotic therapy is essential and should focus on likely pathogens. Early management should also include drainage of fluid collections such as intraabdominal, intrapelvic, or soft tissue abscesses, since antibiotics alone will not eradicate the infection. Antiendotoxin antibodies, anti–tumor necrosis factor antibodies, interleukin-1 receptor antagonists, and nonsteroidal anti-inflammatory drugs remain investigational. Corticosteroids are not efficacious.

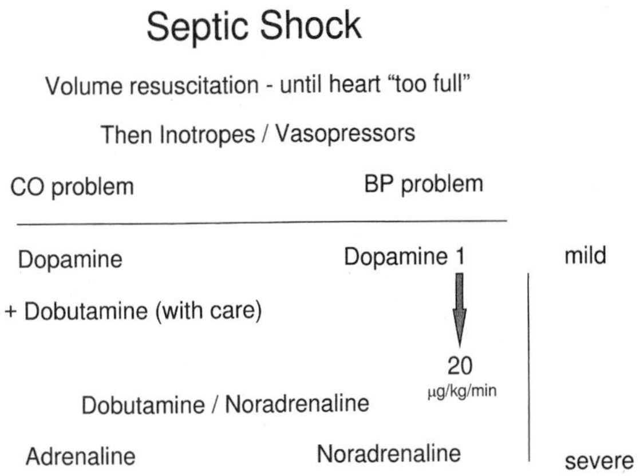
Septic Shock
Volume resuscitation - until heart "too full"
Then Inotropes / Vasopressors
CO problem
BP problem
Dopamine
Dopamine 1
mild
+ Dobutamine (with care)
20
μg/kg/min
Dobutamine / Noradrenaline
Adrenaline
Noradrenaline
severe

FIGURE 23-1 An approach to inotropic drug and vasoactive use in septic shock is illustrated. Initial volume resuscitation is rapidly taken to the endpoint of the heart "too full" to ensure that intravascular hypovolemia does not contribute further to the shock state. The patient is then reevaluated. If evidence of multiple organ hypoperfusion persists, inotropic vasoactive drugs should be used. If cardiac output and oxygen delivery are low or normal and blood pressure is adequate, dopamine (up to 5 μg/kg per minute) is started. Further increases in cardiac output can be accomplished using dobutamine (up to 20 μg/kg per minute). Be aware that if dobutamine is started before adequate volume resuscitation has corrected hypovolemia, significant further hypotension will occur. In contrast, if cardiac output is excessively high yet blood pressure is very low, noradrenaline can be started. Vasoconstrictor therapy with noradrenaline must be assessed by measuring the physiologic response (increased urine output, improved mentation, decreased lactate concentration), as the increase in blood pressure alone does not indicate therapeutic success. In fact, the increase in blood pressure will decrease cardiac output, so that increasing blood pressure beyond what is necessary to effect a salutary physiologic response is detrimental. If vasoconstriction does not improve the physiologic endpoints, it should be discontinued. A range of presentations combining various degrees of "low cardiac output" and "excessively low blood pressure" is typical of septic shock. Therefore, in severe shock, it is reasonable to combine dobutamine (for cardiac output) with noradrenaline (to maintain the minimum pressure required for physiologic flow distribution) or, in occasional instances, combined agents such as dopamine (up to 20 μg/kg per minute) or adrenaline. In every case the infusion rate is titrated down to the lowest rate that maintains the physiologic goal.

OTHER TYPES OF SHOCK

Anaphylactic shock should be considered in patients presenting with the appropriate clinical context of drug or contact exposure, ingestion, or insect bite. Signs and symptoms may include rhinorrhea, shortness of breath, cough, wheeze, stridor, chest tightness, cyanosis, dizziness, nonpitting edema, general skin itchiness, a feeling of impending doom, and hypotension. The release of histamine and other mediators leads to depressed systolic function, marked arterial vasodilation, and increased vascular permeability. Venous tone and therefore venous return are reduced, leading to hypotension. Therapy is fluid resuscitation and epinephrine, 0.05 to 0.1 mg intravenously every 1 to 5 minutes, as needed, and antihistamines and steroid as adjunctive therapy. Laryngeal edema may accompany anaphylaxis and may require early intubation if stridor is noted. Ultimately, removal of the offending agent or agents is definitive therapy.

Patients with neurogenic shock develop decreased vascular tone, particularly of the venous capacitance bed. Therapy consists of fluid resuscitation and catecholamines until circulating volume is repleted.

Adrenal insufficiency may result in shock or may be an important contributor to other forms of shock. Adrenal crisis occurs most commonly in patients who are suddenly withdrawn from chronic steroid therapy or who develop critical illness while receiving small but suppressive doses of corticosteriods. Less common causes include adrenal infarction or infection, such as meningococcemia. Although eosinophilia, hyponatremia, and hyperkalemia may be present these findings are not necessary to make the diagnosis. Often the hypotension of adrenal crisis is relatively refractory to fluid management until hormonal replacement is initiated. Diagnosis should be established by measuring serum cortisol and conducting a corticotropin stimulation test, with presumptive dexamethasone therapy, while awaiting results. Once the test is completed, hydrocortisone, 100 mg intravenously every 6 hours, should be substituted.

For a more detailed discussion, see Chaps. 19 and 20 in *Principles of Critical Care,* 2d ed.

Chapter 24

HYPOVOLEMIC SHOCK

GREGORY A. SCHMIDT

Pathophysiology

Hypovolemia is the state in which intravascular volume is insufficient to maintain systemic perfusion (cardiac output). The determinants of venous return (which equals cardiac output) are the mean systemic pressure (Pms), itself a function of the intravascular volume and the vascular capacitance; the right atrial pressure (Pra); and the resistance to venous return (Figs. 24-1, 24-2, and 24-3). A fall in intravascular volume reduces Pms, thereby reducing cardiac output. Systemic responses to hypovolemia include a reduction in venous compliance (venoconstriction) and Pra (through enhanced ventricular contractility) and, in the longer term, the retention of sodium by the kidneys. When these compensatory mechanisms are insufficient to maintain systemic perfusion, clinical abnormalities arise (Table 24-1). In the extreme case, hypovolemia causes shock and death (see Chap. 23).

Hypovolemia represents a final common path of innumerable primary disorders, including those listed in Table 24-2. In some patients intravascular fluid is lost directly from the body, while in others it may be sequestered within the third space. Patients with sepsis and other conditions may not have lost intravascular volume at all yet are hypovolemic owing to dilation of the venous circulation. At times, the left ventricle (LV) may be unable to fill for reasons unrelated to the systemic volume state, as in cardiac tamponade (Chap. 30), acute right heart syndromes (Chap. 29), severe LV diastolic dysfunction (Chap. 27), or valvular disease (Chap. 31), among others. Whether these patients are considered "hypovolemic" or not is a semantic issue, but the clinical and echocardiographic findings (in part) may mimic those of hypovolemia.

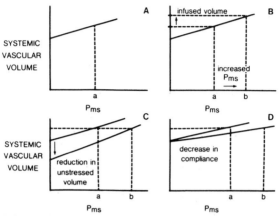

FIGURE 24-1 Mean systemic pressure (Pms) can be increased by the addition of stressed volume to the systemic vascular circuit (*a*). This can occur in three ways: *b*, an infusion of volume into the systemic vasculature; *c*, a reduction in the unstressed volume of the vasculature at constant intravascular volume, which occurs with baroreceptor reflexes, hypoxemia, elevation of the legs, or use of MAST trousers; and *d*, a decrease in systemic vascular compliance, which often accompanies baroreceptor reflexes. (Reproduced, with permission, from Goldberg H, and Rabson J: Control of the cardiac output by the systemic vessels. Am J Cardiol 47:696, 1981.)

Diagnosing Hypovolemia

Hypovolemia is confirmed when clinical abnormalities respond to fluids, yet predicting in advance whether an individual patient will respond positively is difficult. In one study of intensive care unit (ICU) patients with clinical signs suspicious for hypovolemia, the best predictor was the pulmonary wedge pressure (Ppw). Less useful were the central venous pressure and the right ventricular end-diastolic volume index (assessed with a modified pulmonary artery catheter). Even the correlation with Ppw was not very good, probably because one never knows the functional left ventricular compliance (the complex relationship between transmural pressure and ventricular volume), and the pleural pres-

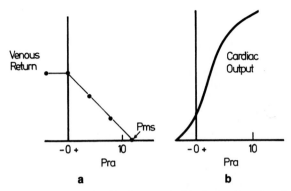

FIGURE 24-2   Relationships between Pra (abscissa) and: *a*, VR; and *b*, QT. In *a*, VR is 0 when Pra is equal to Pms; as Pra is decreased progressively, VR *increases* until Pra equals 0 along the VR curve, the slope of which is 1/RVR. At lower values of Pra, VR does not increase further, because of flow limitation in the collapsible great veins as they enter the thorax. In contrast, *b* shows that QT *decreases* as Pra decreases along the cardiac function curve, because end-diastolic volume decreases.

sure is generally not known. Because of these limitations, the "gold standard" for the diagnosis of hypovolemia is the response to fluids. Nearly every patient with suspected hypovolemia should be given a fluid challenge to test the hypothesis that the clinical abnormalities do, indeed, stem from hypovolemia, regardless of the Pra or Ppw. In critical settings, empiric fluid therapy should rarely if ever be delayed until central catheters can be inserted.

TABLE 24-1   Clinical Manifestations of Hypovolemia

Hypotension
Tachycardia
Oliguria, azotemia
Cool extremities, decreased capillary refill
Impaired mentation
Lactic acidosis

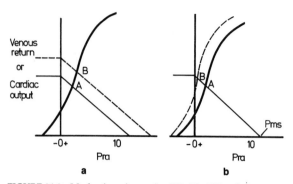

FIGURE 24-3 Mechanisms increasing VR. The VR and $\dot{Q}_T$ curves from Fig. 24-2 are replotted on the same axes (see continuous lines intersecting at point A). This intersection marks the unique value of Pra where VR equals $\dot{Q}_T$ in both Fig. 24-3a and b. When this value of $\dot{Q}_T$ is insufficient, VR can be increased by increasing Pms without changing RVR, indicated by the interrupted VR curve intersecting the unchanged $\dot{Q}_T$ curve at a higher $\dot{Q}_T$ and Pra (see B in Fig. 24-3a). In Fig. 24-3b, VR is increased from A to B by increased cardiac function (see interrupted cardiac function curve intersecting the original VR curve at B). Accordingly, inotropic agents that increase contractility can produce modest increases in VR by lowering Pra, but further increases are limited by compression of the great veins at lower values of Pra (see Fig. 24-3b); note that such enhanced cardiac function displaces central blood volume into the peripheral circulation, tending to increase Pms and so promote further increases in VR, as depicted in Fig. 24-3a. Often such inotropic agents (dopamine, epinephrine) also raise Pms by venoconstriction.

Treatment

The treatment of hypovolemia is, of course, restitution of the intravascular volume, generally through intravenous infusion of one of the fluids listed in Table 24-3. Despite many clinical studies and active debate, the selection of fluid remains more a matter of individual preference than science. Further, how to restore the intravascular volume likely varies depending on the particular patient. For example, in a well-known prospective trial of patients with penetrating trauma and a systolic blood pressure less than 90 mmHg, half were

TABLE 24-2   Causes of Hypovolemia

Loss of volume
  Traumatic hemorrhage
  Gastrointestinal hemorrhage
  Burns
  Vomiting
  Diarrhea
  Diuresis
Redistribution of volume (third-spacing)
  Sepsis
  Pancreatitis
  Systemic inflammatory response syndrome
  Cirrhosis
  Trauma
  Toxins
Increased venous capacitance
  Sepsis
  Drugs
  Spinal cord injury
  Anaphylaxis

---

randomized to conventional fluid resuscitation beginning in the field and continued until surgery while the other half had intravenous cannulas inserted but were given no fluid until they reached the operating room. The delayed-resuscitation group had better survival and shorter length of stay. Other studies have shown that choice of resuscitation fluid may affect microvascular blood flow, splanchnic perfusion, ventricular function, and vascular tone.

Crystalloid fluids remain in the vasculature for a very brief time. After a fluid challenge, about one-quarter of the infused fluid remains intravascularly after 1 h, even in normal subjects who have normal capillary permeability. Colloid fluids have the potential to stay within the vessels, minimizing fluid requirements and secondary tissue edema. On the other hand, if the microvasculature is leaky, colloids will pass through the vessel wall, enter the tissues, and act to draw further fluid into the interstitium. Colloids suffer from additional limitations: they are more expensive than crystalloids and may cause allergic reactions or coagulation disturbances. Although colloids are effective in restoring intravascular volume, no

TABLE 24-3　Choice of Fluids

Crystalloid
　Normal saline
　Lactated Ringer's
　Hypertonic saline (5% is available in the United States; 7.5% has
　　been used in clinical trials)
Colloid
　Albumin (5 and 25%)
　Dextran (D40 and D70)
　Hetastarch
　Pentastarch
　Gelofusine
Blood
　Fresh frozen plasma
　Whole blood
　Packed red blood cells

---

studies have demonstrated the superiority of any colloid as compared with crystalloid. Indeed, a metanalysis of available trials demonstrated an increased risk of mortality attributable to colloids.

Hypertonic saline has been advocated for treatment of patients with trauma, aortic aneurysmal rupture, head injury, sepsis, burns, and right ventricular infarction. Potentially beneficial effects, in addition to hyperosmolality (which tends to draw fluid out of the interstitium), include modulation of vessel tone, ventricular contractility, and improved immune function. Clinical trials to date do not support its use, however.

Blood products should be used for volume replacement only when the particular blood component is indicated, such as the transfusion of packed red blood cells for anemia (or acute massive hemorrhage) or fresh frozen plasma for coagulopathy. Once the blood product deficiency is corrected, further fluid therapy should consist of crystalloid.

When fluid is given for suspected hypovolemia, it should be infused rapidly, preferably through a large-bore catheter. The typical volume challenge given to critically ill patients is 500 mL of normal saline, but this small amount has a trivial impact on systemic hemodynamics and echocardiographic indices of ventricular filling. Whether larger volumes would be superior has not been studied. In general, a discrete, large-volume bolus should be given quickly while following relevant clinical measures of the response. If a patient fails to respond, either the amount of volume was insufficient or the hypothesis ("This patient is hypovolemic") was incorrect. Alternative explanations for the patient's clinical findings should be sought.

Ancillary therapies for hemodynamically significant hypovolemia include measures to reduce venous capacitance, such as military antishock trousers (MAST) and leg elevation, vasoactive drugs, and ventilator manipulations to reduce the pleural pressure (such as using small tidal volumes and reducing PEEP to the minimum level needed for adequate oxygenation). Vasoactive drugs are a poor substitute for effective volume replacement. When very large volumes of fluid are infused intravenously, a fluid warmer should be used to prevent cold-related coagulopathy.

For a more detailed discussion, see Chaps. 19 and 20 in *Principles of Critical Care*, 2d ed.

Chapter 25

SEPTIC SHOCK

BRIAN GEHLBACH

What Is Septic Shock?

BACKGROUND

Serious infection is a leading cause of mortality in most intensive care units (ICUs). Septic shock, defined as high-cardiac-output shock secondary to the vasodilatory effects of infection, carries a mortality of approximately 50%. The incidence of this problem has risen with the advent of chronic indwelling venous catheters, the continued introduction of new invasive procedures, advances in immunosuppression for organ transplantation, and medicine's ability to support increasing numbers of patients with single-organ failure.

DEFINITIONS

A familiarity with definitions is useful. SIRS, or systemic inflammatory response syndrome, refers to the body's response to any of a number of insults, including pancreatitis, trauma, or infection. By consensus, one or more of the following acute perturbations exist: (1) temperature $> 38°C$ or $< 36°C$; (2) pulse > 90; (3) respirations > 20 or $Pa_{CO_2} < 32$ mmHg; and (4) WBC $> 12,000/mm^3$, $< 4000/mm^3$, or $> 10\%$ immature forms. Sepsis is the SIRS secondary to infection. Severe sepsis includes hypotension, hypoperfusion, or organ dysfunction; septic shock is severe sepsis characterized by hypotension refractory to fluid administration and potentially accompanied by lactic acidosis, oliguria, or altered mental status.

PATHOGENESIS

Septic shock is typically caused by pyogenic bacteria, particularly gram-negative rods, which have endotoxin as a component of their cell walls. However, gram-positive cocci, fungi, mycobacteria, protozoa, rickettsia, and viruses are all capable of causing septic shock. To summarize the molecular events leading to the clinical effects of septic shock is a formidable task. Briefly, recognition of infectious organisms by mononuclear phagocytes causes the release of numerous cytokines such as interleukin-1 (IL-1) and tumor necrosis factor alpha (TNF-α). Intercellular signaling causes a cascade of events resulting in WBC activation and release from the bone marrow, fever, and migration of immune cells to the focus of infection. The complement system may be activated, leading to further leukocyte activation and chemotaxis. The release of proinflammatory mediators leads to increased vascular permeability and vasodilation. The coagulation and fibrinolytic systems may be activated. Systemic illness results either from an inability to contain an intense local infection, invasion of the intravascular space by the infecting organism with subsequent systemic activation, or by failure of normal counterregulatory components of the immune system.

PATHOPHYSIOLOGY

Cardiovascular effects occur early. Vasodilation reduces systemic vascular resistance, which results in a fall in the blood pressure if not accompanied by a compensatory increase in cardiac output. Some patients with early sepsis maintain an adequate blood pressure by increasing cardiac output through decreased resistance to venous return, which occurs as a consequence of systemic vasodilation. When loss of effective circulating volume becomes excessive, either through venous pooling of blood as a consequence of excessive venodilation or because of increased tissue permeability, hypotension results. This may occur more readily in the patient with diminished cardiovascular reserve. In fact, those patients with septic shock who are able to defend their blood pressure by augmenting cardiac output are more likely to survive. Myocardial depression occurs in sepsis but is not a prominent early feature.

There is conflicting evidence as to whether, despite supranormal delivery of oxygenated blood to the body as a whole, there are regional or even microcirculatory deficiencies in oxygen and nutrient delivery and utilization. Certainly end-organ dysfunction associated with hypotension would suggest a failure to supply vital organs adequately. Elevated lactate levels, commonly associated with septic shock, have also been used as evidence for ongoing anaerobic metabolism. However, lactic acidosis in septic shock is associated with a normal lactate:pyruvate ratio, arguing against this hypothesis. Similarly, the resuscitation of patients in septic shock often does not improve the lactic acidosis. Recent work has implicated potential cellular defects in sepsis responsible for elevated lactate levels. Finally, a number of trials designed to maximize oxygen delivery in patients with septic shock failed to show a survival benefit. Conceivably, the narrowed arteriovenous oxygen content difference in septic shock reflects a high cardiac output state without cellular hypoxia, while the multiorgan dysfunction is due to metabolic and immunologic effects of sepsis.

A number of other organ abnormalities may occur in septic shock. The lungs may develop low-pressure pulmonary edema, or acute respiratory distress syndrome (ARDS). Disseminated intravascular coagulation is not infrequent and carries a high mortality. Prerenal azotemia, as indicated by oliguria and rising creatinine, may occur. Gastrointestinal barrier function may fail, possibly secondary to regional ischemia, and result in translocation of bacteria with subsequent bacteremia. Central nervous system (CNS) dysfunction, manifest as encephalopathy, is common.

At the Bedside

CLINICAL PRESENTATION

The patient with sepsis commonly presents with obvious evidence of serious infection along with typical signs of sepsis, including fever or hypothermia, tachycardia, tachypnea, warm skin, mental status changes, and oliguria. The elderly or immunocompromised may present more subtly, often lacking fever or a readily apparent source of infection. Associated laboratory abnormalities include leukocytosis or leukopenia with increased numbers of immature cells, thrombocytopenia, and renal insufficiency. Blood gases may reveal respiratory alkalosis, metabolic acidosis, or mild hypoxemia.

The lactate level may be elevated as a consequence of hypoperfusion, dead gut, or ill-defined metabolic derangements found in sepsis.

Shock as a consequence of sepsis must be differentiated from other broad categories of shock; namely, hypovolemic and cardiogenic shock. The distinction clinically rests upon the ability of the physician to differentiate between high- and low-cardiac-output shock. Low-cardiac-output shock, either from hypovolemia or cardiac dysfunction, is associated with a narrowed pulse pressure, cool extremities, and delayed nail-bed return. Conversely, high-cardiac-output shock results in a widened pulse pressure, a much reduced diastolic pressure, warm extremities, and rapid nail-bed return. Evidence of gastrointestinal hemorrhage strengthens the diagnosis of hypovolemic shock, just as fever and cloudy urine support sepsis as the cause of shock.

If the clinical distinction between high- and low-cardiac-output shock is uncertain, it is useful to ask what does not fit with the scheme above and to use right heart catheterization and/or echocardiography to answer the question. The commonest reason for conflicting findings is that more than one mechanism for shock is present—e.g., in the elderly and dehydrated male with urosepsis, or the patient with pneumococcal bacteremia and cardiac dysfunction.

INITIAL RESUSCITATION (AT THE BEDSIDE)

The care of the patient with septic shock can be complex and labor-intensive. When one is called to evaluate such a patient, the first step is to concentrate on basic principles of resuscitation and *then* to perform a detailed evaluation. Prompt resuscitation is critical for preserving cerebral and renal function; it should be administered rationally and with specific goals in mind for each intervention. It is important to avoid the common practice of initiating many halfhearted therapies simultaneously; a bedside approach emphasizing hypothesis formation and immediate testing through measured interventions is far superior.

The primary survey of the patient with shock of any etiology is centered on restoration of the circulation and maintenance of the airway (the ABCs). A brief directed physical exam should be performed, emphasizing the security of the airway, the adequacy of respiration, and the presence and nature of shock (high- or low-output). Intravenous access should be established, ideally with 16-gauge intravenous lines. Except in cases of obvious volume overload, fluid boluses should be administered immediately. If hypervolemia is not suspected, 1 L of normal saline should be administered over 10 minutes and the patient's circulation reexamined. If the patient remains in shock, the therapy should be repeated. Failure to respond after several liters of normal saline may indicate the need for further investigation as to the cause of shock and/or vasoactive drug administration.

Respiratory support is critical. Oxygen should be administered by face mask to the alert patient. The patient with an insecure airway secondary to diminished sensorium should be intubated, as should patients with hypotension refractory to acute volume expansion. Intubation in the latter situation prevents the development of respiratory muscle fatigue generated by excessive metabolic demands (acidemia) on inadequately perfused muscles. In fact, studies in animals provide more support for the efficacy of mechanical ventilation in prolonging the survival of septic patients than for norepinephrine or dopamine.

Finally, the initial examination should include an evaluation of common potential infectious foci: the CNS, lungs, abdomen, genitourinary system, and indwelling catheter sites. A brief examination at this point is important for the time it saves in diagnosing and treating certain obvious and life-threatening conditions: meningitis, urosepsis, and appendicitis, for instance. Often the focus is not immediately apparent, necessitating additional examination and testing. Although the prompt institution of effective antimicrobial therapy is crucial, cardiorespiratory support should not be withheld while detailed investigations ensue.

Once the patient's circulation has been attended to, a more detailed evaluation is appropriate. At this time the clinician should perform a detailed physical examination with attention to potential foci of infection, evidence of end-organ dysfunction, and the response to initial resuscitation efforts. Any potentially infected fluid (i.e., pleural, ascitic, cerebrospinal, etc.) should be sampled and sent for Gram stain and culture.

Chest radiographs are always indicated, as are abdominal films in the presence of vomiting or abdominal pain. Blood and urine cultures are mandatory. Additional basic evaluation should include CBC, electrolytes, BUN, creatinine, liver function, PT/PTT, urinalysis, and lactate. Arterial blood gases are often helpful.

Details of Management

MAGIC BULLETS

As scientists' understanding of the immune system's response to severe infection has evolved, numerous agents have been designed to interrupt various steps in the host response in order to prevent or arrest septic shock. To date more than a dozen pharmacologic agents have been tested in randomized, placebo-controlled clinical trials, and none has convincingly shown any benefit. These include corticosteroids, antibodies to TNF-α, TNF receptor:Fc fusion protein, antibody to endotoxin, and others. Although new agents are continually being tested (i.e., nitric oxide–synthase inhibitors), there is no magic bullet for septic shock at this time, and therapy is supportive.

IDENTIFYING AND TREATING
THE SOURCE URGENTLY

Most infections arise from the CNS, chest, genitourinary system, an intraabdominal viscus, or soft tissues. In considering the source of infection, a familiarity with common organisms and their presentations is helpful (Table 25-1).

The most common infection in the chest is acute bacterial community-acquired pneumonia. *Streptococcus pneumoniae* is highly prevalent and pyogenic. Other highly pyogenic organisms causing pneumonia and shock include enteric gram-negative bacilli, *Legionella pneumophila*, and *Staphylococcus aureus*. An empyema may be present, necessitating drainage for control of sepsis. Lung abscesses are necrotizing infections commonly resulting from aspiration of anaerobic bacteria but also arising from *Staph. aureus*, *Pseudomonas aeruginosa*, *Klebsiella pneumoniae*, *Mycobacterium tuberculosis*, and group A streptococci. Other chest infections commonly result from invasive procedures. These include mediastinitis following cardiac surgery and following esophageal perforation during esophagogastroduodenoscopy.

CNS infections can be divided into those occurring in normal hosts, those associated with neurosurgical procedures or devices, and those associated with immunocompromised states. Meningitis is the most common CNS infection associated with shock, and the most likely serious CNS infection in normal hosts. The most prevalent organisms in community-acquired adult meningitis are *Strep. pneumoniae, Neisseria meningitidis,* and *Haemophilus influenzae.* Fever, nuchal rigidity, photophobia, and depressed sensorium are likely to be present. Petechial rash is often found in meningococcemia, which presents fulminantly and sometimes before the development of meningismus. Patients who have undergone neurosurgical procedures are at risk for meningitis from hospital-acquired organisms, including *Staph. aureus, P. aeruginosa,* and enteric gram-negative bacilli. Opportunistic infections such as those caused by viruses and fungi certainly may be life-threatening, but are uncommon causes of shock.

Skin and soft tissue infections are most commonly caused by *Staph. aureus* and *Strep. pyogenes,* with *Strep. pneumoniae,* other streptococci, and gram-negative bacilli found less often. Gram-negative bacilli are important causes of infection in hospitalized patients and intravenous drug users. Anaerobic cellulitis causes extensive destruction at the site of devitalized tissue but is not a common cause of systemic toxicity as long as the diagnosis is made sufficiently early. Necrotizing fasciitis usually develops in chronically ill patients following minor trauma or in surgical wounds or decubitus ulcers. Limb necrosis occurs rapidly, and systemic toxicity may be severe. Polymicrobic infection from mixed anaerobic and aerobic organisms predominates, though *Strep. pyogenes* is increasingly isolated. Surgical debridement and drainage are mandatory.

Intraabdominal infections may arise from gastrointestinal or genitourinary sources. Gastrointestinal sources include the biliary tract, bowel, pancreas, or spontaneously infected peritoneal fluid. Suppurative cholangitis occurs in the presence of obstructed bile ducts and requires drainage either surgically, percutaneously, or endoscopically. Septic shock secondary to bowel disease usually results from perforation with

TABLE 25-1 Major Bacterial Infection Syndromes Associated with Septic Shock

Infection Syndrome	Common Bacterial Pathogens
Primary bacteremia	
Community-acquired infection in the normal host	*Staphylococcus aureus*
	Streptococcus pneumoniae
	Neisseria meningitidis
	Salmonella species
IV drug abusers, infected IV access in hospital and granulocytopenia	*S. aureus*
	Pseudomonas aeruginosa
	Enterobacteriaceae
Bacteremic meningitis	*N. meningitidis*
	S. pneumoniae
Acute bacterial pneumonia	
Community-acquired	*S. pneumoniae*
	S. aureus
	Enterobacteriaceae
	Legionella pneumophila
Hospital-acquired	Enterobacteriaceae
	P. aeruginosa
	S. aureus
	Legionella species

Mediastinitis	Mixed aerobic and anaerobic bacteria
Intraabdominal sepsis and urosepsis	
Supporative cholangitis and cholecystitis	Mixed enteric aerobic and anaerobic bacteria, including the Enterobacteriaceae, streptococci, and *Bacteroides fragilis* groups
Peritonitis (from perforation)	
Mesenteric ischemia	
Abscess (peritoneal, pancreatic, perihepatic, etc.)	
Septic abortion, endometritis	
Pyelonephritis, pyonephrosis, renal and perinephric abscess	Enterobacteriaceae Enterococcus Pseudomonas species
Skin and soft tissue infections	
Simple cellulitis or erysipelas with bacteremia	*S. aureus* *Streptococcus pyogenes*
Cellulitis in IV drug users	*P. aeruginosa* *S. aureus*
Necrotizing cellulitides and fasciitis	Mixed enteric aerobic and anaerobic bacteria (following major skin breakdown and contamination) *S. pyogenes* (occurring primarily or following trivial skin breaks)

301

resulting fecal peritonitis. Primary peritonitis occurs in the setting of cirrhosis of the liver, peritoneal dialysis, or congestive heart failure. Mesenteric ischemia classically presents with pain out of proportion to examination findings and with significant lactic acidosis. Potential infectious agents for all of these syndromes include enteric gram-negative bacilli, mixed enteric anaerobic bacteria such as *Clostridia* and *Bacteroides fragilis,* and aerophilic streptococci. Genitourinary sources include pyelonephritis, usually associated with obstruction. Emphysematous pyelonephritis typically occurs in patients with uncontrolled diabetes and urinary obstruction. Gram-negative organisms such as *Escherichia coli* predominate, but enterococci are not uncommon. Infections associated with pregnancy or parturition include endometritis and septic abortion. Gram-negative rods, anaerobes, and gram-positive cocci are all potential causes. Recovery of the patient with septic abortion relies on adequate evacuation of the uterus.

Septic shock without obvious localizing signs or symptoms may occur. There are several possibilities in these patients. The first is primary bacteremia, such as that associated with endocarditis or splenic dysfunction or removal. The normal host typically is infected with *Staph. aureus, Strep. pneumoniae,* or *N. meningitidis.* Patients lacking spleens are at risk for these infections plus those caused by *H. influenzae* and *Salmonella.* Bacteremia from *Staph. aureus, P. aeruginosa,* and Enterobacteriaceae occurs in injection drug users and in patients with indwelling vascular catheters. Patients receiving cytotoxic chemotherapy for malignancy are at particular risk for primary bacteremia, either as a consequence of catheter infection or from bacterial translocation occurring in the gastrointestinal tract. Alternatively, the absence of an obvious focus of infection may reflect the host's inability to mount an effective immune response, as occurs in aging, malnourishment, or with immunosuppressive drug use. Finally, noninfectious causes for septic-like shock should be considered, as discussed below.

Urgent empirical antimicrobial therapy should be directed at all potential infectious sources of more than trivial probability. Table 25-2 gives suggested regimens for the most frequently encountered life-threatening infections. When empiric therapy is necessary, it is useful to consider both host and environmental factors in selecting an antibiotic regimen. For example, the patient with known terminal complement deficiency should be covered for *N. meningitidis,* just as an individual with a biliary drain should be given antibiotics with adequate anaerobic activity. Similarly, environmental factors influence the choice of antibiotic. The patient who develops fever, tachypnea, and consolidation on chest examination 10 days after admission has acquired pneumonia in the hospital and should be covered for enteric gram-negative organisms and *P. aeruginosa.* As a rule of thumb, all antibiotic regimens for the patient in septic shock should include coverage for *Staph. aureus* and common enteric gram-negative organisms.

SURGICAL INTERVENTION

Surgical management is the cornerstone of therapy for many infections. Examples include (1) an obstructed hollow viscus, (2) empyema, (3) mediastinitis, (4) necrotizing fasciitis, (5) bowel infarction, and (6) septic abortion. Antibiotics and cardiovascular support are *adjunctive* therapies, serving only to support the patient while definitive surgical management is undertaken. The suspicion of any of these conditions should prompt urgent surgical consultation, as the patient is unlikely to improve until the focus of infection is either drained, removed, or debrided. In most cases this intervention should be delayed only until such time as the patient has undergone essential resuscitation and should not wait for the antibiotics to cure the patient. In many cases an extensive operation need not be performed initially; an infected gallbladder may be drained percutaneously or a necrotizing soft-tissue infection debrided at the bedside. This allows the unstable patient to remain in the ICU while still allowing pus or devitalized tissue to be removed.

CARDIOVASCULAR SUPPORT WITH VOLUME, VASOACTIVE DRUGS, AND MECHANICAL VENTILATION

The goal of cardiovascular support is to augment the perfusion of vital organs such as the brain, gut, and kidney while limiting the adverse effects of fluid and vasoactive

TABLE 25-2 Empiric Antimicrobial Therapy for Septic Shock

Suspected Source of Sepsis	Recommended Antimicrobial Regimen	Alternative Agents
Primary bacteremia (no source evident) Normal host	Third-generation cephalosporin: Cefotaxime 2 g IV q6h or Ceftriaxone 2 g IV q12h or Ceftizoxime 2 g IV q8h	Nafcillin and gentamicin, chloramphenicol and gentamicin, piperacillin/tazobactam, imipenem
IV drug user	Ceftazidime 2 g IV q8h and Nafcillin 2 g IV q4h	Piperacillin/tazobactam or imipenem and gentamicin
Immunocompromised host	Piperacillin 3 g IV q4h and Gentamicin 1.5 mg/kg IV q8h	Ceftazidime and nafcillin, imipenem and gentamicin
Bacteremic meningitis	Third-generation cephalosporin as above	Ampicillin, chloramphenicol
Cellulitis/erysipelas	Nafcillin 2 g IV q4h	Cefazolin, vancomycin, clindamycin
Streptococcal necrotizing fasciitis or toxic shock syndrome	Clindamycin 600 mg IV q8h	Penicillin or a cephalosporin
Acute bacterial pneumonia Community-acquired	Third-generation cephalosporin as above ± erythromycin 1 g IV q6h	Clinamycin and cotrimoxazole Piperacillin/tazobactam or imipenem ± erythromycin

Hospital-acquired	Ceftazidime 2 g IV q8h and gentamicin 1.5 mg/kg IV q8h ± erythromycin 1 g IV q6h	Clindamycin and ciprofloxacin Piperacillin/taxobactam or imipenem and gentamicin ± erythromycin
Mixed aerobic/anaerobic infections Intraabdominal infections Mediastinitis Fulminant aspiration pneumonia Necrotizing cellulitides and fasciitis Septic abortion, endometritis	Third-generation cephalosporin and clindamycin 600 mg IV q8h OR Metronidazole 500 mg IV q8h and ampicillin 2 g IV q4h and gentamicin 1.5 mg/kg IV q8h	Imipenem or piperacillin/tazobactam and gentamicin, cefoxitin and gentamicin, clindamycin and cotrimoxazole
Urinary tract infection	Ampicillin 2 g IV q4h and gentamicin 1.5 mg/kg IV q8h	Third-generation cephalosporin ± gentamicin

drug administration. Each intervention should be measured for its effects not only on the blood pressure but also on the perfusion of vital organ systems. For the kidney, urine output and serum creatinine are useful indicators of adequate perfusion. For the gut, tolerance of tube feedings and mucosal perfusion as measured by gastric tonometry are helpful. For the brain, the sensorium is followed.

Because septic shock decreases effective circulating volume by increasing venous capacitance via systemic vasodilation as well as by increasing vascular permeability, large volumes of fluid are required to reestablish and maintain effective circulating volume during initial resuscitation. Often, 3 L of normal saline administered in 20 to 30 minutes does not raise the blood pressure, while twice that volume begins to elevate the jugular venous pulse (or pulmonary capillary wedge pressure, if this is monitored). Volume resuscitation may include transfusion of packed red blood cells, particularly for patients with poor cardiovascular or respiratory reserve and a hemoglobin concentration of 10.0 g/dL or less. An undesired side effect of volume infusion is edema accumulation in soft tissues. This edema may complicate patient management by impairing gas exchange in the lung, preventing adequate gastrointestinal absorption of medicines and nutrients, interfering with wound healing, and making the establishment of intravenous access difficult. Once vascular permeability has been restored, the edema can be aggressively mobilized with colloid infusions, diuresis, or ultrafiltration.

If the blood pressure remains low or organ hypoperfusion persists despite restoration of an adequate circulating volume, vasoactive drugs are administered. Most studies of the effects of vasoactive drugs have measured such secondary endpoints as total body oxygen delivery or consumption and have ignored their effects on regional blood flow. Thus, dopamine has enjoyed a long run as the agent of choice for septic shock due to its ability to increase systemic vascular resistance without decreasing cardiac output as well as for its perceived ability to increase renal blood flow. Dobutamine was also utilized in patients with cardiac dysfunction, and norepinephrine was avoided because of its deleterious effects on renal and splanchnic blood flow in normal subjects. However, recent studies have provided new insight into the regional effects of these drugs. Although dopamine is capable of increasing urine volumes, it does not improve renal function as measured by creatinine clearance, nor does it raise intramucosal gastric pH. Other studies have suggested that dopamine and epinephrine adversely affect splanchnic blood flow as compared with dobutamine and norepinephrine.

Thus, dobutamine and norepinephrine are now the drugs of choice for the treatment of septic shock (Fig. 25-1). Dobutamine may be used first, particularly in the patient with suspected cardiac dysfunction. Starting doses of 2.5 μg/kg per minute are used and titrated at increments of the same until an adequate circulation is restored, no further benefit is achieved, or a dose of 10 μg/kg/min is reached. At this point norepinephrine is begun, starting at 0.1 μg/kg/min. Doses of dobutamine in excess of 10 μg/kg/min may be used but are associated with greater arrhythmogenesis. Norepinephrine must be administered through a central line to prevent tissue necrosis in the event of extravasation. Vasopressin and angiotensin have been shown to increase blood pressure in septic patients in recent small studies. One study of vasopressin found surprisingly low levels of this hormone in septic patients. Infusion of small amounts of vasopressin to achieve "normal" levels generated a significant increase in blood pressure. This potential deficiency of vasopressin in septic shock deserves further investigation.

The role of mechanical ventilation in the treatment of septic shock should not be overlooked, since this therapy may (1) reduce the load on inadequately perfused respiratory muscles; (2) decrease total body oxygen consumption, also through respiratory muscle rest; (3) protect the airway in the patient with deteriorating mental status; (4) allow for the delivery of higher concentrations of oxygen and PEEP in the patient with hypoxemic respiratory failure; and (5) facilitate respiratory compensation of the anion gap metabolic acidosis so common in septic shock.

Bicarbonate therapy in lactic acidosis from septic shock enjoyed widespread popularity until the last 15 years or so. Since then its two purported salutory effects—restoring myocardial contractility and reducing ventilatory load in the acidemic patient—have not been demonstrated in numerous

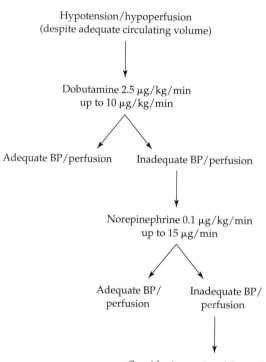

FIGURE 25-1 The use of vasoactive drugs in septic shock.

animal models and a few trials in humans. Bicarbonate therapy is not superior to saline administration in improving cardiac output and may worsen intracellular acidosis as well as ventilatory demands through the generation of increased CO_2 through bicarbonate metabolism. At this time bicarbonate therapy should be reserved for patients in whom increased bicarbonate losses are operative, as in renal tubular acidosis or diarrhea. At this time it is not recommended for use in lactic acidosis.

The overreliance of physicians on pulmonary artery (PA) catheters has been criticized, especially given several studies showing no effect or even a negative effect of this monitoring device on patient outcome. The use of pulmonary artery catheters can still be defended in the management of shock, but only when used rationally and with clear goals in mind. Patients with septic shock for whom PA catheters may be useful include (1) those with significant coexisting cardiac or renal disease, prohibiting the indiscriminant use of fluids; (2) patients who fail to respond to empiric therapy of septic shock with aggressive fluid resuscitation and/or vasoactive drug administration; and (3) patients in whom confounding causes of shock are suspected.

Management of body temperature in the septic patient deserves comment. In most cases, hypothermia is mild and best treated by blankets. Most patients with fever require no specific therapy either. However, patients with life-threatening tissue hypoxia as judged by an abnormally low mixed venous oxygen saturation may be compromised by the inordinate metabolic demands of fevers in excess of 40°C. These patients should be given acetaminophen. Cooling the patient with fans or tepid baths may be deleterious by producing shivering. If cooling of the patient is still desired, meperidine 25 to 50 mg IV or IM may be given to inhibit shivering and allow continued cooling. Muscle relaxation (in the sedated patient) may allow cooling without shivering as well as further reduce the work of breathing in the mechanically ventilated patient.

SUPPORT OF OTHER ORGANS

Renal dysfunction is common in septic shock. Preservation of renal function does not rely on one specific therapy but rather on preservation of adequate perfusion and avoidance of additional insults. Aminoglycosides and intravenous contrast are two examples of poorly tolerated incremental insults in the septic patient and should be used with caution. Electrolyte abnormalities, including hyponatremia and hypocalcemia, are common. The former is usually of the euvolemic or hypervolemic variety and can often be corrected by reconstituting the patient's numerous intravenous infusions in half-normal or normal saline rather than in D_5W. Ionized

TABLE 25-3   Causes of Persistent Vasodilatory Shock

Wrong source/missed source
Wrong antibiotic or dose
Sequestered space with inadequate drainage (pleura, sinuses,
   intraabdominal abscess)
New infection
Noninfectious cause (Table 25-4)

---

hypocalcemia, unlike hypocalcemia resulting from hypoalbuminemia, is relatively uncommon and should probably not
be treated in the asymptomatic patient, given recent studies
showing a potentially negative effect of therapy on outcome.

Hematologic support is limited in scope. Although thrombocytopenia secondary to reduced platelet survival is common, significant bleeding from this alone is uncommon.
Platelet transfusion should be reserved for those patients with
active bleeding and platelet counts below $50,000/\mu L$ or when
the platelet count is under $10,000/\mu L$. Correction of anemia
is dictated by cardiovascular reserve, as described above. Disseminated intravascular coagulation may complicate septic
shock; it is dealt with in Chap. 48.

Nutritional support should be instituted early. The route
should always be enteral, if possible, as long as the source of
sepsis is not in the gastrointestinal system. This may be accomplished most easily by the passage of a feeding tube into
the duodenum. Many factors confound enteral feeding, including the use of opiates for pain control and sedation, im-

TABLE 25-4   Noninfectious Causes of High-Cardiac-
Output Shock

Liver failure
Arteriovenous shunts (Paget's disease, dialysis, grafts)
Thyroid storm
Adrenal insufficiency
Severe pancreatitis
Anaphylaxis
Delirium tremens

---

paired absorption of medicines and nutrients from edematous gut secondary to fluid administration, and the presence of an ileus from sepsis itself. If enteral feeding is contraindicated or unsuccessful, parenteral nutrition should be supplied. Nonetheless, the initiation of parenteral nutrition should not dissuade the physician from frequent attempts to use the gut for feeding. Metoclopropamide or cisapride may be useful agents when gastric emptying is delayed.

WHEN THE PATIENT DOES NOT IMPROVE

Unfortunately, seemingly definitive antibiosis, cardiovascular support, and surgical therapy (if indicated) may result in a persistently septic patient. At this time a fresh look at the diagnosis and management should ensue. Possibilities for failure to respond include (Table 25-3) (1) wrong source/missed source, (2) wrong antibiotic or dose, (3) infection in a sequestered space (i.e., pleural space, sinuses, or intraabdominal abscess), (4) the development of a new infection, or (5) failure to recognize a noninfectious cause (in part or sum) of shock—for example, coexisting cardiac or hypovolemic shock, or vasodilatory shock from some noninfectious cause (Table 25-4).

Conclusions

As the search for a magic bullet for septic shock continues, the contemporary management of this highly prevalent and fatal disorder remains labor-intensive. The mainstays of therapy include recognition and removal of infected material, antibiotic therapy, cardiovascular support with fluid and vasoactive drug administration, mechanical ventilation, and supportive therapy to prevent further organ system failure until such time as the infection is controlled.

For a more detailed discussion, see Chaps. 20 and 42 in *Principles of Critical Care*, 2d ed.

Chapter 26

ISCHEMIC HEART DISEASE AND THROMBOLYTIC THERAPY

IVOR S. DOUGLAS

In patients with noncardiac critical illness, the common manifestations of myocardial ischemia and infarction may be subtle or absent. Severe multisystem illnesses precipitate substantial disturbances in myocardial oxygen demand and supply. The critical care physician must maintain a high index of suspicion for myocardial ischemia in the hemodynamically unstable patient in the intensive care unit (ICU) setting. This chapter reviews the diagnosis and management of myocardial ischemic syndromes and acute myocardial infarction, with particular emphasis on the critically ill patient.

Appreciation of *heart rate, myocardial wall stress,* and *contractility* directs pathophysiologic assessments and appropriate therapeutic interventions.

Myocardial Ischemia

DIAGNOSIS OF MYOCARDIAL ISCHEMIA

The *clinical* identification of myocardial ischemia in the ICU is frequently limited by an atypical presentation and limited communication with sedated, cognitively compromised, and often intubated patients. When identified, myocardial ischemia is most commonly manifest as constant substernal *chest tightness* or pressure, typically left-sided, which may radiate to the throat, jaw, or left arm. Accompanying dysautonomic features of *dyspnea* and *diaphoresis* are not infrequently confused with other sources of distress in these patients, including

TABLE 26-1 Nonischemic Causes of Chest Pain

Pericarditis
Pleuritis or pneumothorax
Dissecting aortic aneurysm
Pulmonary embolism
Gastroesophageal reflux
Peptic ulcer disease
Perihepatitis and biliary disease
Herpes zoster
Tietze's syndrome (costochondritis)

---

respiratory compromise and septic states. Nonischemic chest pain (see Table 26-1) frequently confuses the evaluation.

Silent myocardial ischemia results from brief durations of coronary insufficiency and altered pain perception. Episodes of silent ST segment depression may be associated with ischemia, impaired LV function, and dysrhythmia and should prompt evaluation.

Examination of the precordium may demonstrate the presence of a fourth heart sound, the emergence of a mitral regurgitant murmur, a third heart sound, an elevated jugular venous pressure, or pulmonary crackles. The absence of a third heart sound does not preclude increased left ventricular end-diastolic pressure (LVEDP).

Chest x-ray may demonstrate features of upper-lobe vascular redistribution, Kerley B lines, azygos vein prominence, or presence of noncardiac pathology (e.g., pneumothorax). The combined prognostic implications of these signs of elevated LVEDP are formulated as the Killip classification (Table 26-2).

The *electrocardiographic* (ECG) abnormalities in myocardial ischemia are widely variable. T-wave changes in the leads reflecting the anatomic area of myocardium in jeopardy are the first ECG changes. If the occlusion of the coronary vessel is complete, the T wave is peaked. Previously flattened or inverted T waves may revert, masking ischemic changes— the so-called pseudonormalization of T waves. Hyperacute ST-segment elevation is indicative of transmural ischemia.

TABLE 26-2 Killip Classification of Myocardial Infarction

Class	I	IIa	IIb	III	IV
Clinical findings	No crackles No S3	Crackles < 50% No S3	Crackles < 50% S3 present	Crackles > 50% Pulmonary edema	Shock
Percent of patients per class	30–40	20–30	10–20	5–10	10
30-day MR (OR vs. Killip I)	2–4	3–5	10–15	4.4 (CI, 3.3–5.7)	7.9 (CI, 5.9–10.5)
in-hospital MR,[a] (%)				45	80–90

[a]Pre–thrombolytic era mortality.

ABBREVIATIONS: MR, mortality rate; OR, odds ratio.

Complexes with ST depression may be associated with less discrete areas of jeopardized myocardium and may not evolve typical Q waves despite extensive myocardial injury (non–Q wave infarction). Q waves represent ECG windows through underlying infarcted myocardium. Posterior and right ventricular infarctions are often "silent" on the 12-lead ECG. Right ventricular precordial lead (V_{3R} to V_{5R}) and/or posterior thoracic lead (V_9 to V_{11}) traces should always be obtained in the presence of inferior distribution infarction (II, III, aVF).

Conduction disturbances reflecting sinoatrial (SA) or atrioventricular (AV) nodal ischemia—such as first-degree AV block, sinus or junctional bradycardia, or complete heart block with a narrow QRS complex—are associated with occlusion of the right coronary artery. Occlusion of the left anterior descending coronary artery may lead to right bundle branch block (RBBB), LBBB, or bifasicular block. Ventricular ectopic beats, bigeminy, and ventricular arrhythmias are common during ischemic episodes. Supraventricular arrhythmias can also occur in ischemic syndromes. Atrial fibrillation accompanies acute myocardial infarction (MI) approximately 10 to 15% of the time.

Enzyme diagnosis of myocardial ischemic syndromes is summarized in Table 26-3. Cardiac troponins provide extremely sensitive and specific enzymatic markers of myocardial injury. Troponins T and I are released from ischemic or infarcted cardiac myocytes and are detectable in serum 3 to 12 hours after the onset of ischemia. False-positive elevations are seen in renal failure.

Creatine kinase (CK) remains a most useful and reliable enzyme determination for MI. CK released from the myocardium begins to appear in the plasma within 4 to 8 hours after onset of infarction. To be diagnostic for MI, total plasma CK must be above the upper limit of normal and must be at least 3.0% MB fraction. Therapeutic interventions should not be delayed pending assay results. Some of the causes of false-positive elevations of CK-MB include myocarditis, pericarditis, myocardial trauma, hyperthermia, hypothermia, renal failure, hypothyroidism, subarachnoid hemorrhage, rhabdomyolysis, abdominal surgery, and tumors.

TABLE 26-3   Molecular Markers of Myocardial Necrosis

	Times to initial increase (range)	Time to peak (mean)	Time to Return to Normal Range	Typical Sampling Schedule after Onset
Myoglobin	1–4 h	6–7 h	24 h	Frequent: 1–2 hourly
cTN-I	3–12 h	24 h	5–10 days	Once; On admission
cTN-T	3–12 h	12 h–2 days	5–14 days	Once; On admission
CK-MB	3–12 h	24 h	48–72 h	On admission and q3 hourly—12 h
LDH	10 h	24–48 h	10–14 h	Once > 24 h
AST	3–12 h	36–48 h	48–72 h	Once > 24 h

ABBREVIATIONS: cTN-I, cardiac troponin I; cTN-T, cardiac troponin T; CK-MB, creatine kinase MB isoenzyme; LDH, lactate dehydrogenase; AST, aspartate transaminase.

SOURCE: Donnelly R, Millar-Craig MW Cardiac troponins: IT upgrade for the heart. *Lancet* 351:537-9.

Serum lactate dehydrogenase (LDH) is of utility in diagnosing infarction when the normal pattern of LDH isoenzyme 2 > LDH isoenzyme 1 is inverted ("flip" to LDH1 > LDH2). LDH and aspartate transaminases (ASTs) are less specific markers but may indicate more remote infarction.

Transthoracic or transesophageal echocardiography can detect discrete segmental wall-motion abnormalities of the left ventricle, suggesting ischemia or mitral regurgitation secondary to papillary muscle dysfunction, and can rule out other diagnoses, such as right ventricular infarction, aortic dissection, cardiac tamponade, mural thrombus, and pericarditis (see Chap. 35).

Radionuclide studies of myocardial perfusion, utilizing technetium 99m sestamibi or thallium 201, are important adjuncts to the diagnosis of myocardial ischemic syndromes in the critically ill. Studies may be performed in conjunction with dipyridamole, adenosine, or dobutamine pharmacologic stress to accentuate regional areas of abnormal perfusion. Radionuclide angiography and evaluation of regional wall motion can augment this approach.

Treatment of Unstable Angina

Anginal chest pain or anginal equivalent of recent onset, occurring at rest or not responding to previous doses of antianginal medications, is characterized as unstable angina. There is a moderately high probability of the development of a MI within the next few days. Therapy is aimed at optimizing heart rate, myocardial wall stress, and contractility to improve myocardial metabolism. The "open artery" principle is vital in improving the outcome after MI. Flow in the obstructed vessel should be restored without delay, and patency should be maintained to improve the patient's prognosis and reduce morbidity.

Antiplatelet therapy underpins the immediate management of acute coronary syndromes, including unstable angina. Aspirin for patients presenting with unstable angina reduces the incidence of refractory angina, MI, and cardiac death. It should be used routinely in all patients with unstable angina. A single soluble tablet of 164 or 325 mg, taken immediately and daily thereafter, is sufficient to effectively inhibit platelet activity. Patients intolerant of aspirin may be started on ticlopidine 250 mg twice per day as a substitute. Monitoring for GI intolerance and neutropenia is essential. Concomitant administration of glycoprotein IIb/IIIa receptor antagonists with aspirin and heparin is being investigated.

Nitroglycerin (NTG) is efficacious, with a rapid onset of action, and is a mainstay of therapy for unstable angina. NTG decreases myocardial wall stress by decreasing preload. At higher doses, afterload reduction and epicardial coronary dilation are seen. *Sublingual* doses of 0.4 mg may be administered every 50 to 10 minutes to a total of three doses, if required, to control pain. Frequent blood pressure checks are required. Should hypotension develop, the patient is placed in the Trendelenburg position and given intravenous saline boluses. *Topical* nitroglycerin ointment, 0.5 to 2 in. every 6 to 8 hours, may be applied after angina has resolved with sublingual doses. If pain persists despite three sublingual NTG tablets and initiation of β-blocker therapy (when possible), *intravenous* nitroglycerin may be initiated, commencing at 10 to 20 μg/min and titrated upward at 10- to 20-μg/min increments every 5 to 10 minutes until pain resolves or the systemic systolic pressure is 95 to 110 mmHg. Maximal therapeutic dosing is 400 μg/min. Isosorbide dinitrate in doses up to 3 mg every 5 to 10 minutes is also efficacious.

Narcotics can be given as the dose of nitroglycerin is being titrated upward. Morphine acts as a potent venodilator, thus decreasing left ventricular preload, and is of marked benefit when pulmonary edema is present. Morphine can increase vagal tone, which, in the setting of inferior wall MI, can lead to bradycardia. Hydromorphone (1 to 3 mg) is more potent than morphine and less vagotonic.

Beta blockade is of critical importance, especially in the setting of angina with tachycardia and hypertension. Negative inotropic and chronotropic effects confer substantial benefit on myocardial oxygen consumption, which correlates with measurable reductions in progression to acute myocardial infarction (AMI). Beta blockers are relatively contraindicated in patients with marginal blood pressure, bradycardia, atrioventricular (AV) conduction disturbances, left ventricular failure, and *active* asthmatic bronchospasm. Short-acting esmolol is useful in patients with the potential for hemodynamic instability. Otherwise, metoprolol at a dose of 15 mg intravenously over 15 to 20 minutes in 5-mg increments until the heart rate is between 60 and 70 beats per minute is preferred provided that the systolic blood pressure does not fall below 95 mmHg. Thereafter, 25 to 50 mg every 6 hours is given orally.

Calcium-channel blockers (CCBs) may relieve the component of epicardial coronary artery occlusion due to vasospasm by direct dilation of vascular smooth muscle. The role of CCBs remains extremely controversial in coronary artery disease (CAD) because of the adverse outcomes seen in MI. CCBs should be avoided in patients with pulmonary edema or evidence of LV dysfunction. Nifedipine is preferred for vasospasm and when angina persists despite nitrates, β blockers, and narcotics because it has the least cardiodepressant action (along with nicardipine). Nifedipine must *not* be used without concomitant β blockade. A rapid fall in blood pressure can occur with nifedipine, so hypotension should be anticipated. Diltiazem has been used favorably for the management of unstable angina, and is at least as efficacious as NTG. The illicit use of cocaine causes coronary vasospasm and angina and responds well to treatment with CCBs. The role of amlodipine in unstable angina is unclear.

Heparin is as effective as aspirin for both treating patients with unstable angina and in preventing MI. Patients with unstable angina treated with aspirin who continue to have ischemic episodes should receive heparin. Initial heparin dosage is 80 U/kg bolus and IV infusion of 18 U/kg per hour. The aPTT is obtained 6 hours after beginning infusion with the goal of keeping the aPTT between 46 and 70 seconds. Heparin therapy is generally continued for at least 5 days (Table 26-4).

The low-molecular-weight heparins, (e.g., enoxaparin) appear to be superior to unfractionated heparin in reducing progression to MI, recurrent angina, or death. However, substantial cost and lack of standardized dosing and measurement of intensity of anticoagulation preclude the routine use of these agents at present.

Thrombolytic therapy for unstable angina has not demonstrated added benefit over treatment with aspirin alone. Be-

TABLE 26-4   Management of Heparin Infusion
for Unstable Angina

aPTT <=35	80 U/kg bolus	increase drip 4 units/kg per hour
aPTT 35–45	40 U/kg bolus	increase drip 2 units/kg per hour
aPTT 46–70	No change	
aPTT 71–90		reduce drip 2 units/kg per hour
aPTT > 90	Hold heparin for 1 hour	reduce drip 3 units/kg per hour

cause of the significant risk of bleeding with thrombolytic agents, their routine use in unstable angina cannot be recommended at this time.

After patients are hemodynamically stable on an appropriate initial medical regimen, consideration should be given to early invasive management. *Coronary angiography* should be reserved for patients in whom a possible revascularization—coronary artery bypass graft (CABG) surgery or angioplasty procedure—is considered viable in the near future. In cases in which the patient stabilizes readily with pharmacologic agents and aspirin/heparin, there is no need for early angiography. In unstable patients or those with crescendo angina, early intervention may identify those patients with high-grade left main or three-vessel disease that may benefit from emergent CABG. Tendency to a more conservative approach is borne out by most randomized controlled trials. Careful patient selection is critical.

An *intraaortic balloon pump* (IABP) is indicated in unstable angina when the angina and attendant ECG abnormalities are persistent and refractory to maximal pharmacologic therapy. It is particularly indicated in this situation when coronary angiography or possible revascularization cannot be performed within a reasonably short time or as a method to control progressive unstable angina to allow coronary angiography to be performed safely. Potential complications of IABP include aortic dissection, femoral artery laceration, hematomas, femoral neuropathies, renal failure from renal artery occlusion, arterial thrombi and emboli, limb ischemia, and line sepsis. Once inserted, the patient should be placed on full doses of heparin by constant infusion. Prophylactic administration of antibiotics, such as oxacillin or a cephalosporin, is usually instituted.

OTHER THERAPIES

If measured during the first 24 hours of unstable angina, elevated cholesterol levels are thought to represent premorbid levels. Initiation of cholesterol-lowering therapy by the administration of HMG-CoA reductase inhibitors may further improve outcomes and is under investigation.

Acute Myocardial Infarction

Symptoms suggestive of MI are usually similar to those of ordinary angina, but the intensity and duration of symptoms are greater. In the ICU, infarction may frequently be misinterpreted to reflect hypovolemic or septic shock. Indeed, MI may coexist with and exacerbate these entities. The initial treatment with oxygen, antiplatelet agents, nitrates, and narcotics to relieve pain is similar to that of angina.

THERAPEUTIC APPROACH

β blockers have been shown to have substantial salutary effects in Q-wave infarctions, but not in non-Q-wave infarctions. Administration of 15 mg metoprolol intravenously over 15 to 20 minutes and 50 mg orally every 6 hours thereafter has been shown to reduce mortality and to preserve myocardial function postinfarction. Contraindications include overt cardiac failure, second degree AV block, hypotension, sinus bradycardia, and, of course, cardiogenic shock. A history of bronchospastic pulmonary disease is a relative contraindication.

Thrombolytic therapy has been shown to be an unquestionable cornerstone of management. Maximal benefit is demonstrable if it is initiated within 4 to 6 hours of symptom onset. The two principal thrombolytic agents in use today are streptokinase (SK) and tissue plasminogen activator (TPA). Another less commonly used thrombolytic agent is acylated plasminogen streptokinase activator complex (APSAC). Accelerated regimens of TPA have been shown to confer a small but clinically significant survival advantage over SK at the expense of a slight increase in stroke incidence. Most benefit is derived in younger patients with extensive anterior wall MI less than 4 hours after symptom onset.

Absolute contraindications include any active or recent bleeding (other than menstruation), intracranial neoplasm, AV malformation or aneurysm, stroke or neurosurgery within the preceding 6 months, or head trauma within 14 days. Relative contraindications include major thoracic or abdominal surgery within 10 days, diabetic retinopathy, pregnancy, coagulation disorders, bacterial endocarditis, uncontrolled hypertension (above 200/110 mmHg), and prolonged or traumatic cardiopulmonary resuscitation. Thrombolytic agents should be used only if angina is excluded and there is firm ECG evidence for infarction: at least 1 to 2 mm ST elevation in at least two contiguous leads. When the diagnosis of MI is in doubt, emergent echocardiography may be helpful. Correlative data—including ECG, echocardiographic and enzymatic data—govern thrombolytic therapy for suspected, atypical infarction (non-Q-wave MI, ST-segment depressions, or possible posterior wall MI).

TPA is given as a 15-mg bolus intravenously followed by 50 mg over the first 30 minutes by constant infusion. Then, 60 mg is administered over the next 60 minutes. This "accelerated" regimen has been suggested to achieve more rapid restoration of coronary flow.

Streptokinase is administered over 1 hour to a total of 1,500,000 U by constant infusion. Immediately prior to intravenous SK, 100 mg hydrocortisone is commonly administered, since SK is derived from a potentially antigenic bacterial source. Its administration may result in anaphylactic reactions. APSAC is given as a 30-mg bolus over 2 to 4 minutes and, like SK, is antigenic and generates a profound systemic lytic state, leading some to feel that it offers no advantage over SK.

Aspirin 325 mg should be started concomitantly with thrombolytic therapy and continued as 325 mg orally daily thereafter. Heparin should be initiated at the completion of thrombolytic therapy. Dosage is 80 U/kg bolus and IV infusion of 18 U/kg per hour. The aPTT is obtained 6 hours after beginning infusion with the goal of keeping the aPTT between 46 and 70 seconds. It is continued for 3 to 7 days or until coronary angiography is performed. β blockers should be initiated in concert with thrombolytic therapy according to the protocol previously given.

The role of immediate coronary angiography and infarct-related arterial angioplasty is controversial. This "direct approach" is the standard of care in a growing number of large institutions. Proponents argue that immediate reperfusion rates of 90 to 95% are substantially superior to the 70 to 80% rates with thrombolytics. Additional unquantified benefit derives from ancillary techniques such as direct thrombus extraction (TEC), rotablation, endovascular ultrasound and laser, and endovascular stenting.

Evolving Myocardial Infarction

After these interventions in the first 6 hours, the goals of treatment of acute MI are to monitor and prevent lethal ventricular arrhythmias and to treat hemodynamic instability.

Patients are placed on intravenous nitroglycerin infusion as described for unstable angina. CCBs may be continued or increased if angina recurs. Nifedipine and nicardipine have the most vasodilating effect and least cardiodepressant effect. Diltiazem and verapamil slow conduction in the AV node and therefore should be used cautiously in combination with β blockers and in patients with inferior wall MIs. Diltiazem has been proven to benefit patients with non-Q-wave MIs who do not have evidence of congestive heart failure. It is given at a dose of 30 to 60 mg every 6 to 8 hours.

Left ventricular thrombus develops following approximately 30 to 40% of anterior wall MIs, and 10 to 15% of these embolize. Therefore, in patients with no contraindications to heparin therapy, routine anticoagulation is recommended.

Intense activation of the sympathetic and renin-angiotensin systems mediates remodeling of the left ventricle in the periinfarct period. Evolution to chronic heart failure and progression to death has been substantially ameliorated by the initiation of angiotensin converting enzyme (ACE) inhibitors. Patients with asymptomatic as well as severe LV dysfunction benefit. Initiation doses of captopril (12.5 mg tid) ramipril (2.5 mg qd) or other ACE inhibitors on the first to third postinfarct days should be followed by prompt titration to maximally tolerable doses. ACE receptor antagonists (losartan) alone or in combination with ACE inhibitors may be suitable alternatives for those intolerant of ACE inhibitors.

ARRHYTHMIA MONITORING

The incidence of sustained ventricular tachycardia or fibrillation is highest within the first 3 to 4 hours, but may occur at any time. The prophylactic use of lidocaine is controversial and indicated only in the presence of "warning" ventricular dysrythmias after MI. A loading dose of 50 to 100 mg should be administered, followed by a drip to 1 to 2 mg/min. If complex ectopy persists, additional boluses may be given to a total of 220 mg, with adjustment in the drip, to a total of 4 mg/min. If frequent ectopy persists or if salvos of nonsustained ventricular tachycardia persist, procainamide is added at a loading dose of 1000 mg at a rate of 20 to 50 mg/min followed by a drip of 1 to 4 mg/min. Procainamide is the initial drug of choice if there is coexisting ventricular tachycardia and sustained supraventricular tachycardia. Breakthrough ventricular tachycardia/fibrillation resistant to these drugs should be treated with bretylium, started at a 500-mg loading dose over 30 minutes followed by a 1- to 4-mg/min drip.

Acidosis, hypoxemia, and hypokalemia may cause ectopy. Magnesium depletion is also an important cause of persistent ectopy and may justify therapy despite normal serum levels; 2 to 4 g $MgSO_4$ is administered in divided doses over 24 hours when ectopy persists provided that renal failure is not present. This has been shown not to reduce mortality.

HEMODYNAMIC MONITORING

Invasive hemodynamic monitoring with systemic and pulmonary artery (PA) catheterization is indicated whenever hemodynamic instability is present that does not improve relatively quickly with simple therapeutic maneuvers (e.g., saline bolus, intravenous loop diuretics, nitroglycerin). A PA catheter is indicated when pulmonary edema is suspected, when intravenous inotropes or vasodilators are used, and when the cardiac versus pulmonary origin of hypoxemia and infiltrates on chest x-ray cannot be differentiated clinically. PA catheters are not indicated in uncomplicated MIs or when minor pulmonary edema can be managed with small doses of diuretics and nitrates. The use of PA catheters is controversial and confounded by lack of standardization in the insertion, monitoring and interpretation. Since many patients with acute MI are candidates for thrombolytic and anticoagulant therapy, it is prudent to use insertion sites for a PA and peripheral arterial catheters that are easily compressible should significant bleeding occur.

PHARMACOLOGIC SUPPORT FOR THE FAILING LEFT VENTRICLE

Pump failure due to acute MI is manifest clinically by a weak pulse, poor peripheral perfusion with cool and cyanotic limbs, obtundation, and oliguria. Blood pressure (taken by cuff) is usually low, and there are variable degrees of pulmonary congestion. A third heart sound may be audible. Overall treatment of the failing ventricle emphasizes reducing preload, decreasing afterload, and increasing cardiac contractility. Decreasing resistance to outflow is particularly beneficial in mitral regurgitation and with ventricular septal defects.

Intravenous nitroglycerin is an ideal agent to use for both preload and afterload reduction. It is administered according to the protocol previously described. The other intravenous nitrate preparation is nitroprusside, which is a more potent vasodilator than nitroglycerin. Nitroprusside may cause diversion of blood flow from ischemic to nonischemic zones because of its very potent vasodilating properties ("coronary steal" phenomenon). Nitroprusside is metabolized to thiocyanate, a metabolic poison that can accumulate after 48 hours of infusion (sooner in the face of renal dysfunction). If nitroglycerin at reasonably high doses (300 to 600 μg/min) does not adequately reduce afterload, nitroprusside is started at 0.5 μg/kg/min and gradually increased. Serum thiocyanate levels should be determined after 24 hours; if these are found to exceed 10 mg/dL, nitroprusside should be discontinued.

Diuretics are used to treat pulmonary edema resulting from an elevated pulmonary capillary wedge pressure (PCWP). Isosorbide dinitrate 3 mg every 5 to 10 minutes in conjunction with furosemide 40 mg IV is an effective regimen for severe pulmonary edema. When furosemide or bumetanide at high doses (40 to 80 mg every 6 to 8 hours for furosemide and 1 to 2 mg every 6 to 8 hours for bumetanide) do not produce adequate diuresis, oral doses of metolazone (5 to 10 mg daily) may be added. Serum potassium and magnesium levels must be closely monitored.

Dobutamine is an intravenous inotrope that may be needed to augment cardiac output. It is initiated at 5 μg/kg/min and may be increased to 10 to 20 μg/kg/min. Since it is an adrenergic agonist, dobutamine can be arrhythmogenic. The role of dopamine is limited, but it *may* be beneficial in low doses (2 to 5 μg/kg/min) to augment renal blood flow and urine output.

Amrinone, a phosphodiesterase inhibitor, is an alternate inotropic agent that also acts as a vasodilator and decreases afterload. It is started with a loading dose of 0.75 mg/kg over 15 to 30 minutes, followed by constant infusion at 5 to 15 μg/kg/min. Ventricular arrhythmias, elevation of liver transaminase levels, and thrombocytopenia are potential complications.

Digoxin therapy for congestive heart failure complicating acute MI is controversial, but its use to control ventricular rate in atrial fibrillation is unequivocally beneficial. Digoxin may be loaded with 0.25 to 0.5 mg intravenously initially, followed by an additional 0.5 to 0.75 mg in divided doses in the next 24 hours. Subsequent doses should be adjusted if there is renal failure.

Intractable hypotension in the setting of acute MI unresponsive to dobutamine and cessation of nitrates, should be treated with high-dose dopamine. To ensure coronary, cerebral, and splanchnic perfusion, a systolic blood pressure of 90 to 100 mmHg may be achieved with doses of 10 to 20 μg/kg/min. Hypotension refractory to dopamine is treated with norepinephrine starting at 2 to 4 μg/kg/min and titrating upward as needed. If high doses of pressors are needed to support blood pressure, serious consideration must be given to placement of an IABP in an effort to increase cardiac output and reduce myocardial oxygen requirements.

MECHANICAL SUPPORT FOR THE FAILING HEART

In certain centers, circulatory support devices—including left ventricular assist devices, total artificial heart implantation and percutaneous cardiopulmonary bypass circuits—are utilized to improve organ perfusion and provide a bridge to definitive revascularization or cardiac transplantation.

Cardiogenic Shock

This state of profound hemodynamic instability, is characterized by systolic BP < 90 mmHg, cardiac index < 2.2 l/min/m^2, PCWP > 18 mmHg, and urine output < 20 mL/h. Onset may be several hours to days after onset of infarction. Emergency angiography followed by either direct percutaneous coronary angioplasty (PTCA) or emergency coronary artery bypass graft (CABG) surgery should be performed in such patients to reperfuse the myocardium as quickly as possible. If there is a delay in mobilizing the appropriate staff, an IABP should be inserted to stabilize the patient and facilitate catheterization. Where catheterization and PTCA or CABG surgery are not available, thrombolytic therapy should be instituted, perhaps even in patients who are at high risk for bleeding complications, since the alternative to no reperfusion is bleak. Other mechanical defects result in shock and should be excluded in such cases (tamponade, free wall rupture, ventricular septal defect (VSD), or rupture or a papillary muscle) prior to administering thrombolytic therapy. Elective intubation and mechanical ventilation facilitate unloading of respiratory muscles and optimize alveolar oxygenation. Packed red cell infusions should be used to boost the hematocrit to ≥ 35%.

Management of Mechanical Defects

Mechanical defects can occur after acute MI and prompt surgical repair is indicated, because medical treatment alone is associated with extremely high mortality. Sudden and/or progressive hemodynamic deterioration with low cardiac output and/or pulmonary edema should lead to prompt consideration of these defects and rapid institution of diagnostic and therapeutic measures. On physical examination, the presence of a new cardiac murmur indicates the possibility of either ventricular septal defect (VSD), mitral regurgitation, or occasionally ventricular rupture. A precise diagnosis can usually be established by echocardiography.

Use of a balloon flotation catheter is helpful for both diagnosis and monitoring of therapy. With a VSD and left-to-right shunting, a "step-up" in oxygen saturation is seen in the pulmonary artery compared with the right atrium; thermodilution cardiac output and mixed venous oxygen saturation will be falsely elevated. A prominent V wave will often be evident on the PAWP tracing in acute mitral regurgitation. Diastolic pressure equalization connotes ventricular rupture and pericardial tamponade.

Acute mitral valve regurgitation resulting from papillary muscle rupture is associated with 75% mortality within the first 24 hours if the valve is not surgically repaired or replaced. Nitroprusside may help lower pulmonary capillary pressures and improve peripheral organ perfusion. Emergency surgical repair is also indicated for postinfarction VSD and LV free wall rupture when pulmonary edema or cardiogenic shock is present. If feasible, simultaneous CABG improves long-term survival.

Right Ventricular Infarction

Hemodynamically significant RV infarctions occur almost exclusively in the setting of inferior acute MIs. RVMI is associated with a significantly higher mortality (25 to 30%). Severe ischemia results in acute RV dilation, increased intrapericardial pressure, and a reduced LV preload with a shifting of the interventricular septum toward the left ventricle. The clinical triad of hypotension, clear lung fields, and elevated jugular venous pressure with the presence of Kussmaul's sign (distention of the jugular vein on inspiration) in the setting of an inferior MI are useful but insensitive characteristics of RV ischemia.

Treatment priorities include maintenance of RV preload, reduction of RV afterload, inotropic support of the dysfunctional right ventricle, and early reperfusion. Administration of even small doses of nitroglycerin to these patients may further decrease preload, possibly resulting in hypotension. Volume loading may further elevate right-sided filling pressure and RV dilation, resulting in decreased LV output. Dobutamine is necessary to augment both right and left ventricular forward flow in instances when hypotension is present and is clearly superior to fluid boluses. Additionally, norepinephrine may augment RV contractility. When transvenous pacing is required for a conduction disturbance, dual-chamber AV sequential pacing affords better right ventricular contraction than does single-chamber pacing.

Indications for Temporary Pacing in Acute MI

Disturbances of conduction distal to the AV node and His bundle, as occur in complete heart block with a ventricular escape rhythm, are worrisome even if they are tolerated well hemodynamically. Ventricular foci are unstable and their discharge rate may vary widely, with abrupt acceleration to ventricular tachycardia or deceleration to asystole. Any bradyarrhythmia unresponsive to atropine that results in hemodynamic compromise requires pacing. Pacing for left bundle branch block (LBBB) remains controversial. Further indications include third-degree AV block, alternating LBBB and right bundle branch block (RBBB), new bifasicular block, new first-degree AV block, and LBBB or RBBB, new first-degree AV block and preexisting bifasicular block, and type II second-degree AV block. Another indication considered controversial is third-degree AV block or type II second-degree AV block with narrow QRS escape in inferior-wall MI that is tolerated well hemodynamically.

For a more detailed discussion, see Chaps. 20, 21, and 24 in *Principles of Critical Care,* 2d ed.

Chapter 27

VENTRICULAR DYSFUNCTION IN CRITICAL ILLNESS

JOHN McCONVILLE

Ventricular dysfunction is quite common in the intensive care unit (ICU). Often, patients in the medical or surgical ICU have known ventricular dysfunction as the result of a chronic problem—ischemic or alcohol-related cardiomyopathy, for example. In other instances, the complications of multisystem organ failure (MSOF) may result in acute cardiovascular dysfunction. It is important to detect the acute and chronic causes of ventricular dysfunction because its etiology helps to determine what treatment modalities are to be instituted by the clinician. This chapter focuses on the pathophysiology, diagnosis, and treatment of ventricular dysfunction that results from multisystem organ failure.

Physiology

The diagnosis and treatment of cardiac dysfunction in ICU patients requires an understanding of the factors that normally determine cardiac pump function, which is defined by the relationship of the heart's output to its input. In the ICU, cardiac output (L/min) is a readily measured quantity that best estimates the heart's output, while the pressure in the right atrium (Pra) is a readily measured estimate of the heart's input.

The pump function curve of the heart is illustrated as the relationship between cardiac output and Pra over a range of values (Fig. 27-1A). This graph illustrates that increasing Pra results in an increase in the cardiac output. It is important to note that at higher right atrial pressures, an increase in Pra

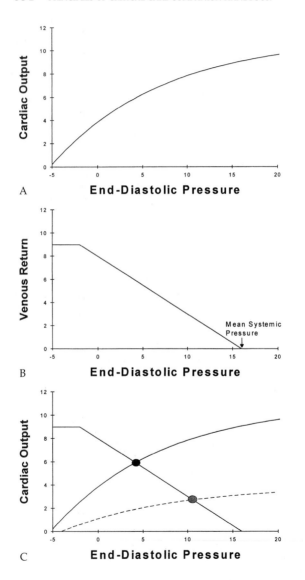

◀ FIGURE 27-1   A. The cardiac function curve relates right atrial pressure (Pra) or end-diastolic pressure (EDP, abscissa) to cardiac output
(*ordinate*). As EDP increases, cardiac output increases, but at high
EDPs, further increases cause less increase in cardiac output. B. The
relationship between EDP (Pra, abscissa) and venous return (*ordinate*) is illustrated. When EDP equals mean systemic pressure (Pms),
there is no pressure gradient (Pms − Pra) driving the blood flow back
to the heart, so venous return is zero. As EDP (Pra) decreases, the
gradient from the veins to the heart to drive blood flow back to the
heart increases so that venous return increases. At very low EDPs
(Pra < 0), central veins collapse and act as Starling resistors so that
further decreases in EDP do not increase venous return. C. The cardiac function curve and the venous return curve are drawn on the
same axes (*continuous lines*). The intersection of the cardiac function
curve and the venous return curve defines the operating point of the
circulation, here at an EDP (Pra) of approximately 5 mmHg and a cardiac output of approximately 5 L/min. The interrupted cardiac function curve illustrates decreased cardiac function, causing reduced cardiac output (about 3 L/min) at a higher EDP (Pra = 10 mmHg).

results in a much smaller rise in cardiac output as compared
with increases in right atrial pressure at lower values at Pra.

Another important determinant of cardiac function is venous return. Ideally, the left ventricle is able to eject as much
blood per minute as the right atrium is receiving from the
major systemic veins. Thus, cardiac output (L/min) is equal
to venous return (L/min). The amount of venous return is
dependent on the mean systemic pressure (Pms), Pra, and the
resistance to venous return (RVR). Thus, as Pra falls, the pressure difference between Pms and Pra increases. If the resistance to venous return remains the same, a decrease in Pra
results in a greater pressure difference between Pms and Pra
and therefore an increase in venous return. This relationship
between Pra and venous return is illustrated in Fig. 27-1B. Of
note, when Pra has increased to the point where it is equal to
Pms, then the pressure *difference* between Pra and Pms is zero;
therefore there is no venous return. The equation that relates
Pra, Pms, RVR, and venous return is:

$$\text{Venous return} = \frac{\text{Pms} - \text{Pra}}{\text{RVR}}$$

If we plot the venous return curve, and the cardiac output versus Pra curve on the same axis, the point at which the curves intersect defines the operating point of the heart for a given right atrial pressure (assuming that in steady state CO = venous return). Figure 27-1C illustrates that any change in the cardiac output or the venous return results in a different operating point of the heart for a particular right atrial pressure. Therefore, in approaching a patient with suspected cardiovascular dysfunction, one should consider both cardiac function *and* venous return abnormalities as potential etiologies for the cardiac dysfunction.

Physical Examination and Diagnostic Tests

Left ventricular (LV) and right ventricular (RV) dysfunction are characterized by elevated ventricular filling pressures in relation to the cardiac output. Initially, clinical examination attempts to identify the presence and severity of depressed cardiac pump function. The physical examination will often enable the clinician to distinguish the contributions of RV and LV dysfunction. For example, a sustained apical impulse suggests left LV hypertrophy or LV aneurysm. In addition, an audible third heart sound is indicative of LV dysfunction with increased LV filling pressure and elevated pressure in the left atrium in the presence of a dilated ventricle. Information about the filling pressure in the left atrium can also be gleaned from the pulmonary examination. Dependent pulmonary crackles on physical examination may be due to LV dysfunction and suggest that LV filling pressures are elevated, usually above 20 to 25 mmHg. It is important to note that the clearance of interstitial edema lags behind reductions in Pla by hours. RV dysfunction can also be detected on physical examination. Distended jugular veins are indicative of elevated right atrial pressures. Typically, the sternal angle is approximately 5 cm above the right atrium when the patient's torso is at a 30- to 45-degree angle. Right ventricular filling pressure is normally no higher than 6 to 8 cmH$_2$O, so that jugular venous distention is usually no higher than 1 to 3 cm above the sternal angle in normal individuals. Thus, elevation of the jugular venous pulsations indicates RV dysfunction.

The pulmonary artery catheter (PAC), also called the right heart catheter, and the echocardiogram are often utilized in the ICU as additional means of obtaining information about the function of the RV and LV. The PAC, utilizing the thermodilution technique, provides an excellent determination of the cardiac output. It is also able to measure the filling pressures of the RV (central venous pressure as an estimate of Pra) and the LV (pulmonary wedge pressure as an estimate of Pla). Therefore, when a patient is found to have decreased ventricular function (depressed cardiac output), the separate contributions of the LV and RV can be distinguished. In addition, the afterload of the RV is best estimated by the pulmonary artery pressure, which can also be obtained from the PAC. Thus, the PAC is able to measure the output of the heart (cardiac output) as well as the input of the heart (right atrial pressure). These measurements allow the clinician to quantify cardiac pump function and then to follow these measurements as different interventions are attempted during the ICU admission (starting vasoactive drugs, for example).

Although the PAC is able to accurately measure the Pra and pulmonary capillary wedge pressure (Pcwp), these measurements are not always a reliable gauge of the RV and LV *volumes.* Abnormal myocardial compliance, elevated positive end-expiratory pressure (PEEP), intrinsic PEEP (PEEPi), and pericardial processes make it difficult for the clinician to draw definitive conclusions about the ventricle's volume status from the PAC values. Figure 27-2 illustrates how PEEP can affect transmural filling pressures. Often, the echocardiogram can be used in conjunction with the PAC to provide additional information about the heart's function and volume status. For example, when a patient is found to have depressed ventricular function, an echocardiogram is able to determine whether this is from decreased contractility or increased diastolic stiffness. A small end-diastolic volume (EDV) when filling pressures are normal or high indicates that increased diastolic stiffness is contributing to depressed ventricular pump function; whereas a large end-systolic volume (ESV) when afterload is low or normal indicates that decreased contractility is contributing to decreased ventricular pump function.

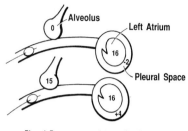

PEEP cm H₂O	Pleural Pressure mmHg	Intracardiac Pressure mmHg	Transmural Pressure mmHg
0	-2	16	18
15	+4	16	12

FIGURE 27-2   The effect of positive end-expiratory pressure (PEEP) on transmural pressure. In this example, 50 percent of PEEP is transmitted to the juxtacardiac space (15 cmH₂O ≈ 12 mmHg). The same wedge pressure of 16 mmHg corresponds to greatly different "transmural" filling pressures.

Decreased Left Ventricular Systolic Function

There are both chronic and acute causes of LV dysfunction. Dilated cardiomyopathy secondary to coronary artery disease is one of the most common chronic causes of poor LV function. Repeated ischemic episodes or infarctions can result in a decreased amount of functional LV muscle mass and subsequently poor LV function. Alcoholic and viral cardiomyopathy are two other important causes of ventricular dysfunction commonly encountered in the medical ICU. Multiple additional causes are listed in Table 27-1.

Often patients are admitted to the ICU with a history of coronary artery disease and well-established ventricular dysfunction. Other patients develop LV dysfunction while in the ICU. These acute causes of worsened LV contractility are important to recognize because they are more likely to be reversible than many of the chronic causes of LV dysfunction. Acute causes of depressed LV contractility include ischemia, hypoxemia, respiratory and metabolic acidosis, ionized hypocalcemia, exogenous toxins such as alcohol, and en-

TABLE 27-1   Chronic Causes of Decreased Contractility
(Dilated Cardiomyopathies)

Coronary artery disease
Idiopathic
Inflammatory (viral, toxoplasmosis, Chagas disease)
Alcoholic
Postpartum
Uremic
Diabetic
Nutritional deficiency (selenium deficiency)
Metabolic disorder (Fabry disease, Gaucher disease)
Toxic [doxorubicin (Adriamycin), cobalt]

---

dogenous toxins such as the circulating depressant factors of
sepsis. Table 27-2 is a list of some of the acute, reversible
causes of decreased contractility.

Management

The first step in treating the ICU patient with new LV dysfunction is to identify the potential causes for depressed contractility. An elevated Pa_{CO_2} of 55 mmHg, in and of itself, may

TABLE 27-2   Acute Reversible Contributors
to Decreased Contractility

Ischemia
Hypoxia
Respiratory acidosis
Metabolic acidosis
Hypocalcemia
Hypophosphatemia
Possibly other electrolyte abnormalities (Mg^{2+}, K^+)
Exogenous substances (alcohol, β blockers, calcium channel
   blockers, antiarrhythmics)
Endogenous substances (endotoxin, histamine, tumor necrosis
   factor, interleukin-1, platelet-activating factor)
Hypo- and hyperthermia

---

not cause significant LV dysfunction. However, when coupled with a Pa_{O_2} of 50 mmHg, a metabolic acidosis, and a temperature of 39.5°C, a moderate respiratory acidosis can be seen as one of the many disturbances that can lead to significant LV dysfunction. Thus, the first step in treating patients with ventricular dysfunction in the ICU setting is to correct any reversible causes. Therefore, when ischemia or hypoxia are present, attempts to correct these abnormalities should be instituted. If acute ischemia is present, treatment with oxygen, aspirin, β blockers, and nitrates to dilate the coronary arteries should be instituted immediately. In addition, attempts to reestablish coronary perfusion with either thrombolytic agents or emergent coronary artery angioplasty/stenting should be pursued. These interventions can often limit further myocardial cell death and prevent significant LV dysfunction.

While it is important to act quickly when a patient develops acute chest pain with ST-segment elevation in the anterior leads, it is also important to act quickly when a patient in the ICU develops hypoxia or acute respiratory acidosis. Correction of these abnormalities can improve the depressed cardiac function that is often found in ICU patients. Thus, the ventilated patient with respiratory acidosis should have alveolar ventilation increased by either an increase in minute ventilation or a decrease in dead space in an effort to correct the respiratory acidosis. Similarly, the underlying cause of a significant metabolic acidosis should be sought, and treatment directed at the underlying abnormality should be initiated. The diabetic patient with a bicarbonate value of 12 and a blood glucose of 700 should be started on intravenous fluids as well as insulin in an effort to improve the metabolic acidosis. It is important to stress that therapy should be directed at the underlying abnormality rather that at correcting an abnormal laboratory value. Infusion of bicarbonate to correct the metabolic acidosis does not correct the underlying problem of diabetic ketoacidosis. There is mounting evidence suggesting that alkali therapy for metabolic acidosis is of no benefit and may be dangerous. Bicarbonate infusion results in an increase in Pa_{CO_2} due to chemical equilibrium of HCO_3^- with H_2O and C_{O_2} unless compensatory hyperventilation is also instituted. Particularly during rapid injection of bicarbonate, local Pa_{CO_2} may climb to extremely high values, so that myocardial intracellular acidosis may transiently be severe. Just as with respiratory acidosis, high Pa_{CO_2} from bicarbonate infusion may cause intracellular acidosis and marked depression of LV myocardial contractility.

Once the acute causes of decreased contractility have been corrected, management strategies can be directed toward optimizing cardiac function. These therapies include maximizing filling pressures of the heart. In the ICU, hypotension and low cardiac output can often be improved with intravenous infusion of fluid or blood products. A fluid bolus is an attempt to move up and to the right on the Starling curve. In other words, the clinician is trying to increase filling pressures of the heart in order to increase ventricular ejection of blood. This strategy is very effective for patients with decreased contractility, but it is often limited by the development of pulmonary edema. In addition to increasing preload, therapy in the patient with chronic LV dysfunction is directed toward improving LV contractility with inotropic agents and reducing afterload with agents that decrease arterial tone.

Increased Diastolic Stiffness

Increased diastolic stiffness of the LV is a common cause of ventricular dysfunction in the critically ill patient. Diastolic dysfunction, as well as depressed LV systolic function, results in a decreased stroke volume (see Fig. 27-3 for an explanation of LV pressure-volume relationships). However, depressed systolic function reduces stroke volume because end-systolic volume (ESV) increases, whereas increased diastolic stiffness reduces stroke volume because end-diastolic volume decreases (Fig. 27-4). Because end-diastolic volume is decreased in patients with increased diastolic stiffness, diastolic dysfunction is commonly thought of as a disorder of ventricular filling. Thus, patients with increased diastolic stiffness often develop worsened overall cardiac function with an increased heart rate because less time is spent in diastole, when the heart is being filled. It is imperative to consider diastolic dysfunction in every ICU patient with cardiac dysfunction, because the treatment of diastolic dysfunction is

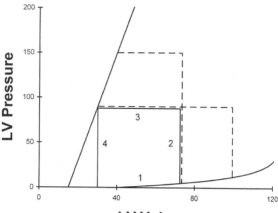

LV Volume

FIGURE 27-3 Left ventricular pressure-volume relationships are illustrated. The continuous thick lines represent a single cardiac cycle as a pressure-volume loop. During diastole, the ventricle fills along a diastolic pressure-volume relationship (*labeled 1*). At the onset of systole, left ventricular pressure rises with no change in volume (*labeled 2*). When left ventricular pressure exceeds aortic pressure, the aortic valve opens, and the left ventricle ejects blood (*labeled 3*) to an end-systolic pressure-volume point. The ventricle then relaxes isovolumically (*labeled 4*). At a higher-pressure afterload, the left ventricle is not able to eject as far (illustrated by the short interrupted lines). Conversely, at a lower afterload, the left ventricle is able to eject further so that all end-systolic points lie along and define the end-systolic pressure-volume relationship (ESPVR, or E_{max}). Increased diastolic filling (here illustrated by the long interrupted lines) results in increased stroke volume from the larger EDV to an ESV that lies on the same ESPVR; accordingly, increased afterload reduces stroke volume unless preload increases to compensate.

vastly different from the treatment of systolic dysfunction. Unfortunately, it is often difficult to make a definitive diagnosis of diastolic dysfunction in most critically ill patients. Often diastolic dysfunction is considered as a potential etiology of ventricular dysfunction only after standard therapies directed at improving systolic dysfunction have failed. In fact,

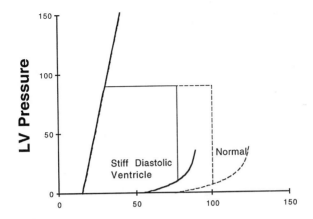

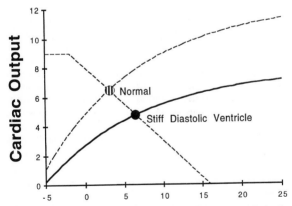

FIGURE 27-4 The bottom panel is a cardiac function curve derived from the pressure-volume relationships illustrated in the top panel. An increase in diastolic stiffness results in a decrease in EDV and in stroke volume at the same EDP, ESP, and E_{max}, so increased diastolic stiffness shifts the cardiac function curve down and to the right (dashed cardiac function curve to the solid cardiac function curve in the lower panel).

diastolic dysfunction is just as common as systolic dysfunction in the critically ill patient. An echocardiogram that reveals a small end-diastolic volume in relation to end-diastolic pressure makes the definitive diagnosis of increased diastolic stiffness. However, the most important step in making the diagnosis of increased diastolic stiffness is considering it as a potential etiology of decreased cardiac output in every patient with cardiac dysfunction in the ICU.

Concentric LV hypertrophy secondary to long-standing hypertension is the most common etiology of increased diastolic stiffness. However, restrictive cardiomyopathies secondary to sarcoidosis, hemachromatosis, amyloidosis, and endomyocardial fibrosis should also be considered as potential causes of increased diastolic stiffness. It is also important to consider the acute, potentially reversible causes of increased diastolic stiffness. Regional or global ischemia results in delayed systolic relaxation, contributing to increased diastolic stiffness. Often the diastolic stiffness associated with acute ischemia will precede the systolic dysfunction resulting from acute ischemia/infarction. In addition to ischemia, anything that causes increased intrathoracic or intrapericardial pressure is a potentially reversible cause of acute diastolic stiffness. A patient who is being mechanically ventilated with PEEP provides an example of how increased intrathoracic pressure can act similarly to increased diastolic stiffness. Positive airway pressure and PEEP are variably transmitted to the heart, depending on the distensibility of the lungs and chest wall. If the lungs are very distensible and the chest wall is relatively rigid (as with a tense abdomen), most of an increase in airway pressure will be transmitted to the heart, so that to maintain the same chamber volumes, the atrial and ventricular pressures have to increase as much. Remember that venous return is dependent on the difference between the mean systemic pressure and the pressure of the right atrium. If a patient is being mechanically ventilated, the positive airway pressure will increase the pressure in the right atrium to the extent that airway pressures are transmitted to the heart. If Pms does not also increase, the increase in Pra will result in a decrease in venous return/cardiac output (assuming that RVR remains constant). This decrease in cardiac output is similar to increased diastolic stiffness in that the cause of the cardiac dysfunction is not poor systolic function but rather decreased filling of the LV. Thus, anything that causes an increase in intrathoracic or intrapericardial pressure is considered a cause of increased diastolic stiffness.

Increased intrathoracic pressure due to pneumothorax or massive pleural effusion may tamponade the heart and thereby result in apparent increased diastolic stiffness. Greatly increased intrabdominal pressure may elevate the diaphragm and similarly increase diastolic stiffness. Because all of these causes of increased intrathoracic or intrapericardial pressure leading to apparent increased diastolic stiffness are treatable, they must be identified or excluded early in critically ill patients. Hypovolemic shock, septic shock, and hypothermia may result in increased diastolic stiffness. The increased diastolic stiffness associated with these types of shock is associated with irreversibility of the shock state and increased mortality.

The acute causes of diastolic dysfunction should be quickly diagnosed and treated. In addition, therapy for acute diastolic dysfunction in the ICU involves maximizing ventricular filling during diastole. This is accomplished with intravenous infusion of volume. The goal of therapy for patients with diastolic dysfunction is to find the optimal filling pressure such that ventricular output is maximized without the subsequent development of excessive pulmonary edema. Also, tachycardia at sufficiently high rates results in an inadequate diastolic filling time, so that stroke volume is reduced because adequate filling does not occur and the contribution to ventricular diastolic filling by the atria is less efficient, particularly in atrial fibrillation. Excessive tachycardias and arrhythmias should be treated quickly in an effort to improve diastolic filling.

Acute-on-Chronic Heart Failure

Heart failure carries a poor prognosis, with survival rates of only 50 percent after 5 years. Mortality is often related to episodes of acute decompensation. A list of precipitating causes of acute decomposition is given in Table 27-3. Therapy of acute-on-chronic heart failure aims to treat intravascular overload, improve gas exchange, reduce afterload, and,

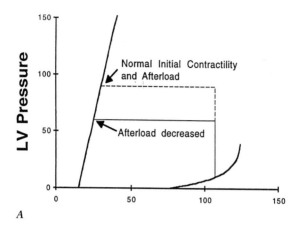

A

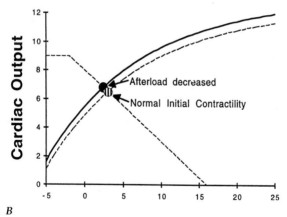

B

FIGURE 27-5 Panels *B* and *D* (*opposite page*) are cardiac function curves derived from the pressure-volume relationships illustrated in panels *A* and *C* (*opposite page*). Panels *A* and *B* show that when contractility is initially normal, then afterload reduction does not improve cardiac output or cardiac function (dashed and solid cardiac function curves in panel *B* are similar) and serves only to produce hypotension. Conversely, panels *C* and *D* show that when

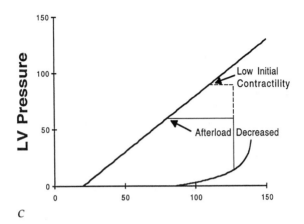

C

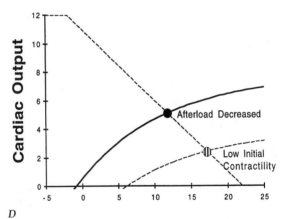

D

FIGURE 27-5 (*Continued*)   contractility is initially reduced (dashed cardiac function curve in panel *D*), then afterload reduction substantially improves cardiac function (solid cardiac function curve in panel *D*). For the same venous return curve (dashed biphasic line in panel *D*), cardiac output increases at a lower LV end-diastolic pressure (black dot compared with striped dot in panel *D*).

TABLE 27-3   Common Precipitating Factors of Acute-on-Chronic Heart Failure

---

Poor compliance with medications
Dietary indiscretion (salt load, alcohol)
Infection
Fever
High environmental temperature
Effect of a new medication (β blocker, calcium-channel blocker, antiarrhythmic, nonsteroidal anti-inflammatory)
Arrhythmia (typically, new atrial fibrillation)
Ischemia or infarction
Valve dysfunction (endocarditis, papillary muscle dysfunction)
Pulmonary embolism
Surgical abdominal event (cholecystitis, pancreatitis, bowel infarct)
Worsening of another disease (diabetes, hepatitis, hyperthyroidism, hypothyroidism)

---

if necessary, augment contractility. Diuretics are utilized in an effort to decrease the pressure in the left atrium (Pla). Furosemide has the additional beneficial quality of causing venodilation, which also helps to reduce Pla. Afterload reduction is also an important therapeutic intervention in patients with depressed LV systolic contractility due to a decrease in the slope of the end-systolic pressure-volume relationship. (Fig. 27-5, upper right-hand graph). Because there is a decrease in the slope of this relationship, small reductions in pressure afterload can result in improved ejection to smaller end-systolic volumes. Intravenous nitroglycerin and nitroprusside are two agents that are commonly used in the ICU setting to reduce left ventricular afterload. These agents are typically used because they can be quickly titrated so that the optimal dose results in maximal cardiac output with adequate blood pressure. Finally, inotropic or vasoactive agents are extremely useful in reversing depressed systolic contractility. Dobutamine, at doses of 2 to 15 $\mu g/kg/min$, acts mainly on β receptors and results in increased ventricular contractility as well as mild peripheral vasodilatation. Dopamine is predominantly a β agonist in doses of 5 to 10 $\mu g/kg/min$, but at higher doses it is an α agonist and therefore increases arterial tone. Amrinone, milrinone, and enoximone are phosphodiesterase inhibitors that probably increase contractility by increasing intracellular calcium during systole. It should be remembered, however, that positive inotropic agents improve contractility at the cost of increased myocardial oxygen demand and therefore may precipitate ischemia.

For a more detailed discussion, see Chap. 21 in *Principles of Critical Care*, 2d ed.

Chapter 28

RHYTHM DISTURBANCES, PACING, AND CARDIOVERSION

EUGENE KAJI

Arrhythmias are commonly observed in the intensive care unit (ICU) setting secondary to the arrhythmogenic stresses encountered in critically ill patients and the continuous cardiac monitoring employed. Management of arrhythmias depends on diagnosis, assessment of the hemodynamic impact, and, most importantly, the effect of treatment on the patient's overall status. Diagnostically, the 12-lead electrocardiogram (ECG) and rhythm strip are of paramount importance. The hemodynamic impact of an arrhythmia is difficult to assess and can depend on both the patient's underlying cardiac function and the arrhythmia itself. The treatment of arrhythmias can be significantly altered by the clinical status of the patient, since liver failure, renal dysfunction, and infections can affect the metabolism of antiarrhythmics and the ability of the cardiologist to opt for interventional procedures.

Bradycardia

Bradycardia management, in principle, is straightforward. If bradycardia causes symptoms or hemodynamic embarrassment, then treatment with medications, temporary trascutaneous or transvenous pacing, and possibly permanent pacing is required. If bradycardia is asymptomatic, then no treatment is necessary unless the exhibited bradycardia portends a poor prognosis (high likelihood of progressing to complete heart block). AV block below the AV node (and sometimes at the level of the AV node) that is secondary to ischemia frequently requires prophylactic temporary pacing.

Sinus bradycardia is the most frequently encountered bradyarrhythmia. Diagnostically, the 12-lead ECG should show a sinus P-wave morphology at a rate less than 60 beats per minute. The hemodynamic impact should be assessed using blood pressure measurements and following the patient's symptoms. If there is hemodynamic compromise secondary to the sinus bradycardia, the rhythm should be treated to increase the heart rate. This may involve transcutaneous pacing or medical treatment with atropine or β-agonists. Transcutaneous pacing should be viewed as a bridge to either temporary or permanent transvenous pacing, since it is poorly tolerated by the patient and somewhat unreliable. Atropine, a vagolytic used to increase the heart rate, can be administered in 0.5-mg doses intravenously to a maximum cumulative dose of 2 mg. Higher doses may cause delirium. Epinephrine may be considered at a dose of 0.5–1 mg every 5 minutes in the treatment of hypotensive bradycardia, since it has both α- and β-effects that deliver pressor and chronotropic effects, respectively. If hypotension is not an issue, isoproterenol, which is a β-agonist without α-effects, can be used at 2 to 20 μg/min. The treatment of sinus bradycardia also involves managing the underlying cause. The etiology of sinus bradycardia includes intrinsic sinus node dysfunction, high vagal tone (athletes, abdominal distension), hypothyroidism, high intracranial pressure (Cushing's reflex), hyperkalemia, and sepsis.

Blocks in the conduction system can occur at the level of the AV node, the left bundle branch, and the right bundle branch. There are three degrees of AV nodal block: first, second, and third degree. First-degree AV block is generally benign and is defined as a PR interval of greater than 200 ms with one-to-one AV conduction. In the absence of bundle branch block, first-degree AV block is generally at the level of the AV node. It can be secondary to ischemia, myocarditis, or medications that depress AV nodal conduction, such as digitalis, β-blockers, or calcium channel blockers. In the presence of bundle branch block, about 50% of patients with first-degree AV block have block below the AV node in the His bundle or bundle branches. Block below the AV node carries a worse prognosis than block at the AV node, and a pacemaker should be considered.

Second-degree AV block is subcategorized into Mobitz type I and II. Mobitz I (Wenckebach) is typically benign, rarely causes hemodynamic compromise, suggests block at the level of the AV node, and is characterized by a constant PP interval, progressively prolonging PR intervals, shortening RR intervals, and eventual loss of AV conduction. The etiology and treatment of Mobitz I is similar to that of first-degree AV block except that temporary pacing might be considered in the presence of ischemia, since Mobitz I may progress to more malignant bradyarrhythmias in this setting. Mobitz II is typically characterized by a constant PP interval with sudden loss of the AV conduction. Mobitz II generally signifies disease below the AV node and is an indication for permanent pacing. In a symptomatic patient, emergent temporary pacing should be considered.

Third-degree AV block, which is also called *complete heart block,* is a complete failure of the atrial impulses to reach the ventricle. There is no relation between the P waves and the R waves on the electrocardiogram (ECG). The causes of complete heart block include ischemia, metabolic derangement, medications, endocarditis, trauma, and congenital block (Table 28-1). If the patient is symptomatic, temporary and subsequent permanent pacing should be considered. Although prophylactic temporary transvenous pacing is reasonable for complete heart block in the setting of an inferior myocardial infarction, permanent pacing may not be necessary if the complete heart block resolves. Even if complete heart block is asymptomatic, pacing should be considered in all cases other than congenital heart block.

Tachycardias

Tachyarrhythmias are diagnosed by 12-lead ECG and rhythm strip. The treatment options include medications to suppress the arrhythmia or control the rate, cardioversion, antitachycardic pacing, and ablation of the arrhythmic focus or pathway. Management is based on the hemodynamic effect and prognosis of the untreated tachyarrhythmia.

TABLE 28-1   Causes of Heart Block

Myocardial infarction or ischemia	Trauma
Cardiomyopathies	Postcardiac surgery
Hypertensive	Infectious diseases
Ischemic	Endocarditis (usually aortic)
Nonischemic, dilated	Syphilis
Drugs	Tuberculosis
Digitalis	Lyme disease
β-blockers	Diphtheria
Calcium-channel blockers	Chagas disease
Phenytoin	Toxoplasmosis
Tricyclic antidepressants	Mumps
Most antiarrhythmics	HIV infection
Increased vagal tone	Inflammatory diseases
Visceral distention	Myocarditis
Pain	Rheumatic fever
Carotid hypersensitivity	Collagen-vascular diseases
Infiltrative processes	Ankylosing spondylitis
Amyloidosis	Rheumatoid arthritis
Sarcoidosis	Polymyositis
Hemochromatosis	Endocrine diseases
Gout	Thyrotoxicosis
Paget disease	Myxedema
Tumors	Addison disease
Degenerative disease	Congenital heart disease
Lev disease	Congenital complete
Lenegre disease	heart block
Calcific aortic stenosis	Poisoning
Muscular dystrophies	Lead
Friedreich ataxia	Organophosphate

Antiarrhythmic Medications

There are four classes of antiarrhythmic medications. Class I refers to sodium channel inhibitors, which are subclassified into Ic (slow release), Ib (fast release), and Ia (intermediate release) (Table 28-2). Class II medications are β-adrenergic blockers, class III are medications that delay repolarization, and class IV drugs are those that inhibit calcium channels. Despite this extensive classification scheme, the efficacy of an antiarrhythmic medication cannot be predicted from the class or mechanism of action; most antiarrhythmics are tried on a trial-and-error basis.

Antiarrhythmics also have troubling side effects, including promotion of arrhythmias, hypotension, negative inotropy, lethargy, impotence, constipation, and hyperthyroidism. Many antiarrhythmics are eliminated via renal or hepatic mechanisms that may necessarily be compromised in an ICU patient. Antiarrhythmics also interact with other medications frequently used in the critically ill patient. To further complicate matters, the therapeutic window of most antiarrhythmics is particularly narrow. Given the limited efficacy of antiarrhythmics, side effects, and drug interactions, medications are used primarily in symptomatic patients or in those with life-threatening arrhythmias that require suppression.

Three antiarrhythmic medications deserve discussion. Classically, lidocaine is the antiarrhythmic of choice for ventricular tachycardia (VT) because of its efficacy in suppressing ischemia-mediated VT. It is hepatically metabolized and interacts with β-blockers and cimetidine. Toxic side effects include seizures, mental status changes, and coma. The lidocaine level should be followed in patients on prolonged lidocaine infusions or with hepatic dysfunction. Procainamide is classically the second-line medication used in VT. It is also used to convert atrial fibrillation pharmacologically. Procainamide is metabolized to an active metabolite, N-acetyl-procainamide (NAPA), which is excreted renally. Both the parent compound and NAPA can predispose to side effects, including torsades de pointes. Patients on procainamide should have their procainamide, NAPA levels, and QT intervals monitored. Particular attention should be paid to patients with renal or hepatic dysfunction. Amiodarone is a class III antiarrhythmic that has gained popularity. It is the only antiarrhythmic that has been shown to produce no *increase* in mortality among patients with structural heart disease. It is effective in suppressing both atrial and ventricular arrhythmias. Amiodarone is metabolized by the cytochrome P450 system, so it can interact with drugs including digoxin, quinidine, procainamide, and warfarin.

TABLE 28-2 FDA-Approved Antiarrhythmic Drugs with Their Indications

Class 1: Drugs that block the fast inward sodium channel

Class 1A

Quinidine	Supraventricular and ventricular arrhythmias
Procainamide	Life-threatening or symptomatic ventricular arrhythmias
Disopyramide	Life-threatening ventricular arrhythmias

Class 1B

Lidocaine	Ventricular arrhythmias
Tocainide	Life-threatening ventricular arrhythmias
Mexiletine	Life-threatening ventricular arrhythmias
Moricizine	Life-threatening ventricular arrhythmias

Class 1C

Flecainide	Paroxysmal supraventricular tachycardias associated with disabling symptoms
	Paroxysmal atrial fibrillation/flutter associated with disabling symptoms
	Life-threatening ventricular arrhythmias
Encainide	Life-threatening ventricular arrhythmias (no longer marketed)
Propafenone	Life-threatening ventricular arrhythmias

Class 2: Drugs that block β-receptors

Propranolol	Paroxysmal atrial tachycardias, particularly those caused by catecholamines or digitalis or Wolff-Parkinson-White syndrome
	Persistent noncompensatory sinus tachycardia that impairs the patient's well-being
	Tachycardias due to thyrotoxicosis
	Atrial flutter/fibrillation when rate cannot be controlled by digoxin alone

	Ventricular tachycardias induced by catecholamines or when other drugs or cardioversion are not indicated or not effective
	Persistent ventricular extrasystoles that impair the well-being of the patient and do not respond to conventional measures
	Tachycardias due to excess catecholamine action during anesthesia
Acebutolol	Ventricular premature beats
Esmolol	Control of ventricular rate in atrial flutter and fibrillation and noncompensatory sinus tachycardia
Class 3: Drugs that delay repolarization	
Bretylium	Ventricular fibrillation and other life-threatening ventricular arrhythmias
Amiodarone	Life-threatening ventricular arrhythmias when other agents have failed
Sotalol	Life-threatening ventricular arrhythmias
Ibutilide	Rapid conversion of atrial fibrillation/flutter
Class 4: Drugs that block calcium channels	
Verapamil	Paroxysmal supraventricular tachycardia
	Control of ventricular rate in atrial flutter and fibrillation, with digoxin
Diltiazem (intravenous)	Temporary control or rapid ventricular rate in atrial fibrillation or flutter (though not to be used in patients with the Wolff-Parkinson-White syndrome)
	Rapid conversion of paroxysmal supraventricular tachycardias
Unclassified Drugs	
Digoxin	Control of ventricular rate in atrial flutter and fibrillation
	Conversion and prevention of paroxysmal supraventricular tachycardia
Adenosine	Rapid conversion of paroxysmal supraventricular tachycardia

Radio-Frequency Catheter Ablation or Surgical Ablation

The advent of radio-frequency catheter ablation has revolutionized the management of many tachyarrhythmias. Arrhythmias are mapped using intracardiac catheters; an ablating catheter is placed in a critical part of the circuit (for example, the point of origin or a necessary path of the arrhythmia). Radio-frequency energy is applied, which burns the myocardium. This technique has been particularly successful in treating Wolff-Parkinson-White syndrome, where the bypass tract from the atria to the ventricle can be ablated, and in treating AV nodal reentrant tachycardias, where the AV node slow pathway can be cauterized. There has been limited success with treating atrial tachycardias by radio-frequency ablation. Ventricular tachycardias that are due to reentrant circuits from previous myocardial infarctions that have been treated with limited success in some tertiary care centers. Treatment for ventricular tachycardias from a single focus in patients without evidence of structural heart disease has been very effective. Recently, there has also been some progress in treating atrial fibrillation using radio-frequency catheter ablation.

Cardiac surgery can also be used to treat malignant arrhythmias. With the advent of radio-frequency catheter ablation, however, the number of surgeries for this reason has significantly decreased. Epicardial and intramyocardial foci are particularly difficult to reach using catheter-based techniques and can be treated surgically if necessary. The tachycardia is mapped during surgery and the region of interest can be excised or frozen by cryosurgery.

Implantable Cardiac Defibrillators

Implantable cardiac defibrillators detect tachyarrhythmias, including ventricular tachycardia, and terminate them with either antitachycardic pacing or defibrillation with 40 J of energy delivered through endocardial or epicardial leads. In patients with ischemic cardiomyopathy with ventricular tachycardia inducible during an electrophysiology study, the placement of an implantable cardiac defibrillator reduces mortality significantly.

Acute Management of Tachycardias

Acute management of arrhythmias centers on emergent and nonemergent treatments. Indications for emergent or urgent treatment include hypotension, pulmonary edema, syncope, and cardiac ischemia. Under these circumstances, electrical cardioversion is appropriate to restore sinus rhythm.

For nonemergent cases, management involves diagnosis and medical treatment. A 12-lead ECG should be obtained to look for P waves and to characterize the QRS complex as wide (more than 120 ms) or narrow (120 ms or less). Narrow-complex tachycardias are frequently supraventricular in origin. While a rhythm strip is being recorded, vagal maneuvers such as carotid sinus massage and the Valsalva maneuver may unmask a hidden P wave that can aid significantly in the diagnosis. Medications such as adenosine will block the AV node, and this will uncover the P wave. Adenosine is also therapeutic for a number of supraventricular tachycardias, including AV nodal reentrant tachycardia and AV reentrant tachycardia. Other AV nodal blocking agents such as verapamil and esmolol can be used for both therapeutic and diagnostic reasons. Wide-complex tachycardias are frequently ventricular in origin. Ventricular tachycardia is more serious in that it frequently degenerates into ventricular fibrillation, which is not compatible with life. The most recent ECG should be compared with an old ECG if available. If the QRS morphology is similar, the tachycardia may be supraventricular. The ECG should be examined closely for AV dissociation, as this would confirm a diagnosis of ventricular tachycardia. Nonemergent ventricular tachycardia should be treated with medications such as lidocaine, procainamide, and amiodarone to restore sinus rhythm.

Supraventricular Tachycardia and Ectopy

Sinus tachycardia is the most frequent arrhythmia in the ICU and is defined as a sinus rate above 100 beats per minute. Almost all sinus tachycardia is an appropriate physiologic response to stress. The medical management, therefore, centers on treating the underlying illness. Very rarely, there can be sinus tachycardia secondary to a reentrant loop involving the sinus node, which is treated effectively by catheter-based ablation.

Atrial Tachyarrhythmias (Table 28-3)

Atrial arrhythmias include atrial fibrillation, atrial flutter, atrial tachycardia, and multifocal atrial tachycardia. The treatment of atrial fibrillation and flutter involves controlling the ventricular response (rate control), anticoagulation, and consideration of cardioversion. Rate control is accomplished using β-blockers and calcium-channel blockers. The negative inotropic effect and propensity to lower blood pressure of these medications are always of concern. It is usually significantly easier to control the rate of atrial fibrillation than that of atrial flutter. Flutter, however, is easily cardioverted. Elective cardioversion should be considered for patients with new-onset atrial flutter or fibrillation. In most cases of flutter and atrial fibrillation that occur in the ICU setting, the rhythm spontaneously reverts to sinus, so conservative therapy is not unreasonable. If spontaneous reversion to sinus rhythm does not occur, cardioversion may be done electrically (usually requiring between 50 and 200 J) or with class Ia or Ic agents. If the atrial fibrillation has persisted for more than 48 hours without anticoagulation, a transesophageal echocardiogram should be considered to assess for atrial thrombus prior to attempted cardioversion, since the presence of a thrombus is a risk factor for pericardioversion stroke. Many forms of atrial flutter can be treated by catheter-based ablation, which can be curative. Pacing can also be used to treat atrial flutter. Entraining the atria through rapid (at about 125 percent of the atrial rate) bursts of pacing will frequently terminate atrial flutter. This technique is particularly useful for patients who have epicardial pacing leads from recent cardiac surgery. Atrial fibrillation is a major risk factor for thromboembolic disease, and numerous trials have demonstrated that anticoagulation reduces mortality and morbidity. If there are no contraindications to anticoagulation, patients with atrial fibrillation should have short-term anticoagulation with heparin. If the atrial fibrillation is persistent or intermittent, patients should be anticoagulated with warfarin to an international normalized ratio (INR) of 2 to 3.

Atrial tachycardia and multifocal atrial tachycardia are usually secondary to underlying disease or pulmonary failure. The treatment, therefore, should center on eradicating the inciting cause. These patients should also have their ventricular response controlled with calcium-channel or β-blockers. Atrial tachycardia is also a common rhythm seen in digitalis toxicity, so this disorder should be considered. If AV conduction block is also present, the likelihood of digitalis toxicity is increased. If significant digitalis toxicity is diagnosed, digitalis antibody may be administered.

Junctional Tachyarrhythmias

There are three common tachyarrhythmias that involve the AV junction. AV nodal reentrant tachycardia and AV accelerated junctional tachycardia involve increased automaticity of the AV node.

The pathophysiology of AV nodal reentrant tachycardia involves two pathways within the AV node. The tachycardia occurs when antegrade conduction occurs down one pathway only to return up the other, creating a self-propagating loop. Since the pathway is in the AV node or perinodal, the atrial and ventricular activation occur nearly simultaneously on the surface ECG, making P waves frequently invisible. The pathophysiology of AV reentrant tachycardias is similar and involves an accessory pathway somewhere in the mitral or tricuspid annulus. The tachycardia occurs when antegrade conduction from the atria to the ventricle occurs down the normal pathway (AV node, bundle of His, and the bundle branches) only to return back to the atria via the accessory pathway to reactivate the atria which starts the process over. The surface ECG during normal sinus rhythm may show preexcitation (delta wave) of the ventricle if the accessory pathway can conduct in an antegrade manner. During the tachycardia, the ECG shows a narrow complex. Most maneuvers that affect the AV node such as vagal stimulation, adenosine, or calcium and β-blockers will terminate both AV nodal reentrant tachycardia and AV reentrant tachycardia, since the circuit involves the AV node. Once the acute arrhythmia is terminated, calcium-channel and β-blockers, which limit recurrence of these arrhythmias, may be administered. Catheter-based ablation of the accessory pathway can be curative.

TABLE 28-3 Doses of Antiarrhythmic Drugs

Drug	Loading Dose	Maintenance Dose	Gastrointestinal Absorption, %	Oral Bioavailability, %	Therapeutic Plasma Concentration
Digoxin	10–15 μg/kg or 0.5–1.0 mg IV/PO, then 0.25 mg prn to total 1.0–2.5 mg	0.125–0.375 mg qd IV/PO	75–90	50–80	0.5–2.0 ng/mL
Adenosine	6–12 mg IV		—	—	—
Verapamil	2.5–10 mg IV over 2–5 min	2.5–5.0 μg/kg per min or 120–480 mg PO qd	90	10–20	15–100 μg/L
Propranolol	0.5–1.0 mg IV q5 min to 0.1–0.2 mg/kg total dose	10–40 mg PO qid-bid to 320 ng PO total dose	95	20–50	50–100 ng/mL
Esmolol	500 μg/kg per min IV	50–300 μg/kg per min IV	—	—	—
Quinidine	5–7 mg/kg IV at 20 mg/min (gluconate) or 600–1000 mg PO (sulfate)	10–30 mg/kg total dose PO divided bid-qid depending on preparation	95	70–80	2.0–5.0 μg/mL
Procainamide	15–20 mg/kg IV at 20 mg/min to total dose 1.0 g or 1000 mg Po	1–4 mg/min IV or 50–100 mg/kg total dose PO divided tid-qid depending on preparation	70–90 NAPA	70–90	Procainamide 5–10 μg/mL 5–10 μg/mL

Drug	Loading Dose	Maintenance Dose			Therapeutic Level
Disopyramide	300 mg PO (immediate release preparation)	400–800 mg/day in divided doses	80–100	80–90	2–4 µg/mL
Lidocaine	1.0 mg/kg IV; 0.5 mg/kg q10 min to total dose 3.0 mg/kg	30–50 µg/kg per min or 1–4 mg/min	—	—	1–5 µg/mL
Flecainide	—	100–200 mg PO bid	95	95	0.2–1.0 µg/mL
Moricizine	—	200–300 mg PO bid	—	38	0.1–0.3 µg/mL
Mexiletine	400 mg PO	150–300 mg tid PO	90	88	0.5–2.0 µg/mL
Propafenone	—	150–300 mg tid PO	95	25–75	0.5–1.5 µg/mL
Bretylium	5 mg/kg IV; repeat bolus 10 mg/kg q 15–30 min to total dose 30 mg/kg	0.5–2.0 mg/min IV	—	—	0.6–20.0 µg/mL
Amiodarone	IV: 150 mg over 10 min followed by 1 mg/min for 6 h, then 0.5 mg/min PO: 800–1600 mg qd PO	200–400 mg/day PO	—	22–88	1.0–2.5 µg/mL
Sotalol	—	80–240 mg bid PO	—	90–100	—
Ibutilide	1–2 mg IV over 10–20 min	—	—	—	—

Accelerated junctional tachycardia is similar to atrial tachycardia and is seen in patients with underlying systemic illness. It is also seen with digitalis toxicity. The pathophysiology involves increased automaticity of the AV node. The ECG reveals either no P waves or inverted P waves due to depolarization of the atrium from below (AV node toward the sinus node). The QRS is narrow or resembles the patient's underlying complex. Junctional tachycardia is unlike AV nodal reentrant and AV reentrant tachycardias in that it does not respond to AV nodal blocking agents or to electrical cardioversion. Generally, accelerated junctional tachycardia will resolve as the underlying systemic illness is treated. Digitalis toxicity can be treated with antibody against digitalis if necessary.

Ventricular Arrhythmias

Premature ventricular complexes (PVC) are common in both health and illness. In the ICU, PVCs are frequently treated unnecessarily. If PVCs cause no hemodynamic compromise and do not trigger more malignant arrhythmias, they can remain untreated. Although PVCs in the context of myocardial ischemia are frequently treated with lidocaine, there is no mortality benefit associated with this practice.

Accelerated Idioventricular Rhythm

Accelerated idioventricular rhythm is secondary to increased automaticity. It is also commonly seen during reperfusion following thrombolytic therapy for myocardial infarction. Accelerated idioventricular rhythm has a rate of 70 to 110 beats per minute and is difficult to distinguish from slow ventricular tachycardia. One difference is that VT is usually abrupt in onset and termination, while accelerated idioventricular rhythm tends to have warm-up and cool-down periods.

Ventricular Tachycardia

Ventricular tachycardia (VT) is defined as greater than three consecutive beats originating in the ventricular tissue. Traditionally, VT is subclassified into sustained versus nonsustained and monomorphic versus polymorphic. Sustained VT persists for more than 30 seconds, while nonsustained VT self-terminates. Monomorphic VT has only a single morphology on the ECG, while polymorphic VT has varied morphology.

There are numerous mechanisms of VT. VT in a patient with a former myocardial infarction is likely secondary to a reentrant loop around the scar. Other kinds of VT include the triggered automaticity from digitalis toxicity, bundle branch reentrant VT seen in patients with dilated cardiomyopathy, torsades de pointes due to early after-depolarizations, and right ventricular outflow tract VT in patients with no obvious structural heart disease.

The management of VT depends on the hemodynamic impact. If there is hemodynamic embarrassment, emergent electrical cardioversion (200 to 360 J) is done to restore sinus rhythm. Cardiopulmonary resuscitation should be instituted. Epinephrine (1-mg bolus every 5 minutes), lidocaine (1-mg/kg bolus followed by 0.5 mg/kg to a total of 3 mg/kg if needed), and bretylium (10 mg/kg) can be administered if electrical cardioversion is not immediately successful. If the patient is hemodynamically stable, the diagnosis should be confirmed with a 12-lead ECG and rhythm strip. The treatment involves lidocaine, procainamide, bretylium, and/or amiodarone. If pacing leads are available, pace termination should be considered. Elective electrical cardioversion may be necessary.

There are some forms of VT that require particular mention. VT in the context of digoxin toxicity should be managed with digoxin antibodies. The dose must be calculated based on the amount of digoxin in the patient. Of note, the serum level of digoxin will rise after administration of the antibody, but these digoxin molecules are bound to antibody and inactive. Torsades de pointes, a polymorphic VT, occurs in patients with prolonged QT intervals and usually self-terminates. If it does not self-terminate, one can consider electrical cardioversion. Most congenital (long-QT) syndromes and central nervous system catastrophes that cause torsades de pointes should be treated with β-blockers, while the acquired form of torsades is treated by removing the inciting medication or metabolic abnormality. The latter type respond to shortening of the QT interval by pacing or isoproterenol infusion. Hyperkalemia can cause VT that is sinusoidal in morphology; in this situation, the underlying hyperkalemia should be treated with insulin, glucose, calcium chloride, and bicarbonate. Electrical cardioversion is usually ineffective.

After normal sinus rhythm is restored, management involves preventing recurrences. Typically, the medication that terminated the original arrhythmia is started. Other inciting medications and metabolic abnormalities should be corrected if possible. These would include electrolyte abnormalities, medication overdoses, and cardiac ischemia. In patients with ischemic cardiomyopathies and sustained VT, electrophysiologic testing should be considered, since a high-risk subgroup of this population has a mortality benefit when an internal cardiac defibrillator is placed.

Pacemakers

Pacemakers have four basic functions: sensing, inhibiting, triggering, and capturing. For example, in a dual-chamber pacemaker with both atrial and ventricular leads, the intra-atrial lead will "sense" the intrinsic atrial depolarization (P wave). The pacemaker will then "inhibit" itself from pacing the atrium; simultaneously, the pacemaker "triggers" itself to pace the ventricle after an appropriate delay. If there is native AV conduction with a native QRS prior to the completion of this delay, the pacemaker will "sense" the ventricular depolarization through the ventricular lead and "inhibit" itself from pacing the ventricle. If there is no native conduction through the AV node, the pacemaker will deliver an electrical stimulus to the ventricle. If the ventricle depolarizes as a consequence of this electrical stimulus, there was "capture" of the ventricle.

Each pacemaker is given a universal three-letter code to denote its type and programming. The first letter denotes the chambers that are paced: A for atrium, V for ventricle, and D for dual chamber. The second letter indicates the chambers that are sensed, using the same convention; O would indicate no sensing. The third letter denotes whether the pacing is inhibited (I), triggered (T), or both (D). In the previous example, both chambers are paced, both chambers are sensed, the atria and ventricle were inhibited, and the ventricle was triggered by the sensed atrial beat. The three-letter code for this pacemaker would be DDD.

There are indications for temporary and permanent pacing. The American College of Cardiology has published guidelines for temporary pacing in the setting of an acute myocardial infarction (Table 28-4). The basic premise for these guidelines is to pace patients prophylactically who have a high likelihood of progression to either complete heart block or asystole and those who are already in complete heart block or asystole. In the absence of cardiac ischemia, temporary pacing is indicated in patients who have hemodynamic compromise or symptoms from a low-output state due to bradycardia. Sinus bradycardia or complete heart block with symptoms would qualify. Temporary pacing is also used to treat torsades de pointes; by rapidly pacing the ventricle (100 beats per minute), the QT interval is shortened, which decreases the likelihood of torsades de pointes. Finally, temporary pacing may be used to terminate reentrant tachycardias. Atrial flutter, AV nodal reentrant and AV reentrant tachycardias, and some ventricular tachycardias can be pace-terminated by burst pacing. Usually, therapeutic pace termination is done in patients who already have either a temporary or permanent pacer in place.

The American College of Cardiology has published guidelines for permanent pacing. The indications for permanent pacing are similar to those for temporary pacing in that symptomatic or hemodynamically significant bradycardias and rhythms that may progress to significant bradycardias should be considered for permanent pacing. In an ICU, the patient's clinical status should also be considered. A terminally ill patient, a patient with a bleeding disorder, or one with an infection would be a poor candidate for placement of a permanent pacemaker.

There are multiple ways to pace temporarily: transvenous, epicardial, transesophageal, and transcutaneous pacing. Transvenous pacing is the most reliable and should be used if there is a significant likelihood of relying on the pacemaker. Temporary pacing leads are generally placed from either the subclavian, internal jugular, or femoral vein under either ECG or fluoroscopic guidance. Usually, only a ventricular lead is placed; however, there are now atrial and ventricular lead systems available. Placement of a transvenous temporary pacer can be complicated by infection, hemorrhage, pneumothorax, arrhythmias, and myocardial puncture. After placement of

TABLE 28-4   Indications for Temporary Pacing in Acute Myocardial Infarction

---

Class I: Usually indicated, always acceptable, and considered useful/effective

Asystole

Complete heart block

Right bundle branch block with left anterior or left posterior hemiblock developing in acute myocardial infarction

Left bundle branch block developing in acute myocardial infarction

Type II second-degree AV block

Symptomatic bradycardia not responsive to atropine

Class IIa: Acceptable, of uncertain efficacy, may be controversial. Weight of evidence favors usefulness/efficacy

Type I second-degree AV block with hypotension not responsive to atropine; during ventricular pacing, if ventriculoatrial conduction causes the atrial contraction to fall within ventricular contraction, atrial or AV sequential pacing may be necessary

Sinus bradycardia with hypotension not responsive to atropine

Recurrent sinus pauses not responsive to atropine

Atrial or ventricular overdrive pacing for incessant ventricular tachycardia

Class IIb: Acceptable, of uncertain efficacy, may be controversial. Not well established by evidence; can be helpful, probably not harmful

Left bundle branch block with first-degree heart block of uncertain duration

Bifascicular block of uncertain duration

Class III: Not indicated; may be harmful

First-degree heart block

Type I second-degree AV block with normal hemodynamics

Accelerated idioventricular rhythm causing AV dissociation

Bundle branch block known to exist before the myocardial infarction

---

the lead, a chest x-ray should be obtained to verify position and absence of a pneumothorax. On a daily basis, the sensing and capturing thresholds should be tested to verify stability of position. Epicardial pacing leads are placed during cardiac surgery to help with the postoperative management of cardiac conduction abnormalities. Usually, both atrial and ventricular leads are placed. Epicardial leads have minimal complications and can frequently be used to diagnose and treat the many supraventricular arrhythmias seen in postoperative cardiac surgery patients. Transesophageal pacing is accomplished by having the patient swallow a lead in a Teflon-coated tablet. The tablet gradually dissolves and the lead can then be optimally positioned in the esophagus. Since the esophagus is directly behind the left atrium, atrial activity (P wave) can be recorded from the esophageal lead. The esophageal lead can be used to pace the atrium but not the ventricle. Transesophageal pacing, therefore, is not appropriate for treatment of complete heart block; it is most effective in paced termination of atrial flutter. Transcutaneous pacing is accomplished by placing large electrodes (patches) on the surface of the chest. Most systems also are equipped to provide direct-current cardioversion if needed; therefore the transcutaneous pacemaker effectively acts both as a defibrillator and pacer. Transcutaneous pacing, however, is painful, so it cannot be used for long periods. Usually, transcutaneous pacing is started emergently while a temporary venous pacer is being placed. If a transcutaneous pacer is placed, it must be checked regularly to ensure appropriate function, since thresholds for capture and sensing can change dramatically within short periods.

Electrical Cardioversion

Electrical cardioversion is effective in treating a wide range of tachyarrhythmias. Most hemodynamically significant arrhythmias should be treated with emergent electrical cardioversion, as discussed above. The only exceptions to this rule are sinus tachycardia, ectopic atrial tachycardias, accelerated junctional rhythms, and arrhythmias due to digitalis intoxication. The first three arrhythmias are due to enhanced automaticity, a mechanism that does not respond to electrical cardioversion. Rhythms due to digitalis intoxication are exacerbated by cardioversion. Elective cardioversion is reserved for arrhythmias that are hemodynamically stable.

Complications of cardioversion are manifold. There is small risk of inducing ventricular fibrillation; however, if the cardioversion is synchronized (in all cases except when defibrillating VF), this risk is minimal. The patient may also have superficial burns incurred from the paddles during defibrillation. An ECG immediately after cardioversion frequently demonstrates ST elevation. Despite this, elevation of the MB fraction of creatinine kinase is rare, although the MM creatinine kinase fraction is routinely elevated. Electrical cardioversion can damage a permanent pacemaker and, rarely, cause malfunction. In the presence of a pacemaker, therefore, the paddles should be placed at least 5 in. from the pulse generator.

For a more detailed discussion, see Chap. 23 in *Principles of Critical Care,* 2d ed.

Chapter 29 _____

ACUTE RIGHT HEART SYNDROMES AND PULMONARY EMBOLISM

JOHN P. KRESS

Shock resulting from cardiac "pump failure" is usually due to left ventricular (LV) dysfunction. However, in a substantial minority of patients, right ventricular (RV) dysfunction is the cause of shock. Causes of acute right heart syndromes (RHS) include acute pulmonary embolism (PE), other causes of acute right heart pressure overload (e.g., acute respiratory distress syndrome, or ARDS), acute deterioration in patients with chronic pulmonary hypertension, and RV infarction.

Right Ventricular Physiology

When the pulmonary vasculature is normal, RV performance has little impact on the maintenance of cardiac output. During acute pulmonary artery (PA) hypertension, RV preload, afterload, and contractile state rise at the same time that heart rate rises. These features all raise RV myocardial oxygen consumption ($\dot{V}_{O_2}$). When an acute RHS is sufficiently severe to cause systemic hypotension, coronary perfusion of the RV may fall. The combination of rising $\dot{V}_{O_2}$ and falling coronary oxygen supply leads to RV ischemia, which reduces RV ejection against the increased PA pressure afterload. As RV pressure rises, the interventricular septum shifts to the left, causing LV diastolic dysfunction. A vicious cycle ensues in which RV ischemia impairs RV ejection, with progressive RV dilation and more LV diastolic dysfunction.

Clinical Clues to Right Heart Syndromes

In the hypoperfused patient, several clinical features should suggest the possibility of an acute RHS (Table 29-1).

TABLE 29-1   Clues to Recognition
of Right Heart Syndromes[a]

Elevated neck veins
Pulsatile liver
Peripheral >> lung edema
Right-sided S3, tricuspid regurgitation
Radiography
Electrocardiography
Echocardiography

---

[a]Suspicion is the key to diagnosis.

Most signs of RHS are not specific; a high index of suspicion is needed, since the treatment of RHS is unique in several regards. Radiographic signs include an enlarged PA or RV, oligemia of a lobe or lung (Westermark sign), and a distended azygos (or other central) vein. Electrocardiography (ECG) may reveal signs of right heart strain/pulmonary hypertension (rightward axis shift, RBBB, right atrial enlargement, RVH, right precordial T-wave inversions, $S_1Q_3T_3$ pattern) but usually shows only sinus tachycardia. Echocardiographic findings of RHS/PE are listed in Table 29-2.

RV infarction can usually be distinguished readily from acute pulmonary hypertension in that high PA pressures are

TABLE 29-2   Echocardiographic Signs of Right Heart
Syndrome/Pulmonary Embolism

Dilated, thin-walled right ventricle
Poorly contracting right ventricle
Tricuspid regurgitation
Pulmonary hypertension estimated from the tricuspid
   regurgitation jet
Leftward shifting of the interventricular septum
Pulmonary artery dilation
Visualized thrombus in RA, RV, or PA
Loss of respirophasic variation in the diameter of the inferior
   vena cava

---

lacking. Echocardiography is so useful in the detection of RHS that it should be obtained early in the hypoperfused patient whenever one of the previously mentioned clinical indicators is present. Causes of acute RHS are listed in Table 29-3.

TABLE 29-3   Causes of the Acute Right Heart Syndrome

Acute pressure overload
  Pulmonary embolism
  ARDS
  Excessive PEEP, tidal volume, and alveolar pressure
  Air, amniotic, fat, and tumor microembolism
  Sepsis (rarely)
  Pulmonary leukostasis, leukoagglutination
  Extensive lung resection
  Drugs (e.g., heparin-protamine reaction)
  Hypoxia
  Post–cardiac surgery/cardiopulmonary bypass
Acute-on-chronic PA hypertension
  Chronic lung diseases
    Emphysema, chronic bronchitis, bronchiectasis, cystic fibrosis
    Restrictive diseases of the lung
    Collagen vascular diseases of the lung
  Thoracic cage deformities
    Kyphoscoliosis, thoracoplasty
  Cardiovascular disorders
    Chronic thromboembolism
    Primary pulmonary hypertension
    Congenital heart diseases
    Pulmonary venoocclusive disease
  Miscellaneous disorders
    Sleep-disordered breathing
    Hyperviscosity syndromes
    Toxins and drugs
    Parasites
    End-stage liver disease
    HIV infection
Right ventricular systolic dysfunction
  RV infarction
  Sepsis
  Toxins

Specific Right Heart Syndromes

ACUTE PULMONARY HYPERTENSION

Acute pulmonary hypertension is caused by an abrupt increase in pulmonary vascular resistance due to vasoconstriction, vascular obstruction, or surgical resection. The prototype of acute pulmonary hypertension is acute pulmonary embolism (discussed further on), but other forms of embolism, microvascular injury (e.g., ARDS), drug effect, and inflammation can raise pulmonary vascular resistance acutely (see Table 29-3).

ACUTE-ON-CHRONIC PULMONARY HYPERTENSION

Patients with preexisting pulmonary vascular disease may present with acute RHS when intercurrent critical illness demands a higher-than-normal cardiac output. When pulmonary hypertension is diagnosed during the course of critical illness, the potential for underlying chronic pulmonary vascular disease should be considered, especially when the history suggests chronic disease, the mean PA pressure is higher than 40 mmHg, or echocardiography shows evidence of RV hypertrophy.

RIGHT VENTRICULAR INFARCTION

This may be seen with inferior myocardial infarction (MI), as well as anterior MIs. RV dilation accompanies significant myocardial injury. One should suspect RV infarction in patients with an inferior MI with increased RA pressure and clear lungs by examination and chest x-ray. Right precordial electrocardiography (ECG) and/or echocardiographic evidence of RV injury can help distinguish RHS due to acute PA hypertension from RHS due to RV infarction.

Treatment of Right Heart Syndromes

Two basic aims of treatment are to reduce systemic $\dot{V}_{O_2}$ while improving oxygen delivery (Table 29-4). The goals of oxygen therapy in RHS are to enhance arterial saturation (Sa_{O_2}) and

TABLE 29-4   Goals of Therapy in the Right Heart
Syndromes

Correct hypoxemia
Find optimal volume
Correct anemia with red blood cell transfusion
Exclude or treat concomitant LV dysfunction
Minimize $\dot{V}_{O_2}$ (sedation, mechanical ventilation, treatment of fever,
   neuromuscular blockade)
Reduce PEEPi and other causes of elevated alveolar pressure

---

block alveolar hypoxic vasoconstriction (AHV). One should
keep $Sa_{O_2} > 96\%$ to ensure alveolar P_{O_2} values sufficient to
block AHV.

FLUID THERAPY

Aggressive fluid administration in patients with acute RHS
may lead to worsening RV systolic function and leftward displacement of the interventricular septum, with LV diastolic
dysfunction. Some patients *are* volume-depleted, so a discrete
fluid challenge (500 mL 0.9% normal saline) is reasonable, especially if the central venous pressure is low. It is important
to pay close attention to indicators of perfusion (renal function, mental status, cardiac output/mixed venous oxyhemoglobin saturation). If no benefit from fluid is detected, attention should shift to vasoactive drugs.

VASOACTIVE DRUG THERAPY

Vasoactive drugs are effective in RHS when they increase cardiac output without significantly worsening systemic hypotension, Sa_{O_2}, or RV ischemia. Vasoactive drugs should be
titrated according to clinical measures of adequacy of perfusion rather than to blood pressure alone. Begin dobutamine
(RV inotropy) at 5 μg/kg/min raising the dose in increments
of 5 μg/kg/min each 10 minutes. If the patient fails to respond to dobutamine (or the response is incomplete), one
may substitute (or add) norepinephrine (which acts as a systemic vasoconstrictor and positive inotrope by raising coronary perfusion pressure to an ischemic RV) infused at 4 to
20 μg/min.

Prostaglandins

Prostaglandin E_1 (PGE_1) is a potent pulmonary vasodilator. Its utility is limited by a propensity to significantly lower systemic blood pressure and increase intrapulmonary shunt. It remains to be shown whether it will be useful in the acute RHS.

Nitric Oxide

Inhaled nitric oxide (NO) is a potent pulmonary vasodilator without systemic hemodynamic effects (it is inactivated by hemoglobin). In patients with ARDS and pulmonary hypertension, it lowers PA pressure and RV end-diastolic volume and increases RV ejection fraction and arterial P_{O_2} without changing mean arterial pressure.

VENTILATOR MANAGEMENT

Hypercapnia and hypoxia raise PA pressure, which may lead to unacceptable hemodynamic deterioration in patients with severe pulmonary hypertension.

The effect of PEEP differs depending on whether atelectatic or flooded lung is recruited or whether relatively normal lung is overdistended. In a study of patients with ARDS, PEEP had little effect on RV function when given in amounts up to that associated with improving respiratory system compliance. At higher levels of PEEP, the dominant effect was to impair RV systolic function.

These effects of mechanical ventilation on RV function suggest the following strategy in patients with acute RHS: (1) give sufficient oxygen to reverse any hypoxic vasoconstriction; (2) avoid hypercapnia; (3) keep PEEP at or below a level at which continued alveolar recruitment can be demonstrated and seek to minimize auto-PEEP; and (4) use the least tidal volume necessary to effect adequate elimination of CO_2. The acute effects of each intervention should be measured to confirm that cardiac output increases.

PULMONARY THROMBOEMBOLISM

PE results from underlying deep venous thrombosis (DVT) in the proximal lower extremities (less commonly from catheter-associated thrombi in the upper extremities). Failure to diagnose PE is a serious management error, since 30 percent of untreated patients die while only 8 percent succumb with effective therapy. Critically ill patients are likely to have limited cardiopulmonary reserve, so that pulmonary emboli may be particularly lethal.

Pathophysiology

PE occurs when thrombi detach and are carried through the great veins to the pulmonary circulation, affecting gas exchange and circulation. Physical obstruction to PA flow creates dead space in the segments served by the affected arteries. Minute ventilation ($\dot{V}E$) usually increases and Pa_{CO_2} typically falls. A widened alveolar-to-arterial gradient for oxygen (A-a)P_{O_2} is often present. However, since hyperventilation is the rule, Pa_{O_2} may not be low. In fact, one-third of patients with proven PE demonstrate a $Pa_{O_2} > 70$ mmHg. Therefore, a normal Pa_{O_2} does not exclude a diagnosis of PE. Hypoxemia is most often due to $\dot{V}/\dot{Q}$ mismatch and is typically responsive to modest increases in FI_{O_2} (by nasal cannula or face mask). Atelectasis due to impaired surfactant production may contribute to hypoxemia. Intracardiac right-to-left shunt due to opening of a probe-patent foramen ovale may be seen occasionally. In addition, the fall in cardiac output ($\dot{Q}T$) that accompanies most pulmonary emboli leads to a fall in mixed venous saturation. Ventilatory failure is usually not a significant problem, since most patients are able to double or triple $\dot{V}E$, if necessary, in order to eliminate CO_2. Although there are exceptions (e.g., some patients with severe chronic obstructive pulmonary disease, or COPD), morbidity and mortality from PE relate to cardiovascular compromise, not respiratory failure. Table 29-5 lists symptoms and signs of PE.

The greatest utility of the chest film is in making (or excluding) alternative diagnoses such as pneumonia, pneumothorax, or aortic dissection. Nevertheless, the typical (albeit nonspecific) findings of basilar atelectasis, elevation of the diaphragm, and pleural effusion should always suggest PE when there is no ready alternative explanation.

TABLE 29-5 Symptoms and Signs
of Pulmonary Embolism

Symptom	Incidence, %
Dyspnea	80
Pleuritic pain	70
Apprehension	60
Cough	50
Symptoms of DVT	35
Hemoptysis	25
Central chest pain	10
Palpitations	10
Syncope	5

Sign	Incidence, %
Tachypnea	90
Fever	50
Tachycardia	50
Increased P_2	50
Signs of DVT	33
Shock	5

Signs from More Invasive Monitoring

An increase in $\dot{V}E$ should prompt consideration of PE. Of course, any cause of rising dead space (airflow obstruction, hypovolemia, PEEP) or CO_2 production (anxiety, pain, fever, sepsis) will also increase $\dot{V}E$. However, when none of these is apparent, especially when other clues are evident, PE becomes more likely.

- *Expired carbon dioxide:* The increment in dead space after PE causes a detectable fall in end-tidal CO_2 (ET_{CO_2}).
- *Pulmonary artery catheter:* The most obvious clues from the PA catheter are increases in RA, RV, and PA pressures and a fall in $\dot{Q}T$. A discrepancy between the PA diastolic pressure and Ppw may provide a clue to PA obstruction.
- *Echocardiography:* See above discussion on acute RHS. Very rarely, echocardiography may demonstrate a thrombus in the RA or RV.

TABLE 29-6   Risk Factors for Pulmonary Embolism

Epidemiologic factors: Obesity, prior thromboembolism, advanced age, malignancy (especially adenocarcinoma), estrogens

Venous stasis: Immobility, paralysis, leg casts, varicose veins, congestive heart failure, prolonged travel, and use of muscle relaxants

Injury: Postsurgical, posttrauma, postpartum

Hypercoagulable states: Proteins C and S and antithrombin-III deficiency, factor V Leiden, antiphospholipid antibody syndromes, polycythemia, macroglobulinemia

Indwelling lines: Central venous and pulmonary artery catheters

---

DIAGNOSIS

A sense of the probability of PE is important, since the critically ill patient is often unable to complain of the usual symptoms of PE, has numerous explanations for tachycardia and tachypnea, is hemodynamically unstable, and is a poor candidate for $\dot{V}/\dot{Q}$ lung scanning. Clinicians must combine an assessment of risk factors (Table 29-6) with a synthesis of the patient's cardiopulmonary physiology.

Diagnostic Tests

In some patients, the pulmonary angiogram can be replaced by the ventilation perfusion $(\dot{V}/\dot{Q})$ lung scan. Unfortunately, $\dot{V}/\dot{Q}$ scanning has limited use in intensive care unit (ICU) patients, since ventilation scanning is technically more challenging in these patients and a normal perfusion scan is less likely, since these patients have so many reasons for pulmonary vascular injury, constriction, or obstruction. Other tests such as noninvasive leg studies, helical CT and MRI of the thorax are discussed below. An integrated approach to the diagnosis of PE is described in Fig. 29-1.

VENTILATION/PERFUSION LUNG SCAN

"High probability" $\dot{V}/\dot{Q}$ scans have a specificity of 85 percent, and the risk of treating this group is felt to be less than the risk and cost of performing pulmonary angiography. Scans of

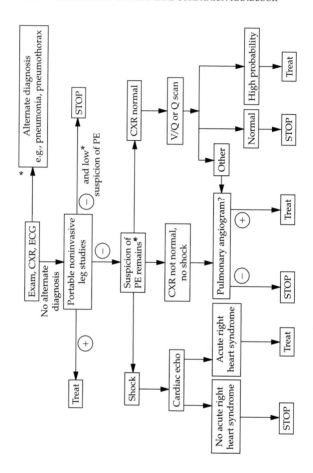

◀FIGURE 29-1   Algorithm for evaluation of a critically ill patient suspected of having a pulmonary embolus. If alternate diagnoses are
not confirmed by examination, chest x-ray, and ECG, noninvasive
leg studies can be requested. If these are of adequate technical quality and are positive, treatment for pulmonary embolism is generally
indicated. If they are negative and the prior suspicion of PE is very
low, no further evaluation for PE is warranted. If the suspicion of
PE remains, angiography is often necessary. This may not be possible for a patient in shock, in whom echocardiography may provide
support for a diagnosis of PE or demonstrate an alternative explanation for shock. Finally, patients with normal chest x-rays should
have perfusion lung scans done when this is technically feasible,
since this may exclude PE from consideration. If the scan is not definitive, however, further evaluation, often angiography, is necessary. Treat = treatment for PE is generally indicated; STOP = PE is
very unlikely and an explanation for the patient's symptoms or signs
should be sought elsewhere.* These decisions hinge critically on
clinical judgement and experience.

"intermediate probability" indicate a 40 percent likelihood of
PE, so that further evaluation to prove or exclude the diagnosis is imperative. Early reports found patients with "low probability" scans to have less than a 5 percent chance of PE, though
subsequent reports found this number to be between 16 and
40 percent; however, if the pretest probability of PE is low
(<20 percent), only 4 percent have PEs. Before obtaining the
scan, the clinical probability of PE should be estimated so as
to limit bias once the scan result is known. Normal scans exclude the diagnosis of PE. "Low probability" scans combined
with a low clinical estimate of PE are strong evidence against
the diagnosis, and an explanation for the patient's symptoms
or signs should be sought elsewhere. All other scan results are
"indeterminate" and should prompt further evaluation.

NONINVASIVE LEG STUDIES

Noninvasive leg studies (impedance plethysmography, venous Dopplers, and B-mode ultrasound) may diagnose DVT
and provide grounds for treatment (usually anticoagulation),
so the question of PE may cease to be important. In a patient
with a high pretest probability of PE, if V/Q scanning is in-

determinate and noninvasive leg studies are negative, one should proceed to helical computed tomography (CT) or pulmonary angiography.

COMPUTER TOMOGRAPHY AND MAGNETIC RESONANCE IMAGING

Recent advances in CT and magnetic resonance imaging (MRI) have rekindled interest in the potential for these relatively noninvasive studies to replace the $\dot{V}/\dot{Q}$ scan and the pulmonary angiogram. Several studies have found high sensitivity and specificity for these studies as compared with pulmonary angiography; however, no studies have been performed on a critically ill patient population. Given the serious limitations of $\dot{V}/\dot{Q}$ scanning, particularly in critically ill patients, helical CT scanning has replaced it in many institutions.

PULMONARY ANGIOGRAPHY

Pulmonary angiography is the definitive test for the diagnosis of PE. Since it is invasive, costly, riskier than $\dot{V}/\dot{Q}$ scanning, and requires the presence of an interventional radiologist, it is usually reserved for patients in whom the diagnosis cannot be made or excluded by less invasive means. However, pulmonary angiography is safer than generally appreciated. Mortality is around 0.2 percent, as shown in several large series.

Treatment

The majority of patients with PE will not die from the clot that leads to diagnosis, since intrinsic fibrinolysis will restore pulmonary blood flow. The primary goal of all therapies for PE is to prevent reembolization. Some patients, however, survive the initial embolus yet remain in shock. These rare patients who succumb to the initial embolus are overrepresented in ICU populations. Therapy to hasten clot resolution is useful in such patients. Supportive care, anticoagulation, vena caval interruption, thrombolysis, fluid and vasoactive drug administration, and, rarely, surgical embolectomy must

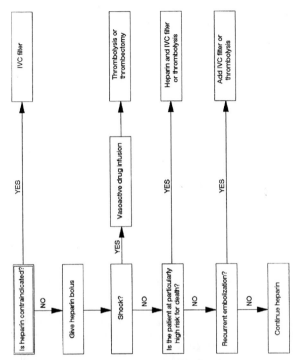

FIGURE 29-2 Treatment of PE in critically ill patients.

all be considered. An integrated approach to the treatment of PE is presented in Fig. 29-2.

Supportive Care

OXYGEN AND BED REST

Bed rest accomplishes two goals—reducing the risk of dislodging further clots from the leg source and reducing oxygen consumption ($\dot{V}_{O_2}$) and thereby the demand for $\dot{Q}T$.

Specific Therapies

ANTICOAGULATION

Heparin is the mainstay of therapy for PE. It is crucial to give sufficient heparin to raise the aPTT to greater than 1.5 times control as soon as possible. Heparin should be instituted once the diagnosis is seriously considered as long as there is no contraindication to anticoagulation. Rapid, adequate anticoagulation is facilitated by a weight-based nomogram with a bolus of 80 U/kg, followed by a continuous infusion of 18 U/kg per hour. Studies suggest that early, adequate anticoagulation leads to improved outcome in patients with PE. *Supra*therapeutic levels of aPTT do not appear to be associated with increased bleeding risks, so one should aim to assure adequate heparin in the first hours of treatment.

Complications of Heparin

The most important complication of heparin is bleeding. The approach to treatment of the patient who bleeds on heparin depends on the severity of the bleeding. Minor bleeding is treated by stopping the heparin (half-life, 90 minutes). Bleeding related to needle sticks may respond to sustained direct pressure. Major bleeding may require neutralization of heparin with protamine sulfate. Fresh frozen plasma is usually ineffective, since circulating heparin inhibits the function of transfused factors. When hemorrhage immediately follows a bolus of heparin, 1 mg protamine per 100 U heparin should be administered. If heparin therapy is ongoing, the dose of protamine should be based on the approximate half-life of heparin. Since protamine, too, is an anticoagulant, the dose should be calculated to only half-correct the estimated circulating heparin. Side effects of protamine include hypotension, shock, dyspnea, and acute pulmonary hypertension upon intravenous injection. This drug should be given very slowly, and a physician experienced with its use should be present. Patients with PE who bleed after receiving heparin will likely require inferior vena caval interruption (VCI).

Low-Molecular-Weight Heparin

Low-molecular-weight heparins (LMWHs) provide a simple, once-daily therapy for venous thromboembolism that does not require monitoring of anticoagulant effect. Several studies have shown LMWHs to be beneficial for treatment of VTE, though experience in the ICU is limited.

Warfarin anticoagulation should be instituted in the first few days [5 mg PO qhs for the first 2 days, then adjustment of dose to achieve an international normalized ratio (INR) between 2.0 and 3.0] and continued to overlap with heparin therapy for at least 5 days. If the patient is clinically unstable, heparin should probably be continued rather than warfarin to facilitate rapid adjustment of anticoagulation if needed.

VENA CAVAL INTERRUPTION

Since most thromboemboli originate in the legs, pelvis, or inferior vena cava (IVC), vena caval interruption (VCI) is effective therapy for PE, since it prevents reembolization and death. Indications for VCI include contraindications to anticoagulation, hemorrhage following anticoagulation, failure of anticoagulation to prevent recurrent embolization, and prophylaxis of patients at extremely high risk.

THROMBOLYTIC THERAPY

Thrombolysis likely improves mortality versus heparin in patients with massive PE and hypoperfusion, and it has been shown to improve RV function (by echocardiographic assessment). Thrombolytic dosing regimens are listed in Table 29-7. Streptokinase is the one agent for which a mortality benefit has been shown, and it is fourfold cheaper than either of the current alternatives. Careful attention should be given to selecting patients appropriately to reduce the rate of hemorrhagic complications (see Table 29-7). It is important to avoid invasive procedures—including those associated with arterial blood gases, arterial catheters, central venous punctures, and pulmonary angiograms—where possible.

TABLE 29-7 Thrombolytic Strategies in Acute
Massive Pulmonary Embolism

Urokinase,[a] bolus of 4400 U/kg, followed by 4400 U/kg per hour
    for 24 hours

Urokinase, bolus of 1 million units over 10 minutes, followed by 2
    million units over 110 minutes

Urokinase, bolus of 15,000 U/kg over 10 minutes

rt-PA, bolus of 0.6 mg/kg over 2–15 minutes

rt-PA, 1 mg/kg over 10 minutes

rt-PA,[a] 100 mg over 2–3 hours

Streptokinase, 1,500,000 U over 1 hour

Streptokinase,[a] 250,000 U over 30 minutes, followed by 100,000 U/h
    for 24 hours

---

[a]Approved by the Food and Drug Administration.

NOTE: Heparin is infused at 1300 U/h when the aPTT falls below twice normal,
then adjusted to keep the aPTT between 1.5 and 2.5 times control.

Various measures of the lytic state correlate poorly with
both efficacy and incidence of bleeding, so routine monitoring is not indicated. Clinical monitoring should include
(1) serial neurologic examinations to detect central nervous
system hemorrhage and (2) frequent vital signs to detect gastrointestinal or retroperitoneal hemorrhage. Patients who
have undergone catheterization should have the groin puncture site examined as well as repeated measurements of thigh
girth made. After the thrombolytic agent is discontinued, heparin is typically begun (without a bolus) when the thrombin
time or the aPTT falls to less than two times control. Heparin
is begun as an intravenous infusion at 1300 U/h and titrated
to a PTT of 1.5 to 2.5 times control. Contraindications to
thrombolytic therapy are listed in Table 29-8.

When serious bleeding occurs (risk ~ 15 percent), the lytic
agent is stopped and large-bore IV access established. Peripheral veins are preferred, and one should use only compressible central veins (jugular, femoral) if needed. Stop heparin if it has been given. Cryoprecipitate (contains fibrinogen
and factor VIII) is the preferred blood product if the lytic state
must be reversed. Start with 10 U and then assay the fibrinogen level. Fresh frozen plasma (as a source of factors V and

TABLE 29-8   Contraindications
to Thrombolytic Therapy

Absolute
  Recent puncture in a noncompressible site
  Active or recent internal bleeding
  Hemorrhagic diathesis
  Recent CNS surgery or active intracranial lesion
  Uncontrolled hypertension (BP > 180/110)
  Known hypersensitivity, or, for streptokinase, use within
    6 months
  Diabetic hemorrhagic retinopathy
  Acute pericarditis
  Recent obstetric delivery
  History of stroke
Relative
  Trauma (including cardiopulmonary resuscitation) or major
    surgery within 10 days
  Pregnancy
  High likelihood of left heart thrombus
  Advanced age
  Liver disease

VIII), platelets, and fibrinolytic drugs (e.g., epsilon aminocaproic acid, 5 g over 30 min) should also be considered in the critically bleeding patient.

EMBOLECTOMY AND MECHANICAL THERAPIES

Additional therapies that are rarely used include surgical embolectomy, catheter suction embolectomy, use of rotational catheter devices, and placement of endovascular stents. Surgical embolectomy is advocated only in those few centers with readily available surgery, anesthesia, and cardiopulmonary bypass teams. Experience with the other procedures mentioned above is extremely limited.

Prophylaxis against Venous Thromboembolism

In the absence of a contraindication, nearly all critically ill patients should receive minidose heparin (5000 U SQ bid/tid).

When heparin is unsafe (e.g., in neurosurgical patients), alternative methods of prophylaxis, such as intermittent pneumatic compression cuffs, should be instituted. In some patients at very high risk of thromboembolism, such as those with acute spinal cord injury, minidose heparin is ineffective and low-molecular-weight heparin is preferred. Finally, although this measure is controversial, some patients at extremely high risk of PE should have consideration given to prophylactic insertion of vena caval filters (see above).

Air Embolism

The syndrome of air (or gas) embolism results when air enters the vasculature, travels to the pulmonary circulation, and causes circulatory or respiratory compromise. For air to enter into the vasculature, there must be an abnormal communication between a vessel and the surrounding air as well as a pressure gradient favoring air entry into the vessel. Table 29-9 lists some of the causes of the air embolism syndrome.

Consequences of air embolism include (1) sudden death (a large volume of air filling the RV), (2) pulmonary hypertension, and (3) paradoxical air embolism with ARDS or patent foramen ovale leading to ischemia of brain, heart, skin (livedo reticularis). The air-blood interface attracts leukocytes, resulting in endothelial injury and capillary leak with low-pressure pulmonary edema. The increase in dead space may impair CO_2 elimination in some patients. A reflex bronchoconstriction may also be seen (Table 29-10).

During upright neurosurgery or when air is seen to enter an intravascular catheter, the diagnosis of air embolism is usually obvious. Other circumstances where it should be considered include (1) states of hypoperfusion, (2) systemic embolization, (3) obtundation, and (4) respiratory failure, particularly when more likely causes are lacking. Many cases are related to central lines (during placement; with catheter disconnection, hub fracture, gas in the line; persistent cutaneous tract after removal). The differential diagnosis of air embolism includes other forms of noncardiogenic pulmonary edema as well as cardiogenic edema. Thus, volume overload, sepsis, and gastric acid aspiration must be excluded.

TABLE 29-9   Etiology of Air Embolism

Surgery- and Trauma-Related	Nonsurgical
Neurosurgery, especially upright	Cardiopulmonary resuscitation
Liver transplantation	Gastrointestinal endoscopy
Total hip replacement	Positive-pressure ventilation
Harrington rod insertion	Barotrauma
Spinal fusion	Infusion computed tomography scan
Pulsed saline irrigation	Scuba diving
Removal of tissue expanders	Self-induced
Transurethral resection, prostate	Orogenital sex
Cesarean section	
Arthroscopy	
Open-heart surgery	
Hysterectomy	
Head and neck trauma	
Dental implant surgery	
Pacemaker insertion	
Tenkhoff catheter placement	
Intraaortic balloon pump	
Bone marrow harvest	
Epidural catheter placement	
Central line placement	
Central line removal	
Percutaneous lung biopsy	
Pulmonary contusion	
Laser bronchoscopy	
Retrograde pyelography	
Hemodialysis	
Percutaneous lithotrypsy	

Management

The goals of treatment are to prevent reembolization while supporting respiration and circulation. In most cases, resolution is prompt. One looks for a source of air entry to close, if possible. Saline administration may raise intravascular pressures and lessen the gradient favoring air entry. When air embolism complicates positive-pressure ventilation, one should lower airway pressures by lowering tidal volumes, reducing PEEP, or intentionally hypoventilating. Oxygen hastens the reabsorption of air from bubbles, so all patients

TABLE 29-10   Manifestations of Air Embolism

Dyspnea, hypoxemia
Confusion, stroke, or peripheral embolization
Hypotension, shock
Diffuse alveolar infiltrates
Increment in airway pressures
Increased dead space, rising V_E
Abrupt fall in $E_{T_{CO_2}}$
Detection of air by echocardiography, Doppler
   monitor, or radiography

---

with significant air embolism should receive 100% oxygen during the initial resuscitation. In animals, prophylactic corticosteroids reduce the degree of lung injury from air embolism; however, steroids have not been shown to be clearly beneficial in humans and should not be given routinely.

TABLE 29-11   Causes of Fat
Embolism Syndrome

Traumatic fat embolism
   Long bone fracture (especially femur)
   Other fractures
   Orthopedic surgery
   Blunt trauma to fatty organs (e.g., liver)
   Liposuction
   Bone marrow biopsy
Nontraumatic fat embolism
   Pancreatitis
   Diabetes mellitus
   Lipid infusions
   Sickle cell crisis
   Burns
   Cardiopulmonary bypass
   Decompression sickness
   Corticosteroid therapy
   Osteomyelitis
   Alcoholic fatty liver
   Acute fatty liver of pregnancy
   Lymphangiography
   Cyclosporine infusion

FAT EMBOLISM

The fat embolism syndrome (FES) is associated with fat particles in the microcirculation of the lung. Some of the causes of FES are presented in Table 29-11.

Clinical Manifestations

There is usually a latent interval of 12 to 72 hours after injury before the syndrome becomes evident. Patients present with ARDS, confusion, obtundation, or coma due to cerebral fat embolism, skin petechiae (upper chest, neck, and face), thrombocytopenia, anemia, and acute RHS (rare). The diagnosis is usually based on the clinical findings in a patient at risk for FES. Prophylaxis and treatment include early fixation of long bone fractures, even in patients with multiple trauma. Prophylactic corticosteroids are more controversial and should not be routinely used (see text).

For a more detailed discussion, see Chaps. 25 and 26 in *Principles of Critical Care,* 2d ed.

Chapter 30

PERICARDIAL DISEASE

EUGENE KAJI

There are two layers of pericardium around the heart: visceral and parietal. In normal adults, there is usually 10 to 15 mL of fluid in the pericardial space between these layers. The pressure in the pericardial space mirrors the pressure in the thoracic cavity: more negative during spontaneous inspiration than expiration. Since the pericardial sac surrounds all four chambers, the force opposing diastolic filling of any given heart chamber is the (normally negligible) pericardial pressure. The net force expanding any heart chamber is, then, the pressure within the chamber minus the pressure outside the chamber (pericardial pressure). As pericardial disease develops, there can be fluid accumulation in the pericardial sac or hardening of the pericardium, which will either increase the pressure opposing diastolic expansion (tamponade) or physically limit the extent of expansion by the chamber (constriction). In short, pericardial disease is characterized by the inability to fill the heart chambers. Common causes of tamponade in the adult population are renal failure (uremia), malignancy, infection (tuberculosis), collagen vascular diseases, and postinfarction (see Table 30-1).

An understanding of the jugular venous tracing is essential to the physical examination of the pericardium. This tracing reflects the right atrial pressure. The atrial pressure waveform has atrial (a) and ventricular (v) components, which are followed by the x and y descents, respectively (Fig. 30-1). The a wave corresponds to the rise in atrial pressure during atrial contraction. Following atrial contraction, there is a gradual decrease in atrial pressure, which is marked by the x descent during atrial relaxation. The v wave follows the x descent and corresponds to the rise in right atrial pressure during ventricular systole when the atrium fills passively while the tricuspid valve is closed. Following ventricular systole, the tricuspid valve opens and there is passive flow from the atrium

TABLE 30-1   Etiology of Pericardial Disease

Etiology	Effusive	Constrictive	Effusive/Constrictive
Idiopathic	X	X	X
Postirradiation			
Early	X	—	—
Late	X	X	X
Postinfarction			
Early	X	—	—
Late	X	X	—
Infection			
Early	X	—	—
Late	X	X	X
Collagen disease (SLE, MCTD, RA)	X	X	—
Renal failure	X	X	—
Postoperative			
Early	X	—	—
Late		X	—
Malignancy	X	—	X

ABBREVIATIONS: SLE, systemic lupus erythematosus; MCTD, mixed connective tissue disease; RA, rheumatoid arthritis.

to the ventricle, which lowers the atrial pressure, resulting in the y descent.

Cardiac Tamponade

In cardiac tamponade (CT), fluid accumulates in the pericardial sac. If fluid is acutely injected into the pericardial sac, the pericardial compliance is limited and the pericardial pressure rises rapidly. Tamponade physiology can develop with volumes as small as 30 to 50 mL. In contrast, large volumes (greater than 1 L) can be accommodated without the development of CT when fluid accumulates slowly, since the pericardium is capable of stretching gradually. As the pericardial pressure rises, the net force expanding each heart chamber decreases and cardiac filling (and, thus, cardiac output) is impeded.

Since the pericardial fluid is generally free-flowing, the pericardial pressure is distributed equally to all four chambers. In addition, the right and left atrial a waves correspond to the right and left ventricular end-diastolic pressure (in the absence of valvular disease). Therefore, in CT, right and left ventricular end-diastolic pressures should be equal and equal to the atrial a waves ("equalization of pressures"). As the tricuspid valve opens, the nearly equal pressures in the right atrium and the right ventricle cause little early diastolic flow across the tricuspid valve, blunting the y descent (Fig. 30-2). In summary, CT is characterized by equalization of pressures, evaluated diastolic pressures, blunted y descent, and impaired early diastolic filling.

The clinical presentation of CT is of a low-cardiac-output syndrome. There is hypotension with peripheral vasoconstriction. Dyspnea develops as the end-diastolic pressures of the ventricular chambers rise and pulmonary edema develops. Auscultation of the heart reveals distant heart sounds due to the pericardial fluid. Palpation of the precordium is quiet for the same reason. A "pulsus paradoxus" greater than 15 mmHg is observed during inspiration in spontaneously breathing patients. This finding is due to ventricular interdependence: when the venous return increases during inspiration, the right ventricle expands, further limiting left ventricular filling. Examination of the neck veins reveals an elevation

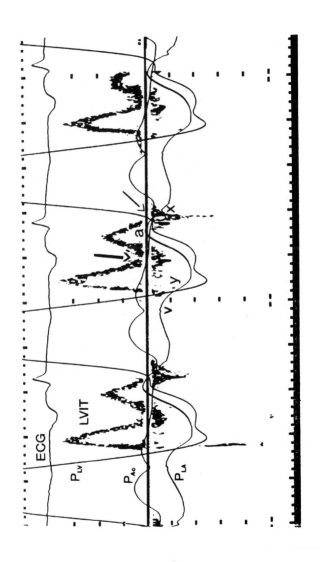

◀ FIGURE 30-1   Simultaneous left atrial, left ventricular, and aortic pressure recordings and ventricular inflow Doppler signal. The *bold arrow* marks the end of passive ventricular filling, when the pressure gradient between atrium and ventricle is small. The *thin arrow* marks AV valve closure and corresponds to the time when ventricular pressure exceeds atrial pressure and transvalvular flow stops. The a and v waves and the x and y descents are as described in the text. P_{la}, P_{lv}, and P_{AO} are the left atrial, left ventricular, and aortic pressures. Note that the left ventricular and aortic pressures are on different scales.

of jugular venous pressure with a blunted y descent. Electrocardiographic signs include diminished voltage and electrical alternans (a beat-to-beat variation in the electrical axis due to the heart swinging in the pericardial fluid). Sinus tachycardia is often observed. Chest x-ray frequently shows a "water bottle" appearance of the heart with a widened apex and narrow base.

Echocardiography is an excellent noninvasive test for the diagnosis of CT, showing pericardial fluid clearly. It can detect hemodynamically significant effusions by identifying diastolic collapse of the right atrium and ventricle (a sign of pericardial pressure being greater than diastolic right atrial or ventricular pressure), lack of respiratory variations in the inferior vena cava (sign of elevated venous pressure), and large variations in the left ventricular inflow pattern (equivalent of pulsus paradoxus). Finally, invasive hemodynamic monitoring with a pulmonary artery catheter will reveal a low cardiac output, elevated filling pressures, and equalization of diastolic pressures.

The ultimate management of tamponade is to relieve the pericardium of the pericardial fluid. Until drainage can be effected, treatment should center around increasing the intracardiac pressures with respect to the intrapericardial pressures by administering fluids. Pericardial drainage can be approached surgically or with a percutaneous catheter. There is no clear consensus on which procedure is better. Pericardiocentesis (needle and catheter placement into the pericardial space) can be lifesaving, with immediate hemodynamic improvement. Unfortunately, the pericardial fluid frequently

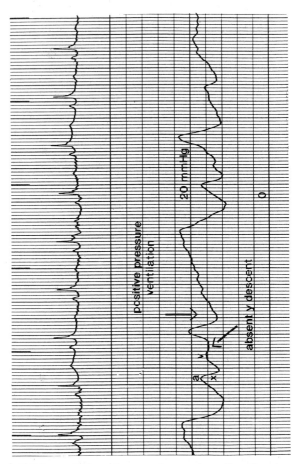

FIGURE 30-2   Right atrial pressure from a patient with cardiac tamponade during mechanical ventilation. Note the absent y descent and the blunting of the waveforms, especially during positive-pressure ventilation.

(50 percent) reaccumulates. Balloon pericardiotomy (a pericardial window created by a balloon) is only available at limited centers. Alternatively, a surgical pericardiostomy offers more definitive therapy and allows a specimen of the pericardium to be obtained for histopathologic examination when the cause of tamponade is unknown.

Constrictive Pericarditis

The basic pathology in constrictive pericarditis (CP) is the rigidity of the pericardium. In CP, unlike tamponade, there is no impedance to early filling and expansion of the heart chambers; however, once the fixed pericardial volume is reached in late diastole, filling ceases. The ventricular waveforms reflect this late diastolic filling limitation with a dip-and-plateau morphology. The diastolic pressure is low in early diastole but rises rapidly to a plateau during late diastole. The right atrial waveform demonstrates a steep y descent, reflecting the ease of early diastolic filling and a rapid rise in pressure during the a wave, reflecting the impaired late diastolic filling. There is a rapid x descent due to atrial relaxation. For reasons identical to those underlying the physiology of tamponade, equalization of pressures is also seen in CP. Kussmaul's sign, a rise in the jugular venous pressure during inspiration, may be seen. In summary, CP is characterized by elevated diastolic pressures, impaired late diastolic filling, Kussmaul's sign, and equalization of pressures.

The clinical presentation of CP is very similar to CT, with a low cardiac output state. There is hypotension, peripheral vasoconstriction, and dyspnea. Unlike the case in tamponade, the heart sounds are normal and the precordium is generally hyperdynamic. There a pericardial knock may be auscultated, which results from the rapid inflow and cessation of blood flow as the maximum diastolic volume is reached. A pulsus paradoxus is observed. Like tamponade, CT has a small aortic pulse pressure. An examination of the neck veins reveals an elevated jugular venous pressure with accentuated x and y descents. The electrocardiogram (ECG) is unrevealing. Sinus tachycardia is present, since the low stroke volume is compensated for by increasing the heart rate. Chest x-ray may show calcification of the pericardium. Echocardiography is less effective in the diagnosis of CP than of tamponade. CP is characterized by M-mode findings of notched interventricular septal motion due to abnormal filling and Doppler findings of diastolic dysfunction. Finally, invasive hemodynamic monitoring with a pulmonary artery catheter will reveal a low cardiac output, elevated filling pressures, accentuated x and y descents, and equalization of diastolic pressures.

Noninvasive treatment of CP is primarily limited to fluid administration. Wide surgical excision is the only effective treatment of CP and most patients improve.

Effusive-Constrictive Pericarditis

This condition is a combination of constrictive pericarditis and cardiac tamponade. Most commonly, there is tamponade physiology in the presence of a pericardial effusion. Once the pericardial effusion is removed, the patient is left with constriction. The most common cause is an underlying malignant process. The disease is initially managed like tamponade and eventually treated with surgical pericardiotomy if the underlying process permits, but the prognosis is poor.

Special Considerations

If indications for anticoagulation exist, the presence of a pericardial effusion or pericarditis is not a contraindication. The only caveat is that prior to needle or surgical treatment, anticoagulation should be withheld if at all possible. Also, the ECG findings of pericarditis should not be confused with those of myocardial ischemia when the decision for anticoagulation is being made.

Renal failure is a common cause of pericardial disease. When pericardial effusions develop in patients with renal failure (an incidence of up to 40 percent of dialysis patients), intensive dialysis should be tried for several days if there is no hemodynamic compromise. If the effusion is large (greater than 250 mL), does not regress with dialysis, or is hemodynamically significant, a subxiphoid pericardiotomy (surgical treatment) is recommended, since most uremic effusions recur despite needle drainage.

Purulent pericarditis is frequently suspected in patients with underlying infection and fortuitously discovered pericardial effusions. The most common causes of purulent pericarditis are lung infections, mediastinitis, endocarditis, prior pericardiotomy, and burns. Despite this, most effusions even in these settings are sterile. If purulent pericarditis is suspected, the diagnosis should be aggressively pursued with a direct pericardiectomy, since needle drainage and subxiphoid windows result in incomplete drainage with a poor clinical response. Purulent pericarditis is rare and should not be routinely suspected as a cause of fever in an uncompromised host.

In the cardiac surgical patient, three kinds of pericardial processes develop. Shortly after surgery, hemodynamic compromise may be caused by bleeding into the pericardial space with resultant tamponade physiology in spite of a surgically "open" pericardium. Some weeks after surgery, pericarditis may develop with a pathophysiology similar to that of Dressler syndrome (pericarditis after myocardial infarction resulting from an autoimmune mechanism). This is best treated with aspirin. Finally, constrictive pericarditis can develop months to years after surgery. This is treated with pericardial excision.

For a more detailed discussion, see Chap. 27 in *Principles of Critical Care*, 2d ed.

Chapter 31

VALVULAR HEART DISEASE

EUGENE KAJI

Valvular lesions are classified as either stenotic or regurgitant and acute or chronic. Stenotic valves limit flow, causing a "fixed" cardiac output, while regurgitant valves produce a volume overload state. Chronic valvular heart disease can remain occult during normal health due to a combination of compensation by the heart and limitation of activity by the patient. With a severe illness, however, the metabolic demands increase and the occult valvular disease becomes manifest. Acute valvular disease is poorly tolerated. The intensive care unit (ICU) physician can diagnose and evaluate the severity of valvular disease using a thorough cardiac examination, reviewing the electrocardiogram (ECG), and incorporating data from the echocardiogram (ECHO) and the catheterization laboratory. Once diagnosed, the valvular lesion can be treated mechanically (surgery or valvuloplasty) or medically.

ECHO has revolutionized the evaluation of valvular lesions. Using Doppler technology, an echocardiographer can estimate the pressure gradient across a stenotic valve. The echocardiographer measures the peak velocity of blood across an orifice. According to the modified Bernoulli equation, the transvalvular pressure gradient in millimeters of mercury is estimated to equal four times the velocity (in meters per second) squared. Echocardiographers can also measure the area of stenotic lesions by direct tracing or using the continuity equation (see *Principles of Critical*, 2d ed, for an explanation of the continuity equation).

The evaluation of valves may also be accurately performed invasively in the cardiac catheterization laboratory. Transvalvular gradients can be measured by directly placing high-fidelity catheters across the valve. Valve areas can be calculated using the Gorlin equation, which relates the measured pressure gradient and the flow of blood across the valve to the area of the valve. Intuitively, for any given flow across an orifice, the greater the measured pressure gradient, the smaller the valve area.

Aortic Stenosis

The etiology of aortic stenosis (AS) is broadly categorized into either congenital malformations of the valve, rheumatic disease, or calcific or degenerative disease. The most common congenital malformation of the aortic valve is a bicuspid valve (the aortic valve is normally tricuspid), which has a prevalence of about 1 to 2 percent in the general population. A bicuspid valve is more prone to premature calcific degeneration; these patients frequently present with aortic stenosis during the fifth decade of life. Rheumatic disease preferentially affects the mitral valve, such that AS due to rheumatic disease is almost uniformly accompanied by rheumatic mitral involvement. With the advent of antibiotics, the incidence of rheumatic disease has significantly decreased. Calcific or degenerative disease primarily affects elderly patients. Many years of turbulent blood flow is thought to cause degeneration and calcification of the valve.

The left ventricle compensates for mild and moderate AS by generating higher ventricular pressures. In order to maintain such pressures, the left ventricle hypertrophies. Initially, the high ventricular pressure is adequate to maintain cardiac output across the stenotic aortic valve. Eventually, as the stenotic lesion progresses, the left ventricle can no longer compensate. At this stage, syncope due to inadequate cardiac output, angina due to increased myocardial demand, or congestive heart failure due to a failing left ventricle may ensue.

Patients with severe AS frequently relate a history of dyspnea on exertion. Remarkably, many patients with severe AS (patients with a valve area less than 0.75 cm^2 or a mean transvalvular gradient of 50 mmHg) may be asymptomatic because of a sedentary lifestyle. In severe AS, the physical examination reveals a loud crescendo/decrescendo systolic murmur that radiates to the neck. The aortic component of the second heart sound is diminished. The carotid upstroke is decreased and delayed. The ECG shows left ventricular hypertrophy. The chest x-ray (CXR) may show aortic valvular calcification and cardiomegaly.

ECHO can accurately measure the transvalvular gradient and valve area. Cardiac catheterization can directly measure gradients and calculate valve areas. In addition, if surgery is contemplated for patients over the age of 40, cardiac catheterization is strongly recommended to evaluate for concomitant coronary artery disease, which can be treated with bypass during the operation.

The management of AS is primarily surgical. Patients with AS and symptoms of angina, syncope, or congestive heart failure should have elective valvular surgery. The medical treatment of AS is limited. The stenotic lesion presents an outflow obstruction that artificially limits the cardiac output (the so-called "fixed output"). As a consequence, medications that reduce afterload are poorly tolerated, since cardiac output cannot be increased to maintain blood pressure. Medications that reduce preload are poorly tolerated, since cardiac contractility may be dependent on the high preload. Patients with end-stage, severe AS frequently present with a failing left ventricle and congestive heart failure. Decreasing preload by diuresis in these patients may require invasive monitoring by Swan-Ganz catheter to follow cardiac output as preload is decreased.

In patients with significant AS in the context of critical illness, management options are severely limited. Critical illness almost certainly demands augmented cardiac output, which may not be possible with an outflow obstruction. Emergency valvular surgery may be necessary, but it frequently carries a prohibitively high mortality rate. An alternative to emergency valve surgery is aortic balloon valvuloplasty. Unfortunately, balloon valvuloplasty is associated with a high rate of restenosis. In light of this, this procedure should be viewed as a bridge to definitive surgery.

Hypertrophic Cardiomyopathy

Although hypertrophic cardiomyopathy (HCM) is not strictly a valvular disorder, it presents an outflow obstruction to the left ventricle that can mimic AS. HCM is a genetic disorder present in approximately 0.2 percent of adults. The most common type results in hypertrophy of the septum. Since the septal wall forms part of the left ventricular outflow tract, extreme septal hypertrophy obstructs outflow from the left ventricle. This obstruction is "dynamic." As the ventricle contracts, the septum thickens and the ventricular chamber size decreases, worsening the obstruction in late systole. The obstruction can cause gradients of greater than 100 mmHg across the left ventricular outflow tract. The hypertrophy of the septum leaves only a small opening for the outflow tract, resulting in high-velocity flow through the tract (similar to the high velocity of water seen when one squeezes the outflow tract of a hose). This increased velocity of flow causes a Venturi effect across the anterior mitral valve leaflet, pulling the leaflet forward resulting in mitral regurgitation. This is the so-called systolic anterior motion, or SAM, of the mitral valve.

Patients with HCM frequently present with exertional chest pain, dyspnea, fatigue, and syncope. Cardiac examination reveals a systolic, crescendo-decrescendo murmur that radiates throughout the precordium but not to the neck. This murmur will increase with a Valsalva maneuver. Due to the Venturi effect causing mitral regurgitation, there may be a systolic, blowing murmur that radiates from the apex to the axilla. The carotid upstroke is normal, but there is an abrupt termination as the obstruction begins. The carotid pressure tracing is described as a "spike and dome." The ECG shows left ventricular hypertrophy and prominent Q waves in the inferolateral leads.

ECHO can document hypertrophy of the septum, measure the severity of the outflow tract gradient, visualize the systolic anterior motion of the mitral valve leaflet, and measure the degree of mitral regurgitation. Catheterization can be used to measure the gradient directly.

The medical management of HCM patients involves decreasing the contractility and chronotropy of the heart. Decreasing contractility will increase the end-systolic volume which will diminish the outflow tract gradient. Slower heart rates permit adequate filling of the heart. Digitalis and beta agonists are contraindicated in HCM patients, since they will increase contractility. Beta blockers and calcium channel blockers are the agents of choice in treating HCM. Surgically, a myomectomy that removes a sizable portion of the septum can be done.

Aortic Insufficiency

Aortic insufficiency (AI) can be due to aortic root dilatation causing secondary AI or to a primary valve problem such as endocarditis. AI can be either chronic or acute. Chronic AI is well tolerated owing to an increased compliance of the left ventricle. The compliance is increased from the prolonged volume overload state; this means that only a minimal increase in left ventricular end-diastolic pressure occurs for a given increase in left ventricular volume. Acute AI, in contrast, is poorly tolerated; the left ventricle and pericardium are unable to accommodate the volume load since the compliance of the left ventricle has not yet increased. A given increase in left ventricular volume results in significant increase in left ventricular end-diastolic pressure. As the left ventricular end-diastolic pressure increases, the left atrial pressure rises, causing pulmonary edema.

Clinically, significant acute AI presents with pulmonary edema, peripheral vasoconstriction, diaphoresis, and cyanosis. The ECG is generally normal and the CXR shows pulmonary edema. In acute AI, the mediastinum on the CXR should be examined closely for signs of an aortic dissection. ECHO can be used to quantitate the amount of AI as well as to identify an etiology (ECHO can accurately diagnose vegetations of endocarditis and aortic dissection). Initially, chronic AI is generally asymptomatic. Eventually, the left ventricle dilates and fails. At this stage, the patient begins to develop signs and symptoms of pulmonary edema. Ideally, the valve should be surgically replaced prior to the development of irreversible left ventricular damage.

The medical management of significant acute AI involves vasodilator therapy with an agent such as sodium nitroprusside. By decreasing the systemic resistance, there will be increased forward flow, reduced regurgitation, and lower left ventricular end diastolic pressures. Agents such as alpha agonists that increase systemic resistance are contraindicated, since this will increase regurgitation. Once stabilized, patients may be converted to an oral vasodilator such as nifedipine.

Mitral Stenosis

The predominant cause of MS is rheumatic heart disease; with the advent of antibiotics, the incidence of mitral stenosis (MS) in this country has been primarily limited to immigrants. Rheumatic heart disease is characterized by an inflammatory process on the valve that causes the fusion of the leaflet commissures. Rarely, calcification of the mitral annulus or submitral apparatus can also cause MS in elderly patients or patients with end-stage renal failure.

As might be intuitively predicted, a stenotic mitral valve increases the required transmitral pressure gradient and the (diastolic) time needed to pass blood from the left atrium to the left ventricle. The increased transmitral gradient increases the left atrial pressure, resulting in pulmonary hypertension and pulmonary edema. With chronically elevated left atrial pressures, this chamber dilates and develops conduction abnormalities resulting in atrial fibrillation. Atrial fibrillation in the context of MS is highly thrombogenic and associated with a high incidence of thromboembolic disease if left untreated. The requirement for increased diastolic time to empty the left atrium results in the need for slow heart rates. Since diastole is shortened as the heart rate increases, the earliest symptom of MS is frequently dyspnea on exertion.

Physical examination of the patient with MS reveals a normal left ventricle, an opening snap heard at the apex, a diastolic rumble at the apex, a louder first heart sound, the findings of pulmonary hypertension including an accentuated pulmonic component of the second heart sound, a right ventricular heave, and a pulmonic insufficiency murmur. The ECG shows left atrial enlargement and right ventricular hypertrophy. CXR may show an enlarged left atrium and mitral annular calcification. ECHO can quantify the mitral valve area, measure the transvalvular gradient, and assess the valve prior to either valve surgery or valvuloplasty. Cardiac catheterization may be used to measure pressures in the heart directly and calculate the valve area using measured transvalvular gradients and cardiac output.

The management of MS centers on decreasing left atrial pressures and increasing the diastolic time. Increased diastolic time will increase time for transmitral flow, which is limited in MS. In an ICU setting, controlling the heart rate with medications to increase diastolic time is crucial. MS patients frequently present with pulmonary edema, and these patients should be treated with aggressive diuresis to lower left atrial pressures. MS can be corrected by either mitral valve replacement surgery, open commisurotomy surgery, or percutaneous balloon valvuloplasty. Unlike aortic stenosis, MS has a durable response to valvuloplasty, making this the procedure of choice in patients who are appropriate for the procedure.

Mitral Regurgitation

Mitral regurgitation (MR) may result from malfunction of the submitral apparatus, mitral annulus, or valve leaflets. The submitral apparatus consists of chordae and papillary muscles. These may rupture or malfunction secondary to ischemia, myxomatous mitral valve prolapse, or infection. The mitral annulus can cause MR by dilation, as seen in dilated cardiomyopathies. The valve leaflets can cause MR by prolapse, malcoaptation, and rheumatic disease.

Initially, the MR results in unloading of the left ventricle into the left atrium, causing an increased ejection fraction. Eventually, the volume overload causes the left ventricle to dilate. Given the unloading into the atrium, even a normal left ventricular ejection fraction indicates a failing ventricle. The volume of MR into the left atrium must be accommodated. If the MR is acute, the left atrium cannot accommodate the volume of the regurgitation without increasing the left atrial pressure. Patients with acute MR therefore present with pulmonary edema. With chronic MR, the left atrium becomes more compliant and enlarges, decreasing the left atrial pressures. As in patients with MS, the enlarged left atrium results in rhythm disturbances such as atrial fibrillation.

The physical examination of the patient with MR is notable for a holosystolic murmur radiating from the apex to the axilla and an S_3. The ECG frequently reveals left atrial enlargement, right ventricular hypertrophy, and atrial fibrillation. The CXR shows cardiomegaly with left ventricular enlargement. ECHO can evaluate the severity of MR as well as the etiology. MR is evaluated in the catheterization laboratory by direct pressure measurements and observing the degree of dye injected into the left ventricle that regurgitates into the left atrium. Since the left atrium cannot accommodate large volumes acutely, MR is poorly tolerated if acute. Chronic MR, however, is well tolerated until left ventricular dysfunction occurs. Unfortunately, the presence of left ventricular dysfunction already indicates significant, irreversible cardiomyopathy in a patient with MR. Definitive treatment (mitral valve replacement) should be planned prior to the onset of left ventricular dysfunction. As the left ventricle fails, the patients develop dyspnea on exertion, which progresses.

Intuitively, the management of MR involves decreasing the afterload to increase forward (to the aorta) flow from the left ventricle and reduce backward (to the left atrium) flow. For chronic MR, oral afterload reducers such as calcium channel blockers and angiotensin converting enzyme (ACE) inhibitors are given. In addition, inotropic agents such as digoxin and preload reduction with diuretics are used in patients with left ventricular dysfunction. Surgical valve replacement or repair of chronic MR should be considered in patients when they become symptomatic or show any signs of left ventricular dysfunction. Once the left ventricular ejection fraction is less than 40 percent in patients with MR, surgery poses a much higher risk and is of unclear benefit. Patients with acute MR are generally less compensated, requiring more aggressive therapy. Afterload reduction can be initiated with intravenous nitroprusside or even an intraaortic balloon pump. Pulmonary edema should be treated with diuretics. Emergency surgical treatment should be considered for patients with hemodynamic compromise.

Prosthetic Valves

Prosthetic valves (PV) come in two varieties: tissue and mechanical. PV in general have three problems: a limited life span, thromboembolic risk, and infectious risk. Tissue valves have the benefit of low thromboembolic risk; anticoagulation is usually required only during the first few months after surgery while the sewing ring is endothelialized. Unfortunately, tissue valves suffer from degeneration, and more than 50 percent have failed by 15 years. Recently, homografts (human donor valves) have done very well in observational trials and may replace other tissue valves in the future. Mechanical valves have the benefit of durability; however, they are highly thrombogenic, requiring chronic anticoagulation. Thrombosis of a mechanical PV can cause acute failure of the valve, requiring emergency surgery. Thrombus on a valve may also embolize, causing cerebral vascular accidents and systemic embolic disease. Finally, both tissue and mechanical valves are highly susceptible to infection. Traditionally, PV endocarditis is divided into early (within 60 days of implantation) or late. Early PV endocarditis is characterized by skin organisms such as *Staphylococcus epidermidis* and *Staph. aureus* from likely contamination of the surgical field. Late PV endocarditis is due to organisms similar to native-valve endocarditis. Unfortunately, PV endocarditis of any type carries a high mortality. Patients are at high risk for valve-ring abscesses, dehiscence of the valve, and perivalvular leaks. Given the propensity for PV to become infected, all patients with PV should have antibiotic prophylaxis for medical and dental procedures.

For a more detailed discussion, see Chap. 28 in *Principles of Critical Care*, 2d ed.

Chapter 32

HYPERTENSIVE CRISIS

MANU JAIN

The term *malignant hypertension* entered the medical vocabulary at a time when there were limited options for the treatment of severe elevations of blood pressure. Given the vast array of antihypertensive medications currently available, *malignant* does not accurately reflect our ability to treat this disease, and the 5-year survival of patients presenting with malignant hypertension is now 75 percent. Today, hypertensive states are often referred to as *hypertensive emergencies* and *hypertensive urgencies,* as outlined in Table 32-1.

Pathophysiology

In animal models there is acute vasoconstriction of the arteries in response to acute elevations in blood pressure, presumably in an attempt to protect the more delicate arterioles. This is protective until a threshold is reached, at which point rupture of the larger vessels occurs at higher pressures. If elevated arterial pressure is maintained for a period of time, chronic vasoconstriction leads to intimal thickening. This has the effect of shifting the curve of blood pressure versus blood flow to the right.

A second, later feature of acute elevations of blood pressure is a necrotizing arteriolitis, which occurs in many vascular beds. It is thought to be both a cause and consequence of the relative ischemia in affected areas. It may be the mechanism by which the relative ischemia of the kidney leads to high renin levels, which can create a positive feedback loop on blood pressure elevation.

Etiology

Although patients with truly malignant hypertension have a higher prevalence of secondary causes, most will still have

TABLE 32-1 Types of Hypertensive States

Hypertensive Emergency (Requires control within hours)	Hypertensive Urgency (Requires control within hours or days)
Severe elevation of blood pressure and evidence of acute end-organ damage	Severe elevation of blood pressure with evidence of subacute end-organ damage
Encephalopathy	
Retinal hemorrhages and exudates	
Papilledema	
Acute cerebrovascular accident	Recent discontinuation of antihypertensive medication
Acute aortic dissection	Need for surgery
Acute LV failure	Immediate postoperative period
Acute myocardial infarction	Renal transplantation
Hematuria	Severe body burns
Acute renal failure	
Other clinical settings	
Bleeding from vascular surgery sites	
Severe epistaxis	
Pheochromocytoma crisis	
Monoamine oxidase inhibitor crisis	

414

essential hypertension. A common scenario predisposing to the development of a hypertensive emergency is the recent discontinuation of antihypertensive medications, such as clonidine, beta blockers, calcium channel blockers, and others. Drug ingestion has become an important cause of severe elevations of blood pressure as well. Cocaine and phencyclidine are two of the most common illicit drugs that do this. Oral contraceptives, monoamine oxidase inhibitors, and phenylpropanolamines are examples of medications that can precipitate elevations of blood pressure.

There is a long list of secondary causes of hypertensive crises. The most common of the secondary causes is renovascular disease. Other causes include pheochromocytoma, IgA nephropathy, vasculitides, and 17-α-hydroxylase deficiency.

Diagnosis

It is important to focus the history toward identifying causes listed in Table 32-2 when a hypertensive crisis is suspected. Symptoms and signs of end-organ damage associated with an extreme elevation of blood pressure are keys to making the diagnosis. Dyspnea, headache, blurred vision, or chest pain may all suggest end-organ damage. The central nervous system (CNS) should be examined for the presence of encephalopathy, a focal sensory or motor loss, retinal hemorrhage, or papilledema. One should look for evidence of

TABLE 32-2   Causes of Hypertensive Crisis

Cessation of Medications	Drug-Induced	Secondary Causes
α blockers (e.g., clonidine)	Cocaine, phencyclidine	Renovascular disease (renal failure, vasculitis, IgA nephropathy)
β blockers, calcium-channel blockers	Monoamine oxidase inhibitors	Pheochromocytoma
Minoxidil	Oral contraceptives	Conn syndrome

congestive heart failure or aortic dissection on the cardiac and pulmonary examinations. The abdomen should be examined carefully for the presence of bruits and or masses (which may provide clues to the etiology to the hypertensive crisis).

Management

The rapidity with which one should bring down the blood pressure is the first decision that must be made in treating a hypertensive crisis. Where the patient should be treated depends on how quickly the blood pressure must be decreased. This decision should be based on factors outlined in Table 32-1. The principle of treatment is to reduce blood pressure to a sufficient degree and for a sufficient time that the autoregulatory curve moves back toward normal. In a true hypertensive emergency, one should begin treatment even if all the monitoring is not yet in place. An important caution is that reduction of blood pressure to "normal" values may be excessive in light of the right-shifted pressure-flow relationship and that this has been associated with organ dysfunction, coma, and death.

The goal of treatment should be to reduce mean arterial pressure [MAP = diastolic blood pressure + (pulse pressure/3)] by 15 percent in the first hour. Over the ensuing 12 hours, the aim should be to reduce the MAP by 25 percent overall or to a MAP of 110 (whichever is higher). It is essential to remain vigilant for signs of ischemic damage as the blood pressure is reduced.

The choice of intravenous antihypertensive agents is growing, but sodium nitroprusside is probably still the drug of choice for initial management. It has a short onset and duration of action and is extremely effective. Nitroprusside should be given intravenously at a dose of 0.5 $\mu g/kg/min$ and increased by 0.5 to 1.0 μg every 3 to 5 minutes until the goal blood pressure is achieved. Toxicity is related to the accumulation of nitroprusside's metabolic products, specifically, thiocyanate and cyanide. Patients with renal or hepatic failure are at especially high risk. Symptoms of toxicity include nausea, fatigue, disorientation, muscle spasms, and acidosis.

Other intravenous medications may be more appropriate in specific clinical situations. Nitroglycerin is useful when angina pectoris is part of hypertensive crisis. When a beta blocker is desired, as in aortic dissection, labetalol can be used. An infusion of the short-acting beta blocker esmolol is also an option. Enalaprilat is useful in situations where impaired cerebral circulation is a concern. Phentolamine is useful for pheochromocytoma crisis. Fenoldopam is a dopamine agonist that has efficacy similar to that of nitroprusside, with fewer side effects, and may be used more widely in the future.

Once an effective dose of nitroprusside has been found, an oral antihypertensive regimen should be selected and started to replace nitroprusside as soon as possible. In choosing which oral antihypertensive agent to use, it is best to avoid prodrugs or drugs that can drop the blood pressure precipitously. Long-acting calcium channel blockers or beta blockers are often good choices. Clonidine, captopril, and prazosin have also been shown to be effective in these situations, and angiotensin II receptor blockers offer still another option. If one cannot gain adequate control with one medication, the addition of a diuretic is a good second choice.

Preeclampsia

Preeclampsia is a pregnancy-induced disorder characterized by hypertension, edema, and proteinuria. Nulliparous women have the highest incidence, but it can occur in multiparous women as well. Presentation is usually after the twentieth week of gestation and most frequently at term. The underlying pathophysiology is not well understood but may relate to poor placental perfusion and maternal vascular endothelial cell dysfunction.

Severe preeclampsia is heralded by a systolic blood pressure > 160 mmHg or a diastolic blood pressure greater than 110. Proteinuria, azotemia, CNS disturbances, seizures, pulmonary edema, right-upper-quadrant pain, elevated liver enzymes, and thrombocytopenia may indicate end-organ damage. A decrease in fetal heart tones may also indicate end-organ damage.

Antihypertensive therapy may be used to prevent maternal vascular damage. The most commonly used parenteral antihypertensive agent in pregnancy, hydralazine, is probably the first choice. Labetalol has also been shown to be safe and effective. Oral nifedipine, diazoxide, and sodium nitroprusside can be used in severe situations but carry significant fetal risks. The definitive treatment is termination of the pregnancy.

For a more detailed discussion, see Chap. 29 in *Principles of Critical Care*, 2d ed.

Chapter 33

AORTIC DISSECTION

MANU JAIN

Aortic dissection (AD) is the most common catastrophe affecting the aorta, with an annual incidence in the United States of approximately 2000 cases. Without treatment, the mortality rate is 1 percent per hour in the first 2 days, with a 3-month mortality rate reaching 90 percent. Rapid recognition and prompt intervention are paramount for a successful outcome. With appropriate treatment, survival rates of over 80 percent can be expected.

Pathogenesis and Classification

Aortic dissections are marked by a dissecting hematoma that separates the intima and the inner layers of the media from the outer medial and adventitial layers. The aorta may be weakened by Marfan or Ehlers-Danlos syndrome, bicuspid aortic valve, coarctation, pregnancy, or iatrogenic injury during cardiac surgery. Alternatively, excessive luminal shear stress, related to hypertension or aortic noncompliance, may precipitate the intimal tear. The tear in the intima allows blood to enter the media and create a false lumen. The hematoma can move in an anterograde or retrograde fashion to rupture into a nonvascular space, occlude aortic branch arteries, or cause acute aortic insufficiency due to prolapse of the aortic cusps.

Aortic dissections are classified as acute if present for less than 2 weeks and chronic if present for longer than 2 weeks. Additionally, aortic dissections are classified on the basis for risk of sudden death. Type A dissections, which are associated with the highest risk of sudden death and represent 60 percent of aortic dissections, involve the ascending aorta. Type B dissections involve only the descending aorta and can generally be managed more conservatively. This classification system replaces the original system proposed by DeBakey.

Clinical Picture

Men have a two to three times higher incidence of AD than women. Over 90 percent of all patients will have a history of hypertension. The signs and symptoms of AD vary depending on the site of the intimal tear and extent of the hematoma dissection; they include manifestations of poor perfusion or occlusions of aortic branches (see Table 33-1). Chest pain is the most common symptom and is often described as having a tearing or a knife-like quality. It can radiate to the back or to the abdomen. Patients can present with either hypertension or hypotension. Hypotension can be a manifestation of a cardiac emergency, such as acute aortic insufficiency or cardiac tamponade, or may simply reflect hemorrhagic hypovolemia. Occasionally the enlarging dissecting aorta can impinge on mediastinal structures, which can lead to Horner syndrome, hoarseness, hemoptysis, hematemesis, stridor, or superior vena cava syndrome. Occasionally, chronic dissections are asymptomatic and discovered incidentally.

Findings on the laboratory examination are nonspecific and rarely helpful. A low hemoglobin may reflect bleeding or hemolysis. An electrocardiogram may show left ventricular hypertrophy as evidence of chronic hypertension.

TABLE 33-1   Clinical Manifestations of Aortic Dissection

Organ	Aortic Branch Occlusion	Signs and Symptoms
CNS Central nervous system	Carotid	Cerebrovascular accident, delirium, coma
Extremities	Iliofemoral or subclavian	Cool, ischemic extremities, pulse deficit
Kidney	Renal	Oliguria or anuria
Heart	Coronary	Ischemia or infarction
Abdomen	Mesenteric	Abdominal pain, intestinal ischemia

Diagnostic Imaging

Standard chest radiography often reveals a widened mediastinum, although this may be absent in 40 percent of type A dissections. Other findings can include an aortic bulge (to the right with a type A and to the left with type B), a double rim of calcification, or a pleural effusion (left larger than right).

More specific investigations include aortography, computed tomography (CT), magnetic resonance imaging (MRI), and echocardiography (transthoracic and transesophageal). Controversy exists as to which is the best method; each has a relatively high sensitivity and specificity. Many authors consider aortography to be the gold standard, but transesophageal echocardiography (TEE) is often the best first test.

Both transthoracic (TTE) and transesophageal echocardiography can accurately evaluate the extent of involvement, presence of aortic insufficiency, pericardial effusion, and left ventricular function. The addition of color-coded Doppler allows better identification of true and false lumens. TEE is more accurate than TTE, with a reported sensitivity and specificity of 98 percent.

Aortography has a sensitivity and specificity in the 90 to 95 percent range for the diagnosis of AD. One advantage that aortography offers is that it can pinpoint the site of the intimal tear. Aortography, however, is invasive and requires the infusion of contrast, so less invasive procedures are preferred initially.

CT can identify true and false lumens, the intimal flap, pericardial and pleural effusions, and the extent of the dissection. It does not provide information about aortic insufficiency or left ventricular function and does require the administration of intravenous contrast. The new third-generation helical CT scans have a specificity approaching 100 percent but the sensitivity (about 83 percent) is less than that of aortography. A negative CT scan in a patient for whom there is a high clinical suspicion should lead to other investigations.

MRI is less well studied than the other modalities but does show promise. It allows excellent visualization of vascular walls and both clotted and flowing blood. The diagnostic accuracy of MRI is estimated to be about 90 percent, but more experience is needed to confirm its reliability.

Management

The optimal management of acute aortic dissection involves the integrated skills and cooperation of an intensivist and a cardiovascular surgeon. The intensivist must optimize monitoring and medical treatment and the surgeon must undertake definitive surgical repair emergently when that becomes necessary. All patients with acute aortic dissections should initially be managed in a critical care setting. They should have continuous cardiac and blood pressure monitoring. Consideration should also be given to placement of central venous pressure and urinary catheters.

The underlying principle in the pharmacologic management of AD is to reduce the systolic blood pressure and the pulse wave (dP/dT). Labetalol is a selective α_1 nonselective β-adrenoreceptor blocker and so reduces dP/dT and systolic blood pressure by vasodilation and decreasing myocardial contractility (Table 33-2). Esmolol is an ultra-short-acting β_1-blocker that is effective in the management of AD. Its rapid onset of action and short duration allows for tight titration of blood pressure. Sodium nitroprusside is a direct smooth muscle relaxant that lowers blood pressure but increases dP/dT, mandating the conjoint use of propranolol. For patients who have an absolute contraindication to β-blockers, trimethaphan camsylate, an autonomic ganglion blocker, may be administered. If "low doses" are being used, the head of the bed can be elevated or the patient's legs dangled over the

TABLE 33-2   Drug Treatment of Aortic Dissection

Drug	Dosing
Labetalol	Bolus: 0.25 mg/kg over 2 min; may repeat every 10 min Continuous: 1–2 mg/min
Esmolol	Bolus: 500 μg/kg over 1 min Continuous: 25–200 μg/kg/min
Sodium nitroprusside	Continuous: 0.5–8.0 μg/kg/min
Propranolol	Bolus: 1–3 mg over 2–3 min; may repeat in 2–3 min
Trimethaphan camsylate	Continuous: Begin 3–4 mg/min

side of the bed to achieve the desired effect. Reserpine or guanethidine may be added to control the sympathoplegic side effects.

The goal of pharmacologic management should be to reduce blood pressure to a level that halts the progression of the dissection. A systolic blood pressure of 90 to 100 mmHg is reasonable as long as organ perfusion is maintained. A clear sensorium, adequate urine output, warm extremities, and the absence of a lactic acidosis are evidence of adequate organ perfusion.

The decision to intervene surgically is complex and must be individualized. Once the decision is made to operate, definitive repair is often needed emergently. Patients with type A dissections should be offered urgent surgical intervention for maximal survival. Relative contraindications to surgery are severe organ dysfunction, such as severe coronary artery disease, severe COPD, age above 80, a moribund patient, cerebrovascular accident (controversial), and paraplegia. Type B dissections are generally best handled by medical management of blood pressure in the intensive care unit; however, a recent small study did report a lower mortality with operative intervention. At this time, surgery for type B dissections should be reserved for progression of dissection despite medical therapy. Evidence for failure of therapy includes increase in size, new aortic insufficiency, new ischemic complications, intractable pain, or a new pleural or pericardial effusion.

Postoperative complications include myocardial infarction, arrhythmia, low-output state, bleeding, renal failure, cerebrovascular accidents, and respiratory compromise. Complications specific to type B dissections include paraplegia or paraparesis, mesenteric ischemia, recurrent laryngeal nerve palsy, and chylothorax. Late complications of both types of dissections include aneurysm formation and recurrent dissection.

For a more detailed discussion, see Chap. 29 in *Principles of Critical Care*, 2d ed.

Chapter 34

PULMONARY ARTERY CATHETERIZATION AND INTERPRETATION

YIPING FU

Insertion of a pulmonary artery catheter (PAC) is one of the most commonly performed procedures in the intensive care unit (ICU). Bedside pulmonary artery (PA) catheterization is widely used in the diagnosis and management of a variety of conditions, including acute myocardial infarction, acute respiratory distress syndrome (ARDS), septic shock, and high-risk surgery. This chapter reviews clinical use of the PAC in the ICU, with particular emphasis upon the principles and common pitfalls of data acquisition, recording, and application.

Indications

The primary conditions for which insertion of a PAC would be considered are listed in Table 34-1. In many instances, patients with these conditions can be managed noninvasively. Often, the PAC is inserted only after a therapeutic trial of volume infusion or diuresis has been unsuccessful. In certain instances, however, the potential consequences of empiric management on gas exchange, blood pressure, or renal function are sufficiently worrisome that more precise definition of the underlying physiology may be required from the outset. The anticipated clinical course is also important, with a projected unstable and variable hemodynamic pattern favoring invasive monitoring. In a number of instances, the etiology of hypotension or pulmonary edema may be reliably diagnosed by two-dimensional Doppler echocardiography. The decision to place a PAC to diagnose these conditions will clearly be

TABLE 34-1 Clinical Uses of Bedside PA Catheterization

DIAGNOSTIC USES	
Condition	Primary data sought
Pulmonary edema	Ppw
Shock	$\dot{Q}T$ and SVR; Ppw; $S\bar{v}_{O_2}$
Oliguric renal failure	Ppw, $\dot{Q}T$
Perplexing lactic acidemia	$\dot{Q}T$, $S\bar{v}_{O_2}$
Pulmonary hypertension	Ppa and PVR; Ppad versus Ppw
Cardiac disorders:	
Ventricular septal defect	Step-up in O_2 saturation (RA to PA)
RV infarction	Pra $\geq$ Ppw
Pericardial tamponade	Pra = Ppw; blunted Y descent
Tricuspid regurgitation	Broad "C-V" wave, Kussmaul sign, deep Y descent
Constrictive pericarditis	Pra = Ppw, Kussmaul sign, deep Y descent
Narrow complex tachyarrhythmia	Mechanical flutter waves (Pra waveform)
Wide complex tachyarrhythmia	Cannon A waves (Pra waveform)
Lymphatic carcinoma	Aspiration cytology
Microvascular thrombi (ARDS)	Angiography
Caloric requirements	$\dot{V}_{O_2}$ (by Fick equation)

MONITORING USES
Assess adequacy of intravascular volume
Hypotension
Oliguria
High-risk surgical patient
Assess effect of change in Ppw on pulmonary edema
Assess therapy for shock
Cardiogenic (vasodilator, inotrope)
Septic (volume, vasopressor, inotrope)
Hypovolemic (volume)
Assess effects of PEEP on $\dot{Q}T$ in ARDS

influenced by the availability of high-quality echocardiography and by the projected need for ongoing invasive monitoring after a diagnosis has been established.

Complications

Complications of PAC insertion include those related to achieving vascular access and those due to the catheter itself (Table 34-2). Other catheter-related complications are considered here.

ARRHYTHMIA

Both atrial and ventricular tachyarrhythmias (VT) can develop as a result of catheter insertion. The incidence of VT is higher in critically ill patients than in those undergoing elective right heart catheterization. Fortunately, VT that occurs during passage through the RV usually terminates as soon as the catheter tip is advanced beyond the pulmonic valve and thus does not require treatment. Prophylactic administration of lidocaine is not recommended.

BUNDLE BRANCH BLOCK

Transient right bundle branch block (RBBB) has been reported to occur in 0.05 to 5 percent of catheterizations. If the patient has preexisting left bundle branch block (LBBB), it is acceptable to have external pacing immediately available rather than routinely placing an intravenous pacemaker prophylactically.

TABLE 34-2   Complications of PA Catheterization

Complications related to central vein cannulation
Complications related to insertion and use of the PA catheter
   Tachyarrhythmias
   Right bundle branch block
   Complete heart block (preexisting left bundle branch block)
   Cardiac perforation
   Thrombosis and embolism
   Pulmonary infarction due to persistent wedging
   Catheter-related sepsis
   Pulmonary artery rupture
   Knotting of the catheter
   Endocarditis, bland and infective
   Pulmonic valve insufficiency
   Balloon fragmentation and embolization

THROMBOSIS

Thrombi usually develop at the site of insertion but may also develop within the heart and PA. These thrombi can lead to clinically apparent pulmonary embolism, but they rarely do so. The catheter itself can cause pulmonary infarction from vascular obstruction, usually without apparent clinical deterioration.

PULMONARY ARTERY RUPTURE

Pulmonary artery rupture, the most serious complication of catheterization, is typically manifest by sudden brisk hemoptysis, from which approximately 50 percent of patients will die. Pulmonary hypertension, cardiopulmonary bypass, and anticoagulation place the patient at increased risk for morbidity and mortality due to PA rupture. Avoidance of distal catheter placement and balloon overinflation and prompt recognition of distal migration may reduce the risk of PA rupture. We recommend always inflating the balloon initially with only half the balloon volume (if the catheter wedges, it is too distal) and only subsequently filling the balloon fully.

Pressure Monitoring

PRESSURE MONITORING SYSTEM

Essential system components required for pressure monitoring include a fluid-filled catheter and connecting tubing, a transducer to convert the mechanical energy from the pressure wave into an electrical signal, and a signal processing unit that conditions and amplifies this electrical signal for display (Fig. 34-1). Two primary features of the pressure monitoring system determine its dynamic response properties: natural resonant frequency and damping coefficient. Modest damping is desirable for optimal fidelity and to suppress unwanted high-frequency vibration ("noise"). It is also essential that the system be "zeroed" (balanced) at the midaxillary line, fourth intercostal space. Because the pulmonary circuit is a low-pressure vascular bed, small errors in transducer position may be clinically significant. Accuracy is not affected by the position of the catheter tip within the chest as long as the catheter is in West zone III.

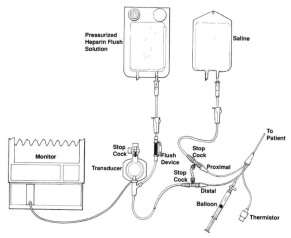

FIGURE 34-1 Standard four-lumen pulmonary artery catheter with pressure tubing, heparinized flush, transducer, and signal processing unit (monitor). Pulmonary arterial or right atrial pressure can be displayed by stopcock adjustment.

CATHETER INSERTION

The preferred vascular access sites for PA catheter placement are the internal jugular and subclavian veins because of ease of cannulation, easier advancement of the catheter across the tricuspid valve, and greater ease in catheter care. The left subclavian is often preferred over the right because of potential problems with catheter kinking with the right subclavian approach. Use of the femoral or antecubital veins introduces more frequent need for fluoroscopy and increased problems with catheter care. Once the site is chosen, vascular access is obtained by insertion of an introducer with a side arm and safety-seal feature. An 8.5 F introducer is adequate for passage of either a 7.0 or 7.5 F catheter.

Before insertion of the catheter, care should be taken to:

1. Assemble and calibrate the pressure monitoring system and clear any air bubbles from the transducer and connecting tubing.

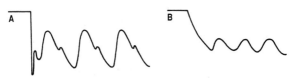

FIGURE 34-2   Rapid-flush test. *A.* Appropriately damped system.
B. Overdamped system.

2. Check the integrity of the balloon by inflating with 1.5 mL
   of air.
3. Connect the appropriate pressure tubing to the distal
   catheter port and flush well.
4. Ensure the expected response to pressure changes on the
   monitoring system by jiggling the catheter tip.
5. Position the sterile sheath over the PAC for later attach-
   ment to the introducer hub.

After the catheter is inserted 15 cm, the rapid-flush test
(described below) is performed to exclude an overdamped
system (Fig. 34-2). The balloon is then inflated with 1.5 mL of
air and the catheter gradually advanced into the right ventricle (RV). The RV is usually reached 30 to 35 cm from the
internal jugular or subclavian access sites. Once an RV tracing is obtained, it is usually not necessary to advance more
than 15 cm to reach the PA. If a PA tracing is not obtained after advancing the cathether 15 cm from the RV, the balloon
should be deflated and the catheter pulled back to the RV, as
feeding excessive catheter promotes coiling and knotting in
the RV. If difficulties persist in reaching PA, fluoroscopy is indicated. The PA tracing is recognized by a rise in diastolic
pressure and by the appearance of a dicrotic notch due to pulmonic valve closure (Fig. 34-3). Once in the PA, the catheter
is advanced until the balloon "wedges," recognized by transition to an atrial waveform and, more reliably, by a fall in
mean pressure. Once it is confirmed that balloon deflation is
followed by transition back to a PA tracing and that reinfla-
tion of the balloon yields a reliable PA occlusion (wedge) pressure (Ppw), the sterile sleeve can be attached to the introducer.
Finally, a chest radiograph is obtained to confirm proper
placement and assess for complications of the procedure.

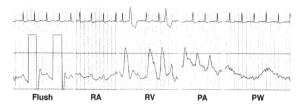

Flush **RA** **RV** **PA** **PW**

FIGURE 34-3 Waveform transition as catheter is advanced from right atrium (RA) to wedge (PW) position. The rapid-flush test before insertion reveals good dynamic responsiveness. Passage from the right ventricle (RV) into the pulmonary artery (PA) is evidenced by a rise in diastolic pressure, and catheter wedging is evidenced by a fall in pressure and appearance of an atrial waveform. Note ventricular ectopy when catheter is in the RV.

A number of factors may cause difficulty in recognizing the characteristic waveforms during catheter insertion. Hypovolemia with reduced stroke volume will diminish pulse pressure and narrow the differences between the diastolic pressures in the RV (RVEDP) and PA (Ppad) and between the mean pressures in the PA (Ppa) and the pulmonary vein (Ppw). As a result, the expected transitions in waveforms are less readily appreciated. The transition from RV to PA may also be more difficult to appreciate when RVEDP approaches Ppad as a result of pericardial tamponade, RV infarction, or overt RV failure. Perhaps most difficult of all is recognizing a wedge in a patient with mitral regurgitation. The expected atrial waveform will never appear, since the large V wave obscures it, but the mean pressure can still be seen to fall (Fig. 34-4).

Large swings in intrathoracic pressure may also hinder the ability to recognize the expected transition in waveforms during catheter insertion. Wide respiratory fluctuations in pressure may even be mistaken for systolic-diastolic excursions. (However, respiratory frequency will not match the heart rate.) If large respiratory fluctuations pose a problem during mechanical ventilation, sedation (or temporary paralysis) may aid delineation of waveforms and will enhance reliability of the measurements obtained.

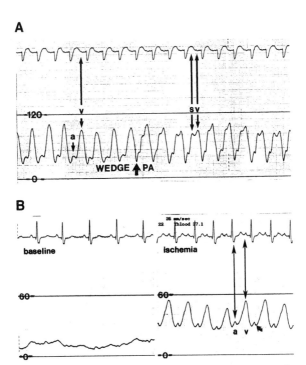

FIGURE 34-4   *A.* Acute mitral regurgitation with giant V wave in pulmonary wedge tracing. The pulmonary artery (PA) tracing has a characteristic bifid appearance due to both a PA systolic wave and the V wave. Note that the V wave occurs later in the cardiac cycle than the PA systolic wave, which is synchronous with the T wave of the electrocardiogram. *B.* Intermittent giant V wave due to ischemia of the papillary muscle. Wedge tracings are from same patient at baseline and during ischemia. Scale is in millimeters of mercury.

WAVEFORMS

Normal pressure waveforms are illustrated in Fig. 34-5. An electrocardiographic lead that clearly demonstrates atrial electrical activity is essential to adequately evaluate pressure waveforms. Common technical difficulties encountered in the generation of pressure waveforms from the PAC include over-

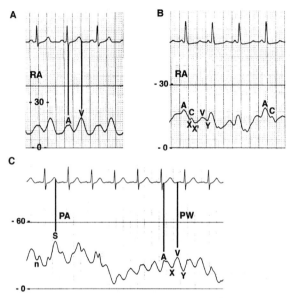

FIGURE 34-5 Pressure waveforms recorded simultaneously with an electrocardiographic lead. *A.* Right atrial (RA) tracing showing timing of A and V waves and X and Y descents. *B.* RA tracing with visible C wave. *C.* Pulmonary artery (PA) showing systolic wave (S) and dicrotic notch (n); wedge (PW) tracing showing A and V waves, X and Y descents. Note the difference in timing of the PA and PW pressure waves with respect to the electrocardiogram. Scale is in millimeters of mercury.

damping, catheter whip, overwedging, and incomplete wedging.

Overdamping decreases systolic pressure and raises diastolic pressure. Extreme overdamping can affect mean values as well. Common causes of overdamping include air bubbles in the transducer or pressure tubing or partial occlusion of the catheter by clot or kinking. A simple bedside test for overdamping is the rapid-flush test (Fig. 34-2). An appropriately damped system will show a rapid fall in pressure with an "overshoot" and prompt return to a crisp PA tracing upon sudden closure of the flush device. In contrast, an overdamped

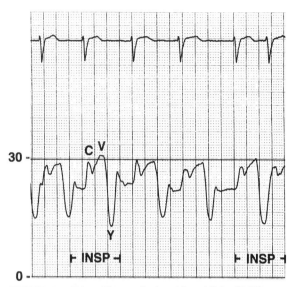

FIGURE 34-6   Tricuspid regurgitation. A broad V (or "C-V") wave and prominent Y descent are apparent in the right atrial tracing. Note that inspiration leads to accentuation of the Y descent and mean right atrial pressure increases slightly (Kussmaul sign).

system will generate a tracing that demonstrates a gradual return to the baseline pressure without an overshoot. Catheter whip is a consequence of the PAC coursing through the right heart, where cardiac contraction may produce "shock transients" or "whip" artifacts. Overwedging, recognizable by a characteristic tracing showing a gradual rise in pressure with balloon inflation, occurs when the catheter tip is closed off from the vessel by balloon herniation over the tip or because the tip is positioned against the vessel wall.

Tricuspid regurgitation is most often due to chronic pulmonary hypertension with dilation of the right ventricle. With tricuspid regurgitation, there is often a characteristically broad V (or "C-V") wave (Fig. 34-6). One of the most consistent findings in the Pra tracing of patients with tricuspid regurgitation is a steep Y descent. The latter often becomes more pronounced with inspiration. The Kussmaul sign, an increase in Pra with inspiration, is also common in patients with severe tricuspid regurgitation.

The Pra tracing in RV infarction often reveals prominent X and Y descents, and these deepen with inspiration or volume loading. With right ventricular infarction, the RV and PA pulse pressures narrow, and with RV failure, the RVEDP may approximate the Ppad. This, together with the frequent presence of tricuspid regurgitation, may lead to difficulties in bedside insertion of the PA catheter, and fluoroscopy may be required. In the setting of a patent foramen ovale, patients with RV infarction may develop significant hypoxemia due to a right-to-left atrial shunt. Profound hypoxemia with a clear chest radiograph and refractory hypotension would also be consistent with major pulmonary embolus. The hemodynamic profile of these two disorders is different, however, in that massive pulmonary embolism is characterized by a significant increase in the Ppad-Ppw gradient, while the latter is unaffected by RV infarction.

Pericardial tamponade results in the characteristic "equalization" of the Pra and Ppw and blunted Y descent (Fig. 34-7). An absent Y descent dictates that echocardiography should be performed to confirm pericardial tamponade, while a well-preserved Y descent argues strongly against this diagnosis.

Constrictive pericarditis and restrictive cardiomyopathy have similar hemodynamic findings (Fig. 34-8). Both disorders may be associated with striking increases in Pra and Ppw due to limitation of cardiac filling. In restrictive cardiomyopathy,

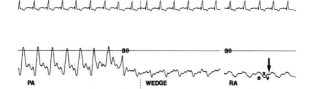

FIGURE 34-7   Pericardial tamponade. Tracings show characteristic equalization of wedge and right atrial pressure and blunting of the Y descent (*arrow*).

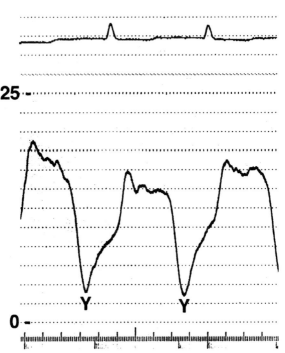

FIGURE 34-8   Constrictive pericarditis. Right atrial tracing (obtained in the cardiac catheterization laboratory) reveals a very prominent Y descent. Paper speed = 50 mm/s.

the Ppw is usually greater than the Pra; while in constrictive pericarditis, the right and left atria exhibit similar pressures. In contrast to pericardial tamponade, the Y descent is prominent and is often deeper than the X descent.

Clinical Use of Pressure Measurements

PULMONARY ARTERY PRESSURE

Pulmonary artery pressure is a function of the flow generated by RV contraction, resistance, within the vascular network, and downstream pressure. Normal values for Ppa are systolic, 15 to 30 mmHg; diastolic, 4 to 12 mmHg; and mean, 9 to 18 mmHg. Factors that increase PVR will cause the Ppad to exceed Ppw and will increase the driving pressure required to sustain flow across the pulmonary circuit. Indeed, a Ppad–Ppw gradient that exceeds 5 mmHg is highly characteristic of acute respiratory distress syndrome (ARDS), sepsis, major pulmonary emboli, excessive PEEP, and other conditions that increase resistance to flow within the pulmonary vasculature. In contrast, pulmonary hypertension due solely to an acutely increased downstream (left atrial) pressure is characterized by preservation of the normal Ppad–Ppw gradient.

An increased $\dot{Q}_T$ alone will not cause pulmonary hypertension. Pulmonary hypertension may result from the combination of only a modest increase in vascular resistance and a major increase in $\dot{Q}_T$ due to sepsis, cirrhosis, or other factors. Measuring $\dot{Q}_T$ and calculating pulmonary vascular resistance (PVR) can assess the relative contributions of blood flow and the pulmonary vasculature to the increase in Ppa. (The PVR = Ppa − Ppw/$\dot{Q}_T$O.)

PULMONARY ARTERY WEDGE PRESSURE

The pulmonary artery wedge pressure (Ppw) is obtained by inflating the catheter balloon with 1 to 1.5 mL of air, thus allowing the catheter tip to advance until it obstructs forward flow within a branch of the PA. The pressure recorded at the catheter tip (Ppw) is equivalent to the pressure in the occluded pulmonary vein at the point (junction, or j point) where it intersects with blood flow from uninterrupted vessels. The Ppw is used clinically as an estimate of hydrostatic pressure (Pcap) in the fluid-exchanging pulmonary capillaries and as a measure of preload. Recorded Ppw should be obtained at end-expiration from a strip recording rather than by the digital estimate. Although only intravascular pressure is routinely measured, it is the transmural pressure (intravascular minus pleural, Ppw − Ppl) that is of most interest.

A Ppw recorded at end-expiration will overestimate the transmural pressure if Ppl is positive at end-expiration. Positive juxtacardiac pressure at end-expiration may occur with an increase in lung volume (applied PEEP, auto-PEEP) or without an increase in lung volume (active exhalation). Removal of PEEP for more than a few seconds to measure Ppw is not generally advisable because the resultant increase in venous return, and perhaps an acute reduction in RV overload, creates a different hemodynamic state than existed when PEEP was present. Also, PEEP withdrawal may lead to worsening oxygenation.

Large errors in Ppw measurement may occur when patients continue to actively expire at end-exhalation. A respiration-related Ppw excursion of 10 to 15 mmHg suggests that end-expiratory Ppw overestimates the true transmural pressure. When this occurs, the use of sedation or paralysis in the mechanically ventilated patient may be necessary for reliable data acquisition.

Pulmonary Artery Wedge Pressure and Pulmonary Edema

The Ppw is commonly used to aid in the diagnosis and management of pulmonary edema. An isolated Ppw reading does not reliably predict whether pulmonary edema occurred on the basis of increased Pcap alone or on the basis of altered permeability, especially when it is recorded after a therapeutic intervention. Acute hydrostatic pulmonary edema frequently occurs, despite normal intravascular volume, on the basis of decreased LV compliance (diastolic dysfunction) due to ischemia or accelerated hypertension. This acute process may have resolved by the time a PAC is inserted. Clarification of the mechanism of pulmonary edema may therefore require a period of clinical observation. The expected Ppw threshold for hydrostatic pulmonary edema, assuming normal permeability, is approximately 22 to 25 mmHg. A higher threshold is common if the Ppw has been chronically elevated. Maintaining the Ppw $\leq$ 18 mmHg should lead to marked improvement in clinical and radiographic evidence of pulmonary edema within 24 hours if permeability is normal. However, hydrostatic pulmonary edema may persist or worsen if there are intermittent elevations in Ppw due to myocardial ischemia.

Although Ppw and Pcap are not equivalent, downward manipulation of Ppw by diuresis, ultrafiltration, or dialysis will reduce Pcap and may markedly benefit gas exchange in patients with ARDS. There is no minimum value for Ppw below which removal of intravascular volume is contraindicated provided that $\dot{Q}_T$ is adequate. If the clinical problem is severely impaired gas exchange requiring high $F_{I_{O_2}}$ or high PEEP, then a trial of Ppw reduction is reasonable as long as $\dot{Q}_T$ and blood pressure remain within acceptable limits. As with all therapeutic manipulations, a measurable and clinically relevant endpoint (e.g., Pa_{O_2}) should be assessed before and after Ppw reduction.

Pulmonary Artery Wedge Pressure and Preload

When afterload and intrinsic contractility are held constant, the forcefulness of ventricular contraction is determined by end-diastolic fiber length (preload). Acute changes in fiber length correlate with changes in left ventricular end-diastolic volume (LVEDV), a function of myocardial compliance and transmural filling pressure (LVEDP-Ppl). Normally, a Ppw closely approximates LVEDLP. However, mean Ppw will overestimate LVEDP when there is mitral valve obstruction or a very large V wave. Conversely, hypervolemia or reduced intrinsic myocardial compliance may cause the mean Ppw to underestimate LVEDP. Even when mean Ppw is a faithful measure of LVEDP, factors that alter left ventricular compliance (hypertrophy, ischemia) or change juxtacardiac pressure (PEEP, active exhalation) will profoundly affect the relationship between Ppw and LVEDV.

The optimal Ppw (for preload) can be defined as the Ppw above which there is minimal increase in stroke volume, or left ventricular stroke work (LVSW). In normal individuals, LVSW often reaches a plateau at a LVEDP of 10 to 12 mmHg. During volume resuscitation from hypovolemic and septic shock, optimal Ppw is often equal to 14 mmHg. By contrast, with acute myocardial infarction or at high levels of PEEP, a Ppw $\geq$ 18 mmHg may be required. Because numerous factors can affect the relation among Ppw and preload, it is useful to define the optimal Ppw through an acute fluid challenge when the adequacy of preload is in question. For example, when the major clinical problem is hypotension or oliguria, the Ppw should be increased with acute volume infusions until it has been clearly demonstrated that no further improvement in $\dot{Q}_T$ can be achieved. Conversely, maintaining a Ppw higher than necessary to achieve adequate $\dot{Q}_T$ may be detrimental in patients who are at high risk for ARDS or who have already shown evidence of vascular congestion or edema on chest x-ray. As a rule, the Ppw in this setting should be kept at the lowest level consistent with near-optimal $\dot{Q}_T$, especially early in the disease process, when edema predominates as a cause of impaired gas exchange. Again, the importance of tailoring hemodynamic interventions to the specific clinical problems at hand cannot be overemphasized.

Cardiac Output Measurement

PRINCIPLES OF MEASUREMENT

The thermodilution technique for measuring $\dot{Q}_T$ is an indicator dilution method in which the indicator is thermal depression ("cold"). Cold fluid is injected through the proximal lumen of the PAC and, after mixing thoroughly in the RV with venous blood returning from the periphery, passes into the PA, where a thermistor at the tip of the catheter senses dynamic changes in temperature. The Stewart-Hamilton formula relates $\dot{Q}_T$ to temperature change over time:

$$\dot{Q}_T = \frac{V\,(T_B - T_I) \times K_1 \times K_2}{\int T_B(t)\,dt}$$

where V = injected volume; T_B = blood temperature; T_I = injectate temperature; $\int T_B(t)\,dt$ = change in blood temperature as a function of time; and K_1 and K_2 are computational constants. Whether iced or room-temperature injectate is being used, the $\dot{Q}_T$td compares favorably with output values obtained by Fick or dye-dilution methods as long as careful technique is used. Errors may occur if the volume or recorded temperature of the injectate is incorrect or if the wrong computational constant for the catheter in use or incorrect injectate temperature is entered into the computer. Errors can also occur due to warming of the injectate because of delay or handling after the syringe is removed from the ice. Prolonged or uneven injections and thermistor contact with the vessel wall are other technical sources of measurement errors.

Clinical conditions resulting in $\dot{Q}$Ttd being an unreliable estimate of cardiac output include cardiac arrhythmias occurring during injection, left-to-right shunts (ASD, VSD), and significant tricuspid regurgitation. Finally, $\dot{Q}$Ttd may vary based on the phase of the respiratory cycle at which the injection is begun. The average of multiple, randomly timed injections probably gives the most accurate assessment in this situation.

Combining assessment of $\dot{Q}$Ttd with measurement of systemic and pulmonary pressures allows calculation of vascular resistances: $SVR = (Pa - Pra)/\dot{Q}T$; $PVR = (Ppa - Ppw)/\dot{Q}T$. To assess the appropriateness of $\dot{Q}T$ to body mass, $\dot{Q}$Ttd is divided by body surface area (BSA) to calculate cardiac index. Unlike flow ($\dot{Q}T$), pulmonary and systemic pressures are not size-dependent. Therefore, to avoid misinterpretation due to variation in body mass, it is also appropriate to compute indices of systemic and pulmonary vascular resistance (SVRI and PVRI) by using cardiac index rather than $\dot{Q}T$ in the resistance calculations.

CLINICAL USE

Assessment of $\dot{Q}$Ttd and vascular resistances may be helpful in the assessment of variety of clinical problems, including hypotension, oliguria, pulmonary hypertension, and unexplained lactic acidosis. Measurement of $\dot{Q}$Ttd is of particular value in the management of septic shock and septic ARDS.

A hyperdynamic state is characterized by a high $\dot{Q}_T$ and a low SVR. Sepsis is the most common cause of hypotension with a low SVR, but other conditions may produce a similar hemodynamic profile. Severe hypotension resulting from excessive arterial vasodilation can occur as a result of acute adrenal insufficiency, thiamine deficiency (beri-beri), severe pancreatitis, or poisoning with a variety of drugs or toxins, including nitrates, calcium-channel blockers, aspirin, tricyclic antidepressants, or cyanide. Large arteriovenous fistulae and cirrhosis are also associated with a very high $\dot{Q}T$ and very low SVR, although blood pressure should remain normal. Failure to include noninfectious processes in the differential diagnosis of a high $\dot{Q}T$-low SVR state may result in misdiagnosis of life-threatening, treatable conditions.

Continuous Cardiac Output

A recent advance in catheter technology has allowed continuous monitoring of $\dot{Q}_Ttd$ The modified PA catheter contains a 10-cm thermal filament that transfers heat directly into the blood using a pseudorandom binary sequence. The amount of heat applied is safe and the upper limit of temperature attained within the filament is 44°C. Temperature change is detected at the catheter tip and is cross-correlated with the input sequence to produce a thermodilution washout curve. The displayed $\dot{Q}_T$ value, an average of 10 separate determinations over the preceding 5 minutes, is updated every 30 seconds. The clinical impact of continuous $\dot{Q}_Ttd$ monitoring is uncertain. It may have greatest utility in clinical situations in which $\dot{Q}_T$ is likely to undergo marked fluctuations, either spontaneously or in response to therapy. From a practical standpoint, it is more convenient.

Mixed Venous Oxygen Saturation

The mixed venous oxygen saturation ($S\bar{v}_{O_2}$) can be measured intermittently by withdrawing a sample of blood from the distal port of the unwedged PA catheter or continuously with a fiberoptic PA catheter that measures O_2 saturation by reflectance oximetry. With either method, technical aspects of the measurement are crucial to obtaining reliable data. Intermittent sampling of $S\bar{v}_{O_2}$ is accomplished by discarding the initial 3 mL of blood, then withdrawing a sample very slowly so as to avoid contamination with capillary blood. The $S\bar{v}_{O_2}$ should be measured by co-oximetry, because the steep slope of the O_2 dissociation curve in the venous range dictates that small errors in measurement of $P\bar{v}_{O_2}$ may result in substantial errors in calculation of $S\bar{v}_{O_2}$.

Oxygen delivery is the product of $\dot{Q}_T$ and arterial O_2 content, the latter being determined by the hemoglobin and arterial O_2 saturation (Sa_{O_2}). The body's O_2 consumption ($\dot{V}_{O_2}$) is determined by the underlying metabolic activity of tissues and is normally independent of O_2 delivery. Thus, as O_2 delivery falls, so too will $S\bar{v}_{O_2}$. Therefore, measurement of $S\bar{v}_{O_2}$ helps assess the adequacy of O_2 delivery in relation to tissue O_2 requirements. Under normal conditions, the $Sa_{O_2} - S\bar{v}_{O_2}$

difference is 20 to 25 percent, yielding an $S\bar{v}_{O_2}$ of 65 to 75 percent when arterial blood is well oxygenated.

Increased $S\bar{v}_{O_2}$ may be seen in a variety of conditions. In sepsis, $S\bar{v}_{O_2}$ is often normal, but in some cases there is extreme peripheral vasodilation and $\dot{Q}T$ increases disproportionately to metabolic demands, resulting in an increase in $S\bar{v}_{O_2}$. Cirrhosis is one of the more common causes of a markedly increased $S\bar{v}_{O_2}$, with values occasionally in excess of 85 percent. A variety of vasodilating agents and left-to-right cardiac shunts also result in an increase in $S\bar{v}_{O_2}$. Last, agents that interfere with mitochondrial cytochrome activity (e.g., cyanide) may produce striking elevation in $S\bar{v}_{O_2}$ due to the tissues' inability to utilize O_2.

Continuous measurement of $S\bar{v}_{O_2}$ with the fiberoptic PA catheter has been advocated as a useful technique for early detection of inadequate $\dot{Q}T$ relative to tissue O_2 demand. Theoretically, continuous $S\bar{v}_{O_2}$ monitoring can lead to more rapid detection of hemodynamic instability than simply monitoring blood pressure and heart rate.

Miscellaneous Diagnostic Applications of the PA Catheter

Additional applications of PA catheter include bedside balloon-occlusion pulmonary angiography, microvascular cytology, evaluation of arrhythmias and intracardiac shunts, and determination of caloric requirements.

For a more detailed discussion, see Chap. 14 in *Principles of Critical Care*, 2d ed.

Chapter 35

ECHOCARDIOGRAPHY

MICHAEL O'CONNOR

Echocardiography has evolved from a rarely performed diagnostic technique into a common one and is increasingly relied upon to guide a wide variety of diagnostic and therapeutic interventions. Echocardiography is noninvasive, readily available in most centers, can be performed at the bedside, and provides a massive amount of information about a patient's heart in a short period of time. As echocardiography has become more commonly available, the advantages of its use have become increasingly apparent in the intensive care unit (ICU). Echocardiography is potentially helpful in an increasing number of clinical situations (Table 35-1). Transthoracic echocardiography and transesophageal echocardiography (TTE and TEE) can be expected to change the management of approximately 25 percent of patients in the ICU.

TTE and TEE can both be used to assess ventricular and atrial volumes, systolic ventricular function, diastolic ventricular function, valvular function, and regional ventricular wall motion. The short-axis view of the left ventricle is the most commonly used when the TEE serves as a monitor, as it allows for the simultaneous assessment of filling volumes and the detection of regional wall motion abnormalities (Fig. 35-1). It is not clear whether echocardiography is more or less sensitive than electrocardiography (ECG) for the detection of myocardial ischemia as evidenced by regional wall motion abnormalities. These abnormalities may occur in the absence of ECG changes, but the vast majority of ECG-documented ischemia is accompanied by echocardiographic evidence of abnormal regional wall motion. Echocardiographic assessment of cardiac performance has improved such that there are now only small differences between echocardiographic assessments of ventricular function and other techniques, such as multiple gated acquisition (MUGA) scanning. Indeed, echocardiography is the most commonly utilized method of seeking diastolic dysfunction.

TABLE 35-1   Indications for Obtaining Echocardiography

Acute myocardial infarction
Shock refractory to conventional therapy
Shock and pulmonary artery pressures that exceed
   40 mmHg in a patient with no prior history of pulmonary
   hypertension
Inadequate circulation in spite of apparently adequate filling
   pressures
New murmur
Peripheral stigmata of endocarditis
Persistently positive blood cultures in spite of adequate
   antibiotic therapy
Suspected tamponade or constrictive pericarditis
Suspected aortic dissection
Suspected right heart failure
Detection of air embolism

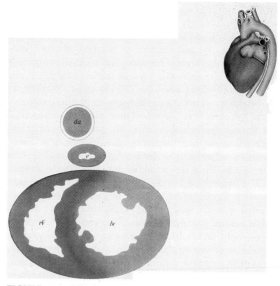

FIGURE 35-1   Short-axis view. Abbreviations: *lv* = left ventricle;
rv = right ventricle; *e* = esophagus; *da* = descending aorta.

Echocardiography is highly useful in the early evaluation of the patient in shock of unknown cause. Because echocardiography is rapidly available and noninvasive, it not only complements pulmonary artery catheterization but can often replace it. Not only can the patient be evaluated for left ventricular dysfunction, but severe hypovolemia, right heart syndromes, and pericardial disease are readily identified.

Echocardiography is increasingly capable of detecting the presence of small thrombi in the atria and is frequently used to assess for the presence of clot immediately prior to the cardioversion of patients in atrial fibrillation. The aortic view (Fig. 35-2) is useful for detecting small vegetations on the aortic valve, and echocardiography, in general, is valuable for assessing valve anatomy and function. TTE and TEE can also be

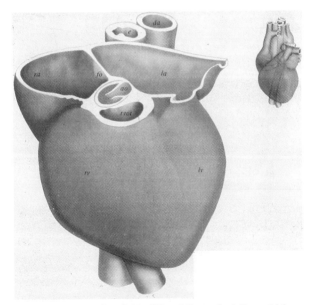

FIGURE 35-2 Aortic view. Abbreviations: *lv*=left ventricle; *rv*=right ventricle; *la*=left atrium; *ra*=right atrium; *e*=esophagus; *da*=descending aorta; *fo*=foramen ovale; *ao*=aortic root; *rvot*=right ventricular outflow tract.

used to detect pericardial effusions, constrictive pericarditis, and intracardiac shunts, including atrial (ASD) and ventricular (VSD) septal and endocardial cushion defects. Echocardiography is the technique of choice for assessing pericardial effusions, as it makes it possible to distinguish hemodynamically significant effusions from those that are not. This is important, as there is little correlation between the size of an effusion and its hemodynamic consequences. Pericardial effusions that are hemodynamically significant cause late diastolic and early systolic collapse of the right atrial free wall. As tamponade evolves, early diastolic collapse of the right ventricle occurs and hypotension ensues. A combination of Doppler studies and the rapid injection of intravenous contrast simultaneously with a four-chamber view of the heart (Fig. 35-3) can reveal the presence of even very small intracardiac shunts.

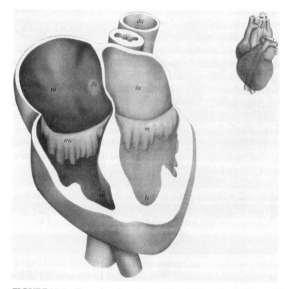

FIGURE 35-3 Four-chamber view. Abbreviations: *lv* = left ventricle; *rv* = right ventricle; *la* = left atrium; *ra* = right atrium; *fo* = foramen ovale; *e* = esophagus; *da* = descending aorta; *tric* = tricuspid valve; *m* = mitral valve.

Doppler waveforms of flows obtained from TTE and TEE can be used for a variety of diagnostic purposes with increasing success, including quantifying the degree of valvular regurgitation, estimating pulmonary artery pressures, detecting diastolic dysfunction, and even gauging cardiac output. Diastolic dysfunction causes decreased ventricular filling during early diastole and increased dependence upon atrial contraction for ventricular filling. This physiology is detectable echocardiographically. In diastolic dysfunction, the Doppler flow across the mitral valve following atrial systole is larger than the early diastolic flow, which is opposite of normal. Echocardiography remains the only way to assess dynamic causes of left ventricular outflow obstruction, such as hypertrophic obstructive cardiomyopathy (HOCM), which can cause otherwise mysterious shock in some patients.

TTE is frequently technically difficult or even impossible to perform in some critically ill patients (Table 35-2). This, in conjunction with the ease of performing TEE in intubated patients, has resulted in the increasingly common use of TEE as the technique of first resort in intubated patients. Images obtained with TEE are typically of higher quality than those ob-

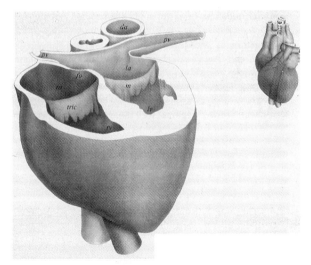

FIGURE 35-4 Alternative four-chamber view.

TABLE 35-2   Factors Associated with Technically Difficult Transthoracic Echocardiography

---

Morbid obesity

Anasarca or chest wall edema

Large lung volumes from COPD or high PEEP

Dressings or appliances on the anterior chest or interposed between the chest wall and the heart (e.g., burns or left ventricular assist device)

Abnormal chest wall anatomy (e.g., open chest)

---

tained by TTE because little or no soft tissue, bone, or air is interposed between the probe and the region of myocardium in question. Some small additional risk of oropharyngeal trauma and esophageal injury is associated with TEE, but these complications are rare in the hands of experienced operators and will diminish as the size of the TEE probes continues to shrink. Because TEE is performed by placing the transducer in the portion of esophagus immediately adjacent to the left atrium, significant quantities of acoustic and thermal energy can be transmitted to the atrium and can rarely cause an atrial arrhythmia (or convert one). Thermal injury of the esophagus is unlikely to occur as a consequence of a diagnostic study but may occur during longer studies, as when TEE is used as a monitor in either the ICU or the operating room. Pressure-related injury to the oropharynx or esophagus may also occur as a consequence of a prolonged study over hours. TEE is commonly used in the operating room to assess the adequacy of ventricular filling and to look for ischemia-related regional wall motion abnormalities. Left ventricular compliance is far more dynamic than previously believed; consequently, direct assessment of the adequacy of filling volumes is increasingly regarded as useful and preferable or complementary to pressure monitoring. TEE also is used to detect the presence and severity of embolic events in patients at risk for them. Although TEE is not used widely for these purposes in the ICU, some believe it is only a matter of time before this occurs.

For a more detailed discussion, see Chap. 21 in *Principles of Critical Care,* 2d ed.

Chapter 36

APPROACH TO SEPSIS
OF UNKNOWN ORIGIN

LISA WOLFE

Not infrequently infection is suspected in a critically ill patient on the basis of a constellation of clinical features consistent with sepsis but without an immediately obvious focus. Two broad categories of patient presentation can be defined. *Primary sepsis* is acute sepsis syndrome or septic shock leading to intensive care admission in a patient without an obvious source of infection. *Secondary sepsis* is newly developing or persistent hemodynamic instability or comprises features of the sepsis syndrome in a patient already being treated for a serious illness in the intensive care unit (ICU).

Approach to Primary Sepsis

SEPSIS DUE TO BACTERIAL INFECTIONS

Hypotension or frank shock with features of sepsis in the absence of localizing findings is a common problem confronting the intensivist. Septic shock may be preceded by vital sign abnormalities and laboratory irregularities that signal progressive infection to the clinician (Table 36-1).

Once circulatory and respiratory stability is achieved and appropriate monitoring is established, the next step is to review the physical examination, history, and basic laboratory data (Table 36-2). If this is unrevealing, one must next think about a common problem presenting in an uncommon manner. Severe intravascular volume depletion may delay the appearance of an infiltrate on chest radiograph in a patient with pneumonia. Head CT and lumbar puncture may be indicated for mild symptoms of confusion or moderate obtundation to rule out central nervous system infection in cases without the

TABLE 36-1   Clinical Features Associated with Sepsis

Clinical examination
  Fever or hypothermia
  Unexplained tachypnea
  Tachycardia and hypotension (low systemic vascular resistance,
    if calculated)
  Oliguria
  Confusion, mental obtundation
Laboratory examination
  Leukocytosis or left-shifted leukopenia
  Thrombocytopenia
  Respiratory alkalosis, unexplained hypoxemia
  Mild to moderate cholestasis or elevation of hepatic
    transaminases
  Hyperglycemia
  Lactic acidosis

---

usual meningeal signs. Urinary tract infection with sepsis but no localizing signs may occur, especially in the elderly, if there is ureteric obstruction, perinephric abscess, or prostatitis. Many intraabdominal processes, including mesenteric ischemia, may not be easily identifiable at the time of the initial evaluation. Repeated physical examination of the abdomen at frequent intervals is important. Even relatively subtle abdominal findings should prompt the intensivist to obtain abdominal radiographs and consultation with a general surgeon. Ultrasound or CT of the abdomen and angiography are further imaging studies to be considered. In the absence of one of the initially missed diagnoses noted above, sepsis in previously well individuals is most commonly due to one of the primary bacteremia syndromes or to acute bacterial endocarditis.

Staphylococcus remains the most common cause of primary sepsis in most hospitals. Diabetes mellitus, chronic renal failure, and parenteral drug abuse are associated with increased risk of this infection. Endocarditis must always be considered in staphylococcal bacteremia. Because of its frequency and poor prognosis if untreated, empiric antimicrobial therapy for life-threatening sepsis of unknown origin should always include coverage for this organism.

TABLE 36-2   Basic Initial Investigation for Suspected
Sepsis in Seriously Ill Patients

Basic initial investigation
  History and physical examination
  Complete blood cell count
  Chest radiograph
  Urinalysis and urine culture
  Blood Culture
Additional investigation (where indicated)
  Intracranial infection suspected: lumbar puncture, preceded by
    computed tomography (CT) scan of head if indication is other
    than meningismus
  Respiratory infection suspected: sputum or endotracheal
    secretions for Gram stain and culture; radiograph of nasal
    sinuses (followed by needle aspiration if sinusitis
    demonstrated); needle aspirate of pleural fluid
  Wound infection or intraabdominal infection suspected: Gram
    stain and culture of wound drainage, needle aspirate of
    peritoneal fluid collection or abscess; imaging of abdominal
    contents (ultrasound or CT, depending on suspect organ)
  Bone or joint infection suspected: radiograph and/or bone scan;
    needle aspiration for Gram stain and culture of suspect joint
  Complicated urinary tract infection suspected: ultrasound or CT
    scan of kidneys and perinephric space
  Primary bacteremia suspected: remove and culture
    semiquantitatively all indwelling vascular catheters; cardiac
    ultrasound (transesophageal approach preferred for suspect
    endocarditis)

Meningococcemia, pneumococcal bacteremia, and *Salmonella* bacteremia are other important causes of sepsis that may not be evident from initial evaluation.

NONBACTERIAL CAUSES OF SEPSIS

Most of the nonbacterial pathogens causing primary sepsis occur in geographically definable areas, so travel history from the patient or family is important. Malaria, Rocky Mountain spotted fever, viral hemorrhagic fever, and viral hepatitis are examples of illnesses caused by such pathogens.

TABLE 36-3   Noninfectious Causes of Apparent Sepsis in Critically Ill Patients

---

Drug-related syndromes
   Acute intoxications and poisonings: cocaine, phenothiazines, organophosphates
   Drug withdrawal syndromes
   Neuroleptic malignant syndrome
   Allergic drug reactions
Anaphylaxis
Systemic vasculitides
   Hypersensitivity angiitis
   Systemic lupus erythematosus
   Polyarteritis nodosa
Acute pancreatitis
Extensive tissue injury
   Crush injury
   Rhabdomyolysis
   Vascular occlusion with tissue necrosis
Heat stroke

NONINFECTIOUS CAUSES OF APPARENT SEPSIS (TABLE 36-3)

Drug-related syndromes (acute intoxications or poisonings, drug withdrawal, neuroleptic malignant syndrome, allergic drug reactions), anaphylaxis, systemic vasculitides (hypersensitivity angiitis, systemic lupus erythematosus, polyarteritis nodosa), acute pancreatitis, extensive tissue injury (crush injury, rhabdomyolysis, vascular occlusion with tissue necrosis), and heat stroke are processes that mimic sepsis in critically ill patients.

OCCULT SEPSIS IN PATIENTS WITH UNDERLYING MEDICAL ILLNESS

The patient's underlying medical illness is often the single most important determinant of the clinical approach to sepsis of unknown origin. Diabetes mellitus predisposes to staphylococcal bacteremia, gram-negative sepsis, rhinocerebral mucormycosis, and candidemia. Chronic renal disease predisposes to staphylococcal bacteremia and pyogenic infections due to encapsulated organisms such as pneumococcus and *Haemophilus influenzae.* Asplenia is strongly associated with increased risk of primary bacteremia, particularly due to pneumococcus, *H. influenzae,* and to a lesser extent meningococcus and *Staph. aureus.* Functional asplenia in sickle cell anemia also increases risk of primary sepsis with these organisms and also with *Salmonella.*

EMPIRIC ANTIMICROBIAL THERAPY

Suspected infection producing life-threatening illness leading to admission to the intensive care unit (ICU) should be treated early with effective antimicrobial therapy to avoid septic shock and its complications. In most cases, the basic medical evaluation outlined above will point in the direction of one or more of the categories shown in Table 36-4. Based on this, an antimicrobial regimen can be selected. When a probable source is not found, a second-generation cephalosporin is generally advised. Extension of this regimen can then be considered by examining the possibility of central nervous system infection, anaerobic infection, infection with a relatively resistant gram-negative bacillus, or infection with an organism not susceptible to conventional antimicrobials, mandating addition of erythromycin, a tetracycline, or quinine.

Approach to Secondary Sepsis

PERSISTENT FEVER IN PATIENTS ON ANTIMICROBIAL THERAPY

Persistent fever despite antimicrobial and sometimes surgical therapy is a common problem that requires a systematic approach. Fever may take longer to resolve when the mass of inflamed tissue is larger. While fever due to infected intravascular catheters usually resolves within 24 h of catheter removal and institution of appropriate therapy, fever from severe systemic infections such as staphylococcal endocarditis may persist for 5 to 7 days. The clinician should reevaluate all the manifestations of sepsis present (white blood cell count, platelet count, temperature, level of consciousness,

TABLE 36-4 Antimicrobial Therapy for Sepsis of Unknown Etiology

Suspected Source of Sepsis	Usual Pathogens	Suggested Antimicrobial Regimens	Alternative Antimicrobial Regimens
None evident Normal host	*Staph. aureus*, streptococci, Enterobacteriaceae, meningococci	Ceftriaxone 2 g IV q12h or cefotaxime 2 g IV q6h	Imipenem/cilastatin 1 g IV q6h or piperacillin/tazobactam 3.375 g IV q6h or chloramphenicol 750 mg IV q6h
Immuno-compromised host	Enterobacteriaceae, *Pseudomonas* spp., *Staph. aureus*, *Staph. epidermidis*, streptococci	Piperacillin 3 g IV q4h and gentamicin 1.5 mg/kg IV q8h[a]	Ceftazadime 2 g IV q8h and vancomycin 500 mg IV q6h
Skin: (cellulitis, IV drug abuse)	*Staph. aureus*, streptococci, *Pseudomonas* spp.	Nafcillin 2 g IV q4h and gentamicin 1.5 mg/kg IV q8h[a]	Clindamycin 600 mg IV q8h or vancomycin 500 mg IV q6h and gentamicin 1.5 mg/kg IV q8h
Lung	*Streptococcus pneumoniae*, *Staph. aureus*, Enterobacteriaceae, *Legionella pneumophila*	Cefuroxime 1.5 g IV q8h or cefotaxime 2 g IV q6h or ceftriaxone 2 g IV q24h and erythromycin 1 g IV q6h[a]	Cotrimoxazole: 2.5 mg/kg TMP +12.5 mg/kg SMX IV q6h and erythromycin 1 g IV q6h[a]
Intracranial Meningitis	*Strep. pneumoniae*, meningococcus, *Listeria monocytogenes*, *H. influenzae*, Enterobacteriaceae	Cefotaxime 2 g IV q6h or ceftriaxone 2 g IV q12h *and* ampicillin 2 g IV q4h[a]	Chloramphenicol 1 g IV q6h and cotrimoxazole: 5 mg/kg TMP +25 mg/kg SMX IV q6h

Abscess	Bacteroides spp. and other anaerobes, Enterobacteriaceae, Staph. aureus	Metronidazole 750 mg IV q8h and ceftriaxone 2 g IV q12h	Chloramphenicol 750 mg IV q6h
Intraabdominal and female genital tract	Enterobacteriaceae, Bacteroides fragilis and other anaerobes	Metronidazole 500 mg IV q8h and ampicillin 2 g IV q6h and gentamicin 1.5 mg/kg IV q8h, or clindamycin 600 mg IV q8h and gentamicin 1.5 mg/kg IV q8h	Ceftriaxone 2 g IV q24h and clindamycin 600 mg IV q8h or Metronidazole 500 mg IV q8h, or piperacillin/tazobactam 3.374 g IV q6h or imipenem/cilastatin 1 g IV q6h
Urinary tract	Enterobacteriaceae, enterococcus, coagulase-negative staphylococci	Ampicillin 1 g IV q4h and gentamicin 1.5 mg/kg IV q8h	Cotrimoxazole 2.5 mg/kg TMP +12.5 mg/kg SMX IV q6h or cefotaxime 2 g IV q6h
Nonbacterial sepsis suspected	Rocky Mountain spotted fever	Doxycycline 100 mg IV q12h	Chloramphenical 750 mg IV q6h
	Human ehrlichiosis	Doxycycline 100 mg IV q12h	Rifampin 600 mg IV or PO q24h
	Viral sepsis		
	Herpesviruses	Acyclovir or ganciclovir[a]	
	Hemorrhagic fever	Ribavirin	
	Influenza	Ribavirin	
	Malaria	Quinine	

NOTE: Abbreviations: q4h, q6h, q8h, q12h, q24h = every 4, 6, 8, 12, or 24 hours.

[a] In hospitals or communities with significant prevalence of methicillin-resistant *Staphylococcus aureus* or high-level β-lactam-resistant pneumococci, vancomycin 1 g IV q12h should be added to the antimicrobial regimen.

TABLE 36-5   Major Nosocomial Infections Complicating Intensive Care for Critical Illness

Site	Diagnosis	Usual Pathogens	Predisposing Factors
Head and neck			
	Maxillary or frontal sinusitis	*Staph. aureus*, Enterobacteriaceae, *H. influenzae*	Nasotracheal endotracheal tube, large-bore NG tube, facial trauma
	Suppurative parotitis	*Staph. aureus*, Enterobacteriaceae	Dehydration, poor oral hygiene
	Intracranial pressure monitor infection	Coagulase negative staphylococci, *Staph. aureus*	Long-duration intracranial pressure monitoring, frequent line manipulation
Chest	Pneumonia	Enterobacteriaceae, *Staph. aureus*, *Pseudomonas* spp.	Endotracheal intubation, depressed level of consciousness, use of antacids or H_2 blockers, aspiration
Skin and vascular access sites			
	Vascular catheter infection and suppurative phlebitis	Coagulase negative staphylococci, *Staph. aureus*, Enterobacteriaceae, *Candida* spp.	Poor aseptic technique; occlusive site dressing; frequent catheter manipulation; location: groin, axilla, antecubital fossa; skin infection/contamination: burns, impetiginized rash
	Wound infection Clean surgery	*Staph. aureus*, *Strep. pyogenes*, coagulase negative staphylococci, *Candida* spp.	Protracted surgery; aseptic technique breaks; hematoma, prostheses

Category	Condition	Organisms	Risk factors
Abdomen	Contaminated abdominal surgery	Enterobacteriaceae, *B. fragilis* and other anaerobes (early) and Coagulase-negative staphylococci, Enterococci, resistant gram-negatives and *Candida* spp. (late)	Gross contamination, no antibiotic prophylaxis, inadequate drainage and debridement, malnutrition
	Infected decubiti	Enterobacteriaceae, *B. fragilis* and other anaerobes, *Staph. aureus*	Fecal soilage, poor perfusion or venous stasis, necrotic tissue not debrided
	Pseudomembranous colitis	*Clostridium difficile*	Prior antimicrobial therapy
	Acalculous cholecystitis	Enterobacteriaceae, enterococci, *B. fragilis* and other anaerobes	Protracted critical illness
	Intraabdominal abscess	Enterobacteriaceae, *B. fragilis* and other anaerobes	Perforated viscus, contaminated abdominal surgery, pancreatitis, malnutrition
Musculoskeletal	Posttraumatic osteomyelitis	*Staph. aureus*, Enterobacteriaceae	Compound fracture, frank wound contamination, foreign body, poor arterial perfusion, prostheses used for fixation with contaminated wound
	Septic arthritis	*Staph. aureus*, Enterobacteriaceae	Prior bacteremia, overlying cellulitis or skin breakdown, joint surgery or prosthesis in place
Urinary tract infection	Acute pyelonephritis	Enterobacteriaceae, enterococcus	Indwelling urinary catheter, diabetes mellitus, anatomic urologic abnormality or nephrolithiasis

hemodynamic stability). This evaluation should also include consideration of potential noninfectious causes of fever and the possibility of a new infection at another site.

The most important cause of antimicrobial treatment failure is lack of penetration of the antimicrobial to the site of the infection. The most important factor causing poor penetration is absence of blood supply to the site of infection, as occurs with abscess, necrotic tissue, and bony sequestra. Incorrect initial choice of drugs and development of secondary antimicrobial resistance are the other causes of failure of antibiotic therapy. If there is no demonstrable resistant pathogen based on all culture results and if the original regimen chosen was in fact appropriate to the clinical situation (see Table 36-4), it is generally not useful simply to change to different drugs; they are at least as likely to be the wrong ones as the initial choice. Obtaining repeat bacteriology from the site of the infection to guide antimicrobial therapy is usually a better approach.

INFECTIOUS COMPLICATIONS OF CRITICAL ILLNESS

There are a number of infections which are either peculiar to the ICU or particularly difficult to diagnose in the critically ill. These require a systematic and directed approach that comes from specifically considering these entities and excluding them in turn. The usual pathogens and predisposing factors are listed in Table 36-5.

NONINFECTIOUS CAUSES OF FEVER OR SEPSIS SYNDROME

The most common noninfectious cause of persistent low-grade fever, elevation of the white blood cell count, and mild to moderate "septic" hemodynamics is the host response to tissue injury. Large hematomas, traumatic injury to soft tissue, tissue ischemia, and pulmonary contusion, atelectasis, or chemical pneumonitis are examples of this. Drug fever may also be a diagnosis of exclusion that follows a careful evaluation for infection, and the diagnosis must be reconsidered at least daily.

EMPIRIC ANTIMICROBIAL THERAPY

In secondary sepsis, there are usually one or more candidate sources for the sepsis. Antimicrobial coverage should include *Staph. aureus* and enteric aerobic gram-negative bacilli regardless of the suspected source of sepsis, while coverage for other bacteria (anaerobes, *Legionella* spp., etc.) will depend on the suspected sources of sepsis. Entirely empiric therapy for fungi is generally not warranted except in neutropenic patients in whom antibacterial therapy is failing or in cases where there is some evidence to support a diagnosis of invasive fungal infection.

For a more detailed discussion, see Chap. 41 in *Principles of Critical Care*, 2d ed.

Chapter 37 _____

AIDS IN THE INTENSIVE CARE UNIT

KIM JOSEN

Human Immunodeficiency Virus (HIV) Infection

HIV is an RNA retrovirus in the lentivirus family. It predominantly infects T-helper lymphocytes (CD4+ cells) but also monocytes, macrophages, dendritic Langerhan cells, microglial cells, B lymphocytes, and bone marrow stem cells.

The basic mode of transmission is through exposure to infected bodily fluids. Worldwide, heterosexual contact is the most common mode of transmission. In the United States, one-half of reported cases are among homosexual men. The second most common cause of infection is through blood products, including shared needles and syringes for injection drug users as well as from mother to fetus. Currently, the risk of HIV infection from screened blood products is between 1 in 450,000 and 1 in 660,000 donations. The risk of infection following accidental skin puncture from an HIV-contaminated needle or sharp object is approximately 0.3 percent. The risk of seroconversion following mucous membrane exposure is probably around 0.1 percent. Given the small but definite risk to health care providers, it is essential to observe universal precautions.

Untreated, HIV causes a progressive deterioration of the immune system over 7 to 12 years. Although HIV infection leads to chronic disease, it is still a universally fatal illness. As the CD4+ cells become dysfunctional and depleted, the patient may develop opportunistic bacterial, fungal, viral, and protozoal infections. HIV-infected patients are also at risk for opportunistic neoplasms, including non-Hodgkins lymphoma (NHL), Kaposi sarcoma (KS), and bronchogenic carcinoma. The CD4+ cell count and viral load are essential in determining a differential diagnosis for new symptoms of disease as well as for prognosis and for monitoring response to antiretroviral therapy.

The current recommendation for the treatment of HIV infection is a combination of two to three antiretroviral drugs. The current categories of drugs include nucleoside analogs, nonnucleoside antiretrovirals, and protease inhibitors. The goal of antiretroviral therapy is maximal suppression of the HIV load. Unfortunately, the regimen is demanding and the drugs cause a number of side effects and drug interactions. Table 37-1 provides a brief overview of the current antiretroviral therapies. Health care workers who experience accidental exposure are advised to start combination therapy immediately while awaiting the results of HIV testing. Antiretroviral therapy should be continued throughout the duration of acute illness whenever possible. If the therapy must be held, it is important to stop all of the drugs in order to prevent the emergence of resistant viral strains.

Acute Respiratory Failure

GENERAL APPROACH

Respiratory failure accounts for about 65 percent of ICU admissions in the HIV-infected population. The most common cause of respiratory failure in the HIV-infected patient is *Pneumocystis carinii* pneumonia (PCP), followed by bacterial pneumonia. Table 37-2 outlines some of the common causes of respiratory failure in the intensive care unit (ICU). It is important to note that polymicrobial infections frequently occur in HIV-infected patients.

The initial evaluation of the HIV-infected patient in respiratory failure consists of a complete history and physical, documenting the duration and character of current symptoms, use of chemoprophylaxis, sick contacts, and history of opportunistic infections. The physical exam may reveal clues to the diagnosis. For example, purple nodules over the skin and mucous membranes should raise the possibility of pulmonary Kaposi sarcoma (KS). Palpable lymphadenopathy may be a sign of NHL. The laboratory studies should include the most recent CD4+ cell count, blood cultures, routine chemistries, a complete blood count, arterial blood gases, and chest radiographs. Sputum should be collected to test for the presence of bacterial, fungal, mycobacterial, and *P. carinii* infection. If the patient has a nonproductive cough, sputum may be induced with hypertonic saline. If the patient has more severe respiratory disease, he or she may require a bronchoscopy with bronchoalveolar lavage (BAL) and possibly transbronchial biopsy in order to establish a diagnosis. Figure 37-1 demonstrates an algorithm to establish a differential diagnosis in patients with respiratory distress in the ICU.

Prompt empiric treatment should include treatment for *P. carinii* and bacterial pathogens, including *Streptococcus pneumoniae*, *Staphylococcus aureus*, *Haemophilus influenzae B*, and gram-negative bacilli. A macrolide should be added to cover *Legionella*, *Chlamydia*, and *Mycoplasma* when these microorganisms are in the differential diagnosis of pneumonia. Treatment should be adjusted once a definitive diagnosis is established.

PNEUMOCYSTIS CARINII PNEUMONIA

Pneumocystis carinii is a ubiquitous fungus that may cause infection in severely immunocompromised hosts when the CD4+ cell count drops below $200/\mu L$. Although there is effective chemoprophylaxis, breakthrough infections can occur. Infection may also happen in patients who are previously undiagnosed as HIV-infected. Clinical features include dyspnea, nonproductive cough, and fever; these progress over several days to weeks. Physical examination may reveal a patient in respiratory distress with minimal adventitous breath sounds. The classic chest radiograph of *Pneumocystis carinii* pneumonia (PCP) shows diffuse interstitial infiltrates, although alveolar opacities, cystic changes, cavities, and pneumothoraces can also occur. The microbiologic burden in cystic PCP is generally so great that the diagnosis is relatively easy to make with the demonstration of PCP in the sputum of BAL. Table 37-3 summarizes some of the treatment options for PCP and other opportunistic infections in the ICU. The addition of prednisone in selected cases of PCP has contributed to a decreased mortality from this infection. In patients with a Pa_{O_2}

TABLE 37-1 Anti-HIV Drug Characteristics and Common Drug Interactions[a]

Nucleoside Reverse Transcriptase Inhibitors

	Zidovudine (AZT, ZDV, Retrovir)	Didanosine (ddI, Videx)	Zalcitabine (ddC, HIVID)	Stavudine (d4T, Zerit)	Lamivudine (3TC, Epivir)
Dose	200 mg tid or 300 mg bid	>60 kg: 200 mg bid or <60 kg: 125 mg bid	.75 mg tid	>60 kg: 40 mg bid or <60 kg: 30 mg bid	150 mg bid or <50 kg: 2 mg/kg
Common adverse effects	Bone marrow suppression, nausea, headache, insomina	Pancreatitis, nausea, diarrhea Peripheral Neuropathy	Peripheral Neuropathy Stomatitis	Peripheral Neuropathy	Minimal Toxicity
Common drug interactions	Hydroxyurea				

Nonnucleoside reverse transcriptase inhibitors

	Nevirapine (Viramune)	Delavirdine (Rescriptor)
Dose	200 mg q d × 14 d, then 200 mg bid	400 mg tid
Common adverse effects	Rash, transaminase, hepatitis	Rash, headache
Common drug interactions	Induces cytochrome p450 enzymes Rifampin, Rifabutin, Oral contraceptives Midazolam, Triazolam Protease inhibitors	Inhibits cytochrome p450 enzymes Terfenadine, Astemizole Amphetamines, Anticonvulsants, Antacids, Clarithromycin, Warfarin Quinidine, Dapsone, Indinavir, Saquinavir, Ergot

Protease inhibitors

	Indinavir (Crixivan)	Ritonavir (Norvir)	Saquinavir-HCG (Invirase)	Saquinavir-SGC (Fortovase)	Nelfinavir (Viracept)
Dose	800 mg q8h, 1 h before or 2 h after meals	600 mg q 12 h with food	600 mg tid with large meal	1200 mg tid with large meal	750 mg tid with food
Common adverse effects	Nephrolithiasis, nausea, hyperbilirubinemia, headache, rash, asthenia, blurred vision, metallic taste, thrombocytopenia hyperglycemia	Nausea, vomiting, diarrhea, headache, hepatitis, paresthesia, taste perversion, hyperglycemia transaminase elevation, hyperglycemia	Nausea, diarrhea, headache, transaminase elevation, hyperglycemia	Nausea, diarrhea, dyspepsia, abdominal pain, headache, transaminase elevation, hyperglycemia	Diarrhea, hyperglycemia
Common drug interactions	Inhibits cytochrome p450 enzymes Rifampin, terfenadine, astemizole, cisapride, triazolam, midazolam, ergot alkaloids, ketoconazole, delavirdine, nelfinavir	Inhibits cytochrome p450 enzymes ethinyl estradiol theophylline, sulfamethoxazole, zidovudine, clarithromycin, desipramine	Inhibits cytochrome p450 enzymes ritonavir, ketoconazole, nelfinavir, delavirdine, rifampin, rifabutin, terfenadine, astemizole, cisapride, ergot alkaloids, triazolam, midazolam	Inhibits cytochrome p450 enzymes ritonavir, ketoconazole, nelfinavir, delavirdine, rifampin, rifabutin, terfenadine, astemizole, cisapride, ergot alkaloids, triazolam, midazolam	Inhibits cytochrome p450 enzyme triazolam, midazolam, ergot alkaloids, terfenadine, astemizole, cisapride, ethinyl estradiol, norethinadrone, rifabutin, saquinavir, indinavir, rifampin

Ergot derivatives, Alprazolam, Midazolam, Triazolam Rifabutin, Rifampin

[a] Brand names are given in parentheses following the generic names.

Source: Adapted from "Guidelines for the Use of Antiretroviral Agents in HIV-Infected Adults and Adolescents," *Annals of Internal Medicine*, June 1998; 128(12):1077-1100. With permission.

TABLE 37-2   Etiology of Respiratory Failure
in the HIV-Infected Patient

Bacteria	***Viruses***
Streptococcus pneumoniae[a]	*Cytomegalovirus*
Staphylococcus aureus[a]	*Adenovirus*
Haemophilus influenzae[a]	*Herpes-simplex*
Legionella sp.	*Varicella-Zoster virus*
Mycoplasma pneumoniae	
Moraxella catarrhalis	***Protozoa***
Mycobacterium avium-intracellulare	*Toxoplasma gondii*
Mycobacterium tuberculosis	
Other Mycobacterial infections	***Fungi***
Nocardia asteroides	*Pneumocystis carinii*[a]
Rhodococcus	*Aspergillus fumigatus*
Salmonella	*Histoplasma capsulatum*
	Cryptococcus neoformans
Noninfectious	*Coccidioides immitis*
Bronchogenic carcinoma	*Blastomyces dematitidis*
Lymphoid interstitial pneumonitis	
Non-Hodgkin's lymphoma	***Nematodes***
Pneumothorax	*Strongyloides stercoralis*
Kaposi's sarcoma	
Bronchiolitis obliterans organizing pneumonia	
Primary pulmonary hypertension	
Nonspecific interstitial pneumonitis	

[a]Most Common

of less than 70 torr and an alveolar-arterial gradient greater than 35, prednisone (40 mg twice daily for 7 days, 40 mg once daily for 7 days, 20 mg once daily for 7 days) should be added to the antimicrobial therapy. Failure to see clinical improvement after 1 week of therapy suggests PCP resistance; an alternative therapy should be considered. Patients with PCP who respond to treatment have a mortality of less than 50 percent, while those who require mechanical ventilatory support have a predicted mortality of over 90 percent.

BACTERIAL PNEUMONIA

The clinical presentation of bacterial pneumonia in the HIV-infected patient is similar to that of the immune-competent

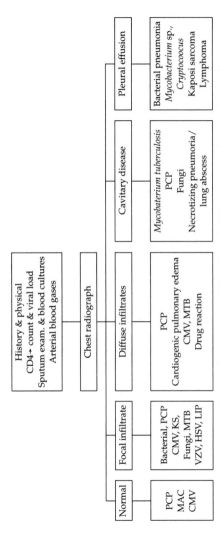

FIGURE 37-1 Differential diagnosis of respiratory failure in the AIDS patient. PCP, *Pneumocystis carinii* pneumonia; CMV, cytomegalovirus; MAC, *Mycobacterium avium-intracellulare*; LIP, lymphocytic interstitial pneumonitis; KS, Kaposi sarcoma; VZV, varicella zoster virus; HSV, herpes simplex virus.

TABLE 37-3 Treatment of Common Oportunistic Pathogens in the ICU

		Drug	Dose	Duration	Alternative treatment
Respiratory infections	Pneumocystis carinii pneumonia	TMP-SMX	20 mg & 100 mg IV q6h	14–21 d	Pentamidine 4 mg/kg IV qd or clindamycin (450 mg IV) primaquine (15–30 mg po q d)
	Mycobacterium tuberculosis	INH	300 mg po q d	9 mo	Empiric treatment for MDR-TB may include an aminoglycoside plus fluoroquinolone plus ethambutol and pyrazinamide and INH and rifampin plus cycloserine or ethionamide or amino salicylic acid
		Rifampin	10 mg/kg po q d	9 mo	
		Pyrazinamide	20–30 mg/kg po q d	2 mo	
		Ethambutol	25 mg/kg po q d	2 mo	
		Pyridoxine	50 mg po q d	9 mo	
	Mycobacterium avium intracellulare	Clarithromycin	1000 mg po q 12 h	lifelong	azithromycin 500 mg po qd
		Ethambutol	25 mg/kg po q d	lifelong	
		Rifabutin	300 mg po q d	lifelong	Rifampin 600 mg po qd ciprofloxacin 750 mg po bid
	CMV pneumonia	Ganciclovir (initial)	10 mg/kg IV q 12 h	12–21 d	Foscarnet 90 mg/kg IV q 12h
		Ganciclovir (maintenance)	5 mg/kg IV q d	lifelong	Foscarnet 90 mg/kg IV q d or ganciclovir 6 mg/kg 5d/week
CNS infections	Cryptococcal Meningitis	Amphotericin	0.7 mg/kg IV q d	2–3 weeks	Fluconazole 800–2000 mg/d, plus flucytosine 100 mg/kg 6 6h
		Flucytosine	100 mg/kg po/iv q 6 h	2–3 weeks	
		Fluconazole	200 mg po q d	lifelong	

		Drug	Dose	Duration / Total dose	
	Toxoplasma gondii (CNS lesion)	Pyrimethamine	200 mg po × 1	loading dose	Pyrimethamine plus clindamycin 900–1200 mg IV q 6 h until improvement clinically, followed by 450 mg po q 6 h
		Pyrimethamine	50–75 mg po q d	4–6 weeks	
		Sulfadiazine	100 mg/kg po q 6h	4–6 weeks	Pyrimethamine plus clindamycin 300–450 mg po q d
		Pyrimethamine (maintenance)	25 mg po q d	lifelong	
Fungal infections	Candidiasis Oropharyngeal	Clotrimazole troche	6 × daily (q 4 h)	7–14 d	Nystatin 100,000 U q 4 h
	Esophageal	Fluconazole	200 mg po	loading	Ketoconazole 200–400 mg q d
		Fluconazole	100–200 mg po q d	3 weeks	Fluconazole 400 mg IV q d for 14 d after last positive blood culture
	Candidemia	Amphotericin B	0.5–1.0 mg IV q d	Total dose 1 gram	Fluconazole 400 mg IV q d
	Invasive Candidiasis	Amphotericin B	0.5–1.0 mg IV q d	Total dose 1 gram	
	Histoplasmosis	Amphotericin B	0.5–1.0 mg IV q d	Total dose 1 gram	Itraconzole 300 mg po bid for 3 d for 12 w
		Itraconazole	200 mg po bid	lifelong	Amphotericin B biweekly
Intestinal infections	Cryptosporidium	No proven therapy			
	Giardia lamblia	Metronidazole	750 mg po q d	5 d	Albendazole 400 mg po q d for 5 d
	Entamoeba histolytica	Metronidazole (initial)	750 mg IV/po q 8 h	10 d	
		Iodoquinol	1.95 g po q 8 h	20 d	

host. The chest radiograph may reveal a lobar or segmental consolidation. Altered B-lymphocyte activation and neutrophil dysfunction predispose HIV-infected patients to infection with encapsulated organisms. Community-acquired pneumonia in HIV-infected individuals is usually due to *Strep. pneumoniae, H. influenzae B, Staph. aureus,* and gram-negative bacilli. The latter organisms are often the cause of nosocomial pneumonias. HIV-infected patients have a sixfold increase in the incidence of pneumococcal pneumonia and a 100-fold increase in pneumococcal bacteremia as compared with non-HIV-infected hosts. Treatment consists of parenteral antibiotics directed against the offending organism.

OTHER CAUSES OF RESPIRATORY DISTRESS IN THE ICU

Active pulmonary tuberculosis may develop at any time during the course of HIV infection, causing disease in 5 percent of AIDS patients. The risk of reactivation in HIV-infected patients with a positive purified protein derivative (PPD) test occurs at a rate of about 7 to 10 percent per year, comparable to the lifetime risk of a PPD-positive immune-competent host. Most active cases of pneumonia due to *M. tuberculosis* (MTB) are from reactivation of a latent infection, which underscores the importance of chemoprophylaxis in high-risk patients. HIV progresses more rapidly in patients with tuberculosis. The classic symptoms of fevers, night sweats, and weight loss overlap with the symptoms of moderately advanced AIDS. Therefore, a high index of suspicion is required in order to establish an early diagnosis. Early in the course of infection, when the CD4+ cell count is preserved, there may be apical infiltrates and cavitary disease. As the HIV infection progresses, however, reactivated tuberculosis may appear radiographically like a primary infection, as evidenced by mediastinal and hilar adenopathy, pleural effusions, mid–low zone infiltrates, or a miliary pattern. Notably, as many as 25 percent of cases of tuberculosis are complicated by coexistent PCP. Therapy for tuberculosis and other opportunistic infections is outlined in Table 37-3.

Mycobacterium avium-intracellulare (MAC) is a ubiquitous organism found in water and soil. The organism is thought to enter the host via the gastrointestinal and respiratory tracts. Typically, disseminated infection occurs when the CD4+ cell count falls below $50/\mu L$. HIV-infected patients presenting with fevers, night sweats, weight loss, and an elevated alkaline phosphatase should be evaluated for MAC. The acid-fast bacilli (AFB) are identified in the blood (85 percent), bone marrow, lymph nodes, and liver. A minority of patients will have an abnormal chest radiograph, which may reveal bilateral lower-lobe interstitial infiltrates, alveolar or nodular infiltrates, and hilar and mediastinal adenopathy. The diagnosis of pulmonary MAC infection relies on the demonstration of two positive sputums or one positive BAL for AFB and subsequent positive culture for MAC.

Cytomegalovirus (CMV) pneumonitis in the setting of HIV infection is a challenging diagnosis to establish. It requires hypoxemia, diffuse interstitial infiltrates, and evidence of cytopathic lung tissue involvement. The significance of finding CMV in the BAL without cytopathic changes remains controversial. Additionally, other causes of pneumonitis must be excluded in order to conclude that the pneumonia is secondary to CMV. Although previous studies have suggested that CMV pneumonitis is rare, recent autopsy studies show that one-third to one-half of AIDS patients dying from respiratory failure had CMV pneumonitis. Unfortunately, CMV penumonia responds poorly to antiviral treatment (ganciclovir, foscarnet, and immunoglobulin).

Kaposi sarcoma (KS) involves the lungs in up to 25 percent of patients with mucocutaneous disease and uncommonly involves the lungs in the absence of skin and mucous membrane disease. Patients may present with symptoms of respiratory tract infection, including fever, nonproductive cough, progressive dyspnea, wheezing, hoarseness, and hemoptysis. The chest radiograph usually shows nodular densities around the hilum, with varying degrees of interstitial nodular infiltrates. Computed tomography (CT) of the chest reveals grape-like clusters along the bronchovascular bundles. Lymphadenopathy and pleural effusions are common. The diagnosis can be made bronchoscopically with visualization of red-violaceous lesions in the endobronchial mucosa. Biopsy is rarely required to confirm the diagnosis. Unfortunately, curative therapy for KS does not exist. It should be noted, however, that patients are more likely to die from infection-induced respiratory failure than from this indolent malignancy. It is true, however, that respiratory failure as a result of pulmonary KS portends a poor prognosis. In this setting, palliative care is the appropriate treatment.

Neurologic Disease

The neurologic diseases that occur in the AIDS patient may be primary to the HIV process or secondary to opportunistic infections and neoplasms.

MENINGITIS

As outlined in Table 37-4, meningitis in HIV-infected individuals may be due to several etiologic agents. The clinical presentation and cerebrospinal fluid (CSF) analysis will often lead to a definitive diagnosis.

Cryptococcal meningitis is the most common cause of meningitis in patients with AIDS. This yeast-like fungus causes serious disease in advanced HIV infection when the CD4+ cell count is less than $100/\mu L$. Patients may experience symptoms of fever, nausea and vomiting, mental status changes, headaches, and meningeal signs for weeks to months prior to diagnosis. Frequently patients have complaints of dyspnea, cough, and hemoptysis. A high index of suspicion is necessary in order to diagnose the infection early. There may be an infiltrate on the chest radiograph as well as cavities, effusions, and hilar adenopathy. With an India ink stain, the CSF may reveal the organism. A positive CSF culture is an indication for treatment.

Aseptic meningitis may occur at any time during the course of HIV disease from the human immunodeficiency virus itself. It may be part of the acute seroconversion syndrome or can occur later in the disease. The patient may have headache, meningismus, fever, and cranial neuropathies. The syndrome is usually limited to 2 to 3 weeks but may become a chronic condition.

Fortunately, bacterial meningitis is uncommon in the AIDS patient. The presentation of fevers, mental status changes, and meningismus is similar to that in the immune-competent patient. Treatment requires parenteral antibiotics that cross the blood-brain barrier.

TABLE 37-4 HIV and Meningitis

Agent	Clinical Clues	CSF Findings
Cryptococcus	Cranial nerve palsies Skin lesions Respiratory abnormalities	WBC < 20/μL Glucose and protein normal Cryptococcus antigen positive (> 90 percent) India ink stain positive (50–90 percent)
Aseptic (HIV)	Cranial nerve palsies Acute seroconversion or late HIV manifestation	Mild mononuclear pleocytosis Elevated protein, normal glucose DD; syphilis & lymphomatous meningitis
M. tuberculosis	Subacute/chronic Focal deficits Extrameningeal infections	Lymphocytic pleocytosis Elevated protein, low glucose AFB smear unreliable, consider PCR
Coccidioides	Recent travel to southwestern United States	Lymphocytic pleocytosis usually > 50/μL Elevated protein, low glucose Any positive CSF titer is diagnostic
Bacterial	Rare in HIV-infected patients	Polymorphonuclear pleocytosis Elevated protein, low glucose Gram stain and bacterial antigens may or may not be positive.
Neurosyphilis	Prodromal headache/mental status changes weeks–months Optic neuritis Focal neurologic deficits Positive serum VDRL	Mononuclear pleocytosis Elevated protein, VDRL may or may not be positive

FOCAL NEUROLOGIC DISEASE

Toxoplasma gondii is the etiologic agent causing toxoplasmosis, a protozoal infection that generally occurs asymptomatically early in life. In patients with CD4+ cell counts less than $100/\mu L$, toxoplasmosis may reactivate to cause central nervous system (CNS) and pulmonary infections. Patients who have antibodies to *T. gondii* are 10 times more likely to develop full-blown toxoplasmosis than are seronegative individuals. HIV-infected patients without antibodies to *T. gondii* are still at risk, albeit small, of developing toxoplasmosis. The most common presentation is fever, headache, and focal neurologic deficits. The patient may experience seizure, hemiparesis, and aphasia. The cerebral edema caused by the space-occupying lesions may cause a diffuse encephalopathy consisting of confusion, dementia, lethargy, stupor, and coma. Magnetic resonance imaging (MRI) or CT of the brain may reveal single or multiple ring-enhancing lesions with surrounding edema. There is a predilection for the basal ganglia, cortex, and thalamus. A definitive diagnosis requires a brain biopsy. Given the morbidity associated with this procedure, many physicians opt to treat empirically with antitoxoplasmosis antibiotics for 2 to 4 weeks. If, at the end of this time period, the imaging study fails to show resolution of the mass lesions, a brain biopsy is indicated in order to establish the correct diagnosis.

The main competing diagnosis with CNS toxoplasmosis is primary CNS lymphoma, which tends to occur in the later stages of HIV disease. Primary CNS lymphomas are usually positive for the Epstein-Barr virus. Treatment is palliative and may include radiation and glucocorticoids. The prognosis is poor, with a median survival of 2 to 4 months.

Mycobacterium tuberculosis may also present as a space-occupying lesion. Treatment is the same as for active pulmonary tuberculosis.

Additional Fungal Infections

Candidal infections, for the most part, are limited to the mucous membranes in the HIV-infected host. Deep candidal infections such as endophthalmitis, vertebral osteomyelitis, or disseminated candidiasis generally occur when additional risk factors for invasive candidemia coexist with the HIV infection. These risk factors include neutropenia, prolonged vascular catheterization, broad-spectrum antibiotic use, intravenous drug use, and recent gastrointestinal or cardiac surgery. In addition to antifungal therapy, infected indwelling catheters should be removed. In patients with granulocytopenia, consideration should be given to adding a neutrophil colony-stimulating factor.

Histoplasma capsulatum is a fungus endemic to the Mississippi and Ohio River valleys, Puerto Rico, the Dominican Republic, and South America. The organism exists in the mycelial phase in soil and is found in areas that contain bat and bird droppings. At body temperature, the fungus is found in its yeast form. Histoplasmosis may present as a primary lung infection. As the immune system deteriorates in the HIV-infected patient, reactivation from a latent to a disseminated form of disease may occur. Disseminated histoplasmosis is a marker of advanced HIV disease. Clinically, the patient may have fevers, weight loss, and fatigue lasting for 1 to 2 months prior to diagnosis. The physical examination may reveal lymphadenopathy and hepatosplenomegaly. Bone marrow infection may cause pancytopenia. About 15 percent of patients develop CNS involvement. Few patients have evidence of mucocutaneous disease. Although respiratory symptoms are usually minimal, the chest radiograph is abnormal in half of the infected patients. It may reveal diffuse interstitial infiltrates, small nodules, and lymphadenopathy. Culture of the organism from blood, bone marrow, BAL, or tissue establishes the diagnosis. The fungal polysaccharide antigen may be detectable and quantifiable in blood and urine; however, this test is not readily available commercially.

Gastrointestinal Infections

The most common gastrointestinal (GI) manifestations in the HIV-infected patient are diarrhea (50 percent), malnutrition, and weight loss. GI disorders are rarely the cause of the ICU admission but are frequently present. Patients are at risk for both opportunistic disease and non-HIV-related disorders. Table 37-5 outlines some of the AIDS-related GI disorders

TABLE 37-5   Gastrointestinal Disorders Associated with HIV Infection

Esophageal disorders	*Stomach*	*Hepatobiliary disease*	*Pancreatitis*
Candidiasis	Kaposi's sarcoma	Cryptosporidium	Drug toxicity
HSV	Lymphomas	CMV	(Pentamidine/ddI/ddc)
CMV	Peptic ulcer disease	Kaposi's sarcoma	CMV
Kaposi's sarcoma		Hepatitis virus	MAC
Lymphoma		Mycobacterial	Subclinical
Gastroesophageal reflux		Fungal	hyperamylasemia
disease			
Enteritis	*Colitis*	*Rectal/Anal lesions*	
HIV enteropathy	MAC	HSV	
Cryptosporidium	CMV	Condyloma accuminatum	
Microsporidium	Shigella	Kaposi's sarcoma	
Giardia lamblia	Campylobacter	Intraepithelial neoplasia	
Isospora belli	Entamoeba histolytica	Neisseria gonorrhea	
Salmonella	Clostridium difficile	Chlamydia trachomatis	
Aeromonas hydrophilia	Vibrio parahaemolyticus	Treponema pallidum	
Clostridium perfringens	Plesiomonas shigelloides		

478

along with some of the common etiologies. A careful search for the cause of diarrhea will reveal a diagnosis in 80 percent of patients (Fig. 37-2). HIV-related enteropathy is the likely cause in patients with diarrhea lasting over 1 month without an identifiable source. The treatment of severe diarrhea includes bowel rest, intravenous fluids, electrolyte replacement, and occasionally antimicrobial therapy. If the diarrhea is severe, the patient may require parenteral nutrition. When bacterial organisms are suspected or diagnosed, the use of antimotility agents is discouraged owing to the increased risk of precipitating toxic megacolon.

Hypotension

In HIV-infected individuals, sepsis, hypovolemia, adrenal insufficiency, adverse drug reactions, and autonomic neuropathy may cause hypotension. Although any organism can cause sepsis, it is most commonly due to bacterial and fungal infection. The clinical approach and management include aggressive intravascular volume repletion, antimicrobial therapy, and possibly vasopressor support.

Summary and Conclusions

The understanding and treatment of HIV infection is an evolving science. From the beginning of the AIDS epidemic in the 1980s, there have been dramatic changes in the outcome of some opportunistic diseases. With the addition of aggressive chemoprophylaxis, antiretroviral therapy, and a better understanding of opportunistic infections, survival and quality of life have improved. In fact, HIV, when aggressively treated, is arguably a chronic disease. Many patients will benefit from intensive care, while survival in others is unlikely to be prolonged. For example, mechanical ventilation of a patient with pulmonary KS is not likely to be of benefit in the absence of a cure for KS. On the other hand, aggressive treatment of PCP may result in a quality of life that is identical to that which the patient had prior to the ICU admission. Therefore, rigid guidelines regarding appropriate admissions to the ICU of HIV-infected patients are discouraged. Clearly, the

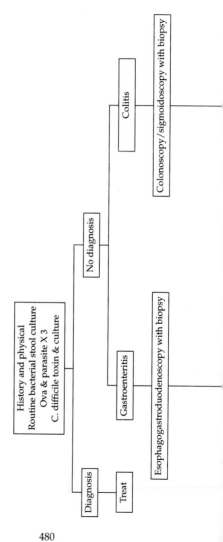

History and physical
Routine bacterial stool culture
Ova & parasite X 3
C. difficile toxin & culture

Diagnosis

No diagnosis

Treat

Gastroenteritis

Colitis

Esophagogastroduodenoscopy with biopsy

Colonoscopy/sigmoidoscopy with biopsy

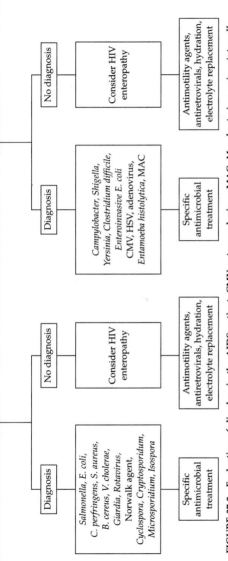

FIGURE 37-2 Evaluation of diarrhea in the AIDS patient. CMV, cytomegalovirus; MAC, *Mycobacterium avium-intracellulare*; VZV, varicella zoster virus; HSV, herpes simplex virus.

outcome of intensive care differs based on the stage of AIDS, multiple organ involvement, and the cause of the acute decompensation in health status.

Finally, it is imperative to involve the patient or the patient's surrogate in discussions regarding intensive care treatment and life support. It is the physician's responsibility to inform the patient of prognostic issues and guide him or her in the decision to receive intensive care or palliative therapy.

For a more detailed discussion, see Chaps. 43 and 44 in *Principles of Critical Care*, 2d ed.

Chapter 38

INFECTIOUS COMPLICATIONS OF INTRAVASCULAR ACCESS DEVICES

WILLIAM M. SANDERS

As progress in critical care has advanced, the number and variety of intravascular devices have multiplied. These include peripheral intravenous catheters, multilumen central venous lines, pulmonary artery catheters, totally implantable devices, and semipermanent central venous access devices such as Hickman, Broviac, and Quinton catheters. While these devices are extremely useful, they are associated with a number of complications including thrombosis, thrombophlebitis, and infection. Bacteremia associated with intravascular devices engenders significant morbidity, increasing mean length of hospitalization by 10 days. The mortality of catheter-related bacteremia is estimated to be 10 to 20 percent.

Risk Factors and Incidence of Infection

The risk factors for development of device-associated infection include those related to the device and those related to the host. Host-related risk factors for the development of catheter-associated infection include age (> 60 years or < 1 year), loss of skin integrity, immunocompromise, distant focus of infection, presence of tracheostomy, and severity of illness. Device-related risk factors include type of the device material as well as the type of the device. Steel, polyurethane, Teflon, and silicone are more resistant to bacterial adherence than polyethylene and polyvinyl chloride. Increased thrombogenicity of some catheter materials leads to increased bacterial colonization. Antibiotic- or antiseptic-coated catheters can reduce the risk of bacterial colonization.

Peripheral venous catheters are generally associated with a low risk of bacteremia, less than 0.2 percent. The type of material, whether polyethylene, Teflon, or steel, has little influence on the incidence of bacteremia associated with these devices. Because of the widespread use of peripheral venous catheters, local complications, including cellulitis and thrombophlebitis, are common.

Peripheral arterial catheters are associated with bacteremia with an incidence of about 1 percent, while significant colonization occurs in about 5 percent. Higher rates of colonization occur if there is catheterization by cutdown, inflammation at the site, or the catheter is in place longer than 4 days.

Studies of bacteremia associated with uncuffed central venous catheters placed in the subclavian or internal jugular site show the incidence to be between 1 and 5 percent and the rate of significant colonization to be between 5 and 30 percent. The rate of catheter-associated bacteremia from pulmonary artery catheters is similar to the rate of bacteremia from central venous catheters. Peripherally inserted central catheters (PICC) are associated with bacteremia with an incidence of 1 to 2 percent.

The circumstances of the catheter placement play an important role in the risk of subsequent infection. Catheters placed by cutdown are more likely to become infected than those placed percutaneously. Emergent placement of a catheter substantially increases its risk of causing infection. Jugular venous catheters are more likely to cause infection than those placed in the subclavian vein. Finally, the longer a catheter stays in place, the more likely it will become infected. When a central line or pulmonary artery catheter is left in place for 4 days or longer, the risk of infection rises significantly.

Aseptic technique at the time of insertion and during access of the intravascular device is important in reducing the risk of infection. Aseptic technique should include maximal barrier precautions—mask, sterile gown and gloves, and a large sterile drape. Chlorhexidine skin preparations may reduce infection rates more effectively than topical povidone or 70 percent alcohol. There is evidence that greater operator skill in vascular puncture and fewer attempts at cannulation are also associated with fewer infectious complications. Dressing central venous catheters with gauze rather than transparent impermeable dressings, and using topical antimicrobial ointment can decrease infection rates. Finally, minimizing the frequency of access into the device can decrease the chances of subsequent colonization.

Clinical Diagnosis

Catheter-related infection is often suspected when a patient manifests fever without another apparent source of infection. Other clinical signs of catheter-related infection include erythema, warmth, and tenderness at the catheter site, but these are present in only about 50 percent of cases. Purulent drainage sometimes can be expressed and cultured to look for a predominant organism. A clinical syndrome of sepsis refractory to antibiotic treatment should also alert clinicians to the possibility of catheter-related infection. Often the diagnosis is established only by recognizing improvement in a febrile syndrome after the catheter is removed.

Laboratory Diagnosis

The diagnosis of catheter-related infection is probable when a positive blood culture is found in a patient with no other source of bacteremia. Any blood culture positive for an organism commonly associated with catheter infections (especially *Streptococcus aureus* or *Candida* species) should raise concern for catheter infection. The diagnosis is more definite when a culture from the catheter exit site demonstrates an identical organism (both species and antibiogram). Also, cultures of the subcutaneous portion of a catheter can be performed using a "roll-plate" technique and usually defines significant colonization as ≥ 15 colony-forming units. Another useful diagnostic tool is to perform differential quantitative cultures on blood drawn peripherally and through the catheter. A ≥ 10-fold larger colony count in the culture from the catheter establishes the diagnosis. Cultures of catheter tips in broth are sensitive but prone to contamination and probably should not be done.

Pathophysiology

Infection of an intravascular device most commonly occurs when endogenous microorganisms colonize the catheter insertion site and migrate along the subcutaneous tract to the catheter tip. Some infections may also occur through colonization of the catheter hub during manipulation and entry into the tubing system. The bacteria then migrate down the lumen of the catheter to the tip. The fibrin sheath that forms around the tip of the catheter then becomes a reservoir of bacteria that is partially protected from the body's immune mechanisms and is a nidus for recurrent bacteremia. The presence of visible clot at the catheter tip further increases the likelihood of bacterial colonization. Hematogenous seeding of the catheter tip with bacteria from a distant site of infection is another possible mechanism of colonization.

Contamination of intravenous medications during manufacture is a rare cause of infection. Intravenous medications more commonly become contaminated during manipulation by medical personnel. Some hypertonic solutions and especially lipid emulsions support the growth of microorganisms. Regular replacement of administration sets and infusates can avoid such contamination.

Microbiology

Coagulase negative staphylococcus—especially *S. epidermidis* and *S. aureus*—account for more than 50 percent of catheter-related infections. Enteric gram-negative organisms and yeast, especially *Candida albicans*, are the next most likely pathogens. Other less common pathogens include *Pseudomonas* species, *Corynebacterium jeikeium* and *Malassezia furfur.*

Treatment

Local infections can usually be treated with removal of the line, local care, and topical antibiotics. Extension of cellulitis along the catheter tract is a definite indication for line removal and systemic antibiotics. Bacteremic infections of short-term central venous catheters are best treated with removal of the catheter and systemic antibiotics. The catheter tip should be sent for culture. If the indication for the catheter still remains and the suspicion for catheter-related infection is low, the catheter can be replaced over a wire and the old catheter sent for culture. If the catheter culture is positive, the replacement catheter should be removed and a new site chosen.

Bacteremic infections of cuffed long-term indwelling catheters and tunneled or totally implanted devices can sometimes be treated without removal of the device. Indications for removal of the device include local purulence, cellulitis, septic thrombophlebitis, tricuspid valve endocarditis, or persistent bacteremia. Bacteremia due to *Staph. aureus* should be treated with removal of the device because of the higher rate of recurrent bacteremia and sepsis-related mortality.

Antibiotics should be chosen to cover the organisms identified by culture and sensitivity testing. Empiric antibiotics should include an antistaphylococcal penicillin and an aminoglycoside or a third-generation cephalosporin to cover most gram-positive and gram-negative bacteria. When the pathogen is identified, antibiotic therapy can be specifically targeted. Most line infections should be treated for 5 to 10 days. Treatment of *Staph. aureus* infections should be continued for 14 days to prevent metastatic complications. If methicillin-resistant *Staph. aureus* is prevalent, vancomycin should be used initially. *Candida* species can be treated with a short course of amphotericin B (3 to 7 mg/kg total), or fluconazole (200 to 400 mg/day for 7 to 10 days). Patients with *Candida* bacteremia should be evaluated for metastatic infection including endophthalmitis, which would necessitate a longer course of treatment.

Prevention

The first step in preventing catheter-associated infection is to remove any unnecessary devices. It is helpful to keep track of the date of insertion of all devices. The medical team should perform a daily assessment of the need for the device as well as inspection of the site for evidence of local inflammation. Careful aseptic technique should be observed during insertion as well as when accessing the device. Placement of devices by skilled operators will reduce the likelihood of infection; minimizing the frequency of entry into the tubing system will decrease the chances of introducing bacteria. Appropriate sterile dressings should cover the insertion site and be replaced on a regular basis. In the future new techniques and microbe-resistant materials may aid in preventing catheter-associated infection.

For a more detailed discussion, see Chap. 46 in *Principles of Critical Care*, 2d ed.

Chapter 39

PNEUMONIA

BRIAN GEHLBACH

Pneumonia is the most common infection leading to intensive care unit (ICU) admission as well as the most important nosocomial infection complicating the course of patients admitted to the ICU for other problems. Herein we discuss the diagnosis and management of five broad categories of pneumonia: community-acquired pneumonia, aspiration pneumonia, chronic pneumonia, nosocomial pneumonia, and pulmonary infiltrates in the immunocompromised host. The problem of ventilator-associated pneumonia is particularly relevant to the intensive care setting and receives special attention.

Pathogenesis

Organisms may enter the lung through *aspiration* of oropharyngeal or gastric contents, *inhalation* of organism-containing particles or aerosols, or *hematogenous dissemination* from another site.

Aspiration is by far the most common of these mechanisms in causing pneumonia. The upper airway is frequently colonized by *Streptococcus pneumoniae, Haemophilus influenzae, Staphylococcus aureus,* and mixed aerobic and anaerobic bacteria. Enteric gram-negative organisms such as *Klebsiella pneumoniae* are found much less frequently and are often associated with alcohol abuse, institutionalization, or poor oral hygiene. Pneumonia occurs when an inoculum of pathogenic microbes invades the normally sterile lower respiratory tract. Physical barriers to infection include the glottis, tracheobronchial secretions, the mucociliary tree, and the cough reflex. Humoral defenses include alveolar macrophages and polymorphonuclear neutrophils. Defects in host defenses or the introduction of numerous or highly virulent microbes promotes the development of pneumonia.

Since inhalation results in small numbers of organisms reaching the lung, only highly efficient pathogens are capable of producing infection in this manner. These pathogens include *Legionella, Mycoplasma pneumonia, Chlamydia* spp., *Coxiella burnetti, Mycobacterium tuberculosis,* most respiratory viruses, and most endemic fungal pneumonias.

Hematogenous spread of infection to the lung occurs when the venous circulation deposits organisms in the pulmonary microvasculature. These infections tend to be multifocal and nodular. Pneumonia may occur in the context of previously established infection elsewhere or by direct inoculation of the bloodstream, as occurs in injection drug users. *Staph. aureus* and gram-negative bacilli are the most common pathogens. Rarely, pneumonia occurs when a highly virulent organism gains entry to the bloodstream through the skin and is spread to the lung hematogenously; tularemia, brucellosis, and melioidosis are examples.

Community-Acquired Pneumonia

ACUTE BACTERIAL PNEUMONIA

The patient with acute bacterial pneumonia classically presents with the acute onset of fever or chills, cough, sputum production, and dyspnea. Pleuritic chest pain may also be present. The elderly or debilitated may present more subtly—for example, with confusion or breathlessness only. Physical examination usually reveals an uncomfortable patient with fever, tachycardia, and tachypnea. Crackles are heard over the site of infection, and signs of consolidation (bronchial breath sounds, egophony, and dullness to percussion) may be present. Splinting or chest wall tenderness indicate pleural inflammation. The chest film usually demonstrates consolidation in a lobar or bronchopneumonic pattern. The WBC count is generally elevated, with a predominance of immature forms; normal or suppressed counts may be found in the immunosuppressed or critically ill patient. The majority of severe acute bacterial pneumonia syndromes are caused by *Strep. pneumoniae, H. influenzae, Staph. aureus,* and the Enterobacteriaceae (Table 39-1).

TABLE 39-1   Infectious Etiologic Agents Implicated in Severe Community-Acquired Pneumonia Requiring Intensive Care Support[a]

Etiologic Agent	Percent of Cases Admitted
Acute bacterial pneumonia	65
Streptococcus pneumoniae	40
Haemophilus influenzae	5
Staphylococcus aureus	10
Enterobacteriaceae	10
Atypical pneumonia	20
Legionella pneumophila	10
Mycoplasma pneumoniae	5
Chlamydia psittaci	2
Coxiella burnetii	1
Viral	2
Aspiration pneumonia/lung abscess	10
Chronic pneumonia syndrome	5
Mycobacterium tuberculosis	3
Endemic dimorphic fungi	2

[a]The percentages shown are approximate only, based on published studies from different geographic locations and population bases. Because these percentages represent cases requiring hospital admission and ICU care, pneumonias that more commonly cause severe illness or which occur more commonly in patients with significant underlying disease (*Staph. aureus,* enteric gram-negative bacilli, *Legionella* spp., etc.) are overrepresented compared to unselected community-acquired pneumonia. Also note that most published series include 20–50% for which no etiologic diagnosis was made and which are not included in this table.

The initial evaluation of patients presenting with severe community-acquired pneumonia should include two sets of blood cultures and analysis of sputum with Gram stain and culture. While a positive blood culture for a typical lung pathogen is diagnostic, the results of sputum analysis should be interpreted with caution. In particular, the clinician should be wary of limiting empiric therapy for patients with life-threatening pneumonia based on sputum analysis, as the negative predictive value of this test is poor. The frequent colonization of upper airways with organisms such as *Strep.*

pneumoniae and *Staph. aureus* ensures their frequent isolation in sputum, even in patients with pneumonia caused by other organisms. Sputum analysis is of greater value if there are more than 25 polymorphonuclear cells and fewer than 10 epithelial cells per high-power field. Also, the Gram stain should be given more weight than the culture.

Bronchoscopy is not indicated in the routine evaluation of patients with severe community-acquired pneumonia. Indications for bronchoscopy include (1) lack of response to empiric therapy, (2) unexplained deterioration following initial improvement, and (3) suspicion of a noninfectious cause of pneumonitis (e.g., lupus pneumonitis).

Atypical Pneumonia

The term *atypical pneumonia* was originally applied to the clinical syndrome resulting from *Mycoplasma pneumoniae* infection. This particular infection is characterized by prodromal upper respiratory symptoms followed by the development of low-grade fever and nonproductive cough. Extrapulmonary symptoms such as arthralgias, diarrhea, and skin rash are common. The chest radiograph reveals a unilateral segmental infiltrate or patchy bilateral interstitial infiltrates. Although hospital admission is rarely necessary, intensive care is occasionally required for the complications of respiratory failure, encephalomyelitis, or myocarditis. Diagnosis of mycoplasmal pneumonia is made by serology.

Several other pulmonary infections are commonly categorized as causes of the atypical pneumonia syndrome (Table 39-2). Chief of these in prevalence are infections by viruses and *Legionella pneumophila*. Legionella infection occurs more commonly in those patients exposed to aerosols generated by cooling systems or from sites of soil excavation and in those with underlying lung disease, renal failure, or other immunocompromised states. Although prominent gastrointestinal symptoms or dry cough may suggest legionnaire's disease, presentation may also be similar to that of pneumococcal pneumonia. Both rounded airspace consolidation and patchy infiltrates are commonly seen on chest film. Patients requiring ICU care may present fulminantly, with rapidly progressive pulmonary infiltrates and severe hypoxemia.

TABLE 39-2   Atypical Pneumonia: Infectious Agents That
May Produce Severe Pneumonia with an Atypical
(Nonbacterial) Clinical Presentation

Mycoplasma pneumoniae
Legionella pneumophila
Chlamydia psittaci
Coxiella burnetii
Viral pneumonia (influenza A and B, varicella zoster, RSV, CMV,
  EBV, adenovirus)
Francisella tularensis
Pneumocystis carinii

Influenza A and B are the major viral causes of pneumonia requiring ICU care. Severe influenza occurs in the winter
or early spring and most often afflicts the unvaccinated elderly or institutionalized, particularly those with debilitating
chronic illnesses. The patient initially experiences fever,
malaise, myalgias, headache, sore throat, and harsh cough
with retrosternal chest pain. Dyspnea may be accompanied
by wheezing and cyanosis. The chest film typically shows bilateral interstitial infiltrates. Influenza infection may be complicated by subsequent bacterial infection, with *Staph. aureus*
as the commonest culprit.

Although different from each other in important ways, the
infections that cause the atypical pneumonia syndrome share
several key features: (1) epidemiologic clues suggestive of an
atypical pneumonia pathogen are present, (2) extrapulmonary
manifestations are common, (3) the diagnosis is made primarily serologically, and (4) beta-lactams are ineffective. In
clinical practice, there is considerable overlap between the
acute bacterial pneumonia and atypical pneumonia syndromes, and decision making based on stereotypical presentations alone without regard to epidemiologic factors should
be avoided. Before the causative organism has been identified,
initial therapy for the critically ill patient should be broad.
Suggested empiric regimens are detailed in Table 39-3. Once
an organism has been isolated, more specific therapy may be
applied and unnecessary drugs discontinued. The treatment
of specific organisms is outlined in Table 39-4. Local patterns
of drug resistance may require alternative therapies.

TABLE 39-3 Empiric Antimicrobial Therapy for Critically Ill Patients with Acute Community-Acquired Pneumonia[a]

Clinical Setting	Recommended Antimicrobial Therapy	Alternative Agents
Acute bacterial pneumonia syndrome (including patients with COPD or alcohol abuse)	Cefuroxime 1.5 g IV q8h	Third-generation cephalosporin, co-trimoxazole IV
Institutionalized elderly	Cefotaxime 2 g IV q6h	Imipenem, piperacillin/tazobactam, co-trimoxazole IV
Atypical pneumonia Suspected	*Add to above:* Erythromycin 1 g IV q6h	Ciprofloxacin
Anaerobic aspiration pneumonia/lung abscess	Penicillin G 2 million U IV q4h and metronidazole 750 mg IV q8h	Clindamycin, imipenem, chloramphenicol
Fulminant pneumonia	Cefotaxime 2 g IV q6h and gentamicin 4.5 mg/kg q24h and erythromicin 1 g IV q6h	Piperacillin/tazobactam or imipenem *and* erythromycin

[a]Note that dosages cited are for patients with normal renal function; dosage adjustment for renal insufficiency is required for several of these agents. Monitoring of blood levels is strongly advised for aminoglycosides and chloramphenicol.

494

Aspiration Pneumonia

Frank aspiration of oropharyngeal or gastric contents may present in a number of different ways. Aspiration of large particles causes airway obstruction, which may lead to acute asphyxia or localized atelectasis or hyperinflation. Liquid or small-particle aspiration generally causes a chemical pneumonitis with rapidly resolving pulmonary infiltrates. Aspiration of large quantities of gastric acid is more serious, causing an acute chemical burn with dyspnea, bronchospasm, frothy pulmonary edema, and hypotension, the latter resulting from rapid exudation of intravascular fluid across the injured alveolar walls. Most episodes of aspiration do not require antibiotic therapy, as the number and pathogenecity of aspirated organisms are low. Those patients who do develop pneumonia following aspiration typically do so within a few days to 1 week following the event. A more serious syndrome of fulminant necrotizing pneumonia occurs in patients whose gastric contents have been contaminated with mixed enteric organisms, as occurs with bowel obstruction, adynamic ileus, or following upper abdominal surgery.

The evaluation of patients with suspected aspiration pneumonia is primarily clinical. Since most aspiration pneumonias occurring in the community are caused by normal oral flora, culture of these specimens will be reported as "normal flora." Thus, the diagnosis of aspiration pneumonia can generally be made when a patient at risk presents with a clinical syndrome consistent with aspiration and examination of expectorated sputum demonstrates only normal flora. Bronchoscopy is recommended when the diagnosis is uncertain, the patient fails to respond to empiric therapy, or suspicion exists for an endobronchial lesion—for example, in patients lacking known risk factors for aspiration pneumonia. Treatment of the critically ill patient consists of clindamycin or penicillin and metronidazole. Acute necrotizing pneumonia secondary to aspiration of feculent gastric contents is caused by aerobic gram-negative and anaerobic organisms. Acceptable regimens include piperacillin/tazobactam with gentamicin, clindamycin plus a third-generation cephalosporin, or imipenem with gentamicin. Note that aspiration pneumonia occurring in the hospitalized patient is associated with a broader range of potential pathogens and is discussed below.

TABLE 39-4 Antimicrobial Therapy for Acute Bacterial or Atypical Pneumonia of Known Etiology in Critically Ill Patients[a]

	Recommended Antimicrobial Therapy	Alternative Antimicrobial Agents
Streptococcus pneumoniae and other streptococci	Penicillin G 1 million U IV q4h	Cefazolin, clindamycin, or vancomycin
Staphylococcus aureus Methicillin-sensitive	Nafcillin 2 g IV q4h	Cefazolin, clindamycin, or vancomycin
Methicillin-resistant	Vancomycin 500 mg IV q6h	—
Haemophilus influenzae β lactamase–negative	Ampicillin 2 g IV q6h	Cefuroxime, co-trimoxazole
β lactamase–positive	Cefuroxime 1.5 g IV q8h	Co-trimoxazole, chloramphenicol
Moraxella catarrhalis	Cefuroxime 1.5 g IV q8h	Co-trimoxazole
Enterobacteriaceae (*Klebsiella, E. coli, Enterobacter* spp., etc.)	Cefotaxime 2 g IV q6h and gentamicin 4.5 mg/kg q24h	Piperacillin/Tazobactam or Imipenem, and gentamicin, co-trimoxazole, ciprofloxacin
Pseudomonas aeruginosa	Piperacillin 3 g IV q4h and tobramycin 4.5 mg/kg q24h	Imipenem or ceftazadime *and* tobramycin, ciprofloxacin +/− β lactam

Anaerobic pneumonia / lung abscess	Penicillin 2 million U IV q4h and metronidazole 750 mg IV q8h	Clindamycin, chloramphenicol
Legionella pneumophila	Erythromycin 1 g IV q6h and rifampin 600 mg IV daily	Ciprofloxacin or ofloxacin, co-trimoxazole and rifampin
Mycoplasma pneumoniae	Erythromycin 1 g IV q6h	Tetracycline
Chlamydia psittaci	Doxycycline 100 mg IV q12h	Erythromycin
Coxiella burnetii	Doxycycline 100 mg IV q12h	Erythromycin and rifampin
Yersinia pestis	Streptomycin 30 mg kg IM qd	Chloramphenicol, tetracycline
Francisella tularensis	Gentamicin 1.5 mg kg IV q8h	Chloramphenicol, tetracycline
Influenza A or RSV (severe with respiratory failure)	Ribavirin aerosol 1 g/day over 12–18 h	—
Varicella zoster	Acyclovir 10 mg/kg IV q8h	

[a]Note that all drug dosages cited are for patients with normal renal function; dosage adjustment for renal insufficiency is required for a number of the agents listed. Monitoring of blood drug levels is strongly advised for the aminoglycosides, vancomycin, and chloramphenicol.

Chronic Pneumonia

Chronic pneumonia is diagnosed when a patient experiences 3 weeks or more of persistent or progressive pulmonary symptoms associated with a radiographic infiltrate. The patient typically appears chronically ill, often with obvious constitutional symptoms such as fatigue and weight loss. Laboratory abnormalities may include anemia and hypoalbuminemia.

Table 39-5 lists some of the more frequently encountered causes of the chronic pneumonia syndrome. These disorders are relatively uncommonly encountered in the ICU because the chronically progressive symptoms generally cause the patient to seek medical attention long before intensive care is required. Those who do present to the ICU typically do so with respiratory failure and extensive bilateral infiltrates.

TABLE 39-5   Infectious and Noninfectious Etiologies of Chronic Pneumonia

---

Bacterial and mycobacterial infections
  Tuberculosis
  Chronic cavitary bacterial pneumonia (*Klebsiella pneumoniae,*
    Pseudomonas aeruginosa, others)
  Actinomycosis
  Nocardiosis
  Melioidosis
  Aspiration-induced anaerobic pneumonia and lung abscess
Fungal infections
  Blastomycosis
  Coccidiodomycosis
  Paracoccidiodomycosis
  Histoplasmosis
  Cryptococcosis
  Chronic necrotizing aspergillosis
Noninfectious causes
  Systemic vasculitides
  Malignancy
  Interstitial pneumonitis (fibrosing alveolitis) and other idio-
    pathic infiltrative pulmonary diseases)
  Bronchiolitis obliterans with organizing pneumonia (BOOP)
  Lymphomatoid granulomatosis
  Sarcoidosis
  Toxic exposure and drug reactions

Although classic radiographic patterns may suggest one diagnosis over another, the heterogeneity of radiographic manifestations in these disorders generally precludes definitive diagnosis. Evaluation of patients with chronic pneumonia begins with careful history taking, often from collateral sources. Sputum should be sampled repeatedly and sent for bacterial, mycobacterial, and fungal culture. Cytologic examination may also be helpful. Evaluation of extrapulmonary sites of involvement may be useful; for example, vasculitis or malignancy may be diagnosed through biopsy of involved skin or lymph nodes, respectively. Immunologically mediated diseases such as Wegener's granulomatosis and Goodpasture's syndrome may be diagnosed through antineutrophilic cytoplasmic antibodies (ANCA) and antiglomerular basement membrane antibodies respectively.

Lacking a definite diagnosis after initial testing, including examination of respiratory secretions and potentially involved extrapulmonary sites, most critically ill patients should proceed to open-lung biopsy, as the range of possible diagnoses is simply too great to attempt to manage the patient empirically. Treatment regimens for the most common fungal pneumonias are listed in Table 39-6.

Pulmonary Infiltrates in the Immunocompromised Host

Immunocompromised hosts are subject to a bewildering array of infections. The approach to diagnosis is simplified if the differential diagnosis is constructed based on the nature of the patient's immunodeficiency. The major categories of immunodeficiency are (1) deficient humoral immunity, (2) deficient phagocytic cell function, and (3) deficient cell-mediated immunity (see Table 39-7). Combined immunodeficiencies are also possible, as in patients receiving cytotoxic chemotherapy.

Additional clues to diagnosis come from the timing of the illness with respect to the onset and duration of immunosuppression. For example, patients who become granulocytopenic from cytotoxic chemotherapy are infected primarily with bacteria in the first 2 to 3 weeks following treatment. Similarly, a patient who develops diffuse pulmonary infiltrates 1 to

TABLE 39-6   Treatment Regimens for Fungal Pneumonia Associated with Critical Illness in the Nonimmunocompromised Host

Etiologic Agent	Recommended Antimicrobial Therapy
Blastomyces dermatitidis	Amphotericin B 0.5–0.8 mg/kg IV qd to total dose of 2–2.5 g
Histoplasma capsulatum	As above
Coccidioides immitis (without CNS involvement)	Amphotericin B 0.5–0.8 mg/kg IV qd to total dose of 3–4 g
Cryptococcus neoformans	Amphotericin B 0.3–0.5 mg/kg IV qd and flucytosine 150 mg/kg daily in four divided doses for 6 weeks

3 months after organ transplantation should be evaluated for cytomegalovirus (CMV) infection, which is highly prevalent during this time period. AIDS-related illnesses such as *Pneumocystis carinii* pneumonia (PCP) and pneumonia due to *Mycobacterium avium-intracellulare* are associated with threshold levels of cell-mediated immunity as measured by CD4+ cell counts.

The history and physical examination should be comprehensive; extrapulmonary manifestations may suggest the diagnosis. Disseminated *Aspergillus* infection may produce necrotic skin lesions, while ecthyma gangrenosum is associated with bacteremia, particularly from *Pseudomonas*. While the chest film seldom establishes the diagnosis, certain patterns may be helpful in context. Localized infiltrates are generally caused by inhaled or aspirated pathogens, as occurs in bacterial or fungal pneumonia. Diffuse infiltrates are caused by pathogens that either reach the lung hematogenously in large numbers or have spread rapidly along the respiratory mucosa early in the course of the illness, such as that due to CMV or PCP. Noninfectious causes of pulmonary infiltrates are numerous and are listed in Table 39-8.

Initial investigations should include blood cultures and Gram stain and culture of respiratory specimens. Selected patients should undergo culture of blood for CMV or examination of sputum for acid-fast bacilli and fungi. Pleural fluid

TABLE 39-7   The More Common Opportunistic Pulmonary Infections of the Immunocompromised Host[a]

Immunodeficiency	Predominant Pulmonary Infections	Most Frequent Clinical Setting
Humoral immunodeficiency	Pyogenic bacterial pneumonias	Hypogammaglobulinemia Chronic lymphocytic leukemia Multiple myeloma
Phagocytic cell deficiency	Bacterial pneumonia Fungal pneumonias Aspergillosis Candidemia with pulmonary involvement Cryptococcosis	Chemotherapy-induced granulocytopenia Acute myelogenous leukemia
Cell-mediated immunodeficiency	*Pneumocystis carinii* pneumonia Legionellosis Nocardiosis CMV pneumonia Cryptococcosis Mycobacteriosis	Lymphoma or acute lymphocytic leukemia undergoing chemotherapy High-dose corticosteroid therapy Organ transplantation AIDS

[a]Note that these categories are not mutually exclusive. Bone marrow transplant recipients, for example, suffer mainly from bacterial and fungal infections associated with phagocytic cell deficits early after transplant; but after marrow recovery these patients mainly develop infections related to chronic suppression of cell-mediated immunity.

TABLE 39-8   Noninfectious Causes of Pulmonary
Infiltrates in the Immunocompromised Host and the
Clinical Settings in Which They Are Most Frequently Seen

Noninfectious Diagnosis	Clinical Settings
Diffuse pulmonary infiltrates	
Interstitial pneumonitis due to cytotoxic drug therapy	Bleomycin (> 150 mg total) or non-dose-related reaction to bleomycin, cyclophosphamide, methotrexate, and others
Cardiogenic pulmonary edema	Preexisting cardiac disease Chemotherapy with daunorubicin or doxorubicin
Lymphangitic carcinomatosis	Carcinoma poorly responsive to therapy
Leukemic infiltration of lung	Uncontrolled acute leukemia
Acute low-pressure pulmonary edema (diffuse alveolar damage)	Leukemic cell lysis after chemotherapy Leukoagglutination reaction following transfusion
Focal pulmonary infiltrates	
Pulmonary metastasis	Untreated or poorly responsive primary carcinoma
Atelectasis	Endobronchial lesion Chest wall or upper abdominal pain Depressed cough or respiration (narcotics)
Pulmonary infarction (pulmonary thromboembolism)	Hypercoagulable state owing to carcinoma or paraproteinemia, immobility, venous obstruction
Radiation pneumonitis	Recent (4–12 weeks) radiotherapy with lung exposure

should be tapped and cultured for bacteria, fungi, viruses,
and acid-fast bacilli (AFB). Skin lesions should be biopsied;
specimens from other extrapulmonary sites should be collected and sent for culture. Patients with diffuse infiltrates
and predominantly cell-mediated immunodeficiency are at
particularly high risk for PCP and/or CMV pneumonia and
should undergo early bronchoscopy with bronchoalveolar

lavage (BAL) (and biopsy if CMV is suspected). Those patients with localized pulmonary infiltrates who fail to respond to treatment for bacterial pneumonia or who have features suggesting an alternative diagnosis such as fungal pneumonia should also be considered for bronchoscopy. Though the issue is controversial, all patients who continue to deteriorate without an established diagnosis should be considered for surgical lung biopsy.

Empiric treatment should include broad-spectrum antibiotics such as an antipseudomonal penicillin/β lactamase inhibitor combination plus erythromycin. Trimethoprim-sulfamethoxazole should be given if PCP is suspected and amphotericin initiated empirically in the patient with prolonged granulocytopenia and respiratory deterioration. Unnecessary drugs may be discontinued once a diagnosis has been established. Table 39-9 lists accepted antimicrobial regimens for various opportunistic lung infections.

Hospital-Acquired Pneumonia Including Ventilator-Associated Pneumonia

Hospital-acquired pneumonia (HAP) is defined as pneumonia occurring more than 48 hours after hospital admission. Ventilator-associated pneumonia (VAP), a subset of HAP occurring more than 48 hours after the institution of mechanical ventilation, complicates the course of roughly 10 to 20 percent of all patients undergoing mechanical ventilation. HAP is a major cause of morbidity and mortality in ICU patients, underscoring the importance of a rational strategy aimed at preventing, diagnosing, and treating this problem.

PATHOGENESIS

Inoculation of the lower respiratory tract may occur by a number of mechanisms in the hospitalized patient, chief among which is microaspiration of colonized oropharyngeal secretions. Other mechanisms include frank aspiration of large volumes of gastric contents, inhalation of microbes directly through inspired gases, hematogenous dissemination from distant sites of infection, and possibly translocation from the gastrointestinal tract.

TABLE 39-9 Antimicrobial Therapy for Opportunistic Lung Infections in Critically Ill Immunocompromised Patients[a]

Pulmonary Infection	Antimicrobial Regimen
Pneumocystis carinii pneumonia	Co-trimoxazole 5 mg/kg TMP and 25 mg/kg SMX IV q6h *or* pentamidine 4 mg/kg IV q24h
Nocardia asteroides pneumonia or abscess	Sulfonamide 2 g q6h (IV if available) *or* co-trimoxazole (as above) ± amikacin 5 mg/kg IV q8h
Aspergillosis	Amphotericin B 0.6–1.0 mg/kg IV q24h to total dose of 2.0 g *and*, if permitted by degree of myelosuppression, flucytosine 150 mg/kg IV or PO per day initially, reducing dose to achieve 1 h predose blood levels of 50–75 μg/mL
Candidal pneumonia due to associated candidemia	Amphotericin B 0.3–0.6 mg/kg IV q24h *or* fluconazole 400 mg IV q24h
CMV pneumonia	Ganciclovir 2.5 mg/kg IV q8h *and* CMV immune globulin 400–500 mg/kg on alternate days (4–10 doses)
Varicella zoster, disseminated, with pneumonia	Acyclovir 10 mg/kg IV q8h

[a]Treatment regimens for the more common acute bacterial pneumonias as shown in Tables 39-4 and 39-6, and for the dimorphic fungi in Table 39-6.
TMP, trimethoprim; SMX, sulfamethoxazole.

Host risk factors for HAP and airway colonization are similar and include duration of hospitalization, prolonged use of antibiotics, malnutrition, coma, shock, renal failure, preexisting lung disease, diabetes, alcoholism, and tobacco use. Certain therapeutic interventions are associated with HAP. Nasogastric tubes and enteral feeding may lead to HAP via reflux and aspiration, a problem exacerbated by feeding in the supine position. Surgery, particularly thoracic or abdominal procedures, increases the risk of nosocomial pneumonia. Immunosuppressives impair systemic host defenses. Antacids and H2 blockers may increase gastric colonization by enteric gram-negative bacilli, though whether this leads to a meaningful increase in HAP remains controversial. Contaminated respiratory equipment and the unwashed hands of medical personnel expose patients to additional sources of pathogens. Finally, endotracheal intubation impairs mucociliary clearance and damages the epithelial surface of the lower airways, promoting bacterial adherence. Duration of mechanical ventilation and reintubation are highly associated with VAP.

ETIOLOGIC AGENTS

The agents responsible for HAP vary among institutions. Nonetheless, certain generalizations can be made (Table 39-10). Patients developing pneumonia in the first week after admission are usually infected with organisms that they brought into the hospital, such as *Strep. pneumoniae*, *Staph. aureus*, and *H. influenzae*. Later infection is increasingly associated with enteric gram-negative bacilli as well as with methicillin-resistant *Staph. aureus*. Anaerobes are implicated when there has been recent abdominal surgery or witnessed aspiration. Infection with *Pseudomonas* or *Acinetobacter* is associated with prior antibiotic therapy as well as with poor survival.

DIAGNOSIS

Studies of HAP have been hampered by the absence of a gold standard for its diagnosis. Various clinical and invasive strategies have been studied; each approach is discussed below.

The clinical diagnosis of HAP is made when a patient develops a new radiographic infiltrate that is thought to be

TABLE 39-10   Bacterial Causes of Nosocomial Pneumonia
in Patients Requiring Intensive Care[a]

Organism	Frequency (% of Cases)
Enterobacteriaceae (*Klebsiella*, *E. coli*, *Enterobacter*, *Proteus*, *Acinetobacter*, *Serratia*, etc.)	30–50
Staphylococcus aureus	10–30
Pseudomonas aeruginosa	10–20
Streptococci (including *Streptococcus pneumoniae*)	10–15
Legionella spp.	5–15
Haemophilus influenzae	2–10
Moraxella (*Branhamella*) *catarrhalis*	2–10
Anaerobes	2–5

[a]Ranges shown are derived from a number of studies from different geographic areas and different patient populations. Incidence of each infection varies greatly depending on local circumstances.

infectious in origin. Fever, sputum production, and leuko-cytosis are supportive of an infectious etiology. Unfortu-nately, hospitalized patients often lack some or all of these features or have other conditions that resemble pneumonia. Pulmonary infiltrates may be secondary to atelectasis, he-morrhage, or pulmonary edema. Fever and leukocytosis are similarly nonspecific in the critically ill patient. Purulent sputum may reflect tracheobronchitis, a condition that is not associated with a poor prognosis and may not warrant an-tibiotic therapy. The lack of specificity of the clinical ap-proach, particularly in mechanically ventilated patients, leads to the overuse of broad-spectrum antibiotics and may distract the clinician from pursuing other causes of pul-monary deterioration.

An invasive approach to the diagnosis of HAP may em-ploy several techniques. The protected specimen brush (PSB) technique uses a fiberoptic bronchoscope to reach the area of interest. A double-catheter brush with telescoping cannulas and a distal occluding plug is advanced and wedged, after which distal secretions are sampled. The brush is then re-tracted into the inner cannula and the telescoping apparatus withdrawn into the fiberoptic bronchoscope and removed.

This technique permits culturing of secretions without cont-amination from more proximal airways. The secretions are cultured quantitatively, with a cutoff of 10^3 colony-forming units per milliliter generally indicating infection rather than colonization. PSB is probably 80 to 90 percent sensitive at di-agnosing pneumonia in mechanically ventilated patients when this cutoff point is utilized. However, several limitations of this technique exist: (1) culture results are not available for 24 to 48 hours; (2) values within 1 log 10 of the cutoff should be viewed with caution because as many as one-third of pa-tients with suspected pneumonia and values between 10^2 and 10^3 are subsequently diagnosed with pneumonia; (3) both false-negative and false-positive results commonly occur when patients have received new antibiotics prior to bron-choscopy, the former secondary to sterilization of secretions and the latter as a consequence of selection pressure.

BAL is performed by instilling 100 to 150 mL of sterile saline into the lungs after first wedging the bronchoscope in the area of suspected infection. The fluid is then aspirated and sent for examination. One advantage of this technique is that the fluid may be examined microscopically immediately after the procedure. The presence of more than 5 percent in-fected BAL cells (cells containing intracellular bacteria) indi-cates infection and thus the need for empiric antibiotic ther-apy pending culture results. BAL quantitative cultures of 10^5 or greater generally indicate infection, although the specificity of BAL cultures has been questioned. Also problematic is the difficulty of performing this procedure in patients with se-vere obstructive lung disease.

While empiric therapy is appropriate for most nonintu-bated patients with HAP, we recommend an invasive ap-proach to the diagnosis of VAP in most situations (Fig. 39-1). We feel this is justified given the difficulty of diagnosing pneumonia in ventilated patients as well as the ease with which bronchoscopy can be performed in the intubated pa-tient. Specimens should be obtained by PSB as well as by BAL. The BAL fluid is immediately examined; if more than 5 per-cent of cells harbor intracellular bacteria, empiric antimicro-bial therapy is initiated, covering the most likely and life-threatening etiologies, as discussed below. If fewer than 5 percent of cells are infected and the patient does not exhibit

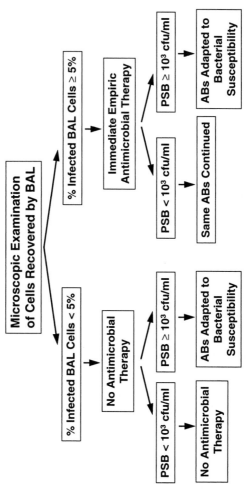

FIGURE 39-1 Therapeutic decision tree, based on results of BAL cell examination and PSB sample cultures, in ventilator-dependent patients clinically thought to have developed nosocomial pneumonia. *(Reproduced with permission from Chastre J, Fagon JY: Invasive diagnostic testing should be routinely used to manage ventilated patients with suspected pneumonia. Am J Respir Crit Care Med 150:570–574, 1994.)*

signs of sepsis, empiric therapy may be withheld pending culture results. PSB cultures $\geq 10^3$ indicate infection and should prompt reexamination of the patient's antimicrobial regimen to ensure adequate coverage. PSB cultures $< 10^3$ combined with a negative BAL microscopic examination justify withholding antimicrobials. Advantages of an invasive approach include the ability to (1) identify organisms not previously considered or else resistant to the current antibiotic regimen; (2) exclude infection and thus limit the indiscriminate use of broad-spectrum antibiotics; and (3) diagnose noninfectious causes of pulmonary infiltrates such as alveolar hemorrhage. Finally, bronchoscopy may reveal organisms which, when present, always indicate infection regardless of quantity. These include *P. carinii, Legionella, Histoplasma, Mycobacterium tuberculosis, Mycoplasma,* and influenza.

Noninvasive alternatives to the diagnosis of VAP have included cultures of endotracheal aspirates. Qualitative culture of endotracheal aspirates is associated with a high percentage of false-positive results caused by upper airway colonization. Quantitative cultures have been examined recently and found to be less sensitive than the combination of PSB and BAL, with a significant number of discordant culture results between the two groups. New nonbronchoscopic methods of obtaining lung specimens include the use of a protected telescoping catheter (PTC), a promising technique that warrants further study.

It should be emphasized that an invasive approach to the diagnosis of VAP does not imply that empiric therapy should be withheld until bronchoscopy is performed, as this delay may result in higher mortality. Rather, empiric therapy and invasive evaluation should both proceed promptly.

TREATMENT

Empiric antibiotic therapy is strongly influenced by the likelihood of infection with resistant gram-negative organisms. Table 39-11 emphasizes this approach to management and includes suggestions for patients at risk for legionellosis, methicillin-resistant *Staph. aureus,* or pneumonia following frank aspiration.

TABLE 39-11 Empiric Antimicrobial Therapy for Nosocomial Pneumonia Associated with Critical Illness[a]

Clinical Setting	Recommended Antimicrobial Therapy	Alternative Antimicrobial Therapy
Acute nosocomial pneumonia (postoperative or complicating medical illness)	Cefotaxime 2 g IV q6h and gentamicin 4.5 mg/kg IV q24h	Co-trimoxazole IV; ciprofloxacin or ofloxacin IV +/− a β lactam
Nosocomial pneumonia with increased risk of resistant aerobic gram-negatives (i.e., prior broad-spectrum antibiotics, acute leukemia, endemic resistant organisms, etc.)	Piperacillin 3 g IV q4h and gentamicin 4.5 mg/kg IV q24h	Gentamicin and imipenem, ceftazadime, or piperacillin/tazobactam; ciprofloxacin or ofloxacin IV +/− a β lactam
Severe pneumonia following aspiration	Clindamycin 900 mg IV q8h and cefotaxime 2 g IV q6h	Clindamycin and co-trimoxazole IV, metronidazole and cefotaxime
Suspect legionellosis (endemic, organ transplant, steroid use) or undiagnosed fulminant pneumonia	Add erythromycin 1g IV q6h ± rifampin 600 mg IV qd to one of above regimens	Ciprofloxacin or ofloxacin
Suspect methicillin-resistant Staphylococcus aureus	Add vancomycin 500 mg IV q6h	

[a]Doses cited are for patients with normal renal function; dosage adjustments for renal insufficiency are required for a number of the listed agents. Monitoring of blood drug levels is strongly advised for aminoglycosides and choramphenicol. Gentamicin is shown as the preferred aminoglycoside, however, where resistance to this agent is common selection of an alternative aminoglycoside may be necessary.

PREVENTION

Prevention of nosocomial pneumonia has been attempted through (1) infection control, (2) control of host risk factors, and (3) the use of novel respiratory equipment. Infection control emphasizes good handwashing, outbreak surveillance, and education of medical personnel. Reduction of host risk involves the judicious use of noninvasive ventilation, the timely removal of nasogastric tubes, and elevation of the heads of ventilated patients. Selective digestive decontamination (SDD) of the oropharynx and gastrointestinal tract using topical, enteral, and/or parenteral antibiotics in patients at high risk for VAP is of dubious benefit; although the incidence of gram-negative pneumonia appears to be decreased, there is no survival benefit and only a minor reduction in duration of mechanical ventilation or ICU stay. Also, SDD may increase the selection of resistant organisms. Finally, careful attention to respiratory equipment (e.g., the removal of tubing condensate, circuit changes for ventilators with humidifiers, etc.) may reduce VAP. Equipment that allows continuous or intermittent aspiration of subglottic secretions may delay the development of VAP but does not prevent late pneumonia caused by *P. aeruginosa* or Enterobacteriaceae or reduce mortality.

For a more detailed discussion, see Chaps. 38 and 47 in *Principles of Critical Care*, 2d ed.

Chapter 40

ENDOCARDITIS AND OTHER INTRAVASCULAR INFECTIONS IN THE CRITICALLY ILL

IKEADI MAURICE NDUKWU

The possibility of intravascular infection should be considered in all critically ill patients with bacteremia or fungemia of uncertain origin, particularly with (1) known intravascular or endocardial abnormalities or intravascular devices present, (2) fever or hemodynamic instability of unclear origin, and (3) signs of inflammation related to an indwelling intravascular device. Intravascular infections in the absence of any foreign device include infective endocarditis on a native valve, mycotic aneurysm, cavernous sinus thrombosis, postanginal sepsis, septic pelvic vein thrombophlebitis, and pylephlebitis. Prosthetic device–related infections include prosthetic valve endocarditis, cardiac pacemaker infections, peripheral and central line infections, and arterial device–induced infections.

Native Valve Endocarditis

The pathogenesis of infective endocarditis (IE) on a native valve involves transient bloodstream invasion by microorganisms, followed by adherence of the organisms to the endocardial surface, and their multiplication within a layer of platelets and fibrin, which is relatively inaccessible to host phagocytic defenses. The risk of developing IE in a native valve depends on the species and concentration of microorganisms in the blood, the presence or absence of antimicrobial agents in serum at the time of bacteremia, fungemia, and the characteristics of the endocardium. *Staphylococcus aureus,* enterococci, and other streptococci are very adherent to the endocardium, thus increasing their ability to cause IE. *Staph. aureus,* often found on the skin, is a common cause of acute bacterial endocarditis, particularly in patients without significant underlying valvular heart disease. Fever and murmur are found in at least 85 percent of patients presenting with IE. Skin lesions such as petechiae, Osler's nodes, and Janeway lesions are frequently found in IE. Roth spots in the optic fundus and splinter hemorrhages under the nails are vascular lesions that may be present in IE. Systemic consequences of IE include stroke syndrome, renosplenic infarction, and ischemic bowel disease or infarction of the small bowel. Patients with IE may also present with heart failure due to valve malfunction, embolic myocardial infarction, and myocarditis.

DIAGNOSIS

Blood cultures are the most important laboratory tests in the diagnosis of IE. The vast majority of blood cultures obtained when a patient is not receiving antimicrobial therapy will be positive. The causes of culture-negative endocarditis are prior antibiotics and endocarditis due to fastidious organisms, including anaerobes, nutritionally deficient streptococci, *Coxiella burnetti, Legionella pneumophila, Chlamydia psittaci, Chlamydia pneumoniae,* members of the HACEK (*Haemophilus* species, *Actinobacillus actinomycetemcomitans, Cardiobacterium hominis, Eikenella corrodens,* and *Kingella kingae*) group, and various fungi. Echocardiography is useful in identifying vegetations or local complications of IE. Transesophageal echocardiography (TEE) is more sensitive and specific in the detection of IE heart valve lesions than transthoracic echocardiography. The sensitivity of TEE in the diagnosis of native valve endocarditis (NVE) is 90 to 99 percent, with a specificity of 90 percent. A TEE should be obtained in patients with sterile blood cultures, an equivocal 2D echocardiogram, or a complicated clinical course.

TREATMENT

Empiric therapy for patients with possible IE should be initiated when one of the following situations is present: (1) the patient is critically ill; (2) antimicrobial therapy will be necessary for some other infectious disorder; (3) early valve replacement is contemplated because of valve malfunction; and (4) IE is clinically suspected and one or more blood cultures are positive for an etiologic microorganism. NVE is most commonly associated with streptococci, *Staph. aureus,* or enterococci. Once the organism is identified, the antibiotic regimen should be based on the minimal inhibitory concentration of that antimicrobial agent (Table 40-1).

The distribution of valvular lesions is as follows: aortic, 35 to 50 percent; mitral, 50 percent; tricuspid, 10 percent; and pulmonic, 1 percent. Valve replacement may be lifesaving in patients with IE. Indications for urgent valve replacement include severe heart failure, valvular obstruction, fungal endocarditis, ineffective antimicrobial therapy, and the presence of an unstable prosthetic device.

PROGNOSIS

The prognosis of IE is dependent on the relative pathogenicity of the infecting organism, the location of the infected valve, and the presence of complications of the infection. *Staph. aureus* typically produces a severe and destructive endocarditis that is fatal in about 50 percent of cases when the infection occurs on the aortic or mitral valve. *Pseudomonas aeruginosa* carries a poor prognosis largely related to the limited activity of available antimicrobials against it. Complications associated with a worse prognosis include severe cardiac failure or shock, major arterial emboli, myocardial abscess formation, and associated major organ system failure.

ANTIMICROBIAL PROPHYLAXIS

Certain medical procedures and cardiac abnormalities are known to place patients at increased risk for the development of IE. Dental extraction, periodontal surgery, lower gastrointestinal procedures, and genitourinary procedures are most frequently associated with bacteremia. Cardiac abnormalities that predispose patients to IE include aortic and mitral valve disease, ventricular septal defects, patent ductus arteriosus, coarctation of the aorta, prosthetic valves, and valves that

TABLE 40-1 Antimicrobial Therapy for Infective Endocarditis and Other Intravascular Infections[a]

Organism	Recommended Therapy	For Penicillin-Allergic Patients
1. Penicillin-sensitive streptococci (MIC < 0.1)	Penicillin G 10–20 million U IV qd for 4 weeks plus[c] aminoglycoside for first 2 weeks: [streptomycin 7.5 mg/kg (500 mg) IM q12h or gentamicin 1.0 mg/kg (80 mg) IM IV q8h]	Cefazolin 2 g IV 18h for 4 weeks[b] plus aminoglycoside for 2 weeks or ceftriaxone 2 g IV qd for 4 weeks
2. Relatively "resistant" streptococci (penicillin MIC 0.2–0.5)	Penicillin G 20 million U/day for 4 weeks plus aminoglycoside[d] for 4 weeks	Cefazolin 2 g IV q8h for 4 weeks[b] plus aminoglycoside for 4 weeks
3. Resistant streptococci and enterococci (MIC > 0.5)	Penicillin G 20–30 million U IV qd for 6 weeks (ampicillin 12 g IV qd is alternative) plus aminoglycoside[d] for 6 weeks[b]	Vancomycin 30 mg/kg (< 2 g) per day plus aminoglycoside[d] for 6 weeks
4. Staphylococci (penicillin-sensitive)	Penicillin G 20 million U IV qd for 6 weeks	Cefazolin 2 g IV q8h for 6 weeks[b]
5. Staphylococci (methicillin-sensitive)—in absence of prosthetic valve	Nafcillin 2.0 g IV q4h for 4–6 weeks[e] or nafcillin 2 g IV q4h plus gentamicin 1 mg/kg q8h for 2 weeks[b]	Cefazolin 2 g IV q8h for 4–6 weeks[b]
6. "Methicillin-resistant" staphylococci	Vancomycin 30 mg/kg IV (< 2 g) per day +/− rifampin 300 mg PO q8h for 6 weeks	Same
7. Staphylococci (methicillin sensitive)—in presence of prosthetic valve	Nafcillin 2.0 g IV q4H for 6–8 weeks plus rifampin 300 mg[f] plus aminoglycoside for 2 weeks	Cefazolin 2 g IV[b] q8h for 6–8 weeks plus rifampin[f] plus aminoglycoside for 2 weeks
8. Staphylococci (methicillin resistant) in presence of prosthetic valve	Vancomycin 30 mg/kg per 24 h IV (< 2 g) for 6–8 weeks, rifampin 300 mg for 6–8 weeks[f] plus aminoglycoside for 2 weeks	

9. *Corynebacterium*	Penicillin G 20–30 million U IV qd for 6 weeks plus aminoglycoside for 6 weeks	Vancomycin 30 mg/kg (< 2 g) qd IV for 6 weeks
10. Gram-negative bacilli		
a. Enterobacteriaceae	Therapy should be directed by in vitro susceptibilities	Same
b. *Pseudomonas*	Therapy should be directed by in vitro susceptibilities, though usual regimen includes tobramycin (8 mg/kg per day) plus extended-spectrum penicillin	Same, though ceftazidime plus tobramycin (8 mg/kg per day) frequently used
c. HACEK group	Ampicillin 2.0 g IV q4h is commonly used, though therapy should be directed by in vitro susceptibilities (aminoglycoside frequently used in combination)	Third-generation cephalosporins (e.g., ceftriaxone 2 g IV qd for 4 weeks)
11. Rickettsiae		
Coxiella burnetti	Tetracycline 500 mg PO q6h for at least 1 year plus trimethoprim 480 mg plus sulfamethoxazole 2400 mg qd until there is no clinical evidence of disease or phase I antibody titer is < 1:128	Same
12. Fungi	Amphotericin B plus surgery	Same
13. Culture-negative endocarditis	Penicillin G 20 million U IV qd for 6 weeks plus an aminoglycoside for 2 weeks	Cephalothin 2.0 g IV[b] q4h for 6 weeks

[a]Duration of treatment given applies to native valve infective endocarditis only.

[b]If patient sensitivity to penicillin is of the immediate hypersensitivity type, vancomycin is recommended.

[c]Aqueous crystalline penicillin G should be used alone in patients over 65 years of age or who have renal disease or hearing impairment.

[d]Choice of aminoglycoside should depend on in vitro susceptibilities.

[e]Addition of an aminoglycoside is optional.

[f]Use of rifampin in coagulase-negative staphylococcal infection is recommended. The value of rifampin in coagulase-positive staphylococcal infections is controversial.

[g]Vancomycin is indicated in coagulase-negative strains; consult when treating vancomycin-resistant strains.

[h]Optional in uncomplicated right sided IE in intravenous drug users.

have previously been infected. Mitral valve prolapse, with re-dundancy of the valve seen on echocardiography or evidence of mitral regurgitation, also predisposes the patient to IE. The specific antimicrobial agents chosen for prophylaxis are de-pendent on the specific procedure to be performed, the car-diac abnormality present, and the presence or absence of penicillin allergy (Table 40-2).

Mycotic Aneurysm

Mycotic aneurysms are aneurysmal dilations of arteries caused by infection of the vessel wall, with consequent weak-ening of the vessel structure. This is most common in patients with IE and usually involves vessels of smaller caliber. The proposed pathogenesis involves embolic localization of a valvular vegetation with extension of suppuration from the lumen circumferentially into the vessel wall; embolization of the vasa vasorum by infected material from the valve; and, in the absence of underlying IE, mycotic aneurysm occurring after transient bacteremia, with seeding of a previously dam-aged site in a larger artery.

CLINICAL FEATURES

Intracranial mycotic aneurysms are most commonly encoun-tered in patients who already carry a diagnosis of IE. Symp-toms and signs consistent with subarchnoid or intracerebral hemorrhage with sudden onset of headache, decrease in level of consciousness, and focal neurologic signs are seen with aneurysmal rupture. Mycotic aneurysms of visceral arteries have a variable presentation based on the organ involved. In the case of the small bowel, there may be colicky abdominal pain and symptoms of small bowel obstruction. Hepatic ar-terial aneurysms present similarly to ascending cholangitis with fever, right-upper-quadrant pain, and jaundice. Mycotic aneurysms of the external iliac artery may present with pain in the lower anterior abdomen, quadriceps wasting, dimin-ished deep tendon reflexes, and arterial insufficiency of the ipsilateral lower extremity. Mycotic aneurysms of the ab-dominal aorta may present with chronic pain and fever. In as many as one-third of patients with abdominal aortic

TABLE 40-2 Endocarditis Prophylaxis

Procedure—Parenteral Regimens	Standard Regimen	Standard Oral Regimen for PCN Allergic Patients	Alternative
Dental or respiratory tract procedure	Amoxicillin 3.0 g PO 1 h before, then 1.5 g 6 h later	Erythromycin 1.0 g PO 2 h before, 30 min before, then 500 mg 6 h later *or* clindamycin 300 mg PO 1 h before, then 150 mg 6 h later	Ampicillin 2.0 g IV or IM then 1.0 g 6 h later *or* clindamycin 300 mg IV 30 min before, then 150 mg 6 h later *or* vancomycin 1.0 g IV over 1 h starting 1 h before procedure; no repeat dose necessary
Gastrointestinal or genitourinary tract procedure	Ampicillin 2.0 g IV or IM, plus gentamicin 1.5 mg/kg body weight IV or IM given 30 min before, repeat 8 h later		Vancomycin 1.0 g IV slowly over 1 h, plus gentamicin 1.5 mg/kg body weight IV or IM given 1 h before, repeat 8 h later

519

aneurysms, there is extension into the lumbar or thoracic vertebrae, with resultant osteomyelitis. Aortoenteric fistula may occur if an aneurysm erodes into the bowel lumen.

DIAGNOSIS

In patients with IE, clinical suspicion of a mycotic aneurysm usually arises after an episode of new neurologic symptoms. Computer tomography (CT) followed by cerebral angiography is the best diagnostic strategy. The role of magnetic resonance imaging in the diagnosis of mycotic aneurysm remains to be studied. The diagnosis of mycotic aneurysm of the abdominal aorta is aided by high clinical suspicion, evidence of bacteremia, and radiologic examination. Abdominal CT, angiography, and bone scanning are useful imaging modalities.

MANAGEMENT

The management of mycotic aneurysm depends on the organ involved. For peripheral intracranial aneurysms, clipping is probably indicated. For deep lesions, for which a surgical approach is felt to be hazardous, antimicrobial therapy alone is advisable because many aneurysms will resolve spontaneously with medical treatment. In the case of abdominal aortic aneurysms, surgical resection of the involved aorta is almost always necessary.

Cavernous Sinus Thrombosis

Cavernous sinus thrombosis usually results from direct spread of bacteria from a contiguous focus of infection. Routes of extension include septic thrombophlebitis of the angular and ophthalmic veins from facial cellulitis, along the lateral sinus and petrosal sinuses from middle ear infections, via the pterygoid venous plexus from a peritonsillar abscess, following a dental infection from osteomyelitis of the maxilla or from a cervical abscess, and along the venous plexus surrounding the internal carotid artery from the middle ear or jugular bulb.

Staph. aureus and streptococci are the most common organisms seen in cavernous sinus thrombosis. Patients generally present early after onset of external ophthalmoplegia with decreased sensation around the eye. The physical examination reveals periorbital edema and chemosis. As the illness progresses, meningismus, altered mental status, and cranial nerve palsies (especially of cranial nerves III, IV, V, and VI) become evident. Examination of the fundus often reveals striking venous congestion. The differential diagnosis of cavernous sinus thrombosis includes orbital cellulitis and rhinocerebral phycomycosis (mucormycosis). Bilateral involvement, as well as fifth-nerve palsy, a fixed, dilated pupil, and signs of meningitis are all more likely in cavernous sinus thrombosis than orbital cellulitis. The diagnosis may be made by clinical features; ultrasound of the orbit; CT, MRI, and MRA scan; carotid angiography; and orbital venography. Lumbar puncture is necessary following negative brain CT.

Successful management of cavernous sinus thrombosis depends on early, effective antimicrobial therapy (see Table 40-1).

Prosthetic Valve Endocarditis

Prosthetic heart valves (PVE) become infected in approximately 2 percent of patients. One-third of these infections occur in the first few months after valve implantation because of intraoperative inoculation or seeding of microorganisms on the new device or following transient bacteremia associated with indwelling lines used in the perioperative period. Increased risk of PVE include IE of the native valve prior to valve resection and replacement, use of a mechanical valvular device as opposed to a tissue heterograft or homograft, a history of intravenous drug abuse, male gender (possibly because of the greater likelihood of superficial cellulitis as a result of shaving prior to surgery), and longer cardiopulmonary bypass time.

Two-thirds of cases of PVE occur 60 days or more after replacement. The pathogenesis of this late-onset PVE resembles that of the NVE. *Staph. epidermidis* is common in early PVE, and microorganisms found in patients with late PVE tend to be similar to those seen in native valve disease (Table 40-3).

TABLE 40-3   Etiology of Valve Endocarditis and Intravascular Infections

Microorganism	Native (%)	Early PVE,[a] %	Late PVE, %	Pacemaker (%)	Vascular Graft (%)
Strep. epidermidis	6	30	20	42	10
Staph. aureus	25	20	11	35	15
Streptococci					30
Group D streptococci	7	5	12	—	
Strep. viridans	55				
Gram-negative bacilli	6	20	12	—	30
Corynebacterium					
(not *C. diphtheriae*)	—	8	3	—	3
Fungi	1	10	5	—	2
Other or culture-negative	7	3	12	23	10

[a]PVE is prosthetic valve endocarditis.

Patients with PVE have a high incidence of cardiac complications. Clinical evidence of these cardiac complications may include new and changing regurgitant murmurs caused by paravalvular leak from dehiscence of the valve ring, intraventricular and atrioventricular conduction defects resulting from extension of a paravalvular abscess into the interventricular septum, and muffling of prosthetic heart sounds or new stenotic murmurs related to malfunction of the valve caused by a vegetation.

Diagnosis of early PVE is made difficult by unrelated bacteremia during the immediate postoperative period. However, blood cultures yielding staphylococci, "diphtheroids," and yeasts are more likely to represent true prosthetic valve infection than is gram-negative bacteremia, which is more likely due to indwelling venous catheter infection. In patients with late PVE caused by staphylococci or streptococci, bacteria are usually recovered consistently from blood cultures provided that the patient has not received prior antimicrobial therapy. The echocardiogram and the cinefluoroscopic examination may be of some help in patients with PVE. Transesophageal echocardiography (TEE) is superior to transthoracic echocardiography (TTE) in visualizing the mitral valve; visualization of aortic valve prostheses with TEE is less clear. A cinefluorogram that reveals more than a 7-degree rocking of the prosthesis is very suggestive of valve dehiscence. CT scan of brain should be performed when there are neurologic symptoms, and cerebral angiography is indicated when CT findings do not adequately explain the neurologic symptoms.

When the infecting microorganism has not been identified, initial therapy should include vancomycin and gentamicin to cover the likely possibilities of *Staph. epidermidis,* *Staph. aureus,* and streptococci (Table 40-1). Relative indications for valve replacement in PVE include early PVE, nonstreptococcal late PVE, and periprosthetic leak. Patients with PVE should be treated for 6 to 8 weeks in most instances whether or not the valve is removed. If microorganisms can be cultured at the time of valve replacement, we recommend 6 to 8 additional weeks of therapy beginning at that time.

Cardiac Pacemaker Infections

Approximately 4 percent of pacemakers become infected at some point after placement. Generator box infections, infection of the electrode along its subcutaneous course, and bacteremic infection of the intravascular portion of the electrode—with or without associated endocarditis—each contribute approximately one-third to the overall infection problem. Predisposing factors include diabetes mellitus, cancer, corticosteroid therapy, and skin erosion adjacent to a generator pouch. Pacemaker infections may occur early (3 to 6 months) or late (more than 6 months) after implant. Early infections are generally attributed to wound contamination by skin organisms at the time of implantation; late infection, particularly of the intravascular electrode, is often due to transient bacteremia with adherence of organisms to the surface of the device. *Staph. epidermidis* and *Staph. aureus* are the most common microorganisms isolated from patients with pacemaker infection.

Chills, fever, and other constitutional symptoms without another evident source is the usual presentation of pacemaker infection. In the absence of other sources of infection, the diagnosis of pacemaker infection may be made by inspecting the generator pocket and the subcutaneous electrodes, along with obtaining blood cultures. Persistent bacteremia in a patient with an intravascular pacemaker suggests intravascular electrode infection or IE. An initial trial of intravenous antimicrobial therapy (Table 40-1) for 4 to 6 weeks is warranted if pacemaker removal is not an option. If the decision is made to remove the pacemaker, then the new transvenous generator should be located in a deeper pocket. Two weeks of antimicrobial therapy after removal of the device is probably sufficient in the case of most generator pocket infections due to pyogenic microorganisms unless there is metastatic disease or secondary NVE, in which case the usual duration of treatment for NVE is given after the device is removed.

Arterial Graft Infections

Arterial grafts have an infection rate that has varied between 2 and 6 percent, with a mortality rate as high as 50 percent. The pathogenesis of graft infection is analogous to that of prosthetic valve disease. Graft infections present a mean of 8 months after implantation, but late infection may occur as long as 7 to 10 years after graft placement. Susceptibility of arterial graft to infection is dependent on donor material and site: autogenous vein grafts are the least susceptible to infection; woven Dacron is less susceptible than knitted Dacron, which appears to be most susceptible to infection. Grafts that cross the femoral area seem to be at greatest risk for infection, possibly due to contamination by bowel flora at the time of implantation. Gram-positive microorganisms are the most common cause of graft infections, particularly in the groin or popliteal area (Table 40-3).

Intraluminal infection may present as fever and nonspecific constitutional complaints due to bacteremia. Extraluminal infection may present with evidence of local graft infection with erythema, tenderness, and swelling over the graft site, with systemic inflammatory symptoms without definite localizing findings, or with graft occlusion. Rapid swelling suggests disruption of the suture line, with bleeding and false aneurysm formation, and almost always implies graft infection. Graft thrombosis should be suspected when signs and symptoms of peripheral arterial insufficiency develop. Exteriorization of the graft secondary to breakdown of tissue overlying the graft is pathognomonic of infection. Abdominal aortic graft infection may lead to mass effect with evidence of ureteral obstruction or hydronephrosis, symptoms and signs of lower extremity ischemia, or the development of an aortoduodenal fistula. Diagnosis of graft infection can be made clinically and with blood cultures, scanning with indium- or technetium-labeled white blood cells, or CT scanning for soft tissue edema or false aneurysm formation.

Management of an infected intravascular graft almost always requires specific antimicrobial therapy (Table 40-1), chosen on the basis of the presumed or demonstrated infecting microorganism, as well as graft removal.

AN APPROACH TO PATIENTS WITH FEVER AND SUSPECTED INTRAVASCULAR INFECTION

Patients with otherwise unexplained positive blood cultures in the presence of an intravascular device must be presumed to

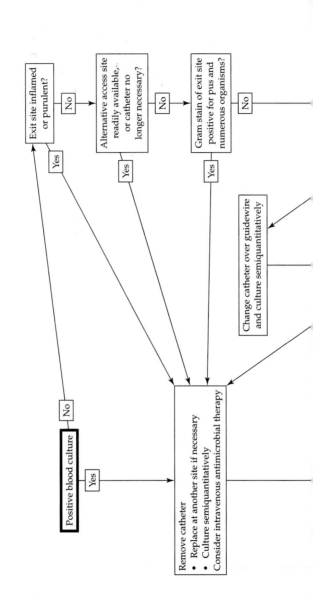

526

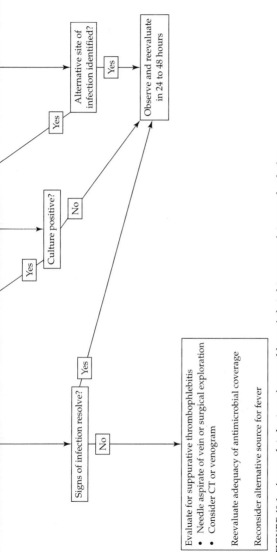

Alternative site of infection identified?

Yes

Culture positive?

Yes

No

Yes

Observe and reevaluate in 24 to 48 hours

Signs of infection resolve?

Yes

No

Evaluate for suppurative thrombophlebitis
• Needle aspirate of vein or surgical exploration
• Consider CT or venogram

Reevaluate adequacy of antimicrobial coverage

Reconsider alternative source for fever

FIGURE 40-1 Approach to bacteremia caused by an infected temporary intravascular device.

527

have an infection of the device. When the device is a temporary one—such as a peripheral intravenous line, central venous catheter, or temporary pacemaker—it should be removed. If pus can be expressed from the puncture site or there is persistent bacteremia, surgical exploration of the peripheral veins is indicated. Tunneled central venous catheters call for a more selective approach (see Fig. 40-1).

For a more detailed discussion, see Chap. 45 in *Principles of Critical Care*, 2d ed.

Chapter 41

INFECTIONS OF THE CENTRAL NERVOUS SYSTEM

DELBERT DORSCHEID

Presented here is a summary of the major CNS infections, including meningitis, brain abscess, subdural empyema, epidural abscess, suppurative thrombophlebitis, and encephalitis.

Meningitis

Today, even after the development of a vaccine for *Haemophilus influenzae*, this organism accounts for about 5 percent of isolates in patients above 6 years of age. When isolated, this organism should suggest the following predisposing factors: sinusitis, otitis media, epiglottitis, pneumonia, diabetes mellitus, alcoholism, asplenic states, and other immune-compromised conditions. *Neisseria meningitidis* may cause epidemics of meningitis in both adults and children. Asymptomatic carriers are the usual causes of the infection. *Streptococcus pneumoniae* is the most common cause of meningitis in individuals over 30 years of age and is associated with the following risks: pneumonia, otitis media, mastoiditis, sinusitis, endocarditis, and head trauma with cerebrospinal fluid (CSF) leak. *Listeria monocytogenes* is responsible for only about 1.9 percent of all cases of bacterial meningitis, but as it goes unrecognized, it is associated with a high mortality rate. Risks include age (neonates, elderly), alcoholism, cancer, and other immunocompromised states. *Staphylococcus epidermidis* is the most common cause of meningitis in individuals with CSF shunts, and *Staphylcoccus aureus* is most frequently the isolate in the immediate postneurosurgical period.

Clinical presentation in the adult includes fever, headache, meningismus (accompanied by either the Kernig or Brudzinski sign), and signs of cerebral dysfunction. These signs and symptoms are found in more than 80 percent of cases. Associated complaints include nausea, vomiting, photophobia, rigors, diaphoresis, and myalgias. Seizures (in about 30 percent of cases) and cranial nerve palsies (in 10 to 20 percent of cases) are additional signs, but evidence for papilledema should suggest another diagnosis, such as an intracranial mass.

Special consideration must be given to the elderly with mental status changes. Even if the patient has alternative medical diagnoses to explain the mental state (liver or cardiac diseases, diabetes) one should always exclude an infection of the central nervous system (CNS) by spinal fluid analysis. Similarly, a post-neurosurgical or trauma patient may have signs of meningitis due to the primary condition, but if new fever emerges, an examination of the cerebrospinal fluid (CSF) may be indicated.

DIAGNOSIS

The "gold standard" for diagnosis is lumbar puncture and CSF analysis. Initial opening pressure is often elevated and values over 600 mm H_2O suggest the presence of cerebral edema, suppurative foci, or communicating hydrocephalus. Xanthochromia (pale yellow-orange discoloration of the CSF) is usually indicative of an old inflammatory process or subarachnoid bleeding. The usual CSF white blood cell (WBC) count in bacterial meningitis is 100 to 10,000/mm, with a majority of neutrophils, but 10 percent of cases exhibit a lymphocyte predominance. A low CSF WBC with organisms cultured or seen on stain carries a poor prognosis. All CSF analysis should include a Gram stain and culture as a routine. The Gram stain will provide rapid identification of the causative organism in 60 to 90 percent of bacterial meningitis cases and cultures are positive in 70 to 90 percent of untreated cases. Chemical analysis of CSF in meningitis demonstrates an elevated protein and decreased glucose (< 40 mg/dL) in 60 to 90 percent of cases. Rapid tests, such as the direct fluorescent antibody (DFA) and latex agglutination tests, are available for many pathogens and can provide useful information about negative CSF smears.

TREATMENT

Appropriate empiric therapy may be guided from the CSF analysis, including the Gram stain, with additional consideration for factors such as age and the patient's underlying status. Antibiotics are the definitive therapy and their administration should not be delayed in cases of presumed meningitis. If a patient demonstrates a focal neurologic examination, lumbar puncture is delayed until CT scan has excluded the possibility of an intracranial mass, but antibiotics must be given if meningitis is considered. Empiric therapy for presumed bacterial meningitis is outlined in Table 41-1. If the patient has had recent neurosurgery or head trauma, empiric treatment should include ceftazidime and vancomycin because of the possibility of diptheroids, gram-negative bacilli, and *Staphylococcus* as infecting organisms. The results of any positive microbiologic studies should always dictate a focused antibiotic regimen. Suggestions for specific bacteria are listed in Table 41-2, with dosages in Table 41-3. Since resistant pneumococcus is a growing problem, susceptibility testing should be performed on all isolates and knowledge of one's own institutional resistance profile will assist the empiric choice of antibiotics. Treatment duration must be determined on an individual basis, given the clinical response of the particular patient and the causative bacteria. In general, 10 to 14 days for nonmeningococcal meningitis, 21 days for gram-negative bacilli, and 7 days for meningococcal and *H. influenzae* meningitis are useful guidelines.

Brain Abscess

There are three main mechanisms for the development of a brain abscess. The most common is contiguous spread from an infected middle ear, mastoid air cells, or paranasal sinuses. Hematogenous spread from distant sites of infection usually results in the formation of multiple foci of intracranial infection and presents with a higher mortality rather than does spread from contiguous sites. The usual primary sources of blood-borne CNS infection are chronic pyogenic lung diseases such as cystic fibrosis, empyema, bronchiectasis, and lung abscess. Finally, brain abscess can be a sequela of head trauma or neurosurgery. Of note is that about 20 percent of all cases are cryptogenic. *Streptococcus* sp. account for 60 to 70 percent of all cases, *Staph. aureus* for 10 to 15 percent, and anaerobes or mixed flora for 20 to 30 percent of cases where an organism is identified.

TABLE 41-1 Empirical Therapy of Purulent Meningitis[a]

Age	Standard Therapy	Alternative Therapies
0–3 weeks	Ampicillin plus cefotaxime	Ampicillin plus an aminoglycoside[c]
4–12 weeks	Ampicillin plus a third-generation cephalosporin[b]	Ampicillin plus chloramphenicol
3 months to 18 years	Third-generation cephalosporin[b]	Ampicillin plus chloramphenicol
18–50 years	Penicillin G or ampicillin	Third-generation cephalosporin[b]
> 50 years	Ampicillin plus a third-generation cephalosporin[b]	Ampicillin plus an aminoglycoside[c]; trimethoprim/sulfamethoxazole

[a]Vancomycin should be added to empirical therapeutic regimens when highly penicillin- or cephalosporin-resistant strains of *S. pneumoniae* are suspected.

[b]Gentamicin, tobramycin, or amikacin.

[c]Cefotaxime or ceftriaxone.

TABLE 41-2   Antimicrobial Therapy of Bacterial Meningitis

Organism	Antibiotic of Choice
Streptococcus penumoniae	
Penicillin MIC < 0.1 μg/mL	Penicillin G or ampicillin
Penicillin MIC 0.1–1.0 μg/mL	Third-generation cephalosporin[a]
Penicillin MIC ≥ 2.0 μg/mL	Vancomycin plus a third-generation cephalosporin[a]
Neisseria meningitidis	Penicillin G or ampicillin
Haemophilus influenzae (β lactamase–negative)	Ampicillin
Haemophilus influenzae (β lactamase–positive)	Third-generation cephalosporin
Enterobacteriacaea	Third-generation cephalosporin
Pseudomonas aeruginosa	Ceftazidime[b]
Streptococcus agalactiae	Penicillin G or ampicillin[b]
Listeria monocytogenes	Ampicillin or penicillin G[b]
Staphylococcus aureus (methicillin-sensitive)	Nafcillin or oxacillin
Staphylococcus aureus (methicillin-resistant)	Vancomycin
Staphylococcus epidermidis	Vancomycin[c]

[a]Cefotaxime or ceftriaxone.
[b]Addition of an aminoglycoside should be considered.
[c]Addition of rifampin may be indicated.

533

TABLE 41-3   Recommended Doses of Antibiotics
for Intracranial Infections in Adults with Normal
Renal Function

Antibiotic	Total Daily Dose in Adults (Dosing Interval)
Penicillin G	24 million U (q4h)
Ampicillin	12 g (q4h)
Nafcillin, oxacillin	9–12 g (q4h)
Chloramphenicol	4–6 g[a] (q6h)
Cefotaxime	8–12 g (q4h)
Ceftriaxone	4 g[b] (q12–24)
Ceftazidime	6–12 g[c] (q8h)
Vancomycin	2–3 g (q8h to q12h)
Gentamicin, tobramycin	3–5 mg/kg (q8h)
Amikacin	15 mg/kg (q8h)
Trimethoprim/sulfamethoxazole	10 mg/kg[d] (q12h)
Metronidazole	30 mg/kg (q6h)

[a]Higher dose recommended for pneumococcal meningitis.
[b]Actual dose studied was 50 mg/kg every 12 h.
[c]Not enough patients studied to make firm recommendations.
[d]Dosage based on trimethoprim component.

The clinical presentation is that of a space-occupying or
mass lesion. Symptoms include headache, nausea and vomiting, nuchal rigidity, and papilledema. Generalized deficits include mental status changes ranging from lethargy to coma.
Seizures occur in about 25 to 30 percent of patients. Fever is
documented in about 50 percent of cases; and when these patients are afebrile, the prognosis is worse and the mortality rate
higher. A classic triad of fever, headache, and focal neurologic
changes is found in less than 50 percent of presentations.

DIAGNOSIS

Computed tomography (CT) has redefined how brain abscess
is evaluated. This imaging allows for simultaneous examination of the brain parenchyma, sinuses, extent of surrounding
edema, and presence of midline shift or hydrocephalus. Even
with clinical improvement, changes may not be seen radiographically until 4 to 6 weeks, and CT resolution may require
4 to 6 months. The use of stereotactic CT-guided aspiration

may facilitate the microbiological diagnosis when samples are sent for Gram stain and culture. Lumbar puncture is contraindicated in situations of suspected brain abscess. Gadolinium-enhanced magnetic resonance imaging (MRI) may provide superior images of the affected soft tissues, but it is often impractical for the critically ill patient and in cases where aspiration is required.

TREATMENT

As for meningitis, when the diagnosis of brain abscess is considered, therapy should not be delayed. Empiric treatment can be initiated either by knowledge of the predisposing condition or by any initial microbiological data until such time when specific organisms and sensitivities have been determined (Tables 41-4 and 41-5). Empirical use of penicillin G should be in the range of 20 to 24 million units per day. Penicillin G should be used in all cases where a third-generation cephalosporin is used and the presumed causative bacteria may include *Streptococcus* species. This approach is justified because, of poor gram-positive coverage by the late-generation cephalosporins. Identification of an organism allows for focused therapy, and if *Bacteroides fragilis* is suspected or identified, metronidazole should be used at a dose of 7.5 mg/kg every 6 h. Treatment duration is often 4 to 6 weeks of high-dose intravenous antibiotics followed by 2 to 6 months of oral antibiotics. Surgical drainage and monitoring of intracranial pressure (ICP) may be required in selected patients, and neurosurgical consultation is warranted in all patients.

Subdural Empyema

Predisposing conditions for this infectious state include otorhinologic and sinus infections that have spread directly into the subdural space either by entry from the valveless emissary veins or an adjacent osteomyelitis. Metastatic or distant hematogenous spread is rare. Clinical presentation includes fever > 39°C in most cases and signs or symptoms of increased ICP, meningeal irritation, or focal cortical inflammation. Focal neurologic findings appear early and usually progress rapidly (over 24 to 36 h); hemiparesis and hemiplegia are the most common findings. If left untreated, this

TABLE 41-4 Empiric Antimicrobial Therapy for Brain Abscess

Predisposing Condition	Antimicrobial Regimen
Otitis media or mastoiditis	Penicillin plus metronidazole plus a third-generation cephalosporin[a]
Sinusitis	Nafcillin or vancomycin[b] plus metronidazole plus a third-generation cephalosporin[a]
Dental sepsis	Penicillin plus metronidazole
Cranial trauma or postneurosurgical state	Vancomycin plus a third-generation cephalosporin[a]
Congenital heart disease	Penicillin plus a third-generation cephalosporin[a]
Unknown	Nafcillin or vancomycin[b] plus metronidazole plus a third-generation cephalosporin[a]

[a]Cefotaxime or ceftriaxone; ceftazidime is used if *P. aeruginosa* is suspected.
[b]Vancomycin is used in the penicillin-allergic patient or when methicillin-resistant *S. aureus* is suspected.

536

TABLE 41-5 Antimicrobial Therapy for Brain Abscess

Organism	Standard Therapy	Alternative Therapies
Streptococcus milleri and other streptococci	Penicillin G	Third-generation cephalosporin,[a] vancomycin
Bacteroides fragilis	Metronidazole	Chloramphenicol, clindamycin
Fusobacterium sp., *Actinomyces*	*Penicillin G*	Metronidazole, chloramphenicol, clindamycin
Staphylococcus aureus	Nafcillin	Vancomycin
Enterobacteriaceae	Third-generation cephalosporin[a]	Aztreonam,[b] trimethoprim sulfamethoxazole
Haemophilus sp.	Third-generation cephalosporin[a]	Aztreonam[b]
Nocardia asteroides	Trimethoprim sulfamethoxazole	Minocycline, third-generation cephalosporin,[a] fluoroquinolone, imipenem (all[b])

[a]Cefotaxime or ceftriaxone.
[b]Limited data available for use of these agents; firm recommendations are not possible at this time.

537

process will rapidly continue to cerebral herniation. Seizures are noted in about 50 percent of patients.

As with brain abscess, if subdural empyema is clinically presumed (meningeal signs and a focal neurologic exam), lumbar puncture is contraindicated. Diagnosis is best made with either CT or MRI with the appropriate contrast infusion. The MRI images are more sensitive in detecting lesions of the central nervous system (CNS), like empyema, which may be undetected by CT. The identification of vascular abnormalities associated with surrounding inflammation by use of cerebral arteriography may be useful in situations where MRI is not available.

Treatment involves both surgical drainage and medical (antibiotic) approaches. The purulent material must be drained by the procedure thought to be best by the neurosurgeon. Empiric antibiotic options include nafcillin or vancomycin plus a third-generation cephalosporin with or without metronidazole (see Table 41-6). Duration of therapy is similar to that for brain abscess.

Spinal Epidural Abscess

The most common predisposing risk factor for spinal epidural abscess is bacteremia. The incidence of epidural abscess is thus high in intravenous drug users and individuals with long-standing intravenous catheters. Epidural abscess may also develop as the result of direct extension from a vertebral ostdeomyelitis. *Staph. aureus* is the major causative organism.

Clinical presentation is dependent upon the time over which the abscess evolved—hours to days for bacteremic spreading versus months for that associated with spinal osteomyelitis. The stages of evolution include focal vetebral pain; foot pain; defects in motor, sensory, or sphincter function; and finally paralysis. Once there are symptoms of motor, sensory, or sphincter dysfunction, the decline to paralysis may be rapid, typically < 24 h. Respiratory muscle function may be involved if the cervical spine is the focus of the abscess. Fever occurs in most patients at some point during the evolution of the abscess.

TABLE 41-6 Empiric Antibiotic Therapy for Subdural Empyema, Epidural Abscess, and Septic Intracranial Thrombophlebitis

Condition	Site of Primary Infection	Antibiotics
Cranial subdural empyema, cranial epidural abscess, or septic intracranial thrombophlebitis	Paranasal sinusitis, otitis media, or mastoiditis	Nafcillin or vancomycin[b] plus metronidazole plus a third-generation cephalosporin
	Cranial surgery	Nafcillin or vancomycin[b] plus a third-generation cephalosporin[a]
	Hematogenous from distant and/or unknown site	Nafcillin or vancomycin[b] plus metronidazole plus a third-generation cephalosporin[a]
Spinal epidural abscess or spinal subdural empyema	Extension of osteomyelitis or paravertebral infection	Nafcillin or vancomycin[b] plus a third-generation cephalosporin[a]
Spinal epidural abscess	Hematogenous spread	Nafcillin or vancomycin[b] plus a third-generation cephalosporin[a]
Spinal subdural empyema	Hematogenous spread	Nafcillin or vancomycin[b]

[a]Cefotaxime or ceftriaxone should be used. If *P. aeruginosa* is suspected, ceftazidime is indicated instead.

[b]Vancomycin is indicated in the penicillin–allergic patient or when methicillin-resistant *S. aureus* is suspected.

SOURCE: Modified from Greenlee. JE: Subdural empyema, in Mandell GL, Bennett JE, Dolin R (eds): *Mandell, Douglas and Bennett's Principles and Practice of Infectious Diseases*, 4th ed. New York, Churchill Livingstone, 1995, p. 900.

As with subdural empyema, a combined medical-surgical approach is needed to ensure complete treatment. Diagnosis and localization can be achieved with either CT or MRI. If these radiographic techniques are not available, myelography is acceptable. After drainage of the purulent material, empiric antimicrobial therapy should include nafcillin or vancomycin; if the patient is an intravenous drug user or has had a recent spinal procedure, gram-negative coverage should be added (see Table 41-6).

For all the focal CNS infections requiring surgical drainage, other adjuvant therapies should be considered. Pre-operative use of mannitol, hyperventilation, and/or dexamethasone may be useful in reducing or preventing increases in ICP prior to the surgical drainage. Steroids may provide significant benefit in situations where the surgical procedure must be delayed or is contraindicated. Any patient whose clinical presentation includes seizures should be started on an appropriate antiepileptic agent.

Suppurative Intracranial Thrombophlebitis

Predisposing conditions include abnormalities of the veins or venous sinus (including cavernous sinus thrombosis related to paranasal sinusitis or facial infections), head and neck infections, or septic dissemination from epidural abscess, subdural empyema, or bacterial meningitis. *Staph. aureus* is the most important and common causative organism. Clinical presentation includes periorbital swelling, headache, drowsiness, diplopia, photophobia, and ptosis. Additional defects include cranial nerve III, IV, and VI abnormalities; papilledema; meningismus; and dilated, sluggish pupils. Fever is noted in about 90 percent of all cases. The diagnostic procedure of choice is MRI, but if this is not available, the use of carotid arteriography with venous studies, including orbital venography, is acceptable.

The choice of empiric antimicrobials should be directed by the presumed antecedent infection (see Table 41-6). The involvement of vascular or neurosurgery may be indicated, particularly in instances where antibiotics have failed. As with any thrombophlebitis, the role of anticoagulants (heparin, for example) is considered controversial.

Encephalomyelitis

The clinical presentation does not usually suggest the etiology of the illness. An important consideration is underlying immune status. Toxoplasmosis is the most common cause of encephalitis in acquired immunodeficiency syndrome (AIDS), but other organisms to be considered in human immunodeficiency virus (HIV) disease are cytomegalovirus (CMV), other herpesviruses, cryptococcus and other fungi, *Mycobacterium, Listeria,* and *Nocardia.* The multiple other causes of encephalitis are cataloged in Table 41-7. The specific clinical syndromes associated with Arbovirus infections are given in Table 41-8. Most patients do not present with specific signs or symptoms but rather display fever, headache, altered mental status, or other behavioral changes. A focal neurologic examination requires empiric antimicrobials and diagnostic radiologic evaluation with either CT or MRI. If there is no evidence of increased ICP or intracranial mass effect, lumbar puncture should be performed. An alternative approach is a cisternal puncture if there is concern for elevated ICP and possible herniation with lumbar puncture. The use of electroencephalography (EEG) can provide useful information with respect to the localization or extent of the infection. If no diagnosis is forthcoming, one must consider a brain biopsy. For AIDS patients, further serologic evaluation for *Toxoplasma* and fungal entities may aid in the choice of empiric treatments [for example, a positive *Toxoplasma* serology would dictate the use of trimethoprim/sulfamethoxazole (Bactrim) in an encephalitic patient].

Herpes encephalitis is the most common cause of fatal nonepidemic encephalitis, and the patients are seldom immunocompromised. Although this diagnosis carries a high mortality rate if untreated, it can be successfully treated with antiviral medications. The clinical presentation of herpes encephalitis is indistinguishable from that seen with other causes of encephalitis. The findings thus include fever, headache, altered level of consciousness, personality changes, dysphasia, and autonomic dysfunction. In about 85 percent of cases, herpesvirus produces focal neurologic defects, although they may be subtle.

TABLE 41-7   Causes of Encephalomyelitis

Viral
  Herpetoviridae
    Herpes simplex virus
    Varicella zoster virus
    Cytomegalovirus
    Epstein-Barr virus
    Human herpesvirus type 6
    Herpes B virus
  Togaviridae
    Alphaviruses
    Eastern equine encephalitis virus
    Western equine encephalitis virus
    Venezuelan equine encephalitis virus
  Flaviviridae
    St. Louis encephalitis virus
    Murray Valley encephalitis virus
    Japanese B encephalitis virus
    Dengue fever virus
  Bunyaviridae
    California (La Crosse) encephalitis virus
  Picornaviridae
    Echovirus
    Coxsackievirus
    Poliovirus
    Hepatitis A virus
  Arenaviridae
    Lymphocytic choriomeningitis virus
    Lassa fever virus
  Rhabdoviridae
    Rabies virus
  Retroviridae
    Human immunodeficiency virus
    Human T-cell lymphotropic virus (myelitis)
  Paramyxoviridae
    Measles virus
    Mumps virus
  Myxoviridae
    Influenza virus
  Rubivirus
    Rubella virus
  Adenoviridae
    Adenovirus
  Filoviridae
    Marburg virus
    Ebola virus

Nonviral
  Bacterial meningitis, brain abscess
  Parameningeal infection
  Infective endocarditis
  Mycobacterium
  Listeria
  Brucellosis
  Mycoplasma
  Coxiella burnetii
  Rickettsia
  Borrelia
  Leptospira
  Treponema pallidum
  Cryptococcus
  Nocardia
  Actinomycosis
  Coccidioides
  Mucormycosis
  Histoplasma
  Toxoplasma
  Plasmodium falciparum
  Trypanosoma
  Acanthamoeba
  Naegleria
  Connective tissue diseases, vasculitis

NOTE: Conditions that may resemble encephalitis include tumor, toxic or metabolic encephalopathy, intracranial hemorrhage or hematoma, and cerebrovascular disease.

TABLE 41-8   Clinical Aspects of Arbovirus Infection

Disease	Clinical Features	Morbidity and Mortality in Patients Who Develop Encephalitis
Eastern equine encephalitis (EEE)	Mainly affects children and the elderly Abrupt onset with fulminant course Seizures are common; diffuse signs	50 – 75% mortality; 30% of survivors have severe sequelae: mental retardation, behavior changes, seizures, and paralysis
Western equine encephalitis	Mainly affects infants and the elderly Subclinical infections are common Similar to EEE but milder (except in infants)	3 – 7% mortality; sequelae less than with EEE
Venezuelan equine encephalitis	Many subclinical infections < 4% develop encephalitis Myalgias are prominent	10 – 20% mortality
St. Louis encephalitis	< 1% infected people develop encephalitis Most severe in elderly May have tremor, seizures, paresis, syndrome of inappropriate antidiuretic hormone, urinary symptoms	5 – 15% mortality; mortality increases with age; neurasthenia may be a persistent problem
Japanese B encephalitis	Most common arbovirus worldwide Mainly among children < 2% of infected develop encephalitis A vaccine is available	10 – 15% mortality, especially among children; up to 70% of survivors have neuropsychiatric sequelae
Murray Valley encephalitis	Patients frequently present in coma Rapid disease progression in infants	20 – 50% mortality; 40 – 100% of survivors have neurologic sequelae
California (La Crosse) encephalitis	Mainly affects boys (ages 3 – 10 years) Fulminant onset with seizures Rapid recovery after 2 – 5 days	< 2% mortality; up to 15% have behavioral problems or recurrent seizures

543

TABLE 41-9   Dose of Intravenous Acyclovir
for Herpes Simplex and Varicella Zoster Encephalitis
according to Renal Function

Creatinine clearance (mL/min per 1.7 m^2)	Dose Schedule
> 50	10 mg/kg every 8 h
25–50	10 mg/kg every 12 h
10–25	10 mg/mg every 24 h
0–10	5 mg/kg every 24 h
Hemodialysis (3 times per week)	5 mg/kg every 24 h
Postdialysis	6.0 mg/kg after dialysis

SOURCE: From Deeter RG, Khanderia U: Recent advances in antiviral therapy. *Clin Pharm* 5:961, 1986.

Diagnostic evaluation includes lumbar puncture, which usually demonstrates an increased WBC with a predominance of leukocytes (10 to 500/mL). Glucose is often normal to elevated, and protein may be evaluated as well. A normal CSF examination should raise concern in this clinical setting for toxic or metabolic encephalopathy. Present laboratory analysis includes DFA and improved culture techniques for the isolation of the various herpesviruses (herpes simplex virus type 2, varicella zoster virus, cytomegalovirus, and Epstein-Barr virus) and the use of herpes-specific oligonucleotide probes for polymerase chain reaction (PCR) identification of the presence of a particular herpesviral genome in the patient's CSF. MRI is the most sensitive imaging modality, but a combination of infused CT and EEG in the early stages of the illness may similarly assist in the diagnosis.

Often, even with improved diagnostic capability, we are left to treat empirically the presumed state of herpes encephalitis. The institution of acyclovir should not be delayed once the diagnosis is considered. The dosing of acyclovir must be adjusted for renal function, as shown in Table 41-9. The duration of therapy is 10 to 14 days, and patients are followed by clinical response and resolution of lesions by MRI.

For a more detailed discussion, see Chaps. 48 and 49 in *Principles of Critical Care*, 2d ed.

INFECTIONS OF THE HEAD AND NECK

KIM JOSEN

Most life-threatening infections of the head and neck originate from dental, oropharyngeal, or otorhinolaryngologic
sources. These infections are less common now than in the
preantibiotic era. Many physicians are unfamiliar with these
infections because they are infrequent and because of the
challenging head and neck anatomy. An understanding of
this anatomy, however, is necessary in order to diagnose,
treat, and anticipate the complications of life-threatening
otorhinolaryngologic infections. Figures and 42-1 and 42-2
demonstrate the potential spaces defined by natural fascial
planes as well as the surrounding sinuses, vessels, and cranial nerves. All of these spaces may communicate with one
another; hence the same process may violate multiple
spaces. Collaboration with an otolaryngologist is important
in managing most head and neck infections in critically ill
patients.

The close proximity of the structures of the head and neck
results in a shared bacterial flora. At most sites, anaerobes
outnumber aerobes by a ratio of 10:1. Immunocompromised
hosts are at risk for gram negative and staphylococcal infections. Table 42-1 is a guide to antibiotic treatment of the various otorhinolaryngologic infections in normal and compromised hosts.

Submandibular Space Infections

LUDWIG'S ANGINA

Ludwig's angina is an abscess in the floor of the mouth, usually originating from an odontogenic infection. The infection

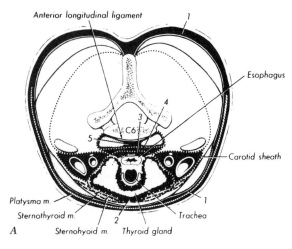

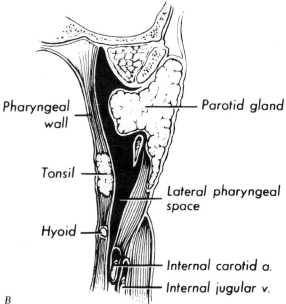

FIGURE 42-1 *(Continued on the opposite page)*

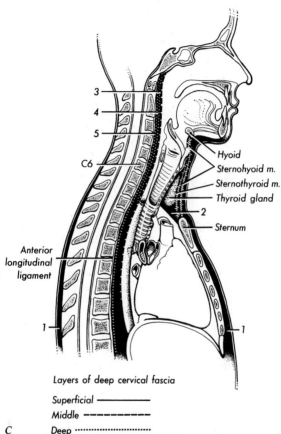

Layers of deep cervical fascia

Superficial ─────────

Middle ─ ─ ─ ─ ─ ─

C   Deep ·······················

FIGURE 42-1 (*Continued*)   Relation of lateral pharyngeal, retropharyngeal, and prevertebral spaces to the posterior and anterior layers of deep cervical fascia: 1, superficial space; 2, pretracheal space; 3, retropharyngeal space; 4, "danger" space; 5, prevertebral space. *A.* Cross section of the neck at the level of thyroid isthmus. *B.* Coronal section in the suprahyoid region of the neck. *C.* midsagittal section of the head and neck. (*From Chow AW: Infections of the oral cavity, neck, and head, in Mandell LA, Bennett JE, Dolin R (eds): Mandell, Douglas, and Bennett's Principles and Practice of Infectious Diseases, 4th ed. New York, Churchill Livingstone, 1995, p. 593.*)

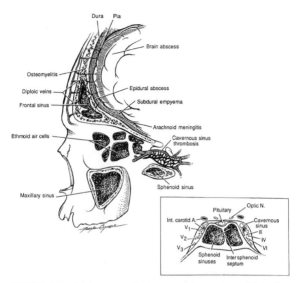

FIGURE 42-2 Major routes for intracranial extension of infection either directly or via the vascular supply. The coronal section demonstrates the structures adjoining the sphenoid sinus. *(From Chow AW, Vortel JJ: Infections of the sinuses and parameningeal structures, in Gorbach SL, Bartlett JG, Blacklow NR (eds): Infectious Diseases. Philadelphia, Saunders, 1992, p. 431.)*

spreads rapidly and bilaterally, causing a gangrenous cellulitis of the submandibular, sublingual, and submental spaces. The patient presents with fever, mouth pain, trismus, drooling, dysphagia, and tachypnea. The tongue swells, causing upward displacement against the palate or posterior displacement into the hypopharynx, thus compromising the airway. The infection may spread at alarming speed; airway obstruction may lead to death. Lateral views of the neck will demonstrate soft tissue swelling and possibly gas. Dental films may reveal the original source of infection. The usual microbes are *Streptococcus,* oral anaerobes, or both. If the infection is caught in the cellulitic phase, however, intravenous

TABLE 42-1 Alternative Empirical Antibiotic Regimens for Life-Threatening Infections of the Head, Neck, and Upper Respiratory Tract

Infection	Antibiotic Regimens	
	Normal Host	Compromised Host
Submandibular, lateral pharyngeal, and retropharyngeal infections	Penicillin G, 2–4 MU IV q4–6h; and clindamycin, 600 mg IV q8h; or metronidazole, 500 mg IV q8h; or cefoxitin, 1–2 g IV q6h	Cefotaxime, 2 g IV q6h; or ceftizoxime, 3 g IV q8h; or piperacillin, 3 g IV q4h; or imipenem, 500 mg IV q6h
Peritonsillar abscess	Penicillin G, 2–4 MU IV q4–6h; and clindamycin, 600 mg IV q8h; or cefoxitin, 1–2 g IV q6h	Cefotaxime, 2 g IV q6h; or ceftizoxime, 3 g IV q8h; or piperacillin, 3 g IV q4h
Pharyngeal diphtheria	Penicillin, 1–3 MU IV q4–6h; or erythromycin, 0.5–1 g IV q6h	Same as for normal host
Acute epiglottitis	Ampicillin plus sulbactam, 1–2 g IV q6h; or cefuroxime, 2 g IV q8h	Cefotaxime, 2 g IV q6h; or ceftriaxone, 1 g IV q12h; or cefotetan, 2 g IV q12h

ABBREVIATIONS: MU, million units; IV, intravenous.

antibiotics and close observation may suffice. Surgery is indicated if clear evidence of suppuration is present or if the patient fails to improve despite adequate medical management. Attention to the airway is paramount. If the patient develops dyspnea, an artificial airway should be placed immediately, preferably using a flexible fiberoptic scope. Tracheostomy may be necessary in order to stabilize the airway safely. Infected teeth should be extracted. The mortality rate is from zero to 4 percent.

Lateral Pharyngeal Space Infections

The danger of a lateral pharyngeal space infection is the proximity to the carotid sheath as well as the ninth to twelfth cranial nerves and sympathetic trunk. Sources most commonly responsible are dental infections, peritonsillar abscess, parotitis, otitis, and mastoiditis. Clinically, there may be trismus, swelling beneath the angle of the mandible, fevers, chills, rigors, and medial bulging of the pharyngeal wall. The infection may spread to the surrounding compartments and mediastinum, in which case surgical debridement is essential. Bacteremia, metastatic abscesses, and central nervous system (CNS) infection are all potential complications. A diagnosis of lateral pharyngeal space infection may be made with the use of a neck CT, gallium scan, or indium scans. *Bacteroides* and *Fusobacterium* are common etiologic agents. Treatment consists of prolonged intravenous antibiotics and possible surgical incision and drainage.

Retropharyngeal Space Infections

Retropharyngeal abscesses are among the most dangerous of the deep neck infections because this space is contiguous with the anterior and posterior mediastinum. In children, the onset is insidious, with fever, irritability, drooling, and possibly meningismus. The mass effect or laryngeal swelling may cause dysphagia and dyspnea. If the abscess progresses, it may cause airway obstruction. Antibiotics alone may be curative if the infection is identified early.

In adults, retropharyngeal space infections result from trauma (a swallowed chicken bone), odontogenic sepsis, and peritonsillar abscess. Computed tomography (CT) of the neck or a lateral neck film may reveal gas in the retropharyngeal area and cervical lordosis, causing anterior displacement of the larynx and trachea. Surgical exploration and drainage should be carried out immediately.

Necrotizing mediastinitis is the most life-threatening complication of retropharyngeal infections. The onset is rapid, affecting the posterior mediastinum and retropharyngeal space. It may rupture into the pleural space, with resulting empyema. Pericardial involvement may cause cardiac tamponade. Surgical intervention is mandatory in order to control the infection.

Suppurative Parotitis

Suppurative parotitis is a loculated abscess of the parotid. The patients at risk are elderly, malnourished, dehydrated, or postoperative. Obstruction of the Stensen duct from sialolithiasis is a major predisposing condition. Essentially any factor that chronically dries the mouth or traumatizes the salivary glands may lead to suppurative parotitis. There is swelling and erythema of the angle of the mandible extending to the pre- and postauricular area. Complications include osteomyelitis of the adjacent facial bones as well as extension into the lateral pharyngeal and prevertebral spaces. Staphylococci are the usual bacterial cause. The patient should be treated with intravenous antistaphylococcal antibiotics and surgical drainage.

Peritonsillar Abscess (Quinsy) and Pharyngeal Diphtheria

PERITONSILLAR ABSCESS

Peritonsillar abscess may affect patients of all ages; however, it is most common between the ages of 15 and 30 years. It is a suppurative complication of recurrent or chronic tonsillitis involving the peritonsillar space. The patient will complain of severe pain radiating to the ear a few days after the onset of tonsillitis. Odynophagia and dysphagia may cause drooling. There may be cervical adenopathy, trismus, and tilting of the head to the involved side. Physical examination reveals unilateral swelling with downward displacement of the tonsil. The uvula will be displaced to the opposite side. Intravenous penicillin should be started in order to cover mixed aerobic and anaerobic bacteria. Needle aspiration or surgical drainage is performed acutely. Failure to aspirate pus is an indication for surgical incision. Complications include airway obstruction, dissection into the lateral pharyngeal space, and aspiration of purulent material.

Acute Epiglottitis and Laryngotracheobronchitis

ACUTE EPIGLOTTITIS

Acute epiglottitis in an adult is a different disease from that seen in children. The bacteria responsible tend to be *Haemophilus influenzae B, Haemophilus parainfluenzae, Streptococcus pneumoniae, Staphylococcus aureus,* and oral anaerobes. Because of the *H. influenza B* vaccine, the occurrence of epiglottitis in children has declined; in most centers, epiglottitis is now more common in adults. Clinically, the patient complains of sore throat and odynophagia. Fever, stridor, and drooling may be present. The voice may be muffled rather than hoarse. A negative lateral soft tissue radiograph of the neck does not exclude the diagnosis. In the adult, the caliber of the airway is larger than in children. Thus, it is preferable for an otolaryngologist to confirm the suspicion of epiglottitis visually. The epiglottis will appear pale, boggy, and edematous, unlike the cherry-red epiglottis seen in children. Also, in adults, the aryepiglottic folds may be inflamed to a greater degree than the epiglottis itself. The management of adult epiglottitis requires admission to an intensive care unit. The patient should be monitored for respiratory distress, inability to handle secretions, and worsening stridor. Some 20 percent of adults will require an artificial airway. A β lactamase–resistant intravenous antibiotic should be started immediately. Because of the proclivity of *H. influenzae B* to infect the meninges, an antibiotic that crosses the blood-brain barrier should be selected.

Pericranial Infections

SINUSITIS

Figure 42-2 demonstrates the proximity of the sinuses to the surrounding structures in the skull. The complications of untreated sinusitis may lead to critical illness, but sinusitis also commonly complicates critical illness. The roof of the frontal and ethmoid sinuses is the anterior cranial fossa. A suppurative infection in these sinuses may lead to a frontal lobe or epidural abscess or to subdural empyema. A frontal or ethmoid sinusitis may lead to superior sagittal sinus thrombosis and orbital complications ranging from periorbital cellulitis to cavernous sinus thrombosis. Ethmoid sinusitis may cause an infection of the retroorbital space. The complications of sphenoid sinusitis are cavernous vein thrombosis, meningitis, temporal lobe abscess, and orbital fissure syndromes. Maxillary sinusitis may extend into adjacent structures, causing osteomyelitis, retroorbital cellulitis, proptosis, and ophthalmoplegia.

Nosocomial sinusitis is a complication of endotracheal and nasogastric intubation. It is present in at least 25 percent of patients who are intubated for more than 5 days. Local trauma to and edema of the sinus ostia as well as prolonged supine positioning may impair sinus drainage, thus creating an ideal environment for infection. The findings of nosocomial sinusitis are subtle. The patient may have an unexplained fever and leukocytosis. A sinus CT may suggest the diagnosis; however, the majority of intubated patients have air-fluid levels and mucosal thickening by 48 hours after intubation. The infection is frequently polymicrobial. When the patient fails to respond to antibiotics and decongestants, a sinus aspirate Gram stain and culture should guide antimicrobial therapy.

RHINOCEREBRAL MUCORMYCOSIS AND MALIGNANT OTITIS EXTERNA

Patients with uncontrolled diabetes or neutropenia are at risk for rhinocerebral mucormycosis, a malignant, destructive infection of the paranasal sinuses. The infection begins in the nasopharynx or nose and spreads to the sinuses, orbit, and central nervous system. These fungi are angioinvasive, causing extensive tissue infarction and thrombosis. The internal carotid artery and cavernous sinus are vulnerable to infection. Clinically, there are black, necrotic areas over the mucosa of the soft palate and nose. There may be proptosis, blindness, and cranial nerve impairment. Meningeal signs may also be present. The patient may become obtunded and comatose. The diagnosis is confirmed by demonstrating nonseptate hyphae in biopsy specimens and culture. The treatment is amphotericin B and surgical debridement. When the infection is treated early, the prognosis is good.

MALIGNANT OTITIS EXTERNA

Pseudomonas aeruginosa is the cause of malignant otitis externa; poorly controlled diabetes is the major risk factor. Clinically, there is otalgia, hearing loss, purulent discharge, edema, and granulation tissue in the external auditory canal. Initially the infection is localized to the external ear, but it may progress to cause a facial palsy and multiple cranial nerve abnormalities. The infection may spread to the temporal and occipital bones. Treatment requires prolonged antibiotics and surgical debridement.

Intracranial Suppuration

BRAIN ABSCESS

A brain abscess begins as a localized cerebritis and develops into a collection of pus surrounded by a vascular capsule. Brain abscesses are classified according to the entry point of infection (Table 42-2).

The clinical presentation of a brain abscess depends on its size and location, the virulence of the microorganism, and the

TABLE 42-2   Brain Abscesses in Adults—Source, Site, and Microorganism

Source	Site of Abscess	Microorganism
Paranasal sinus	Frontal lobe	*Streptococcus* (microaerophilic) Anaerobes
Otogenic	Temporal lobe Cerebellum	*Pseudomonas* Enterobacteriacae
Metastatic spread	Multiple lesions Especially the middle cerebral artery	Depends on original source
Penetrating trauma	Depends on site of wound	*Staph. aureus*
Postoperative		*Staph. epidermidis*

patient's underlying disease. Most patients complain of headache. If the headache is severe and abrupt, it may suggest bacterial meningitis or rupture of the abscess into the ventricular system. Nausea, vomiting, drowsiness, lethargy, and stupor may all signify increased intracranial pressure. Half of the affected patients will have fever. Therefore the absence of fever does not exclude the diagnosis. Depending on the location of infection, some patients will have focal neurologic signs.

In general, the laboratory data are not helpful in diagnosing a brain abscess. The white blood cell count and erythrocyte sedimentation rate may be normal. The utility of a lumbar puncture should be weighed against the risk of brainstem herniation. The cerebrospinal fluid (CSF) may reveal a nonspecific elevation of protein and a pleocytosis. Bacterial culture of the CSF is rarely positive.

Perhaps the most important diagnostic tool is a head CT. Abscesses have a hypodense center surrounded by a contrast-enhancing ring. They tend to form in the watershed areas between vascular distributions. MRI is also an important diagnostic tool, particularly in identifying lesions in the posterior fossa. Serial imaging studies should be used to assess the response to treatment and aid in the timing of surgery.

Stereotactic needle aspiration of the brain abscess provides material for Gram stain and culture. The Gram stain is useful for guiding the initial choice of antibiotics. The antibiotics should be selected for their ability to penetrate the abscess cavity as well as the sensitivities available after culture growth. In addition to surgical drainage, 6 to 8 weeks of parenteral antibiotics are generally recommended in order to eradicate the infection. Patients with small, peripheral lesions who are poor surgical candidates may be successfully treated without surgery. The risks of this nontraditional approach are related to complications of long-term antibiotics as well as the possibility of rupture of the abscess into the ventricular system.

Steroids are generally not recommended in the absence of life-threatening cerebral edema. Rarely, a ventriculostomy catheter may be required to relieve increased intracranial pressure. Some 25 to 50 percent of patients seize during the initial hospitalization. Anticonvulsant treatment should be initiated prophylactically at the time of diagnosis and continued for 3 months postoperatively.

SUBDURAL EMPYEMA AND CRANIAL EPIDURAL ABSCESS

In adults, subdural empyema is the result of a complicated sinusitis, mastoiditis, or otitis media. In the setting of untreated or suboptimally treated sinusitis, the initial signs of subdural empyema may be fever, purulent discharge, headache, or meningismus. Progressive infection can lead to unilateral motor seizures, hemiplegia, hemianesthesia, aphasia, and signs of increased intracranial pressure, ultimately leading to lethargy, stupor, and coma. The CSF will resemble that of aseptic meningitis.

Postcraniotomy patients and those with chronic cranial osteomyelitis are at risk for epidural abscess. There is a more focal inflammatory component than in subdural empyema, and generalized neurologic signs are uncommon. A fifth- and sixth-nerve palsy—resulting from petrous bone infection, presenting as otorrhea, retroorbital headache, and diplopia (secondary to sixth nerve palsy)—constitutes Gradenigo syndrome.

CAVERNOUS SINUS THROMBOSIS

Distinguishing between orbital cellulitis or abscess and a developing cavernous sinus thrombosis is difficult but imperative because cavernous vein thrombosis is a life-threatening condition. It results from the spread of paranasal sinusitis or orbital infections to the valveless orbital veins and ultimately to the cavernous sinus. Clinically there is bilateral orbital chemosis, ophthalmoplegia, retinal engorgement, and high fever. Treatment includes intravenous antibiotics, abscess drainage, and possibly orbital decompression. Despite timely intervention, the condition may progress to meningitis, complete visual loss, and death. Because its role is controversial, heparin is generally not given.

For a more detailed discussion, see Chap. 50 in *Principles of Critical Care,* 2d ed.

Chapter 43

THE ACUTE ABDOMEN AND INTRAABDOMINAL SEPSIS

MICHAEL WALDMAN

The term *acute abdomen* refers to the condition of a patient whose chief presenting symptom is the acute onset of abdominal pain (Table 43-1). The diagnosis depends heavily on an accurate history and a complete physical examination. However, in an intensive care unit (ICU) patient, both of these sources of data may be severely limited owing to varying levels of consciousness, the presence of an endotracheal tube as well as various other lines and tubes, and medications including narcotics, benzodiazepines, and corticosteroids. The intensivist frequently must infer the presence of an acute abdomen from nonspecific findings such as unexplained sepsis, hypovolemia, and abdominal distention. In evaluating a possible acute abdomen, one should approach the patient in the context of the underlying disorder; surgical consultants should be used liberally, and the available screening examinations (computed tomography and/or abdominal ultrasound) should be performed.

Patients in an ICU setting with an acute abdomen frequently have intraabdominal sepsis (IAS), the etiology of which is usually secondary to primary or secondary peritonitis (see Table 43-2). Primary peritonitis is characterized by an infection of the peritoneal cavity without an obvious source. This usually occurs in individuals with ascites secondary to underlying disease states, such as cirrhosis of the liver, congestive heart failure, and end-stage renal disease. Patients typically present with fever and signs of peritoneal irritation. Diagnosis is frequently made from clinical suspicion, as many patients will have no abdominal pain. Although approximately 35 percent of the patients will have negative ascitic fluid cultures, ascitic fluid aspiration is the

TABLE 43-1   Etiology of Acute Abdominal Pain

Inflammatory disorders (e.g., cholecystitis, diverticulitis,
  perforated peptic ulcer)
Colics
  Biliary
  Renal
  Intestinal obstruction
Vascular lesions
  Mesenteric ischemia
  Ruptured abdominal aortic aneurysm
  Intraabdominal or retroperitoneal hemorrhage
Urologic or gynecologic disorders
Medical disorders (e.g., lupus serositis, sickle cell crisis)

---

key to confirming the presence of primary peritonitis. An ascitic neutrophil count greater than $250/\mu L$ can be considered diagnostic. In culture-negative patients, there should be a clinical response within 48 hours of initiating appropriate antibiotics associated with a decrease in the ascitic neutrophil count. Ampicillin and an aminoglycoside or a third-generation cephalosporin alone is usually the treatment of choice.

TABLE 43-2   Classification of Intraabdominal Sepsis

Primary peritonitis
  Infected ascitic fluid
  Infected peritoneal dialysis catheter
  Miscellaneous (e.g., tuberculosis)
Secondary peritonitis
  Intraperitoneal
    Biliary tree
    Gastrointestinal tract
    Female reproductive system
  Retroperitoneal
    Pancreas
    Urinary tract
  Visceral abscess
    Liver
    Spleen

Secondary Bacterial Peritonitis

Secondary bacterial peritonitis is caused from contamination from the gut lumen, which leads to pus, gastrointestinal contents, and/or multiple organisms in the ascitic fluid. Generalized peritonitis is caused from bowel perforation, bowel infarction, infected gallbladder, infected pancreatic pseudocyst, or other diseases. Patients are subject to massive fluid loss into the abdomen and rapid absorption of endotoxin, bacteria, and inflammatory mediators into the circulation. Patients are unlikely to respond to antibiotic treatment alone and usually require surgical treatment. Broad-spectrum antibiotics should be given, including anaerobic coverage with either clindamycin or metronidazole. As broad-spectrum antibiotics put the patient at risk to develop candidiasis, pseudomembranous colitis, and drug-resistant organisms, antibiotics should be discontinued as soon as possible. Guidelines to stopping antibiotics include resolution of fever, leukocytosis, hemodynamic compromise, peritoneal signs, and ileus. If fever or leukocytosis persist, a CT scan should be obtained to search for an intraabdominal abscess. If no abscess is identified, antibiotics can be discontinued and a search for an extraperitoneal source of infection should be performed. The mortality of generalized peritonitis is about 30 percent, usually from uncontrolled sepsis.

The intensivist's role in these patients is to guide hemodynamic, ventilatory, and nutritional support, antibiotic therapy, and renal dialysis if necessary. In addition, the critical care physician should be aware of the wide variety of complications that may be seen in a postsurgical patient (see Table 43-3). The patient's wound should be examined daily. The risk for fascial dehiscence is greatest at postoperative days 4 to 8. The earliest sign is usually the drainage of serosanguinous fluid through the incision, which would require an immediate surgical consultation. All pumps and drains should also be inspected for proper function and position. The gastrointestinal tract should be evaluated for its ability to tolerate enteral feedings. In an ICU patient, this frequently requires challenging the gastrointestinal tract with tube feedings and checking residuals every 4 hours. Finally, the intensivist must

TABLE 43-3   Postoperative Complications Specifically
Related to the Surgical Treatment of Peritonitis

Wound complications
  Wound infection
  Necrotizing soft tissue infection
  Fascial dehiscence/evisceration
Gastrointestinal tract complications
  Ileus
  Mechanical obstruction
  Enterocutaneous fistula
  Gastrointestinal bleeding
  Anastomotic disruption or perforation
  Ischemic bowel
  Antibiotic-associated colitis
Complications arising in the peritoneal cavity
  Abscess formation
  Intraabdominal bleeding
Miscellaneous
  Postoperative pancreatitis
  Septicemia
  Acalculous cholecystitis

---

determine if the patient has persistent sepsis and if the source
is intraabdominal (see Table 43-4). If the patient does not show
clinical improvement postoperatively or if there is any deterioration, an abdominal CT scan should be performed. An
early postoperative patient (5 to 7 days) frequently has multiple sterile fluid collections, and computed tomography (CT)
may not be fruitful. These patients will frequently require repeat laparotomy if they deteriorate. If a well-organized abscess is identified, percutaneous drainage is the treatment of
choice.

Biliary Tract Sepsis

Biliary tract sepsis should be considered if sepsis and hyperbilirubinemia coexist. However, most jaundiced ICU patients
do not have biliary sepsis. Infection of the biliary tree usually
stems from acute calculous cholecystitis, acute cholangitis,
and acute acalculous cholecystitis. Calculous cholecystitis is

TABLE 43-4   Anatomic Sites of Bacterial Infection
in Postoperative Peritonitis

Intraabdominal
  Peritoneal fluid
  Peritoneal fibrin
  Extraperitoneal tissues (e.g., hepatic macrophages)
  Visceral abscess
  Within the gastrointestinal tract lumen ("tertiary" peritonitis,
    Clostridium difficile colitis)
  Infected prosthetic vascular graft
  Acalculous cholecystitis
Extraabdominal
  Soft tissue infection
  Pneumonia
  Urosepsis
  Intravascular catheter infection
  Disseminated candidiasis

---

usually treated by cholecystectomy and rarely requires ICU attention unless the patient has other medical conditions.

Acute cholangitis occurs as a bacterial infection within an occluded bile duct system. The clinical triad consists of right-upper-quadrant abdominal pain, jaundice, and fever. Diagnosis can be confirmed by ultrasound endoscopic retrograde cholangiopancreatography (ERCP), or a percutaneous transhepatic cholangiogram (PTC). Treatment consists of biliary tree decompression and broad-spectrum antibiotics covering gram-negative rods as well as anaerobes. If a patient does not improve clinically, it must be assumed that there is inadequate biliary decompression; thus the biliary tree should be reimaged. A CT scan to search for intrahepatic abscesses may also be necessary.

Acute acalculous cholecystitis occurs in 0.5 to 1.5 percent of long-term (> 1 week) ICU patients. Its etiology is unknown, but the gallbladder wall becomes inflamed and infected with enteric organisms while the cystic duct becomes edematous and occluded. It can be quite difficult to diagnose, although CT scans and ultrasound may be helpful with the findings of pericholecystic fluid, intramural gas, or a sloughed mucosal membrane. A negative biliary radionuclide scan effectively rules out the diagnosis. Liver function tests and percutaneous bile aspiration for culture are not helpful.

Frequently laparotomy and direct visualization of the gallbladder are required for diagnosis. In the rare patient who is unable to undergo laparotomy, percutaneous drainage of the gallbladder may be performed, with a cholecystectomy following at a later date.

Visceral Abscesses

Visceral abscesses of the spleen and liver are rare. The causes of hepatic abscesses include trauma, perihepatic sepsis, systemic bacteremia, portal bacteremia, and cholangitis, although at least 20 percent of the cases are cryptogenic. The clinical presentation is sepsis, right-upper-quadrant abdominal pain, and occasional peritoneal signs. CT scan or ultrasound may confirm the diagnosis. Percutaneous drainage is the preferred method of treatment, along with broad-spectrum antibiotics.

Splenic abscesses may form as a result of trauma, direct extension of the septic process (pancreatic abscess), infection of a splenic infarct, or bacteremia. Patients present with left-upper-quadrant pain, a left pleural effusion, or unexplained sepsis. The diagnosis can be confirmed with CT scan or ultrasound. Treatment usually requires splenectomy, although percutaneous drainage may serve as a temporizing measure.

Occult Causes of IAS

Frequently, an ICU patient will have sepsis or multisystem organ failure with no obvious cause. As other sources are ruled out, the abdomen must be considered, even in patients with no prior gastrointestinal disorders. CT is an excellent screening tool, but negative imaging studies do not rule out peritoneal infections. Often diagnostic peritoneal lavage (DPL) is a useful test in patients with occult IAS. Findings of pus, bacteria, or high leukocyte counts may clarify the need for laparotomy. Occult causes of IAS include acute acalculous

TABLE 43-5   Occult Sources
of Intraabdominal Sepsis

Acalculous cholecystitis
Small intraabdominal abscess(es)
Ischemic bowel—short segment
"Tertiary" peritonitis

---

cholecystitis, interloop abscesses, a short segment of ischemic
or necrotic bowel, and bacteremia from increased gut mucosal
permeability (see Table 43-5). Diagnostic laparotomy in the
absence of clinical information pointing to a specific etiology
rarely prevents death.

For a more detailed discussion, see Chaps. 82 and 85 in *Principles of
Critical Care,* 2d ed.

Chapter 44

URINARY TRACT INFECTIONS

IMRE NOTH

Urinary tract infections (UTI) account for 30 to 40 percent of all nosocomial infections. Some 80 percent of UTIs follow urinary catheterization. Significant bacteriuria simply means the presence of $\geq 10^5$ organisms per milliliter urine. Any level of bacteriuria in a catheterized intensive care unit (ICU) patient may indicate that the urinary tract is a cause of sepsis.

Acute Pyelonephritis

Escherichia coli is the most common etiologic agent causing acute pyelonephritis in community-acquired disease. Other prominent organisms include *Staphylococcus saprophyticus* and Enterobacteriaceae such as *Proteus* spp., *Klebsiella* spp., *Enterobacter* spp., and *Enterococcus* spp. While *E. coli* is still the most common cause of acute pyelonephritis in the hospital setting, other pathogens frequently encountered are *Pseudomonas* spp., *Enterococcus* spp., coagulase negative *Staphylococcus,* and *Candida.*

Acute pyelonephritis is a syndrome characterized by fever and signs of renal inflammation, such as costovertebral angle tenderness or flank pain. In septic patients who have had other potential sites investigated, subacute pyelonephritis should be considered as a possible etiology even when other local signs are lacking. Development of urosepsis should prompt an ultrasound examination or other imaging procedures such as computed tomography (CT) in order to exclude obstruction and papillary necrosis or to assess for a suppurative focus such as intrarenal or perinephric abscess. Ultrasound is safe, inexpensive, and obtainable at the bedside. CT is indicated in persistent sepsis as it can more readily distinguish complications of UTI such as cortical abscess, acute focal bacterial nephritis, and perinephric abscess. CT may also assist with percutaneous drainage into suppurative collections or placement of ureteric stents.

Gram stain of urine may be useful to direct therapy. A urinary culture should always be obtained prior to initiating therapy. Blood cultures should also be checked for concomitant bacteremia. Serum creatinine as a measure of renal function should also be assessed.

A wide variety of regimens are available and appropriate for empiric therapy of acute pyelonephritis. A combination of an aminoglycoside and ampicillin is most cost-effective and provides coverage against most aerobic gram-negative bacilli and *Enterococcus* spp. In hospitals where ampicillin resistance is common, vancomycin and an aminoglycoside should be considered. In patients with higher risk of aminoglycoside toxicity, one should consider using an alternative. In unstable critically ill patients, urinary drainage as well as drainage of any suppurative collections is a priority. Acute pyelonephritis requires 10 to 14 days of antimicrobial therapy. Oral agents may be started once systemic toxicity has resolved. Trimethoprim-sulfamethoxizole or a quinolone are commonly used as oral therapy.

Acute focal bacterial nephritis (AFBN) is an infection of one of the lobes of the kidney and frequently may be appreciated only by CT with contrast infusion. Differential diagnosis of this CT finding may include neoplasm, evolving renal infarct, and abscess. Renal abscess may develop when AFBN progresses to suppuration. Usual pathogens are *E. coli*, *K. pneumoniae*, and *Proteus* spp. Treatment classically involved incision and/or drainage, but a trial of antimicrobial therapy is appropriate for many patients. Perinephric abscess arises from intrarenal abscess. Perforation of the renal fascia is possible, leading to retroperitoneal space and peritoneal infection, with 50 percent mortality. Most patients can be treated with antimicrobial agents and pecutaneous drainage.

Urinary Tract Infection due to Candida

Candiduria may reflect renal infection if the patient has neutropenia, loss of mucous membrane integrity, chemotherapy, burns, steroid use, diabetes mellitus, total parenteral nutrition, upper gastrointestinal tract surgery, or broad-spectrum antibacterial therapy. Patients with otherwise unexplained features of sepsis might have candiduria as a source. Primary infection of the urinary tract is generally associated with an indwelling urinary catheter and the presence of broad-spectrum antibiotics. *Candida* casts may be present in urinary sediment. Isolation of *Candida* from respiratory secretions, wound exudate, or throat swabs should heighten concerns for systemic candidiasis.

Renal or disseminated infection requires treatment with systemic amphotericin B therapy in a dose of 0.6 mg/kg per day or fluconazole. Ketoconazole and itraconazole are not appreciably excreted through the kidney and are therefore unacceptable. In stable ICU patients with persistent candiduria, amphotericin B bladder washes (50 mg of amphotericin B in 1000 mL of sterile water administered over 24 hours by a three-way catheter) have been considered standard therapy. However, oral fluconazole for 7 days has been shown to be just as effective. Daily urine cultures should be performed after stopping the washes. Immediate relapse of candiduria is indirect evidence of renal infection and should prompt systemic amphotericin B therapy.

Prostatic Infections

Acute bacterial prostatitis and chronic bacterial prostatitis that have been surgically manipulated or instrumented may be accompanied by sudden onset of high fevers to 40°C, chills and malaise, as well as urgency, frequency, and dysuria. Rectal examination can reveal a very tender and swollen prostate. Usually a concomitant bladder infection is present with the identical pathogen as in the prostatitis and can be isolated from a urine culture. A gram-negative enteric organism is most commonly responsible. Treatment regimens are similar to those for acute pyelonephritis. Follow-up therapy with an oral agent for a total of 6 weeks is prudent to eradicate the responsible organism. A prostatic abscess should be suspected if fevers persist in the face of adequate antimicrobial therapy. Transrectal ultrasonography and CT can help identify such lesions. Definitive therapy for abscess is surgical drainage.

Catheter-Associated Bacteriuria

About 1 percent of patients will acquire bacteriuria from single "in-out" catheterizations. The risk per day is about 5 percent. Age and female sex are also risk factors. Antimicrobial resistance develops as quickly as 4 days after catheterization. Samples should always be obtained by aspiration of urine through the distal catheter or collection port after disinfection. Catheterization is necessary in many ICU patients for monitoring urine output in shock, hemodynamic instability, or polyuric renal failure and relief of lower urinary tract obstruction. Catheterization should not be used to avoid incontinence and contamination of the perineal skin. There is no need for regular scheduled replacements. Necessity of catheter usage should frequently be questioned and the catheter should be removed when feasible. Bacteremia arises in 1 to 5 percent of patients with catheter-associated bacteriuria. These cases are frequently associated with manipulation or instrumentation. Therefore all patients with bacteriuria should be treated prior to instrumentation of the urinary tract. Hospital-acquired bacteriuria may be treated with single-dose therapy in selected female patients provided that the infection is confined to the lower tract, the catheter has been removed, and no clinical suspicion of sepsis is present. Trimethoprim-sulfamethoxazole, an aminoglycoside, a third-generation cephalosporin, ticarcillin-clavulanic acid, piperacillin-tazobactam, or a quinolone to which the organism is susceptible should be used. Infections suspected in the upper urinary tract require 2 weeks of therapy of an appropriate antibiotic. Relapse requires 6 weeks of therapy.

For a more detailed discussion, see Chap. 52 in *Principles of Critical Care*, 2d ed.

Chapter 45

MISCELLANEOUS INFECTIONS

SHANNON CARSON

Tuberculosis

Tuberculosis as the primary cause for admission to the intensive care unit (ICU) is uncommon but not insignificant, occurring in 1 to 3 percent of hospitalized patients with tuberculosis (TB). As many as 20 percent of patients hospitalized with miliary or disseminated TB infection may require ICU care. Mortality from respiratory failure associated with TB infection ranges between 47 and 80 percent, a rate much higher than for nontuberculous pneumonia. Patients with disseminated infection are at higher risk for death than those with respiratory failure due to tuberculous pneumonia. Patients with tuberculosis and respiratory failure have a high incidence of acute respiratory distress syndrome (ARDS), multisystem organ failure, and disseminated intravascular coagulation (DIC), which contribute to their high mortality.

Tuberculosis should be suspected in any patient with known risk factors such as a history of exposure, alcohol or drug abuse, incarceration, or an immunocompromised state, especially individuals infected with human immunodeficiency virus (HIV). Patients presenting with apical infiltrates on chest radiographs, with or without cavitation, or infiltrates in the superior segments of the lower lobes should raise suspicion, as should any patient presenting with a chronic pneumonia that has not responded to conventional antibacterials. It is very important to recognize, however, that immunocompromised patients with reactivated disease often present with radiologic appearances typical of primary disease, including hilar or mediastinal adenopathy, mid- and lower-lung infiltrates, pleural effusions, or a miliary pattern. Up to 10 percent of HIV-infected patients may present with normal chest radiographs and positive sputum culture for TB. Diagnosis is made by acid-fast smear and culture of respiratory secretions. Bronchoscopy with BAL and transbronchial biopsy is often required; open-lung biopsy may be necessary in some cases.

TREATMENT

Tuberculosis in adults should be treated with isoniazid (INH) 300 mg daily and rifampin 600 mg daily (or 450 mg for patients weighing less than 50 kg). Pyrazinamide 20 to 30 mg/kg daily should be included for the first 2 months of therapy. Ethambutol 25 mg/kg daily should also be included if the patient is from an area at increased risk for INH-resistant TB or if the patient has disseminated disease including central nervous system (CNS) manifestations. Critically ill patients may present with difficulties in achieving adequate serum levels of antituberculous medications due to gut dysfunction. If this problem is suspected, INH and rifampin can be given intravenously and streptomycin intramuscularly.

Foreign-born patients or patients previously treated for TB are at increased risk for multidrug-resistant TB (MDR-TB), especially if they are HIV-infected. Multidrug resistance should be suspected in a patient with persistent fevers after 14 days of conventional therapy. Pending susceptibility testing, an empiric regimen for MDR-TB may include a parenteral drug (amikacin, kanamycin, or capreomycin) plus a fluoroquinolone (ciprofloxacin or ofloxacin), plus ethambutol, pyrazinamide, INH, rifampin, and cycloserine (or ethionamide or amino salicylic acid).

Risk factors for nosocomial spread of tuberculosis include close contact with infectious patients, bronchoscopy, endotracheal intubation, endotracheal suctioning during mechanical ventilation, open abscess irrigation, autopsy, and procedures that stimulate coughing. Obviously, care of a critically ill patient on a ventilator presents many of these risk factors. The greatest risk factor for nosocomial transmission is close contact with a patient who is not yet known to be infected. This situation is encountered in the ICU in patients presenting with atypical manifestations or when risk factors are not identified. Miliary patterns that are not recognized on the chest radiograph or patients presenting with advanced illness suggestive of sepsis due to more conventional causes are typical scenarios where diagnosis or suspicion of disease may be delayed or missed altogether. Nosocomial transmission of disease to health care workers has been reported to be as high as 76 percent in such circumstances. Therefore, any patient with risk factors for TB and an abnormal chest radiograph should immediately be isolated in a room that minimizes recirculation of contaminated air. Use of fit-tested high-efficiency particulate air (HEPA) filter respirators by anyone coming into contact with the patient is strongly recommended although not yet proven to be effective.

Tetanus

Tetanus is a toxin-mediated disease caused by *Clostridium tetani* and characterized by trismus, dysphagia, and localized muscle rigidity near a site of injury. It often progresses to severe generalized muscle spasms complicated by respiratory failure and cardiovascular instability. Tetanus occurs primarily in nonimmunized or inadequately immunized patients, especially the poor and the elderly. A history of proper immunization does not entirely exclude the diagnosis of tetanus, however. Tissue necrosis, foreign bodies, or concurrent anaerobic or facultative anaerobic infections allow toxin formation after inoculation of tissues. The toxin is transported to the ventral horns of the spinal cord or motor nuclei of cranial nerves, where it impairs inhibition of motor neurons and interneurons. This results in enhanced excitation and muscular rigidity. Paralysis is less common and usually localized to areas of high toxin concentration.

There are three clinical forms of tetanus; generalized, local, and cephalic. Generalized tetanus is the most common form and is characterized by diffuse muscle rigidity. Localized tetanus is characterized by rigidity of a group of muscles in close proximity to the site of injury. Cephalic tetanus, which is a variant of local tetanus, is defined as trismus plus paralysis of one or more cranial nerves. It is important to realize that both local and cephalic tetanus may progress to generalized tetanus, the latter occurring in approximately 65 percent of cases.

CLINICAL AND LABORATORY MANIFESTATIONS

The common means by which *C. tetani* enters the human host is through lacerations, especially if associated with tissue necrosis or foreign body. Tetanus can also follow burns or animal bites, septic abortion complicated by gangrene of the uterus, skin infections in intravenous drug users and, rarely, otherwise uncomplicated abdominal surgery. However, in 15 to 25 percent of cases, a portal of entry cannot be determined (cryptogenic tetanus). The interval between injury and onset of clinical symptoms is usually from 3 days to 3 weeks but occasionally as long as several months. In general, the shorter the incubation period, the more severe the disease.

Muscle rigidity is the most prominent early symptom of tetanus. Trismus, dysphagia, and opisthotonos caused by rigidity of verterbral muscles are most frequently observed. Muscular spasms are initially tonic, followed first by high-frequency and then low-frequency clonic activity. In very severe tetanus, spasms can occur so frequently that status epilepticus may be suspected and may be forceful enough to cause fractures of long bones and of the spine. Spasm-induced damage to muscles can also result in rhabdomyolysis complicated by acute renal failure. Spasms may be initiated by touch, noise, lights, and swallowing, even in the sleeping patient. Spasms severe enough to require treatment may persist for up to 6 weeks. Apnea occurs when spasms involve the respiratory muscles or larynx.

Manifestations of impaired sympathetic inhibition include tachycardia, labile hypertension alternating with hypotension, peripheral vasoconstriction, fever, and profuse sweating. Overactivity of the parasympathetic nervous system causes increased bronchial and salivary gland secretions, bradycardia, and sinus arrest.

The diagnosis of tetanus is based on clinical manifestations rather than laboratory tests. Tissue cultures are positive in less than 50 percent of patients. The major clinical features on which the diagnosis of tetanus is based are listed in Table 45-1 along with the features of other conditions with which it can be confused.

TABLE 45-1   Differential Diagnosis of Tetanus: Clinical Features

	Tetanus	Strychnine	Neuroleptics	SMS[a]	Rabies	Meningitis
Trismus	+	+	+	+	–	–
Nuchal rigidity	+	+	+	+	–	+
Risus sardonicus	+	+	–	–	–	–
Opisthotonus	+	+	+	–	+	–
Muscle rigidity continuous	+	+	+	–	+	–
Muscle rigidity intermittent	–	–	–	+	+	–
Encephalopathy	–	–	–	–	+	+
Rapid course	–	+	+	–	–	–

[a]Stiff-man syndrome.

575

TREATMENT

Patients with a presumptive diagnosis of tetanus should be admitted to an ICU. The principles of initial treatment of tetanus consist of airway management, sedation, treatment of the portal of entry, antitoxin therapy, administration of appropriate antibiotics, and general supportive measures. Drugs commonly used in the management of tetanus are listed in Table 45-2 together with their indications and doses.

Appropriate management of the airway is the first priority. Patients with diffuse rigidity, especially if unresponsive to benzodiazepine therapy, should be intubated, even in the absence of respiratory compromise. All patients who have already had a generalized spasm or with evidence of respiratory compromise, including patients with severe dysphagia who are in danger of aspiration, should be intubated. An emergency cricothyroidotomy tray should be at the bedside prior to attempted intubation. If paralysis is required to facilitate intubation, a nondepolarizing agent should be used, since depolarizing neuromuscular blocking agents (i.e., succinylcholine) may cause hyperkalemia and cardiac arrest in patients with tetanus.

Patients with muscular rigidity should be sedated with intravenous diazepam and morphine. Pancuronium, atracurium, and vecuronium are safe and effective in controlling tetanic spasms, but neuromuscular blockade may be avoided by use of dantrolene along with sedation.

Aggressive surgical treatment of tetanus-producing wounds results in improved survival. Patients with tetanus should be treated with antitoxin as soon as possible. There is evidence that in patients who have not yet progressed to generalized rigidity and spasms, intrathecal tetanus immune globulin-human (TIG-H) is more effective than intramuscular TIG-H in preventing generalization and can reduce the mortality rate. They should receive a single dose of intrathecal TIG-H (250 IU) via lumbar puncture. Preparations containing no preservatives should be used for intrathecal injections to reduce the incidence of vomiting, which is the most significant side effect. Intramuscular doses of TIG-H ranging from 3000 to 6000 IU have been suggested for patients in whom generalization has already occurred. It is important to

TABLE 45-2 Drugs Used in Medical Management of Tetanus

Medication	Indication	Dose
TIG-H[a]	Local or cephalic tetanus	250 IU intrathecal
TIG-H	Generalized tetanus	3000–6000 IU intramuscular
Penicillin G	Toxin production (given in all cases)	1×10^6 U IV q6h for 10 days
Diazepam	Cardiovascular instability and sedation	2.5–20 mg IV q2–6 h
Morphine	Sedation, spasms and analgesia	2.0–10 mg IV q1h or 1.0–2.0 mg/kg IV q12h
Magnesium sulfate	Cardiovascular instability	70 mg/kg IV load then 1–3 g IV q1h
Vecuronium	Neuromuscular blockade for severe muscle spasms	3–4 mg/h IV
Dantrolene	Rigidity and spasms	0.5–1.0 mg/kg IV q4–6h
Clonidine	Cardiovascular instability	300 µg q8h via nasogastric tube

[a]Tetanus immune globulin-human.

577

administer antitoxin prior to debridement because the toxin may be introduced into the bloodstream during manipulation.

Antibiotics are generally given both to treat infection at the injury site and to eliminate continued toxin production. Penicillin G, 1 million units intravenously every 6 h for 10 days, is the antibiotic of first choice for *C. tetani*. Metronidazole, tetracycline, erythromycin, and chloramphenicol are also effective.

Treatment of cardiovascular instability consists of deep sedation, which, if not successful, is followed by morphine using doses of up to 10 mg/h. Alternatively, successful control of autonomic dysfunction has been achieved using intermittent boluses of morphine, 1 to 2 mg/kg intravenously over 15 min every 12 h. Core body temperature should be monitored and maintained below 41°C. If magnesium sulfate is used, it is important that diazepam and morphine be continued. A loading dose of 70 mg/kg over 5 to 20 min is followed by a continuous infusion titrated to maintain serum magnesium levels between 2.5 and 4.0 mmol/L. This usually requires infusion rates of 1 to 3 g/h. Serum calcium and magnesium levels should be measured every 4 h. Calcium supplements may be required to maintain serum calcium levels above 1.7 mmol/L. Any magnesium-induced cardiac arrhythmias should also be treated with intravenous calcium. Clonidine is indicated for any patient who is not responding to magnesium. Epidural bupivacaine has also been successfully used to control autonomic dysfunction.

Early nutrition, correction of electrolyte disturbances, subcutaneous heparin prophylaxis, and prompt treatment of nosocomial infection are crucial. Finally, it is important to remember that recovery from tetanus does not guarantee natural immunity. Patients should begin their primary immunization series prior to leaving the hospital.

For a more detailed discussion, see Chaps. 47 and 55 in *Principles of Critical Care*, 2d ed.

Chapter 46
CEREBROVASCULAR DISEASE
BABAK MOKHLESI

Approximately 500,000 Americans suffer an acute stroke every year, resulting in almost 200,000 deaths. The role of the intensivist in the management of acute stroke is likely to expand, particularly with the advent of reperfusional therapy.

Cerebrovascular diseases can be divided into three categories: cerebral ischemia and infarction, intracerebral hemorrhage, and subarachnoid hemorrhage (Table 46-1).

Ischemic Stroke

ETIOLOGY AND EPIDEMIOLOGY

Cerebral ischemia and infarction are caused by processes that impair cerebral perfusion. Atherosclerosis of the large arteries from the aortic arch extending rostrally is the most common cause and accounts for approximately 65 to 70 percent of all ischemic strokes. While emboli arising from the heart cause approximately 30 percent of all cerebral infarcts, they assume more importance in intensive care unit (ICU) patients (Table 46-2). Emboli can be secondary to endocarditis, atrial fibrillation, or ventricular mural thrombus. Localized stenosis of one or more cerebral arteries in the setting of systemic hypotension may rarely result in a "watershed" infarction.

CLINICAL, LABORATORY, AND IMAGING DIAGNOSIS

Clinical and Laboratory

Ischemic strokes occur without any warning symptoms in 80 to 90 percent of patients. Transient ischemic attack precedes only 10 to 20 percent of cases. Most patients with thrombotic

TABLE 46-1 Distribution of the Major Cerebrovascular Accidents (CVA)

Type of CVA	Percentage of all Strokes	Cause/Risk Factor	Presentation
Thrombotic	40–50%	Atherosclerosis	Gradual onset, slow progression over minutes to hours
Embolic	30%	Arrhythmias, valvular abnormality, paradoxical (R→L) shunt, cardiac wall motion abnormalities	Maximum deficit at onset, lethargy, coma
Intracerebral hemorrhage	12%	Hypertension, amyloid angiopathy, coagulopathy	Acute onset of focal deficit, headache
Subarachnoid hemorrhage	8%	Berry aneurysm, arteriovenous malformation, trauma	Subtle prodrome, explosive headache, loss of consciousness in 45%

TABLE 46-2   Causes of Embolic Stroke

Arrhythmia
Endocarditis
Ventricular mural thrombus
Paradoxical embolus
Carotid or vertebral artery dissection

stroke have fluctuating symptoms that worsen over minutes to hours. On the other hand, embolic strokes usually present with maximum neurologic deficit at onset.

Thromboembolic stroke generally produces the sudden onset of focal brain dysfunction such as hemiparesis and focal neurologic deficit, including neglect, agnosia, aphasia, cortical blindness, cranial nerve dysfunction, and amnesia. Multiple small brain infarctions may mimic a metabolic or toxic encephalopathy, with depressed consciousness and minimal focal neurologic deficits. It is beyond the scope of this chapter to describe the multiple stroke syndromes based on vascular distribution.

The laboratory evaluation should include a complete blood count and chemistry profile. In the young, a search for a hypercoagulable state or endocarditis should be considered. Lumbar puncture with cerebrospinal fluid examination is extremely important to rule out meningitis if clinically indicated (Table 46-3).

Imaging

The primary goal of imaging is to differentiate between infarction and hemorrhage. Computed tomography (CT) is the

TABLE 46-3   Conditions That May Mimic Stroke

Seizures
Metabolic encephalopathy
Cerebral tumor
Bell's palsy
Hypoglycemia
Vertigo
Subdural hematoma

standard initial evaluation. It is sensitive, rapid, and can be easily performed, even on acutely ill patients. Acute intra-cerebral hemorrhage is easily identified by noncontrast CT. Intravenous contrast increases sensitivity for detecting tumor, subdural hematoma, and abscess. The ability of CT to detect acute ischemic stroke in the first 24 to 48 h is low, as cerebral infarction may not be demonstrated by CT for several days. Emergent CT is mandatory in patients being considered for anticoagulation or thrombolytic therapy. Delayed CT 48 to 72 h after the acute event may be useful to prove the diagnosis.

Cerebral magnetic resonance imaging (MRI) is more sensitive than CT for detection of infarction, especially for lacunar and posterior fossa events, but it is less available; it is also more cumbersome because of longer imaging times and a requirement of nonferromagnetic support and devices.

Echocardiography, especially transesophageal echocardiography, may help to differentiate thrombotic from embolic stroke. It is relatively insensitive in patients with no clinical or electrocardiographic evidence of heart disease. Carotid duplex scanning and transcranial Doppler ultrasonography have little to add to the ICU management or to distinguish cardioembolic from thrombotic atherosclerotic brain infarction. Cerebral angiography carries a morbidity risk of 1 percent but may be useful when there is suspicion of dissection, vasculitis, venous thrombosis, vascular malformations or aneurysm, and in anticipation of emergent endarterectomy.

Therapy

ATHEROTHROMBOTIC INFARCTION

General Management

Meticulous supportive therapy is the basis of all stroke treatment, with close attention to airway and pulmonary management, careful blood pressure management, and treatment of seizures. Patients should have endotracheal intubation if airway protection is in doubt, as when significant bulbar involvement or depressed consciousness is present. Early mobilization will decrease risk of venous thrombosis, pneumonia, and pressure sores. Patients confined to bed should receive subcutaneous heparin or intermittently pumping antithrombotic stockings. Careful fluid replacement may be required, with special attention to avoid hypoosmolarity, which may exacerbate brain edema.

Systemic arterial hypertension is common following acute stroke. In most cases, blood pressure returns to basal levels without treatment in a few days. Because of abnormal cerebral autoregulation of blood flow, any reduction in systemic blood pressure is likely to cause a decrease in cerebral blood flow and increasing ischemia. Since there are no known hazards to the brain from this spontaneous transient elevation in systemic blood pressure, it is better not to treat unless there is evidence of organ damage elsewhere (e.g., myocardial ischemia, congestive heart failure, or dissecting aortic aneurysm). In this case, it requires careful and judicious lowering with constant monitoring of neurologic status. *It should be emphasized that there is no level to which blood pressure can be reduced that does not carry the risk of further neurologic deterioration.*

Anticoagulation

A controlled trial has demonstrated no benefit from anticoagulation with heparin in patients with partial stable stroke. There are limited data that anticoagulation may be of benefit in patients with progressing stroke, even though further progression usually occurs in spite of anticoagulation. This issue is unsolved.

Thrombolytics

In 1995 the National Institute of Neurological Disorders and Stroke IV (NINDS) study of tissue plasminogen activator (t-PA) in its t-PA Stroke Trial demonstrated that intravenous t-PA improves functional status in carefully selected patients with acute ischemic stroke when instituted within 3 h of onset. Because of strict inclusion and exclusion criteria (Table 46-4), less than 5 percent of screened patients were enrolled. The dose of t-PA administered was 0.9 mg/kg (90 mg maximum), 10 percent as initial bolus over 1 min followed by continuous infusion of the remainder over 60 min

TABLE 46-4   Inclusion and Exclusion Criteria
from the NINDS t-PA Stroke Trial

Inclusion criteria
1. Age 18 through 80 years.
2. Clinical diagnosis of ischemic stroke causing a measurable neurologic deficit, defined as impairment of language, motor function, cognition, and/or gaze or vision, or neglect. Ischemic stroke is defined as an event characterized by the sudden onset of an acute focal neurologic deficit presumed to be due to cerebral ischemia after CT has excluded hemorrhage.
3. Time of onset well established to be less than 180 min before treatment would begin.
4. Prior to treatment, the following must be known or obtained: CBC, platelet count, prothrombin time (if the patient has a history of oral anticoagulant therapy in the week prior to treatment initiation), partial thromboplastin time (if the patient has received heparin within 48 h of treatment initiation), blood glucose, CT scan (noncontrast).

Exclusion criteria
1. Minor stroke symptoms or major symptoms that are improving rapidly.
2. Evidence of intracranial hemorrhage on CT scan.
3. Clinical presentation that suggests subarachnoid hemorrhage even if initial CT scan is normal.
4. Female patient who is lactating or known or suspected to be pregnant.
5. Platelet count less than $100,000/\mu L$; prothrombin time greater than 15 seconds; heparin has been given within 48 h and partial thromboplastin time is greater than the upper limit of normal for laboratory; anticoagulants currently being given.
6. Major surgery or serious trauma, excluding head trauma, in the previous 14 days, or head trauma within the previous 3 months.
7. History of gastrointestinal or urinary tract hemorrhage in the previous 21 days.
8. Arterial puncture at a noncompressible site or a lumbar puncture within the previous 7 days.
9. On repeated measurement, systolic blood pressure > 185 mmHg or diastolic blood pressure > 110 mmHg at the time treatment is to begin, or patient requires aggressive treatment to reduce blood pressure to within these limits.
10. Patient has had a stroke in the previous 3 months or has ever had an intracranial hemorrhage considered to put the patient at an increased risk for intracranial hemorrhage.

(Continued)

TABLE 46-4   *(Continued)*

11. Serious medical illness likely to interfere with this trial.
12. Abnormal blood glucose (< 50 or > 400 mg/dL).
13. Clinical presentation consistent with acute myocardial infarction or suggesting postmyocardial infarction pericarditis.
14. Patient cannot, in the judgment of the investigator, be followed for 3 months.
15. Seizure occurred at onset of stroke.

with discontinuation if intracranial hemorrhage was suspected. All patients were observed in the ICU. Anticoagulant or antiplatelet drugs were not allowed for 24 h and blood pressure was kept below 185/110 mmHg. Symptomatic cerebral hemorrhage occurred in 6 to 7 percent of treated patients and less than 1 percent in the control group. Although patients in the treatment arm had improved neurologic function at 3 months, there was no difference in mortality.

CARDIOEMBOLIC INFARCTION

Basic supportive care is the same as for atherothrombotic infarction. In carefully selected patients (Table 46-4), intravenous t-PA within 3 h is of benefit. Anticoagulation is recommended in patients with myocardial infarction, atrial fibrillation, cardiomyopathy, left ventricular aneurysm, or rheumatic valve disease. Recurrent embolic stroke is rare within the first few days. This makes the timing of anticoagulation controversial. Because of risk of hemorrhage, which tends to be highest within the first 2 weeks, some experts recommend postponing heparin therapy as much as 2 weeks.

PROGNOSIS

Early mortality in ischemic stroke is 10 to 15 percent and is due to cerebral edema with herniation or to medullary infarction involving the respiratory center. Causes of delayed death include myocardial infarction, pulmonary embolism, pneumonia, and urosepsis. Another 20 percent of surviving patients require long-term specialized care, and one-third to one-half are left with major disability. Patients who have had one stroke are at increased risk of having a second, particularly those with embolic stroke of cardiac origin.

Most functional recovery returns within 3 months. Preliminary data suggest that thrombolytic therapy may be associated with a better functional recovery.

Intracerebral Hemorrhage

Intracerebral hemorrhages (ICHs) make up 10 percent of all strokes. Hemorrhage into the basal ganglia and cerebellum occurs most commonly in middle-aged patients with long-standing hypertension. Hemorrhage into the subcortical hemispheric white matter occurs more often in younger patients due to arteriovenous malformations. Amyloid angiopathy has become increasingly more important in the elderly and is now recognized as the most common cause of nonhypertensive brain hemorrhage in the elderly. Less common causes include coagulopathy and rupture of intracranial aneurysms.

ICH usually presents with the acute onset of focal neurologic deficits. Increased intracranial pressure (ICP) is suggested by altered mental status, headache, and vomiting. Focal deficits depend on the location and size of the hemorrhage. The picture may progress over a period of minutes to hours. The stroke patient who is lethargic or comatose has probably had a hemorrhagic stroke. Acute ICH is identified by noncontrast CT.

THERAPY

The care of patients with ICH requires the same attention to the principles of general care. As in patients with cerebral infarction, blood pressure is transiently elevated, and because of impaired autoregulation of blood flow, lowering of the blood pressure may induce more ischemia to the areas surrounding the hemorrhage. Increased ICP may further reduce cerebral perfusion, and vasodilatation caused by systemic antihypertensive agents may cause further increases in ICP (for a more detailed discussion of increased ICP management, refer to Chap. 64). Rebleeding may occur in up to one-third of patients, but there is no relation to early arterial hypertension. Special attention should be paid to correction of any apparent coagulopathy. No specific medical therapy has been shown to be of value in patients with ICH. Corticosteroids do not reduce morbidity and mortality. Mannitol and hyperventilation can be effective in managing increased ICP. Decompressive surgery is indicated for significant or life-threatening mass effect unresponsive to medical therapy. Its value is best proven for cerebellar hemorrhage.

PROGNOSIS

Early mortality with intracerebral hemorrhage is high (30 to 40 percent). Most survivors achieve a good functional status or complete recovery, although approximately 20 percent of survivors require long-term care.

Subarachnoid Hemorrhage

Subarachnoid hemorrhage (SAH) often results from the rupture of a saccular berry aneurysm or an arteriovenous malformation. Head trauma is an important and frequent cause of SAH. Although 5 percent of the population harbor aneurysms, the incidence of SAH is low, approximately 30,000 per year.

SAH usually presents as an acute neurologic event, rarely causing focal neurologic findings. Prodromal symptoms are rare. The classic presentation is "the worst headache I've ever had," accompanied by decreased level of consciousness in severe cases.

The CT is falsely negative in as many as 10 to 20 percent of cases. In these patients the diagnosis requires analysis of the cerebrospinal fluid (CSF) by a lumbar puncture. CSF xanthochromia distinguishes bloody CSF from a traumatic tap. Lumbar puncture can be performed safely without a prior neuroimaging study as long as the conditions that cause increased ICP have been excluded by a careful history and neurologic examination. Cerebral angiography confirms the diagnosis and provides the necessary information to plan a surgical approach.

THERAPY

Following rupture of an intracranial aneurysm, three events commonly occur that can cause further brain damage: rebleeding, delayed ischemia (vasospasm), and hydrocephalus. Emergent clipping of a ruptured intracranial aneurysm, acute ventricular drainage for hydrocephalus, and prophylactic treatment for vasospasm by experienced neurosurgical teams have been associated with improved outcome.

Routine Management

Initial evaluation should assess airway, breathing, circulation, and neurologic function. In general, patients with a Glasgow Coma Scale (GCS) score of less than 8 should be intubated in a controlled setting, minimizing patient agitation to reduce the risk of rebleeding. The severity and prognosis of SAH is graded on the basis of clinical and radiographic criteria (Table 46-5). These scales predict the likelihood of vasospasm and death.

Routine management includes anticonvulsants, since seizure occurs in 25 percent of patients; strict bed rest; and prophylaxis for deep venous thrombosis with pneumatic compression stockings. Corticosteroids such as dexamethasone may reduce head and neck pain caused by the irritative effect of blood, but there is no evidence that they are helpful in managing cerebral edema. Fever commonly accompanies SAH and is treated symptomatically with antipyretics. Volume contraction should be avoided by liberal enteral hydration (see below). Nimodipine 60 mg every 4 h for 21 days from the time of hemorrhage is recommended to reduce the incidence and severity of vasospasm and delayed ischemia.

Rebleeding

Rebleeding is most common in the first 24 h. The cumulative risk after 1 week is approximately 20 percent. Mortality of rebleeding is about 50 percent. Avoidance of hypertension, cough, and Valsalva maneuver are crucial. Antifibrinolytics can reduce the risk of rebleeding, but they increase the incidence of hydrocephalus and vasospasm. With early surgery, antifibrinolytics have become less useful. Most experienced teams operate on the majority of patients in grades I to III on

TABLE 46-5   The Hunt-Hess and the World Federation of Neurologic Surgeons Scales

HUNT-HESS SCALE	
Grade	Criteria
I	Asymptomatic or mild headache
II	Moderate to severe headache, nuchal rigidity, with or without cranial nerve deficits
III	Confusion, lethargy, or mild focal symptoms
IV	Stupor and/or hemiparesis
V	Comatose and/or extensor posturing

WORLD FEDERATION OF NEUROLOGIC SURGEONS SCALE		
Grade	Glasgow Coma Scale	Motor Deficits
I	15	Absent
II	14–13	Absent
III	14–13	Present
IV	12–7	Present or absent
V	6–3	Present or absent

FISHER SCALE (BASED ON INITIAL CT APPEARANCE AND QUANTIFICATION OF SUBARACHNOID BLOOD)

1. No SAH on CT
2. Broad diffusion of subarachnoid blood, no clots and no layers of blood greater than 1 mm thick
3. Either localized blood clots in the subarachnoid space or layers of blood greater than 1 mm thick
4. Intraventricular and intracerebral blood present, in absence of significant subarachnoid blood

the Hunt-Hess scale in the first 24 to 48 h. The timing of surgery in patients with grade IV or V on the Hunt-Hess scale remains controversial.

Acute Hydrocephalus

The hallmark of symptomatic hydrocephalus is a diminished level of consciousness. It can develop very quickly after SAH and can be diagnosed reliably with CT. Since less than half the patients with CT evidence of hydrocephalus will deteriorate clinically, ventriculostomy is usually reserved for those with a diminished level of consciousness.

Hyponatremia and Intravascular Volume Contraction

A total of 30 to 50 percent of SAH patients develop this entity when given volumes of fluids intended to meet maintenance levels (also referred to as *cerebral wasting syndrome*). Administration of large volumes (5 to 8 L/day) of normal saline prevents hypovolemia and decreases vasospasm. In SAH patients with hyponatremia, the volume of fluids should never be restricted; instead, only free water should be limited.

Vasospasm

Patients at highest risk for vasospasm are those with Hunt-Hess grades III through V and Fisher grades 3 or 4, with peak risk from days 5 to 10. Vasospasm presents as a decline in the global level of function or a focal neurologic deficit. Angiography and/or transcranial Doppler may be useful to confirm the diagnosis.

Hemodynamic augmentation (hypervolemic/hypertensive therapy) is delivered by intravenous administration of normal saline to achieve an optimal intravascular volume, even though this volume is unknown. Patients should be monitored with pulmonary artery catheters and arterial lines. The mean arterial pressure (MAP) should initially be raised 15 to 20 percent. The MAP is increased progressively until the neurologic deficit is completely resolved or risk of toxicity becomes unacceptable. Dobutamine to increase cardiac output has also been used. It has not yet been determined whether the optimal therapy is to enhance cardiac output, MAP, or both. Once started, it is continued for 3 to 4 days with gradual weaning. Its complications include congestive heart failure and volume overload.

PROGNOSIS

Aneurysmal SAH remains a devastating neurologic problem with up to 25 percent of patients dying within 24 h with or without medical attention. Of those patients that survive, more than half are left with neurologic deficits as a result of the initial hemorrhage or delayed complications. One year mortality approaches 50 to 60 percent. Without surgical repair, the annual rebleed rate is near 3 percent. SAH secondary to head trauma has a better prognosis.

For a more detailed discussion, see Chap. 58 in *Principles of Critical Care*, 2d ed.

Chapter 47

STATUS EPILEPTICUS

SARAH YOUNG

Status epilepticus is a severe form of seizure activity in which seizures do not cease or are so frequent that patients do not recover consciousness between successive episodes. Status epilepticus requires timely diagnosis and management in order to prevent brain damage from recurrent electrical activity and the multiple systemic complications which ensue.

Many types of seizures, including both convulsive and nonconvulsive types, may progress to status epilepticus. (Table 47-1). Nonconvulsive status epilepticus may be very difficult to identify and should be considered in any patient with altered consciousness. The diagnosis can be made promptly by electroencephalography (EEG), and patients should be treated as aggressively as those with tonic-clonic activity to prevent brain damage.

Other conditions that may be confused with status epilepticus include decorticate posturing, tetany, spasticity, spinal seizures, and repetitive movements secondary to psychiatric disorders. An EEG can help distinguish between these conditions and status epilepticus.

The prognosis in status epilepticus depends largely on the underlying condition (Table 47-2). Patients with a history of epilepsy who present with worsening seizure activity usually respond readily to pharmacologic interventions. Patients who have suffered an acute neurologic insult [e.g., trauma, cerebrovascular accident (CVA), central nervous system (CNS) infection, or anoxic damage] can be refractory to many pharmacologic interventions. The longer the duration of seizure activity, the greater the potential for CNS damage. Repeated seizures result in damage to neurons from repetitive electrical activity as well as multiple systemic complications from tonic-clonic activity. Cardiovascular complications include both bradycardia and tachycardia as well as arrhythmias that may be exacerbated by metabolic derangements and drug

TABLE 47-1   Types of Seizures That Can Be Manifest
as Status Epilepticus

Convulsive	Nonconvulsive
GENERALIZED SEIZURES	
Tonic-clonic (grand mal)	Absence (petit mal)
PARTIAL SEIZURES	
Partial seizures (simple or complex) generalizing to tonic-clonic seizures	Simple partial seizures (no change in consciousness)
	Somatomotor (Kojevnikov's)
	Aphasic
	Complex partial seizures (altered consciousness)
	Confusional state

interventions. Respiratory complications range from respiratory arrest to tachypnea secondary to acidemia and hypercarbia. Respiratory arrest may be precipitated by benzodiazepines administered for control of seizure activity or by the underlying CNS pathology. Patients with status epilepticus are also at great risk for aspiration and inability to protect their airway due to their altered consciousness. Rhabdomyolysis with subsequent renal failure is another potential systemic complication. Status epilepticus is often complicated by profound metabolic disturbances such as lactic acidosis, hyperkalemia, hyponatremia, and hypoglycemia as well as autonomic disturbances such as hyperpyrexia and diaphoresis.

Management of status epilepticus requires meticulous attention to the patient's airway, breathing, and circulation (ABCs) (Table 47-3). The patient should be evaluated promptly to determine the need for endotracheal intubation, the adequacy of oxygenation and ventilation, and the existence of any cardiovascular complications. A detailed history should be taken and physical examination performed, focusing on potential causes of the patient's seizure. An EEG and brain imaging should be obtained to help in diagnosis. Magnetic resonance imaging (MRI) is the preferred method of imaging in patients with epilepsy; otherwise, a more readily available computed tomography (CT) scan can be substituted.

TABLE 47-2   Causes of Seizure Activity

Metabolic
  Fever
  Hypoglycemia/hyperglycemia
  Hypocalcemia
  Hypernatremia/hyponatremia
  Uremia
  Hypomagnesemia
  Hepatic failure
  Thyrotoxicosis/hypothyroidism
  Drugs/toxins
    Alcohol withdrawal
    Benzodiazepine withdrawal
    Cocaine
    Amphetamines
    Heroin
    Tricyclic antidepressant
    Lidocaine
    Aminophylline
    Lithium
    Lead
    Mercury
Infectious
  Meningitis
  Encephalitis
CNS lesions
  Trauma
  Brain tumors
    Primary CNS tumors
    Metastatic tumors
  Arteriovenous malformations
  Cerebrovascular disease
  Congenital malformations
Eclampsia
Pseudoseizures

Patients who are febrile or for whom there is a suspicion of bacterial meningitis should undergo lumbar puncture (LP) to rule out bacterial meningitis. A mild cerebrospinal fluid (CSF) pleocytosis is to be expected in patients with seizure activity (Fig. 47-1).

TABLE 47-3 Treatment Protocol with Time Frame of Intervention

Time Frame min	Treatment Protocol
0–5	Assess cardiorespiratory function, obtain history, and perform neurologic and physical examination. Take blood for antiepileptic drug levels, glucose, blood urea nitrogen, electrolytes, metabolic screen, and drug screen. Insert oral airway and administer oxygen only if needed.
6–9	Start intravenous infusion with saline solution. Administer 25 g of glucose and thiamine.
10–30	Administer lorazepam, 4 to 8 mg IV. Begin infusion of fosphenytoin, 20 mg/kg, at a rate no faster than 150 mg/min. This may take 20–40 min. Monitor ECG and blood pressure. If patient is having serial seizures, begin with fosphenytoin IV or IM and use lorazepam, in small doses as needed.
	If seizures persist, give phenobarbital, 10 mg/kg given at 100 mg/min intravenously, or midazolam, 0.2 mg/kg loading dose and maintenance as needed.
	If seizures persist, coma or general anesthesia with agents with which the facility is familiar should be started (pentobarbital, propofol).

As soon as the diagnosis of status epilepticus is made, pharmacologic treatment should begin to prevent the neurologic morbidity associated with sustained seizure activity (Table 47-4). The first line of therapy is benzodiazepines and phenytoin (fosphenytoin). Lorazepam is the preferred benzodiazepine because of its long duration of action in the CNS and acute onset of action. When using benzodiazepines, one must always be alert for respiratory depression, especially in this setting, where the patient's underlying acute event may further suppress respirations. Phenytoin or fosphenytoin should be used in conjunction with lorazepam to maintain its antiseizure effect. Phenytoin is very effective in controlling seizure activity and is now safer to administer in the form of fosphenytoin, a water-soluble disodium phosphate ester that

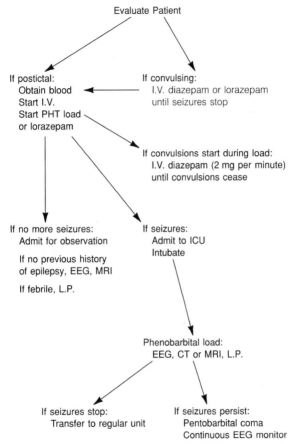

FIGURE 47-1   Diagnostic and treatment flowchart for status epilepticus.

does not need propylene glycol in its formulation. The propylene glycol phenytoin formulations is thought to be responsible for the hypotension and cardiac arrhythmias seen in patients receiving phenytoin. Seizures not controlled by

TABLE 47-4   Pharmacologic Treatment of Status Epilepticus

Drug Therapy	Dose
Lorazepam	4–8 mg IV
Phenytoin	20 mg/kg IV at no greater than 50 mg/min
Phenobarbital	10 mg/kg IV at 100 mg/min
Midazolam	0.2 mg/kg IV, then maintenance drip

phenytoin and lorazepam may be successfully controlled with parenteral phenobarbital.

Finally, status epilepticus refractory to multiple drugs deserves the attention of an experienced neurologist and an intensivist. In their hands, inducing anesthesia with propofol or a midazolam drip may abort seizures. This always requires intubation and mechanical ventilation. Pentobarbital coma has also been used for refractory seizures. After a loading dose of pentobarbital, the pentobarbital dose is titrated to maintain a burst suppression pattern on the EEG. The use of pentobarbital requires frequent EEG monitoring.

For a more detailed discussion, see Chap. 59 in *Principles of Critical Care,* 2d ed.

Chapter 48

COMA, PERSISTENT VEGETATIVE STATE, AND BRAIN DEATH

MATTHEW H. TRUNSKY

Coma is the manifestation of acute brain failure, defined as a state of "unarousable psychologic unresponsiveness in which the subject lies with eyes closed." A causal observer would see the person as sleeping, yet closer inspection would reveal that there was no purposeful response to the environment or to verbal, tactile, and painful stimuli. The ascending reticular activating system (ARAS), which is responsible for controlling the normal sleep/wake cycle, is depressed in the comatose state, either by primary brainstem disorders (e.g., infarction or hemorrhage), transtentorial herniation, or diffuse brain dysfunction arising from toxic and metabolic disorders. Various stages of consciousness including obtundation and stupor exist, but use of these terms is often misleading. Accurate descriptions of the level of consciousness are therefore preferred.

There are other clinical conditions that may be misdiagnosed as coma. The following are included in this category: (1) Hypersomnia, characterized by excessive somnolence. This often occurs as a result of sleep-disordered breathing, narcolepsy, psychiatric disorders, and hypothyroidism. (2) Locked-in syndrome, in which all skeletal muscle is paralyzed. Preserved are consciousness and sensation as well as vertical eye movements, making communication possible. (3) Akinetic mutism, in which patients appear to be awake but have no movement or response to the environment. Careful attention must be paid to ensure that these diagnoses are excluded.

Persistent vegetative state (PVS) is a chronic disease that occurs after severe brain injury. PVS differs from coma in that these patients regain sleep/wake cycles with preserved brainstem function, allowing independent breathing, yet they lack any cognitive function and therefore have no meaningful interaction with their environment. With good nursing care, these patients can live for years. This has raised both legal and ethical concerns.

Acute deterioration in mental status is a medical emergency that requires immediate evaluation. By answering the three following questions, a rapid diagnosis can often be made and the appropriate therapy initiated.

1. Is there a systemic illness causing brain failure?
2. Is there evidence of diffuse or focal brain injury?
3. Is the patient improving or deteriorating?

The most common causes of mental status deterioration in the hospital are metabolic derangements and toxic ingestions (Table 48-1). To evaluate the first question, therefore, a detailed physical examination must be performed with attention focused on identifying signs of infection. Equally important are the laboratory tests (Table 48-2) necessary to evaluate metabolic causes of a decreased level of consciousness. Often, the examination and supporting laboratory data yield the underlying diagnosis.

The second question is addressed by a limited neurologic examination that focuses on the five variables outlined in Table 48-3. The single most important sign that helps to distinguish patients with a metabolic or toxic cause from those who have a structural cause of coma is the presence of a pupillary light response. Other signs suggestive of a metabolic source of coma include confusion, asterixis, myoclonus, and tremor. Central hyperventilation often occurs with metabolic disorders, compensating for an underlying acidosis that often coexists.

Decreased responsiveness with focal and asymmetrical neurologic findings, on the other hand, is generally supportive of a structural supratentorial brain lesion. Careful examination can often help to localize the involved area. These lesions present with specific brainstem findings that precede the onset of coma, and careful cranial nerve examination is especially important when there is concern for a structural mass.

TABLE 48-1   Metabolic Causes of Coma

1. Hypoxia: decreased P_{O_2}, anemia, cyanide poisoning, carbon monoxide poisoning, methemoglobinemia
2. Ischemia: cardiac arrest, shock, blood hyperviscosity, cerebral arterial spasm after subarachnoid hemorrhage, disseminated intravascular coagulation, systemic lupus, multifocal embolism, hypertensive encephalopathy, arteritis
3. Hypoglycemia
4. Cofactor deficiency: thiamine, niacin, pyridoxine, vitamin B_{12}, folate
5. Infections: meningitis, encephalitis, postinfectious demyelinating encephalomyelitis, brain abscess
6. Hepatic or renal failure
7. Systemic diseases: septicemia, paraneoplastic syndromes, hypothyroidism, porphyria
8. Exogenous toxins and drugs: benzodiazepines, opiate analgesics, barbiturates, anticonvulsants, salicylates, ethanol, tricyclic antidepressants, anticholinergics, phenothiazines, amphetamines, cocaine, lithium, monoamine oxidase inhibitors, antihistamines, lysergic acid diethylamide (LSD), paraldehyde, methanol, ethylene glycol, cimetidine, heavy metals, organophosphates, penicillins
9. Fluid and electrolyte disorders: hypo- and hypernatremia, hypo- and hyperosmolality, acid-base disorders, extreme values of calcium, magnesium, phosphorus
10. Hypothermia and heat stroke

TABLE 48-2   Emergency Laboratory Tests for Metabolic Coma

1. Venous blood: hemoglobin, white blood count, platelets, glucose, electrolytes, calcium, blood urea nitrogen, creatinine, osmolality, coagulation studies, liver function tests, muscle enzymes, thyroid and adrenal functions, toxicology screen, blood cultures
2. Arterial blood: pH, P_{CO_2}, P_{O_2}, carboxyhemoglobin, ammonia
3. Urine: toxicology, microscopic examination
4. Gastric aspirate: toxicology
5. Cerebrospinal fluid: cell count and gram stain, protein, glucose, culture, counterimmunoelectrophoresis, viral and fungal antigens, and antibody titers

TABLE 48-3 The Neurologic Examination in Patients with Acute Deterioration in Mental Status

Response	Clinical interpretation
Response to external stimuli	
Follows command, responds to touch	Intact brainstem and cerebral function
Purposeful (attempts to remove noxious stimulus)	Intact brainstem and intact connection to appropriate cerebral hemisphere
Eye opening (spontaneous or response to stimulus)	Preserved function of ARAS in the upper brainstem and hypothalamus
Motor response	
None	Severe brain damage (terminal coma) or severe sedative drug ingestion
Decerebrate (extensor) posturing	Bilateral cerebral hemispheric damage or toxic metabolic brainstem depression
Decorticate (flexor) posturing	Destructive lesion of the midbrain and upper pons or severe metabolic insults
Withdrawal from pain	Purposeful—intact brainstem and cerebral function
Pupillary responses	
Small, reactive pupils	Metabolic brain disease and/or increased intracranial pressure with hypothalamic dysfunction
Pinpoint pupils responsive to naloxone	Narcotic overdose
Bilateral fixed and dilated pupils	Seizures, severe anoxic ischemia, exogenous catecholamines or anticholinergic agents
Midposition and fixed pupils	Sympathetic and parasympathetic failure at the level of the midbrain, seen in brain death
Unilateral, fixed, and dilated pupils	Usually implies damage to ipsilateral third cranial nerve

Eye movements

Spontaneous, roving, horizontal, and conjugate movements	Intact brainstem, but do not require that the frontal or occipital cerebral cortex be functioning
Conjugate lateral deviation of eyes	Massive hemispheric lesion (eyes deviate toward lesion) or pontine lesion (eyes deviate away from lesion)
Dysconjugate deviation of eyes	Nonspecific, seen in coma of many etiologies
Doll's-eye reflex	Normal sleep, coma, PVS—implies intact connections between the afferent sensory nerves in the neck, the vestibular nuclei (medulla), the nuclei of the third and sixth cranial nerves, and medial longitudinal fasciculus
Loss of oculovestibular reflex	Destruction or compression of brainstem, ototoxic drugs, vestibulosuppressant drugs, neuromuscular blocking agents, preexisting vestibular disease

Pattern of breathing (nonintubated, spontaneously breathing patients)

Cheyne-Stokes respirations (phases of hyperpnea regularly alternating with apnea)	Frontal lobe damage, either unilateral or bilateral; also occurs in severe cardiac failure, metabolic brain dysfunction, hypertensive encephalopathy, and occasionally in normal sleep
Central neurogenic hyperventilation	Upper brainstem damage; also occurs with sepsis, metabolic derangements, intoxications (salicylate), psychogenic causes, and CNS infection, hemorrhage, or neoplasm
Apneustic breathing (prolonged pause after full inspiration)	Discrete lesion at the level of the mid- or caudal-pontine level
Ataxic breathing (irregular pattern with random deep and shallow breaths)	Medullary damage, not compatible with long-term survival

ABBREVIATIONS: ARAS, ascending reticular activating system; PVS, persistent vegetative state.

The initial evaluation of coma, therefore, requires careful examination, a search for sepsis, and assessment for potential metabolic derangements. Analysis of blood, urine, sputum, and cerebrospinal fluid is generally indicated. Computed tomography (CT) of the head remains the imaging technique of choice, since this test is excellent for identifying supratentorial lesions as well as intracranial bleeding. While magnetic resonance imaging (MRI) may be more sensitive for identifying some lesions, it is generally more difficult to obtain in a timely fashion and is technically difficult to carry out in intubated patients. Lumbar puncture is essential in the diagnosis of both meningitis and encephalitis and often makes the diagnosis of subarachnoid hemorrhage (SAH), which is generally poorly identified on CT. When concern for increased intracranial pressure exists, CT scanning should precede lumbar puncture; ventriculostomy can then be safely performed. Occasionally, a cerebral angiogram is also used when the diagnosis of SAH due to aneurysm or vascular malformations is likely. Electroencephalography (EEG) is useful to identify metabolic causes of encephalopathy but poor at distinguishing between them. Rarely, an EEG will also diagnose subclinical status epilepticus. With the exception of the somatosensory evoked potential response (SSER), the use of evoked potentials has been unhelpful. These responses may be present in some patients in whom the EEG is isoelectric and has correlated with prognosis in specific groups.

Hypoxic-ischemic encephalopathy is a common cause of coma in the intensive care unit. Chiefly responsible for this are cardiac arrests, during which there is decreased blood flow to the brain. Other causes include severe hypotension, cardiac failure, strangulation, cardiopulmonary bypass, status epilepticus, diffuse cerebral atherosclerosis, increased intracranial pressure, cerebral artery spasm, closed head trauma, hyperviscosity, and hypoxemia. The pathogenesis of the encephalopathy is probably more complex than simply a decreased blood flow. The level of brain injury depends on the mismatch between the brain's metabolic demands and the supply of oxygen and glucose. At colder temperatures, the metabolic demands of the brain are less and the injury may be less severe, while the injury may be worse during states in which the metabolic demand is increased (e.g., status epilepticus). Some data now suggest that an exaggerated hyperemic reperfusion may reduce the extent of brain damage. Investigation with calcium-channel-blocking agents and excitatory amino acid antagonists is currently under way.

The length of time that coma persists is also correlated with the likelihood of survival. Patients who are in coma for less than 12 h often make a full recovery, while those in coma longer than 1 week generally fail to recover consciousness. Early prognostic signs that predict a poor recovery after cardiopulmonary resuscitation (CPR) include lack of corneal reflexes and pupillary responses.

The treatment of coma is emergent, and there are several supportive measures that must be initiated while the evaluation is taking place. An airway is mandatory, both to provide adequate oxygenation as well as to assure protection from aspiration, a potentially fatal complication. Care must be taken to avoid injury to the cervical spine in patients with trauma and arthritis. Equally important is the maintenance of an adequate blood pressure and circulating volume. Hypotension clearly potentiates cerebral ischemia, while hypervolemia, especially of hypotonic solutions, may increase intracranial pressure. In shock, it may be necessary to use vasopressors and inotropic agents.

Several therapies should be offered to all patients when the cause of coma is unknown (Table 48-4). Glucose (50 mL of 50% glucose) along with thiamine (100 mg IM or IV) should be administered quickly. Seizures, regardless of cause, must be stopped. Increased intracranial pressure must be treated

Table 48-4   Emergency Treatment for Coma

1. Protect airway and provide oxygen
2. Evaluate for trauma and stabilize spine
3. Support and maintain circulation
4. Administer glucose, thiamine, and naloxone
5. Treat intracranial hypertension
6. Stop epileptic seizures
7. Treat infections
8. Treat hypothermia
9. Correct electrolyte and acid-base disorders
10. Give specific antidote for identified toxins

aggressively with mannitol and hyperventilation treated acutely and then monitored continuously. Sources and mechanisms of shock should be sought promptly and treated aggressively and hyperthermia reversed. Indeed, mild hypothermia exerts a protective effect on the brain. Prophylactic antibiotics may be considered, although they have not been proven to improve survival. Specific interventions such as surgery (for subdural hematoma) and antidotes (for drug poisonings) should be initiated in the appropriate setting.

There is no accurate way to identify which patients with coma will evolve to a persistent vegetative state. However, the clinical course of PVS depends in part on its cause. A classification system exists which describes three broad categories: (1) acute traumatic and nontraumatic brain injuries, (2) degenerative and metabolic disorders, and (3) severe congenital malformations of the central nervous system. In general, recovery from a posttraumatic PVS is unlikely after 12 months and from a nontraumatic PVS after 3 months. Similarly, patients with degenerative or congenital reasons for PVS are unlikely to recover. The life expectancy for patients in PVS is 2 to 5 years, and survival beyond 10 years is uncommon.

Brain death was defined by the President's Commission in 1981. The Uniform Determination of Death Act states that "an individual who has sustained either (1) irreversible cessation of circulatory and respiratory functions, or (2) irreversible cessation of all functions of the entire brain, including the brain stem, is dead. A determination of death must be made in accordance with accepted medical standards." Even with this definition, however, there is still much confusion regarding how to declare death.

With all of the technology available to physicians, the diagnosis of brain death (i.e., death) still remains one that is made clinically. Two preconditions for this declaration must exist. First, the cause of coma must be known. Second, the known cause must be adequate to explain the coma. Yet intensivists must pay careful attention to other possible preconditions (e.g., hypothermia or overdose of sedative medications) that require serial evaluations or confirmatory testing.

The determination of death by neurologic criteria must demonstrate several clinical features. Patients must not have any response to stimuli including loud noises, bright lights, or pain. Decerebrate and decorticate posturing requires intact brainstem functioning and is therefore incompatible with the diagnosis of death. Additionally, brainstem functions including the pupillary light response, and oculocephalic, oculovestibular, corneal, and oropharyngeal reflexes must all be absent. Apnea testing, during which adequate oxygenation is maintained, is positive if the Pa_{CO_2} increases to > 60 torr without an attempt to breathe by the patient.

Irreversibility can often be suggested by CT scan. However, care must be taken to exclude several diagnoses that cause diffuse damage to the brain, such as cerebral hypoxia, uremia, hepatic failure, drug intoxication, meningitis, and encephalitis. In these circumstances, confirmatory testing may be required.

The possibility of recovery must also be excluded. The most common conditions that cause coma and are reversible include hypothermia, drug intoxications, severe hypotension, and neuromuscular paralysis. Therefore, the determination of brain death cannot be made until the patient has a core body temperature > 35°C and until all possibly offending drugs have been metabolized or removed. Finally, an appropriate period of observation is necessary before making the determination of brain death. Depending on the underlying cause, 12 to 24 h is generally adequate.

Several confirmatory tests exist when the diagnosis of brain death remains in doubt. The EEG remains a standard test for the diagnosis of brain death in many hospitals but is not necessary when the clinical diagnosis is certain. However, if concern about the diagnosis remains, the EEG is useful and may help to exclude sedative drug intoxication when the CT scan is normal. Four-vessel cerebral angiography showing complete absence of cerebral circulation is an absolute confirmation of brain death. Radioisotope brain scanning may also be helpful by documenting absent blood flow, but it cannot image the vertebrobasilar circulation. Transcranial Doppler sonography can provide noninvasive confirmation of the absence of blood flow but is technically unsuccessful in about 10 percent of patients because of skull thickness. This test is also incapable of imaging the vertebrobasilar system.

It is crucial for intensive care physicians to be familiar with brain death criteria as well as the specific policies of their own hospitals. Organs that could be made available for transplantation are lost every day because of confusion about the diagnosis of brain death. Furthermore, many physicians are uncomfortable about approaching families to request permission for organ donation. Families often have difficulty accepting the diagnosis of death because the ventilator continues to operate and the cardiac monitors continue to show a viable cardiac rhythm. While families require time to process the information, physicians should be firm in their diagnosis and explain that the "machines" function only as organ support, not as life support. Religious guidance may be helpful both in allowing the family to process the loss as well as in securing organs for donation. In the event that organ donation is refused by the family, the ventilator should be discontinued in a timely fashion.

For a more detailed discussion, see Chap. 61 in *Principles of Critical Care,* 2d ed.

Chapter 49

BLEEDING DISORDERS
WILLIAM M. SANDERS

Bedside and Laboratory Diagnosis of Coagulopathies

The diagnosis of a bleeding disorder begins with a careful history and physical examination followed by appropriate screening laboratory tests. The history can provide information about preexisting congenital or acquired bleeding diathesis as well as preexisting organ dysfunction that can predispose to bleeding—such as liver or kidney disease. A list of medications recently taken is essential—especially anticoagulants and platelet inhibitors such as nonsteroidal anti-inflammatory drugs (NSAIDs)—and may point directly to the cause of the coagulopathy.

The physical examination can reveal whether bleeding is strictly a local, possibly surgical problem or a manifestation of a systemic bleeding diathesis requiring further investigation. If multiple bruising or bleeding sites are identified or if the extent of bleeding exceeds the known injury or trauma, a systemic bleeding diathesis should be suspected. The physical exam may also provide clues as to the nature of the bleeding diathesis. Vascular and platelet disorders are characterized by *immediate bleeding*—continued, prolonged bleeding after injury as well as pronounced petechial and mucosal manifestations. Problems of fibrin generation or fibrinolysis manifest in *delayed bleeding*—rebleeding after hemostasis with prominent ecchymoses, deep muscle bleeding, and hemarthrosis. Complex coagulopathies, such as disseminated intravascular coagulation, may manifest both immediate and delayed bleeding.

Several considerations are important in the initial evaluation of a bleeding patient. First, coagulopathy should not be invoked as the cause of bleeding until uncomplicated vascular injury as a result of trauma or surgery is ruled out. Second, brisk bleeding is rarely due to coagulopathy alone and should prompt a search for a surgically correctable lesion. Third, clinically significant hemorrhage is often the result of coagulopathy superimposed on a trauma or injury, such as a peptic ulcer. Fourth, screening laboratory tests of patients in the intensive care unit may predict who is at risk for bleeding complications due to either preexisting lesions or invasive procedures.

Appropriate screening laboratory tests for a bleeding disorder in a critically ill patient should include a platelet count, an examination of the peripheral smear looking for schistocytes and platelet number and appearance, and a measurement of bleeding time, prothrombin time (PT), activated partial thromboplastin time (PTT), thrombin time, fibrin degradation products (FDP), and a D-dimer assay. These tests should be done simultaneously rather than sequentially (Table 49-1).

Defects in the formation of a platelet plug after vascular injury prolong the bleeding time. Defects in the clotting cascade hamper the formation of a definitive fibrin plug and can often be detected as a prolongation of in vitro clotting times, such as the PT and PTT. The thrombin time depends on the final step of the clotting cascade (the conversion of fibrinogen to fibrin) and can detect abnormalities of fibrinogen as well as the presence of inhibitors of fibrin formation such as heparin. Excessive fibrinogenolysis and fibrinolysis can lead to clot instability and are manifest by an increase in FDP and D-dimer. D-dimer is specific for fibrinolysis and indicates that a consolidated clot rather than fibrinogen is being degraded (Fig. 49-1). It is helpful to review systematically the coagulation cascade when evaluating a patient with coagulopathy, as disorders can present with specific coagulation test profiles (Table 49-1).

Vascular Disorders

Vasculitis can be due to a variety of causes including drugs, infections, neoplasm, and connective tissue disease. Vascular fragility in these disorders leads to increased risk of bleeding. Physical exam findings of palpable purpura should prompt the suspicion of vasculitis. Cutaneous vasculitis results in a prolonged bleeding time and may increase the risk of invasive procedures, especially if there is an incision through the involved area. The diagnosis of vasculitis can be confirmed by a punch biopsy of the purpuric lesion. Drug-induced vasculitis should be treated by removing the offending agent. If the vasculitis is due to a systemic disorder, the underlying disease should be ameliorated if possible.

Vascular malformations may bleed when inadvertently injured. Patients with congenital diseases such as hereditary hemorrhagic telangiectasia (Osler-Weber-Rendu disease) may have cutaneous, mucosal, and deep visceral malformations, which are prone to bleeding. Moreover, the disease may coexist with other coagulopathies such as hemophilia A or von Willebrand disease. Some patients with congenital cavernous hemangiomas may have a coagulopathy due to consumption of platelets and coagulation factors in stagnant vascular spaces. Their coagulation profile may resemble that of disseminated intravascular coagulation (DIC).

Microcirculatory obstruction sometimes occurs in the acute nonlymphocytic leukemias due to the stasis of myeloblasts in the small vessels and may manifest as purpura. The organs most affected are the brain, lung, and skin. The clinical presentation can resemble DIC, thrombotic thrombocytopenic purpura (TTP), heparin-induced thrombocytopenia, or fat embolism.

Thrombocytopenias

The platelet count reflects the balance of platelet production and the removal of platelets from the circulation. The bone marrow normally has the capacity to increase its production by six- to eightfold and can compensate for abnormally reduced platelet half-life due to consumption or destruction. The rate of platelet production by the marrow can be assessed by the examination of Wright-stained peripheral blood smear, looking for young, large, basophilic platelets and from measurements of mean platelet volume.

TABLE 49-1 Screening Coagulation Test Profiles in Selected Typical, Fully Manifest Bleeding Disorders

Disorder	Platelet No.	Bleeding Time	PT	PTT	TT	FDP Level	D-Dimer Level	Other
Vasculitis	N	I	N	N	N	N	N	Palpable purpura
Telangiectasia	N	N	N	N	N	N	N	Cutaneous and visceral lesions
Immune thrombocytopenia	D	I	N	N	N	N	N	Antiplatelet antibodies
Thrombotic thrombocytopenic purpura	D	I	N	N	N	N	N	Schistocytes, renal failure
Thrombocythemia	I	I or N	N	N	N	N	N	Large platelets
Thrombocytopathy	I, N, or D	I	N	N	N	N	N	Impaired platelet aggregation
Hypofibrinogenemia	N	N	I	I	I	N	N	Liver dysfunction
Hemophilia A	N	N	N	I	N	N	N	Low VIII:C levels
von Willebrand's disease	N	I	N	I	N	N	N	Low levels of VIII:C, and ristocetin cofactor

Disorder							Comments
Vitamin K deficiency	N	N	I	I	N	N or I	
Advanced liver disease	N or D	N or I	I	I	I	N or I	Elevated VIII:C level, short euglobulin lysis time
Disseminated intravascular coagulation	D	I	I	I	I	I	Schistocytes, low fibrinogen and VIII:C levels, normal euglobulin lysis time
Heparin therapy	N	N	I	I	N	N	Low antithrombin III level, positive circulating anticoagulant test
Warfarin therapy	N	N	I	I	N	N	Negative circulating anticoagulant test
Thrombolytic therapy	N	N	I	I	I	I	Low fibrinogen level, short euglobulin lysis time

ABBREVIATIONS: N, normal; I, increased; D, decreased; TT, thrombin time.

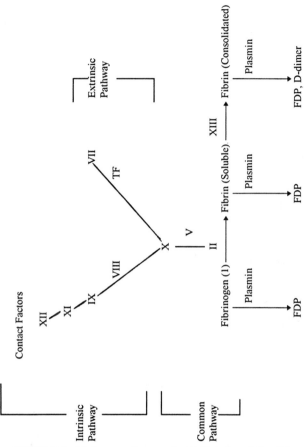

FIGURE 49-1 Fibrin generation cascade and fibrin degradation. TF, tissue factor; FDP, fibrin degradation products.

UNDERPRODUCTION STATES

Hypoplastic Marrow

Numerous agents can suppress the bone marrow or cause a selective decrease in megakaryocyte number. These include drugs, chemotherapy, radiation, environmental toxins, infections, and immune processes. Idiopathic hypoplastic or aplastic marrow can also result in reduced megakaryocyte number. Bone marrow biopsy may show decreased cellularity involving all cell lines or a selective decrease in megakaryocytes.

Ineffective Marrow

Ineffective marrow states result when there is normal marrow production but abnormal release of precursors into the circulation. A common cause of ineffective marrow is folate deficiency, which can come about from decreased folate intake in the diet as well as from increased metabolic requirement for folate. Ineffective marrow can arise when tumor or granuloma replaces the marrow or when it is impaired by azotemia, hypothyroidism, or a variety of inflammatory conditions.

SHORTENED PLATELET SURVIVAL

Certain disease states can decrease the half-life of platelets in the circulation, which is normally 5 days. These include fever, bleeding and sepsis. Other disorders involve immune-mediated platelet destruction, hypersplenism, and consumptive coagulopathy. Bone marrow biopsy usually shows increased or normal numbers of megakaryocytes. The peripheral smear contains many young platelets, which appear large and basophilic.

Idiopathic Thrombocytopenic Purpura (ITP)

ITP is characterized by antiplatelet antibodies, which can sometimes be detected in the patient's serum. Often drugs induce these autoantibodies, and removal of the potential offending agents is the first step in treatment. Common drugs implicated in ITP are furosemide, ranitidine, sulfonamides, heparin, and rifampin. Lymphoma, collagen vascular disease, and viral infections including human immunodeficiency virus (HIV) are also associated with ITP. Infusion of exogenous platelets is of limited benefit, because the half-life of infused platelets is also shortened. If the platelet count is dangerously low ($< 20,000/mL$) or bleeding is a problem, corticosteroids and intravenous γ-globulin (0.4 to 1.0 g/kg/day for 3 to

5 days) are usually effective. Other therapies include splenectomy, splenic irradiation, danazol, colchicine, and cytotoxic
agents. However, these therapies are usually more appropriate in subacute and chronic management.

Thrombotic Thrombocytopenic Purpura (TTP)

The clinical presentation of TTP is classically characterized by
the pentad of thrombocytopenia, microangiopathic hemolytic
anemia, fever, neurologic abnormalities, and renal insufficiency. In TTP, intravascular platelet aggregation causes vasoocclusion and thrombocytopenia. Diseases associated with
TTP include HIV infection and malignancy. Chemotherapy,
particularly mitomycin, can precipitate TTP. Laboratory studies reveal profound thrombocytopenia ($< 50,000/\mu L$), usually normal coagulation studies, renal dysfunction, and evidence of hemolysis, including elevated LDH and bilirubin as
well as schistocytes on peripheral smear. Coombs' test is negative in TTP. Plasma exchange is the therapy of choice for TTP
and should be started immediately. High-dose corticosteroids
may also contribute to significant improvement. Other therapies include antiplatelet agents, vincristine, and splenectomy. Transfusion of platelets is contraindicated in TTP, as it
may exacerbate the vasooclusive pathophysiology.

Heparin-Induced Thrombocytopenia

While heparin-induced thrombocytopenia (HIT) appears in
approximately 1 to 3 percent of patients exposed to heparin,
the use of this medicine is ubiquitous in the intensive care
unit (ICU); therefore the incidence of HIT is relatively high.
Immune-mediated heparin-induced thrombocytopenia usually appears 5 to 7 days after first exposure to heparin. The
clinical picture may range from asymptomatic to dramatic,
life-threatening thrombosis, both venous and arterial. Bleeding is a less frequent manifestation. If HIT is suspected, all
exposure to heparin must be discontinued. This includes discontinuation of all heparin flushes and removal of heparin-
coated catheters. Low-molecular-weight heparins may be less
likely to cause HIT but should also be stopped. Laboratory
confirmation may be performed, but often the syndrome must
be diagnosed promptly on clinical grounds. Platelet transfu-

sions may contribute to thrombotic complications and should be avoided unless there is clinically significant bleeding.

Hypersplenism

Thrombocytopenia may result when platelets are sequestered in an enlarged spleen. Hypersplenism is associated with hepatic cirrhosis, splenic vein occlusion, lymphoma, leukemia, and sarcoidosis. The bone marrow is usually hypercellular and contains increased numbers of megakaryocytes. The peripheral smear shows large basophilic platelets in decreased number. Bedside ultrasound can confirm splenic enlargement. Splenectomy may be indicated if there is risk of splenic rupture or if platelet counts are dangerously low. In leukemia or lymphoma, radiation of the enlarged spleen often provides temporary improvement in spleen size and platelet number.

Thrombocytosis/Thrombocytopenia

Reactive thrombocytosis is commonly seen in patients in the ICU and is attributable to inflammation, bleeding, surgery, hemolysis, and malignancy. Platelet counts are usually less than 1 million/μL, and there are no serious sequelae. Much higher counts (greater than 1 million/μL) can be seen in the myeloproliferative disorders and can lead to clinically significant bleeding and thrombosis. When bleeding is a problem or invasive procedures are anticipated, platelet counts should be reduced to below 500,000/μL. This can be achieved through plateletpheresis. Chemotherapy with hydroxyurea or busulfan can be used to maintain normal platelet counts or to prevent secondary reactive thrombocytosis after surgery. Inadvertent splenectomy during abdominal surgery should be carefully avoided, since it may result in marked, life-threatening thrombocytosis and vasoocclusive events.

Thrombocytopathy

Qualitative platelet abnormalities are common in critically ill patients. A number of medical disorders can cause platelet dysfunction, including uremia, myeloproliferative disorders, dysproteinemia (e.g., Waldenström's macroglobulinemia), and DIC. Mechanical devices such as bypass pumps and intraaortic balloon pumps can damage platelets and impair their function. Drugs such as NSAIDs, aspirin, alcohol, and penicillins can also cause prolongation of the bleeding time. Disordered platelet function usually resolves when the causative agent is removed or the underlying disease is treated. Uremic platelet dysfunction should be treated first with adequate dialysis. DDAVP (0.3 mg/kg intravenously every 6 to 12 h) can reduce the bleeding time in uremia, but tachyphylaxis develops in 1 to 2 days. Additional treatments include corticosteroids, cryoprecipitate, platelet transfusion, and conjugated estrogens.

Disorders of Fibrin Generation

Abnormal fibrin generation can result from deficiencies in coagulation factors as well as from factor inhibitors. Considering the values of PT and PTT in combination can identify the site of deficiency in the cascade (Table 49-2). Mixing the patient's serum with pooled normal serum can identify whether the prolongation of clotting time is due to a factor deficiency or the presence of factor inhibitors. If mixing results in correction of the clotting time, a deficiency is present. If the clotting time remains prolonged, an inhibitor is present.

ISOLATED FACTOR DEFICIENCIES

Hypofibrinogenemia

Low functional fibrinogen levels can result from decreased hepatic synthesis or increased removal from the circulation, as in DIC. Finding a low functional fibrinogen level relative to the level of antigenic fibrinogen may identify dysfibrinogenemia. Bleeding is unusual above a functional level of 100 mg/dL, but the anticoagulant effects of fibrin spit product in high titer may increase bleeding risk. Fibrinogen may be replaced with fresh frozen plasma (FFP). Cryoprecipitate is more effective, and 1 Cryopack will raise fibrinogen levels approximately 4 mg/dL in a 70-kg patient. Fibrinogen levels should be measured every 6 to 12 h to determine the need for further transfusion.

TABLE 49-2 Use of Combined PT and PTT Results to Determine Site(s) of Fibrin Generation Cascade Defects

	PT Normal	PT Elevated
PTT Normal	Result 1	Result 2
PTT Elevated	Result 3	Result 4

Result 1:	Normal results on screening tests of cascade (factor levels at least 30 to 35% of normal)
Result 2:	Isolated low factor VII level—may be due to congenital deficiency or early liver disease, vitamin K deficiency, or warfarin effect
Result 3:	Intrinsic pathway abnormality—low levels of factors VIII, IX, XI, or XII; typical pattern in hemophilia A and von Willebrand's disease
Result 4:	Due to common pathway abnormality—factors I (fibrinogen), II, V, X—and/or combined intrinsic and extrinsic pathway defects. Seen in advanced liver disease, vitamin K deficiency, full warfarin and heparin effects, and DIC

Hemophilia A and B

Critical illness in a patient with hemophilia A (factor VIII deficiency) necessitates prompt correction of the preexisting coagulopathy, particularly when other bleeding disorders supervene. When significant bleeding is present or major surgery is anticipated, the presence of a factor VIII inhibitor should first be excluded, then factor VIII should be replaced with concentrate to 100% of normal (1 U/mL) or higher. Subsequent dosing is dictated by bleeding and the monitoring of levels, usually every 8 to 12 h. In hemophilia B, deficient factor IX is replaced with FFP or factor IX concentrate.

von Willebrand's Factor (VWF)

The bleeding diathesis of VWF deficiency is clinically similar to disorders of platelet function. Findings include prolonged bleeding time, moderately prolonged PTT, and mildly decreased factor VIII coagulant (VIII:C). Diminished levels of ristocetin cofactor and von Willebrand's antigen may also be found. The most common form of this disorder (type I) results from a defect in secretion of normal VWF from vascular endothelial cells. Patients with type II secrete a qualitatively abnormal VWF, while type III patients have a recessively inherited deficiency in VWF synthesis. DDAVP may be used in type I patients to displace VWF from endothelial cells, but the effect is short-lived. Cryoprecipitate may be used for more long-term treatment and for types II and III deficiency. Desmopressin should not be used in type II VWF deficiency, as it can lead to platelet aggregation and thrombocytopenia.

Other Factor Deficiencies

Other inherited deficiencies of coagulation factors are relatively rare, and most are treated with FFP or prothrombin complex. Acquired deficiencies of factor VII are common and frequently associated with deficiencies of other factors, particularly II, V, IX, and X. These acquired deficiencies may result from vitamin K deficiency, liver disease, or warfarin therapy. Vitamin K supplementation usually corrects the coagulopathy. Oral administration of vitamin K is preferred over intravenous dosing, which can cause anaphylaxis.

INHIBITORS

Factor VIII Inhibitors

The most commonly encountered inhibitors are those directed against factor VIII. They are most frequently discovered in hemophiliac patients on factor replacement therapy. They can also be found in the elderly, in postpartum patients, in lymphoma, and in autoimmune disorders. Factor VIII inhibitor levels are quantified in Bethesda units, and a level > 10 U/mL indicates a more potent inhibitor. Hemophiliacs should be tested for the presence of inhibitors when bleeding is a problem in order to predict the response to replacement therapy. Patients with low levels of inhibitor can be treated with factor VIII concentrate, while high titers may need to be treated with prothrombin complex concentrate, which bypasses the factor VIII–dependent step. Other therapies include immunosuppressant agents, plasma processing columns, and high-dose intravenous immunoglobulin.

Lupus Anticoagulant

The lupus anticoagulant may be identified in patients with systemic lupus erythematosus (SLE), drug-induced lupus syndrome, various autoimmune disorders, and in otherwise normal individuals. It is usually detected as an elevated PTT, and about 25 percent of patients will have clinically significant hypercoagulability.

Complex Coagulopathies

DISSEMINATED INTRAVASCULAR COAGULATION

DIC is common in the ICU. It is characterized as a consumptive coagulopathy with abnormal clotting and vasoocclusion as well as bleeding due to the consumption of clotting factors. It is precipitated most commonly by sepsis, tissue injury, and malignancy. It may present as an asymptomatic laboratory abnormality or life-threatening thrombosis and hemorrhage. The microangiopathic hemolytic anemia of DIC may lead to significant organ dysfunction and is usually apparent on peripheral blood smear. Other laboratory findings include coagulopathy indicated by elevated PT and PTT, increased fibrin/fibrinogen degradation products (FDP) and D-dimer levels, thrombocytopenia, hypofibrinogenemia, and decreased factor levels (particularly factor VIII).

DIC usually resolves as the underlying disorder responds to therapy. If hemorrhagic complications supervene, judicious blood product support is indicated with packed red blood cells (RBCs), platelets, FFP, and cryoprecipitate. Heparin is indicated when there are significant thrombotic complications, such as purpura fulminans, massive thromboembolism, and acute promyelocytic leukemia. The initial dose of heparin is

5 U/kg per hour. This is increased to 10 U/kg per hour if FDP levels do not decline within 24 h. A lack of response to heparin may result from deficiency of antithrombin III, which can be repleted with FFP.

MASSIVE TRANSFUSION

When patients are transfused with one to two blood volumes of stored RBCs, a complex coagulopathy may develop, characterized most prominently by a thrombocytopenia due to both dilution and consumption of platelets in the circulation. Other coagulation factors may be diluted as well. Treatment includes transfusion of platelets and FFP.

Liver Disease

Significant coagulopathy can develop when the liver fails to synthesize adequate amounts of clotting factors. Hypersplenism can be present and lead to thrombocytopenia. Often one must distinguish coagulopathy due to liver disease from DIC. In DIC, euglobulin lysis times are normal, factor VIII:C is low, and D-dimer is elevated. In liver disease, euglobulin lysis time is short and factor VIII:C is elevated.

Therapy consists of administering vitamin K and replacing factors, usually with FFP. If volume of infusion must be limited, prothrombin complex may be used; however, it contains only the vitamin K–dependent factors, not all of the coagulation factors made in the liver.

Guidelines for Invasive Procedures in Coagulopathic Patients

Invasive procedures should be performed only when absolutely necessary in coagulopathic patients. Procedures should be as limited as possible and should be performed under direct vision, so hemostasis can be assured. A complete evaluation of coagulation parameters should be done prior to the procedure in order to anticipate potential bleeding problems and need for therapy. If treatment is administered prior to the procedure, one should check that the coagulopathy has corrected appropriately. Sometimes the timing of procedures must be coordinated with other departments of the hospital, such as the blood bank, so that an adequate supply of replacement products can be available promptly. The patient should be monitored for both early and late bleeding, and members of the health care team should be alerted to potential bleeding problems and educated about the appropriate therapy based on the patient's previous history. Serial reassessment of coagulation status may be necessary as new medical problems may intervene and their initial response to therapy may change.

SPECIFIC COAGULOPATHIES

Thrombocytopenia

For limited procedures such as peripheral line insertions or needle biopsies performed under direct vision platelet counts of 50,000 to 80,000/μL are probably adequate. For major surgery, central line insertion, or closed-space needle biopsy counts of 80,000 to 100,000 are preferred. Lumbar puncture can usually be performed with platelet counts of 50,000/μL.

Thrombocythemia

In patients with thrombocythemia, platelet counts should be lowered below 500,000/μL if possible. The bleeding time can be a helpful measure of the risk of bleeding in these patients; however, in patients with myeloproliferative disorders, bleeding can be unpredictable even with normal platelet counts and bleeding times. Therefore, procedures should be performed only when absolutely necessary.

Anticoagulants

Heparin should be stopped approximately 6 h prior to invasive procedures. When anticoagulation needs to be reversed urgently, protamine can be used. Warfarin anticoagulation usually normalizes in 2 or more days after stopping the drug. FFP can be used to correct the coagulopathy urgently. Vitamin K can be given orally or intravenously but can lead to a state of warfarin resistance when anticoagulation must be resumed. Heparin may be used temporarily to protect the patient from clotting, as warfarin anticoagulation wears off and again while oral anticoagulation is being resumed. It should be stopped for approximately 6 h prior to a procedure.

For a more detailed discussion, see Chaps. 64 and 65 in *Principles of Critical Care*, 2d ed.

Chapter 50

ACUTE LEUKEMIA

JOHN McCONVILLE

Acute leukemia is a malignant proliferation of bone marrow or lymphoid cells that is uniformly fatal when left untreated. The acute leukemias include acute myeloid (nonlymphocytic) leukemia (AML) and acute lymphoblastic leukemia (ALL) as well as the blastic transformation of chronic myelogenous leukemia (CML) and the myelodysplastic syndromes (MDS). Therapy-related AML occurs following treatment with chemotherapy or radiotherapy for an earlier cancer or other disease (see Table 50-1 for a classification of acute leukemia and associated clinical features). With the use of intensive chemotherapy and extensive supportive care, many patients, especially children and younger adults, can be cured of their leukemia. The likelihood of a cure depends on the type of leukemia and its stage as well as the medical problems existing prior to the diagnosis of acute leukemia. This chapter focuses on the metabolic, infectious, and infiltrative complications necessitating ICU admission that occur as a result of acute leukemia or its treatment.

Management

Initial management of acute leukemia involves induction chemotherapy. The goal of the initial chemotherapy regimen is to induce a complete remission, defined by the absence of detectable leukemia in the bone marrow and blood, the regeneration of normal marrow elements, and the return to normal levels of all three blood cell lines for at least a month. After the blood counts have recovered from induction chemotherapy, the patient undergoes consolidation. The goal of consolidation chemotherapy is to destroy any clonal leukemia cells that are still present after induction chemotherapy. The timing, dosage, and type of consolidation chemotherapy is dependent on how

TABLE 50-1 French-American-British (FAB) Classification of Acute Leukemias and Their Clinical Features

FAB Subtype	Type	Characteristic Clinical Features
Acute lymphoblastic leukemia (ALL)		
L1	Small cells; homogeneous	T- or B-cell immunophenotype
L2	Large cells; heterogeneous	T- or B-cell immunophenotype
L3	Large cells; homogeneous (Burkitt type)	CNS involvement; lactic acidosis, organomegaly; mature B-cell immunophenotype
Acute myeloid leukemia (AML)		
M0	Undifferentiated acute myeloid leukemia (AML)	Myeloid immunophenotype but no myeloperoxidase activity
M1	Acute myeloblastic leukemia without maturation (AML)	—
M2	Acute myeloblastic leukemia with maturation (AML)	Auer rods; granulocytic sarcomas
M3	Acute promyelocytic leukemia—hypergranular (APL)	DIC, low WBC count
M3V	Acute promyelocytic leukemia—microgranular (APL)	DIC, high WBC count

626

M4	Acute myelomonocytic leukemia (AMMoL)	Auer rods
M4Eo	Acute myelomonocytic leukemia with abnormal eosinophils (AMMoL-M4Eo)	Granulocytic sarcomas
M5a	Acute monoblastic leukemia—poorly differentiated (AMoL)	CS involvement, gingival hypertrophy, granulocytic sarcomas
M5b	Acute monocytic leukemia—well-differentiated (AMoL)	Skin involvement, granulocytic sarcomas
M6	Acute erythroleukemia (AEL)	—
M7	Acute megakaryoblastic leukemia (AMegaL)	Low WBC count, normal or increased platelet levels in approximately 30% of cases
Chronic myelogenous leukemia (CML)—blast phase		
—	Lymphoid blast phase	TdT-positive; B-cell immunophenotype
—	Myeloid blast phase	Leukostasis, organomegaly, granulocytic sarcomas, bone pain, fever
Therapy-related acute myeloid leukemia (t-AML)		
Primary myelodysplastic syndrome (MDS)		
—	Refractory anemia with excess blasts in transformation (RAEB-T)	20–30% bone marrow blast cells

627

the patient tolerated induction chemotherapy and the type of leukemia. Occasionally, patients will receive maintenance chemotherapy, which does not cause significant myelosuppression, in an effort to maintain remission. Allogeneic bone marrow transplantation is available for patients who relapse after a successful induction.

Infection

Patients with leukemia are immunocompromised by both their disease and their treatment. Immature leukemia cells are ineffective barriers to infection. The leukemic patient presenting with a white cell count of 100,000 is every bit as immunocompromised as the leukemic patient who has a negligible white cell count 7 days after induction chemotherapy. Leukemic patients, in addition to being more susceptible to infection, manifest several factors that make the diagnosis of infection more difficult. First, many patients with leukemia are so immunocompromised, either from the leukemia itself or from chemotherapy, that they are unable to mount a significant inflammatory response even to severe infections. Thus, a neutropenic patient (the absolute number of mature neutrophils in addition to the number of bands being less than 500) with a perirectal abscess may not complain of significant pain or have erythema, tenderness, or swelling on exam. Second, leukemic patients often have a temperature above 38.5°C (101.5°F) with no identifiable source of infection. Because even a seemingly insignificant infection, such as a small cellulitis, can quickly develop into bacteremia, septic shock, and death, it is the standard of care that intravenous antibiotic treatment be initiated immediately in any neutropenic patient who has a fever above 38.5°C (101.5°F). Typically, ceftazidime as a single agent or a semisynthetic penicillin plus an aminoglycoside is started as empiric treatment. Initial attempts to identify a source of infection should include a chest x-ray as well as urine, sputum, and blood cultures. If the patient has a chronic indwelling catheter, such as a double- or triple-lumen Hickman, blood cultures should be taken from each port as well as from peripheral sites. In addition, the skin around the catheter should be carefully examined for signs of infection. Should initial cultures reveal a pathogen, antibiotic therapy should be adjusted for maximal bactericidal activity based on susceptibility testing in vitro. Often, no pathogen is ever identified in febrile leukemic patients. However, broad-spectrum antibiotics should be continued until the patient is no longer neutropenic, even if the patient subsequently becomes afebrile. Because chemotherapy damages mucosal barriers, these patients are susceptible to endogenous pathogens. Most common are gram-negative enteric bacteria, gram-positive cocci, and fungi such as *Candida* and *Aspergillus* species. Patients with ALL also are susceptible to *Pneumocystis,* mycobacterial and viral infections.

Typhlitis is an infection that occurs in neutropenic patients and deserves special mention. Typhlitis is a necrotizing enterocolitis of the terminal ileum, appendix, cecum, and right colon that occurs in granulocytopenic patients. Symptoms and signs are similar to those of inflammatory bowel disease: nausea, vomiting, abdominal pain and tenderness, profuse watery or bloody diarrhea, and fever. The intestinal mucosa is ulcerated, allowing invasion of enteric organisms into and through the bowel wall. Ileus and bowel dilatation result. Bowel perforation and peritonitis may follow. Most patients are best managed with aggressive medical treatment: broad-spectrum antibiotics; transfusion of packed red blood cells, platelets, and fresh frozen plasma; maintenance of normal serum electrolytes; and bowel rest with nasogastric suction. Narcotic analgesics and paralytic agents should be avoided because they increase the risk of ileus. Patients with clear evidence of perforation require surgery. Radiographic evidence of air within the bowel wall (pneumatosis intestinalis) does not in itself necessitate surgery, nor should a granulocytopenic patient who is otherwise doing well necessarily undergo laparotomy for intraperitoneal free air.

Granulocyte transfusions are rarely necessary for patients receiving chemotherapy for acute leukemia. However, over the past several years, the hematopoietic growth factors filgrastim (granulocyte colony-stimulating factor, or G-CSF) and sargramostim (granulocyte-macrophage colony-stimulating factor, or GM-CSF) have become available in the United States. Unfortunately, randomized controlled trials have not demonstrated significant clinical benefits from using myeloid growth factors in patients with AML. In addition, the current data do not support the routine use of colony-stimulating factors as adjuncts to antibiotic therapy in febrile neutropenic patients. For adults with ALL however, clinical trials have demonstrated statistically significant shortening of the duration of neutropenia following remission-induction chemotherapy when G-CSF was used.

Hyperleukocytosis

A small number of patients with leukemia have an extraordinary elevation of circulating leukocytes. Hyperleukocytosis (greater than 100,000 blast cells per microliter) is a true medical emergency, but the risks of circulatory complications begin to rise at counts above 50,000 cells per microliter. Immature leukocytes are much larger and less deformable than erythrocytes. The high oxygen consumption and invasiveness of these leukemic cells may interact with slow flow through capillaries, leading to hypoxia and vascular end-organ damage. Leukostasis and hypoxia in the capillary beds can induce respiratory distress, cardiac arrhythmias, and central nervous system (CNS) symptoms leading to coma. It is the increased blood viscosity and hypoxia that leads to damage of end organs and makes hyperleukocytosis with leukostasis a medical emergency.

The incidence of leukostasis is highest among CML patients in the blast phase, followed by that in patients with AML. These two types of leukemia have the highest incidence of leukostasis because leukemic myeloblasts are much greater in size than the leukemic lymphocytes seen in ALL and CLL. Although in some cases the increased leukocrit causes an increase in the blood viscosity, in most cases the whole-blood viscosity will not be increased above normal because of the accompanying anemia. This is why some patients with a white blood cell (WBC) count above 100,000 do not have symptoms associated with hyperleukostasis.

The treatment of leukostasis involves hydration, monitoring end-organ function closely for signs of compromise, and initiating therapy to decrease the WBC count. Hydration with normal saline will help to decrease the whole-blood viscosity and improve perfusion of vital organs. Monitoring closely for end-organ damage secondary to increased viscosity is also essential. Close attention should be paid to urine output as a marker of renal function. Pulse oximetry can be used as a crude measure of cardiopulmonary function, and cerebral perfusion can be assessed by examination of the retinal vessels and mental status. Finally, if signs and symptoms of end-organ damage are present, attempts should be made to reduce the WBC count acutely. A single efficient leukapheresis can decrease the leukocyte count by approximately 50 percent within 2 to 3 h. If specific chemotherapy cannot be started immediately, oral hydroxyurea should be given in a dose of 2 g every 6 h. If necessary, a single dose of irradiation (400 cGy) can be used to treat respiratory distress with hypoxia or mental status changes if these symptoms are believed to be secondary to leukostasis. Of note, prophylactic platelet transfusions must be given to prevent bleeding as the circulation is restored to hypoxic tissues (see Table 50-2).

Anemia, Thrombocytopenia, and Disseminated Intravascular Coagulation

Patients with leukemia are characterized by bone marrow failure, due either to replacement of the bone marrow by leukemic cells or to chemotherapy-induced hypoplasia. Red blood cell transfusions are given to maintain a hematocrit of approximately 30 percent. Platelets should be transfused prophylactically to maintain a platelet count $> 10,000/\mu L$ in an effort to decrease the risk of spontaneous hemorrhage, such as stroke or gastrointestinal hemorrhage. No salicylates or other drugs that interfere with platelet function should be given to a thrombocytopenic patient. The use of single-donor platelets collected by apheresis will decrease the rate of alloimmunization in leukemic patients.

Disseminated intravascular coagulation (DIC) is frequently present when the diagnosis of acute promyelocytic leukemia is made. DIC can also accompany any leukemia or infection in which there is rapid cell turnover and cell lysis. The initiating event in DIC is not clearly understood, but the coagulation cascade appears to be initiated by the release of intracellular thromboplastic material. The syndrome is characterized by the consumption of plasma coagulation proteins

TABLE 50-2   Diagnosis and Management of Leukostasis Syndrome

---

- Leukostasis begins to occur when the peripheral blast count rises above 50,000/μL.
- Blast counts greater than 100,000/μL should be treated as a medical emergency.
- The signs and symptoms of leukostasis are due to increased blood viscosity and are manifestations of decreased small vessel perfusion of end organs: mental status alterations (CNS), respiratory failure (pulmonary capillaries), renal failure (renal glomeruli), and cardiac arrhythmias (cardiac microvasculature).
- Cerebral perfusion should be assessed by examination of the retinal vessels and mental status; renal perfusion should be assessed by careful measurement of urine output; perfusion of the heart and lungs should be assessed by cardiopulmonary monitoring (pulse oximetry).
- Hydration should be maintained vigorously with saline infusion to decrease viscosity.
- Since the viscosity of blood is a function of both the leukocrit and the hematocrit, red blood cell transfusions should be withheld until the WBC count has been reduced (unless the patient is severely anemic).
- If specific chemotherapy will not be started immediately, then oral hydroxyurea should be given in a dose of 2 g every 6 h.
- A temporary large-bore catheter should be placed and leukapheresis begun as soon as possible; leukapheresis should be continued daily until the WBC count is below 100,000/μL.
- Specific chemotherapy should be begun as soon as the patient is stable.
- For mental status changes due to leukostasis, cranial irradiation with a single dose of 400 cGy should be considered.
- Respiratory compromise with hypoxemia due to leukostasis (not infection) can be treated with 400 cGy of thoracic irradiation and supplemental oxygen.

---

and platelets. DIC results in an elevated PT, PTT, and thrombin time as well as a decrease in plasma fibrinogen and an elevation in fibrin split products and D-dimer. Clinically, patients present with a combination of bleeding and/or thrombotic complications. The DIC in leukemia patients is most severe shortly after chemotherapy begins.

Management of DIC is always directed at correcting the underlying disorder, whether due to leukemia, infection, trauma, or an obstetric complication. Also, the consumption of coagulation proteins by fibrin formation and its associated secondary fibrinolysis can be brought under control by continuous infusion of heparin at 5 U/h. The heparin infusion is typically well tolerated, even by patients who are thrombocytopenic. Heparin infusion allows consumed coagulation factors to be replaced without concern about adding more substrate for further intravascular coagulation. Typically, coagulation factors are supplemented in the form of cryoprecipitate or fresh frozen plasma. Cryoprecipitate infusions should be used to maintain the fibrinogen concentration at 100 mg/dL. If, after 24 h of heparin therapy, the fibrinogen has not stabilized and the level of fibrin degradation products has not decreased, the heparin infusion may be increased to 10 U/kg per hour.

Recently, all-*trans*-retinoic acid (tretinoin, ATRA) has emerged as a remarkably effective agent for inducing complete remission in patients with acute promyelocytic leukemia (AML-M3). In addition, patients treated with ATRA usually do not have an exacerbation of DIC, as can happen with standard chemotherapy. In fact, resolution of DIC often occurs within 24 to 48 h. Thus, a subgroup of patients who are at increased risk of developing DIC, those patients with AML-M3, can be treated with ATRA at the time of diagnosis in an effort to reduce the development of DIC complications. However, ATRA does have its own unique toxicities. The two most significant toxicities of ATRA are hyperleukocytosis and the retinoic acid syndrome. Acute promyelocytic patients receiving ATRA sometimes exhibit a progressive leukocytosis, which may become marked. This occurs because ATRA causes the differentiation of the leukemic blasts in the bone marrow, resulting in the accumulation of maturing forms in the peripheral blood. Early institution of concurrent chemotherapy at full doses or hydroxyurea has been used to treat those patients who develop a WBC count greater than 20,000 to 30,000 after treatment with ATRA. In addition, the retinoic acid syndrome occurs in approximately 25 percent of patients receiving ATRA and is characterized by fever, rapidly progressive respiratory distress with diffuse pulmonary infiltrates on chest radiograph, pleural effusions, and weight gain. Early consideration of this syndrome coupled with investigations directed at ruling out infection can lead to the prompt initiation of therapy. Typically, patients who develop retinoic acid syndrome are treated with steroids (dexamethasone 10 mg bid). This therapy effectively reverses the syndrome in most patients.

Tissue Infiltration

Leukemia is a systemic disease. Malignant cells circulate through the bloodstream and can infiltrate any tissue. For example, CNS infiltration by leukemic cells occurs in ALL as well as AML. CNS infiltration is more common in ALL and more common in children than adults. The most common symptoms experienced by patients with CNS leukemia are those caused by increased intracranial pressure: vomiting, headache, papilledema, lethergy, and diplopia. Cranial neuropathies can occur from the impingement of cranial nerves by malignant cells as the nerves traverse narrow bony foramina. The diagnosis is established by finding leukemic cells in the CSF. Typically, the CSF pressure is elevated, the glucose concentration is low, and the protein concentration is moderately elevated. CNS leukemia is usually rapidly responsive to irradiation or intrathecal chemotherapy. Dexamethasone can alleviate symptoms of increased intracranial pressure. Cord involvement is best treated with intrathecal methotrexate.

Renal insufficiency is a frequent complication of acute leukemia and may result from a variety of insults, including infiltration of kidneys by leukemic cells, ureteral obstruction by enlarged lymph nodes, and urate nephropathy. In leukemia patients, the production of organic acids together with decreased urine formation from dehydration frequently leads to precipitation of urates within the renal tubules and collecting system, leading to obstruction. Effective management of hyperuricemia and hyperuricosuria in leukemia patients is based on reducing the production of uric acid and at the same time promoting the solubility of uric acid in the urine. An adequate urine flow should be established by oral or intravenous hydration. The blood volume must be expanded and acidosis corrected. Alkalinization of the urine with acetazolamide or sodium bicarbonate makes uric acid more water-soluble and therefore less likely to precipitate out of solution. This reduces the risk of tubular obstruction from uric acid crystal deposition. Allopurinol should also be started in an effort to decrease uric acid nephropathy in the leukemic patient. Allopurinol will effectively inhibit the conversion of xanthine and hypoxanthine to uric acid.

For a more detailed discussion, see Chap. 66 in *Principles of Critical Care,* 2d ed.

Chapter 51

ONCOLOGIC EMERGENCIES

DELBERT DORSCHEID

Complications of malignancies are an increasingly common reason for admission to the intensive care unit (ICU). As therapeutic advances continue and the survival of cancer patients improves, these oncologic emergencies will become ever more common. The nature and complexity of problems that arise in cancer patients require that differential diagnosis be expanded to include etiologies not otherwise seen in patients without cancer. Table 51-1 lists abbreviated differential diagnoses of common signs and symptoms seen in cancer patients. Following in Table 51-2 is a summary of possible causes for those symptoms.

TABLE 51-1   Differential Diagnosis for Common Signs and Symptoms in Cancer Patients

Sign/Symptom	Differential Diagnosis
Nausea and vomiting	Hypercalcemia
	Renal failure
	Brain metastases or brain herniation
	Leptomeningeal carcinomatosis
	Gastric outlet obstruction
	Liver metastases
Abnormal mental status	Hypercalcemia
	Hyponatremia
	Renal failure
	Sepsis
	Leptomeningeal carcinomatosis
	Brain metastases or brain herniation
Hemodynamic instability	Pulmonary embolism
	Pericardial tamponade
	Pericardial constriction
	Brain herniation
	Superior vena cava syndrome
Renal failure	Hypercalcemia
	Tumor lysis syndrome; hyperuricemia
	Urinary obstruction
	Paraneoplastic changes
	Glomerulonephritis

TABLE 51-2 Oncologic Emergencies

Condition	Pathophysiology	Diagnosis	Treatment
Metabolic syndromes Hypercalcemia	Bony metastatis; tumor production of osteoclast activating factor, PTH or PTH-like molecules; symptoms relate to acuity of condition	Clinical symptoms (mental status changes, polydipsia, polyuria); long PR or short QT on ECG; elevated free-[Ca] with low PTH	Restore intravascular volume; decrease bone resorption by use of bisphosphonates to inhibit osteoclastic activity (see Table 51-3); for acute and long-term care (see Table 51-4)
Syndrome of inappropriate antidiuretic hormone	Multifactorial; euvolemia with hypoNa or a hypoosmolar state; ectopic ADH or ADH-like molecule or stimulated ADH release (vincristine, cytoxan)	$U_{Na} > 20$ meq/L $U_{Osm} > 500$ mOsm/kg $S_{Osm} < 280$ mOsm/kg	Eliminate causative tumor; if symptomatic, correct [Na] to 120–125 meq/L using 3% saline and a loop diuretic; if no symptoms, consider free water restriction, demeclocycline, or lithium carbonate
Lactic acidosis	Related to large tumor burdens (leukemias, lymphomas >> solid tumors) usually with hepatic involvement	Exclude all other possible causes (shock, infection, sepsis)	Reduce tumor burden; this may indicate the need for emergent chemotherapy; questionable role for bicarbonate

TABLE 51-2 Oncologic Emergencies *(Continued)*

Condition	Pathophysiology	Diagnosis	Treatment
Tumor Lysis syndrome	Release of cellular contents after chemotherapy given to sensitive tumors (leukemia, lymphomas >> solid tumors); may lead to cardiac arrhythmias or uric acid nephropathy	Hyperkalemia, hyperphosphotemia, hypocalcemia, hyperuricemia	Hydration to maintain 100–200 mL/h of urine output; allopurinol at 300–600 mg/day; urine alkalinization to pH 7.0–7.5; dialysis for renal failure, [K] > 6 meq/L, phosphate > 10 mg/dL, and uric acid > 10 mg/dL
Neurologic syndromes Spinal cord compression	Known metastatic disease (~5% of all cancer-lung > myeloma > prostate > lymphoma > breast) where lesion is the result of direct tumor extension into epidural space, intervertebral space, or compromised blood flow or vertebral body integrity	Local pain; dermatomal or radicular pain with or without weakness and sensory loss below the spinal level of the pain; bowel or bladder dysfunction Spinal x-rays or MRI	Dexamethasone, radiation therapy, and surgical decompression; treatment is not indicated if paraplegia has developed as the cord has little chance for functional recovery

Cerebral herniation	Primary or metastatic tumors (lung, breast, melanoma) causing mass effect and edema, increasing the ICP	Clinical setting and suspicion based on the neurologic exam should indicate what has occurred: *temporal lobe-tentorial* or uncal herniation causes progressive bilateral loss of brainstem reflexes *transtentorial herniation* of diencephalon and brainstem progresses from altered mental status to coma, decorticate posture, flaccid paralysis, irregular and shallow respirations, and fixed midline pupils *cerebellar-foramen magnum* herniation usually results from large frontal or posterior fossa masses leading to respiratory arrest, coma, bradycardia, and absence of DTRs	Based upon empiric clinical diagnosis and intended to reduce ICP; this could include intubation and hyperventilation to P_{CO_2} of 25–30 mmHg; mannitol at 0.25–0.5 g/kg and to maintain S_{osm} of 300–310; dexamethasone; and radiation or decompressive surgery if condition stabilizes

(Continued)

TABLE 51-2 Oncologic Emergencies (Continued)

Condition	Pathophysiology	Diagnosis	Treatment
Leptomeningeal carcinomatosis	Tumor spreads to the meninges, where lymphoma, breast, colon, gastric lesions, and melanoma account for most, either by direct extension or metastasis	Clinical findings of headache, altered mental status, hallucinations, meningeal signs, radiculopathies or cranial nerve palsies Lumbar puncture with elevated CSF pressure, high protein, low glucose, and a monocytic pleocytosis; definitive diagnosis by cytologic examination may require multiple samplings; CT and MRI of limited diagnostic use	Intrathecal chemotherapy via repeated lumbar puncture or Ommaya shunt; radiation as a primary or adjuvant therapy to clinically affected areas
Thoracid syndromes Superior vena cava syndrome	External compression by tumor or invasion of SVC by tumor; luminal thrombus or web	Clinical complaints of dyspnea, headaches, dizziness, head fullness; clinical signs of facial	Supportive measures include treating the hypoxia, elevating the head, and using dexamethasone; if

	formation; tumors involved include lung (50–80%), non-Hogkin's (15%), metastatic breast, and primary mediastinal thrombus is most often the result of central venous catheters	swelling and venous congestion of head/neck /chest, and cyanosis; CXR may show a widened mediastinum and right hilar mass with pleural fluid; CT with contrast could delineate the lesion, but venography may be required	tissue diagnosis is known, then specific chemotherapy and/or radiation may be given. Thrombus can be treated with heparin and /or thrombolytics; stenting may be needed for chronic strictures
Pericardial disease	*Effusions* are the result of pericardial seeding from the primary tumor (~5% of all cancer) where lung and breast are the most common; fluid may accumulate slowly or rapidly and it is this rate and accommodation by the pericardium that determines the development of tamponade	Clinical setting of cancer and hemodynamic instability; dyspnea, head or abdominal fullness; if tamponade then distant heart sounds, hypotension, and increased CVP (Beck's triad), tachycardia and narrow pulse pressure; CXR may show an enlarged cardiac shadow; ECG with low voltage and electrical alternans; ECHO and PA catheter may	Intravenous fluids but the use of pressor agents may worsen cardiac output due to the induced tachycardia; pericardiocentesis or pericardiostomy for recurrent effusions if patient prognosis is adequate

(Continued)

643

TABLE 51-2 Oncologic Emergencies *(Continued)*

Condition	Pathophysiology	Diagnosis	Treatment
		indicate RA and RV end-diastolic collapse with loss of *y* descent and prominent *x* descent with equalization of pressures, these are the most sensitive for diagnosis of tamponade; cytology may yield the cause of the fluid	
	Constrictive pericardial disease is commonly the result of radiation to the chest but may also include the spread of cancer to the pericardial sac, both of which cause thickening; these changes may take place 6–30 months after treatment	Clinical setting to explain slowly developing fluid retention (ascites, edema, dyspnea) and the Kussmaul sign (neck veins do not collapse on inspiration); ECHO shows thickening of pericardium and rapid deceleration of the filling velocity; PA catheter shows the "square-	If the patient is believed to have adequate survival time, perform a pericardiectomy

		root sign" of early filling deceleration (Fig. 51-1)	
Urologic emergencies			
Hematuria	Drug toxicity, infections, urethelial breakdown from chemotherapy; cyclophosphamide is the most common cause	Visualization	Hydration, acrolein, discontinuation of insulting drugs
Obstruction	Retroperitoneal tumors, pelvic masses, or treatment-associated fibrosis; external urethral compression	Foley catheter to assess bladder filling; CT or cytoscopy to evaluate the obstruction	Foley catheters, stents, percutaneous nephostomy tubes
Hyperuricemic nephropathy	Massive tumor lysis with production of uric acid exceeding renal excretion and allowing for the formation of uric acid crystals, which destroy the ducts and collecting tubules	Serum uric acid > 20 mg/dL	Hydration, allopurinol, alkalinization of urine, crystal removal by use of urethral or nephrostomy lavage

ABBREVIATIONS: PTH, parathyroic hormone; ADH, antidiuretic hormone; ECG, electrocardiogram; ICP, intracranial pressure; MRI, magnetic resonance imaging; DTR, deep tendon reflex; CSF, cerebrospinal fluid; SVC, superior vena cava; CT, computed tomography; CVP, central venous pressure; CXR, chest x-ray; ECHO, echocardiography; PA, pulmonary artery; RA, right auricle; LV, left ventricle.

TABLE 51-3   Bisphosphonates Currently Available for Treatment of Malignancy-Associated Hypercalcemia

Bisphosphonate	IV Dose	Duration of Treatment	% of Patients Achieving Normocalcemia
Etidronate	500 mg/day (7.5 mg/kg per day)	3–5 days	30–50
Clodronate	600–1200 mg *or* 300 mg/day	Once 3–5 days	85
Pamidronate	60–90 mg (0.5–1.5 mg/kg)	Once	90

TABLE 51-4   Stepwise Treatment of Hypercalcemia

FIRST-LINE		
1. Normal saline infusion	250–500 mL/h (4–10 L/day)	Replace K^+, Mg^{2+} losses Carefully monitor cardiopulmonary status Consider loop diuretic to enhance calciuresis and prevent fluid overload Maintain saline infusion until normocalcemia is reached
2. Pamidronate	60–90 mg IV over 3–4 h	
3. Calcitonin[a]	8 IU/kg IM or SC every 6 h	

SECOND-LINE		
4. Plicamycin	25 μg/kg, as bolus or IV infusion over 2–4 h	Repeat dose every 3–4 days Increased toxicity with repeated doses Rebound hypercalcemia possible
5. Gallium nitrate	200 mg/(m^2 per day) as continuous IV infusion × 5 days	

LONG-TERM MANAGEMENT	
1. PO intake Pamidronate	2–3 L fluid per day 60–90 mg V over 2–4 h every 2–3 weeks 200–1200 mg PO daily
Clodronate	3200 mg PO daily
Etidronate	10–20 mg/kg PO daily

[a]Calcitonin can be used in conjunction with pamidronate for severe hypercalcemia.

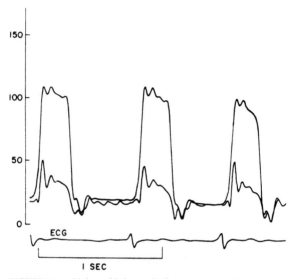

FIGURE 51-1   Right and left ventricular pressure recording in a patient with constrictive pericarditis. The tracing depicts equilibration of right and left ventricular diastolic pressures and the characteristic "square-root sign" of the diastolic waveform.

For a more detailed discussion, see Chap. 67 in *Principles of Critical Care,* 2d ed.

Chapter 52

TOXICITIES OF CHEMOTHERAPY

EDWARD BOTTEI

Basic Principles of Chemotherapeutic Toxicities

First and foremost, drug toxicity from chemotherapeutic agents used in the treatment of malignancies is often a diagnosis of exclusion. The symptoms, findings on physical examination, and laboratory/radiologic studies are often nonspecific. Before being able to attribute the findings to the drugs, the physician must look for and rule out other causes first.

Second, the dose of the drug, the schedule by which the drug is given, and the other drugs given in combination with the drug in question can produce different toxicologic profiles for any given drug. Bolus versus continuous infusion therapy can give different side-effect profiles. High-dose protocols can produce side effects not usually seen with routine dosing. When given in combinations, each individual drug's toxicity can be synergistic with the other drugs' toxicities.

Third, not all toxicities of any given drug are known. This becomes especially important in light of the continuous development of new drugs and in the new combinations of drugs being tested. Also, it is important to remember that individual patients can have idiosyncratic reactions to any drug.

Fourth, treatment for most of the chemotherapeutic drug toxicities includes removal of the drug and supportive care.

Systemic Effects

While almost any drug can cause an acute hypersensitivity reaction, L-asparaginase and paclitaxel are notorious for this side effect. The health care team should be prepared to treat anaphylaxis (appropriate medications at the bedside) before therapy with these two drugs is started. Several drugs are well known for causing fevers without producing a hyper-sensitivity reaction, cytarabine and bleomycin being well known for this.

Myelosuppression

Myelosuppression is seen with many chemotherapeutic regimens. Granulocytes reach their nadir 7 to 14 days after chemotherapy and recover in 21 to 28 days. Granulocyte count can be slower to return to normal if the patient has had pelvic or spinal irradiation. The use of granulocyte and granulocyte macrophage colony-stimulating factors (G-CSF and GM-CSF) can assist in a more rapid recovery of the white blood cell count. Platelets can remain low for several weeks after the recovery of granulocytes. Nitrosoureas and mitomycin C can cause a late and severe thrombocytopenia. In general, the red blood cell count will be somewhat decreased but rarely falls to critical levels. If the patient becomes severely anemic, other sources of blood loss should be sought. All of these effects put together can result in infection and bleeding, two problems that should be carefully watched for.

Mucositis and Diarrhea

Mucosal cells in the GI tract proliferate rapidly and are therefore easily damaged during chemotherapy. Mucositis and diarrhea will range from the mild to to the extreme. High-dose chemotherapy regimens are well known for producing severe mucositis. Candidal and herpes infection at the time of chemotherapy can cause or worsen stomatitis and eosphagitis. In all patients with diarrhea, it is important to look for *Clostridium difficile* in the stool and to treat appropriately if present. The disruption of the mucosal barrier opens a portal for infection. Mouth care is very important to prevent infection and decrease discomfort. Topical anesthesia or parenteral narcotics may be necessary to control the pain. Disruption of the gastrointestinal mucosa compromises nutritional intake and absorption (too painful to eat and recurrent diarrhea); patients frequently need TPN to maintain their nutritional status.

Irinotecan (CPT-11) is notable for causing severe diarrhea without mucositis. It produces two types of diarrhea, the first being associated with a cholinergic surge during or shortly after infusion. This can be treated with atropine. The second type, occurring 6 to 10 days after administration of the drug, is probably a secretory diarrhea from the small intestines. There has been some success at treating this diarrhea with loperamide and octreotide.

Pulmonary Toxicity

Pulmonary symptoms can present as acute pleuritic chest pain, hypersensitivity pneumonitis, noncardiogenic pulmonary edema, pneumonitis, and fibrosis (Table 52-1). Lung toxicity is typically associated with busulfan, bleomycin, and BCNU. These toxicities are usually sporadic rather then dose-related. Methotrexate can cause a lung disease that is believed to be a type of hypersensitivity reaction, but it also causes hilar lymphadenopathy. Lung symptoms can occur after a few cycles of chemotherapy or years after therapy is done. The progression of the symptoms and lung disease can be either slow or rapid. The signs and symptoms are usually nonspecific. Dyspnea is universal, but the commonly found fever and nonproductive cough are not. Patients are sometimes hypoxic. The chest x-ray usually shows diffuse infiltrates but ranges from near normal to complete whiteout. Pathologic specimens reveal diffuse interstitial fibrosis with variable inflammatory infiltrate. This finding is nonspecific, but it can rule out infectious causes. Lungs affected by bleomycin toxicity will also have multiple nodules. Decreased $D_{L_{CO}}$ is commonly found on pulmonary function testing. Steroids are anecdotally helpful.

Bleomycin is associated with a 1 to 2 percent incidence of fatal lung toxicity. Below 450 to 500 mg total dose, the incidence of lung disease is sporadic rather then dose-related. While $D_{L_{CO}}$ can be an indicator of lung damage, stopping bleomycin when the $D_{L_{CO}}$ begins to decline does not necessarily change the course of the lung disease. The risk factors for developing pulmonary complications include age greater then 70 years, having radiation therapy, and cytoxan and methotrexate being given concurrently. Preexisting lung disease is not a risk factor.

ATRA (all trans retinoic acid) produces what is called the retinoic acid syndrome. It is manifest by high fevers, fluid retention, pulmonary infiltrates and respiratory distress. It occurs in 10 to 20 percent of patients with acute promyelocytic leukemia who receive ATRA and is thought to be due

TABLE 52-1 Antineoplastic Drugs That Have Pulmonary Toxicity

Agent	Type of Toxicity	Incidence, %	Comments
Bleomycin	Pneumonitis/fibrosis	2–40	Chest x-ray may be atypical
	Hypersensitivity pneumonitis	Rare	Eosinophilia may be seen on lung biopsy; steroids felt to be useful
	Acute chest pain	Rare	Substernal pressure or pleuritic pain; self-limited over 4–72 h
Busulfan	Pneumonitis/fibrosis	4	Insidious onset after prolonged therapy; poor prognosis
Carmustine (BCNU)	Pneumonitis/fibrosis	20–30	Toxicity is dose-related; common in pretransplantation regimens; effects may appear years after therapy has ended
Cyclophosphamide	Pneumonitis/fibrosis	<1	May potentiate toxicity of bleomycin, BCNU

Drug	Syndrome	%	Comment
High-dose cytarabine	Noncardiogenic pulmonary edema	4–20	Care is supportive, but corticosteroids are occasionally helpful; prognosis is variable
Gemcitabine	Noncardiogenic pulmonary edema	1–5	Care is supportive, but corticosteroids are occasionally helpful; prognosis is variable
Methotrexate	Hypersensitivity pneumonitis	8	Prognosis is good; dramatic response to corticosteroids
	Acute pleuritic pain	Rare	May be associated with pleural effusion or friction rub; subsides over 3–5 days
	Noncardiogenic pulmonary edema	Rare	Few reports, most with intrathecal injection
Mitomycin C	Pneumonitis/fibrosis	3–12	High mortality reported
Procarbazine	Acute hypersensitivity		Onset within hours after drug dose; recovery rapid
Tretinoin (ATRA)	Retinoic acid syndrome	10–20	Corticosteroids suggested
Vinorelbine	Acute dyspnea	5	Readily reversible chest pain

to pulmonary leukostasis. Whether decadron is helpful in treating this syndrome is uncertain.

Cardiac Toxicity

A majority of cardiac events that occur in patients receiving chemotherapy are related to prior heart disease or tumor involvement of the pericardium or myocardium. The one class of drugs that directly affects the heart are the anthracyclines—doxorubicin and daunorubicin (Table 52-2).

Electrocardiographic (ECG) changes are seen in 40 percent of patients receiving doxorubicin. These consist of nonspecific ST and T wave changes, PACs, PVCs, sinus tachycardia, and low QRS voltages. The ECG changes are transient and the result of direct effects of these drugs on the heart. There are also several indirect effects from metabolic and electrolyte changes caused by the anthracyclines.

Paclitaxel, through a direct effect, causes an asymptomatic, reversible sinus bradycardia. Only rarely does paclitaxel cause worse problems, like third-degree heart block. Whether paclitaxel can cause acute myocardial infarctions or atrial and ventricular tachycardias remains a question.

Radiation can speed up atherogenesis in the coronary arteries.

Vinca alkaloids combined with bleomycin will sometimes cause myocardial infarction.

Some 4% of patients receiving 5-fluouracil (5-FU) develop angina, and there have been several reports of patients having myocardial infarction secondary to 5-FU. Nitrates and calcium-channel blockers can be used to treat these problems.

The cardiomyopathy caused by doxorubicin and daunorubicin is part of the myocarditis-pericarditis syndrome these drugs cause. With this, there can be an acute drop in ejection fraction from hours to weeks after infusion. Occasionally the patient will develop a pericardial effusion or severe congestive heart failure (CHF). The classic form of anthracycline-induced cardiomyopathy is subacute in presentation and affects 1 to 10 percent of patients who received 550 mg/m^2 of doxorubicin. It typically shows up 30 to 60 days after treatment but can appear years later. The signs and symptoms include tachycardia, dyspnea, and cardiomegaly. The total dose of anthracycline is the single most important factor in

TABLE 52-2 Antineoplastic Drugs That Have Cardiac Toxicity

Drug	Effect	Incidence, %	Comments
Anthracyclines	Acute ECG changes	Common	Almost always benign and reversible
	Acute myocarditis/pericarditis syndrome	Rare	
	Chronic cardiomyopathy	1–2	May appear years after treatment
Cyclophosphamide	Acute hemorrhagic cardiac necrosis	Unusual	Only in very high doses
5-Fluorouracil	Angina/myocardial infarction	Rare	Usually within hours of drug dose; asymptomatic ECG changes more common
Mitoxantrone	Cardiomyopathy	1–2	Drug is structurally related to anthracyclines, but incidence of cardiomyopathy is probably somewhat less; risk is < 1% if cumulative dose ≤120 mg/m^2
Paclitaxel	Arrhythmias	10–20	Most common is asymptomatic bradycardia
Vinca alkaloids	Angina/myocardial infarction	Rare	Scattered case reports

predicting whether this complication will occur. There is no dose below which cardiomyopathy has not been seen, but the incidence of cardiomyopathy accelerates at the level of 550 mg/m². Very old age and radiation might make the cardiomyopathy worse. Standard therapy for CHF is the treatment. There is a very late form of cardiac toxicity, seen many years after therapy, in patients who were without acute or subacute symptoms. In one study, 57 percent of children who received anthracyclines for pediatric malignancies had some abnormality in heart function.

Cytoxan can cause a severe hemorrhagic myopericarditis with doses greater then 1.5 g/m², the doses used in marrow-ablative treatments. Usually this produces a decrease in QRS amplitude, followed by typical CHF symptoms 7 to 10 days after treatment. Hemorrhagic or serosanguinous pericardial effusion can occur with signs of tamponade. Draining the effusion usually produces no change in clinical status because of the myocardial damage already done. There is also a fulminant course where symptoms occur within 48 h of treatment; these patients usually die from cardiogenic shock.

Neurotoxicity

It is rare for chemotherapeutic drugs to produce neurotoxicity severe enough to lead to the intensive care unit (ICU). Usually neurologic symptoms severe enough to warrant admission to the ICU are caused by local tumor effects or a combination of benzodiazepines, narcotics, antiemetics, and steroids (Table 52-3).

Peripheral neuropathy is a frequent side effect of many chemotherapeutic drugs. Paclitaxel causes stocking-and-glove paresthesias, rarely with motor dysfunction. Cisplatin can cause a sensory peripheral neuropathy that can develop into a severe ataxia. Cisplatin also causes tinnitus, deafness, autonomic neuropathy, seizures, retinal injury, transient cortical blindness, and the l'Hermitte sign.

Of the vinca alkaloids (vincristine, vinblastine, vinorelbine) vincristine is the worst at causing neurologic symptoms. Patients can develop a symmetrical mixed sensorimotor neuropathy that can progress to quadriparesis. It is dose-related and gradual in onset. Rarely will the vincas produce a mononeuropathy. The paresthesias and motor weakness may or may not improve over time. Transient severe muscle pain

(Velban myalgias) is seen mainly in children within hours after treatment. This severe jaw pain might be from a trigeminal neuralgia and can require narcotics. Cranial nerve palsies develop in up to 10 percent of patients. The dysphagia, vocal cord paralysis, ptosis, ophthalmoplegia, and facial nerve involvement can be very abrupt in onset. The symptoms are bilateral and usually resolve when the drug is stopped. Autonomic neuropathy can occur without peripheral findings in vinca-treated patients. Ileus can be severe enough to mimic an acute abdomen, atonic bladder, impotence, and orthostatic hypotension—the common symptoms which usually resolve over several days.

L-asparaginase causes cerebral dysfunction in 25 to 50 percent of the patients treated with this drug. Signs and symptoms include depression, somnolence, confusion, stupor, and coma. Encephalopathy can begin the first day of treatment, clears rapidly after therapy is stopped, and usually produces no focal neurologic abnormalities.

Cytarabine in high doses (2 to 3 g/m^2 bid) produces cerebellar and cerebral changes in 10 to 20 percent of patients. The changes start 5 to 7 days after the beginning of therapy. The cerebellar effects are usually more severe: intention tremor, dysarthria, horizontal nystagmus, and limb and truncal ataxia. The cerebral symptoms include somnolence, disorientation, memory loss, coma, and seizures. These changes can resolve over days to weeks but in some cases are permanent. The intrathecal route is not associated with cerebellar problems.

Methotrexate in high doses of 1 to 7 g/m^2 causes transient CNS syndromes in 2 to 15 percent of patients. The symptoms develop on average about 1 week after treatment. There is an abrupt onset with variable symptoms that include fluctuating mental status, local or generalized seizures, or symptoms resembling those of a stroke. Therapy is supportive and complete recovery usually occurs over several days. Intrathecal methotrexate can cause acute arachnoiditis, which resolves over 12 to 72 h. During this time, though, it can mimic a bacterial meningitis. Very rarely will methotrexate cause an acute reaction with paralysis, cranial nerve palsies, and seizures. Recovery is usually complete.

Renal Toxicity

Cisplatin is the only chemotherapeutic drug that causes renal failure in conventional doses. It causes a focal necrosis of

TABLE 52-3 Antineoplastic Drugs That Have Neurologic Toxicity

Drug	Incidence, %	Comments
		ENCEPHALOPATHY
L-Asparaginase	25–50	Ranges from drowsiness to stupor; onset usually on the day after start of therapy; generally resolves rapidly when therapy is over
High-dose busulfan	15	Acute obtundation, seizures; prophylactic anticonvulsants often used
High-dose carmustine (BCNU)	10	Severe acute or chronic encephalomyelopathy; time of onset variable; usually not reversible
High-dose cytarabine	10–20	Ranges from disorientation to coma; onset usually 5–7 days after start of therapy; prognosis variable
Fludarabine	Rare at conventional doses	Optic neuritis, altered mental status, paralysis. May appear weeks after treatment
Hexamethylmelamine	Variable	Toxicity ranges from depression to hallucinations; usually reversible when drug is withdrawn
Ifosfamide	5–30	Frequency greater with higher doses; ranges from mild somnolence to coma; onset hours after infusion, recovery usually within days
High-dose methotrexate	2–15	Onset usually 1 week after administration; most common presentation is a strokelike syndrome; usually reversible
Mitotane	40	Lethargy, somnolence, dizziness, vertigo
Pentostatin	Rare at conventional doses	Lethargy, seizures, coma
Procarbazine	10	Usually mild drowsiness or depression, rarely stupor or manic psychosis
High-dose Thiotepa	Dose-dependent	Somnolence, seizures, coma; dose-limiting extramedullary toxicity
Vincristine/vinblastine	Rare	SIADH

		ACUTE CEREBELLAR SYNDROME
High-dose cytarabine	10–20	Ranges from mild dysarthria to disabling ataxia; onset is 5–7 days after start of therapy; prognosis is variable
5-Fluorouracil	<1	Usually seen with large bolus doses; reversible in 1–6 weeks
		ACUTE PARAPLEGIA
Intrathecal administration of cytarabine, methotrexate thiotepa	Rare	These are the only drugs normally given intrathecally; all cause acute reversible arachnoiditis fairly often, paralysis exceedingly rarely; paralysis may or may not be reversible
		PERIPHERAL NEUROPATHIES
Cisplatin	Dose-dependent	Ototoxicity; distal sensory neuropathy
Hexamethylmelamine	Variable	Peripheral paresthesias and weakness
Suramin	Dose/schedule-dependent	Distal paresthesias, severe sensorimotor polyneuropathy, flaccid paralysis (Guillain-Barré)
Procarbazine	10–20	Decreased tendon reflexes, mild distal paresthesias
Paclitaxel, docetaxel	Common	Distal sensory neuropathy
Vinca alkaloids	See text	Symmetrical areflexia and distal paresthesias; symmetrical motor weakness starting with dorsiflexors; jaw pain; cranial nerve palsies; paralytic ileus

ABBREVIATION: SIADH, syndrome of inappropriate antidiuretic hormone.

the distal tubules and collecting ducts. Prehydration helps but does not prevent this injury, which can be severe enough to cause acute renal failure (Table 52-4). Adding chronic renal problems or an aminoglycoside to this situation increases the risk of kidney damage. There is a cumulative toxicity as the patient receives more doses of cisplatin. The damage peaks at 1 to 2 weeks. Magnesium wasting occurs with hypocalcemia and hypokalemia also. The patient can also get hyponatremia to the point of orthostatic hypotension.

Methotrexate in high doses of > 50 mg/kg has to be given with careful hydration and alkalinization. Leucovorin rescue should be performed until the serum levels are safe. Renal failure occurs because methotrexate crystals precipitate in the distal nephron. The damage usually resolves in 2 to 3 weeks. If the methotrexate accumulates in a third-space area (pleura, ascites), it can leach out of the third space and into the bloodstream for days to weeks.

Cytoxan causes hemorrhagic cystitis, bladder fibrosis, and bladder cancer. The hemorrhagic cystitis is usually idiosyncratic, but there is a higher incidence with prolonged or high-dose therapy. Ifosfamide can cause even worse urothelial toxicity. The damage is due to cytoxan's metabolism to acrolein, which causes the damage. Sodium 2-mercaptoethane sulfonate (mesna) provides free sulfhydryl groups to neutralize the acrolein. The bleeding is usually self-limited but is worse with thrombocytopenia and can be massive. The hemorrhagic cystitis is treated with continuous bladder irrigation, platelet transfusion, and vigorous hydration.

Mitomycin C produces renal failure with microangiopathic hemolytic anemia. This thrombotic thrombocytopenic purpura (TTP)/hemolytic-uremic syndrome (HUS) picture can happen as a late complication of allogeneic or autologous bone marrow transplantation. Hypertension, renal failure, and anemia predominate, rather than the fever and neurologic signs. Normal plasmapheresis is not as helpful as in idiopathic TTP; instead, plasmapheresis should be performed with a staphylococcal protein A immunoadsorption plasmapheresis column. Steroids, intravenous immunoglobulin, and plasma exchange are all of uncertain benefit.

TABLE 52-4 Antineoplastic Drugs Producing Renal and Electrolyte Abnormalities

Agent	Toxicity	Comments
Cisplatin	Magnesium, calcium, potassium, sodium wasting; renal insufficiency	See text
Cyclophosphamide	Impaired free water excretion	Transient; seen with doses > 50 mg/kg
Ifosfamide	Proximal tubular defect	—
High dose methotrexate	Acute renal failure	Usually reversible
Mitomycin C	Renal failure with microangiopathic hemolytic anemia (HUS/TTP)	Common with cumulative dose > 60 mg
Nitrosoureas (BCNU, CCNU, methyl-CCNU)	Progressive renal failure appearing after large cumulative doses	Decrease in renal size may be noted; effect may occur years after therapy
Streptozotocin	Renal failure, proximal renal tubular acidosis, nephrotic syndrome	Transient proteinuria is earliest manifestation
Suramin	Reversible renal insufficiency	Resolves within 1–6 weeks of discontinuing drug

TABLE 52-5 Cytotoxic Agents That Have Hepatic Toxicity

Drug	Frequency of Toxicity	Comments
L-Asparaginase	Common	Fatty metamorphosis; decreased synthetic function; reversible
Azathioprine	Uncommon	Cholestasis/necrosis; hyperbilirubinemia; variable prognosis
High-dose cytarabine	Common	Elevated bilirubin and transaminases; reversible
Floxuridine (FUDR)	Common	Biliary sclerosis with hepatic intraarterial infusion; chemical hepatitis
Methotrexate	Common	Cirrhosis, fibrosis, fatty metamorphosis; laboratory data may be normal; seen with prolonged daily therapy; variable prognosis
High-dose methotrexate	Common	Elevated transaminase levels, usually reversible in weeks
6-Mercaptopurine	Common	Cholestasis or necrosis; usually reversible
Mithramycin	Common	Necrosis; rarely seen with lower doses used for hypercalcemia
Nitrosoureas (BCNU, CCNU)	Occasional	Generally mild and reversible
Vincristine	Rare	May produce severe damage when combined with radiation to the liver

TABLE 52-6 Toxicities of Interleukin 2

Toxicity	Comments
Febrile reaction complex	Dose-dependent fever and chills are ameliorated with antipyretics and meperidine
Cardiovascular toxicity	Capillary leak syndrome. Rare cases of eosinophilic myocarditis reported
Central nervous system toxicity	Dose-dependent reversible somnolence, disorientation, cognitive deterioration. Appears several days after beginning of a treatment course
Hematopoietic toxicity	Frequent anemia, occasional thrombocytopenia, rare neutropenia; lymphopenia with rebound lymphocytosis, dramatic eosinophilia
Gastrointestinal toxicity	Mild nausea, vomiting, diarrhea. Mucositis is unusual, but may be severe. Profound, reversible cholestasis with hyperbilirubinemia and elevated alkaline phosphatase but normal transaminases
Infectious complications	Increase in staphylococcal bacteremia, often catheter related
Renal toxicity	Oliguria and prerenal azotemia reversible when infusion discontinued
Cutaneous toxicity	Rash ranging from discrete nonpruritic maculopapular lesions to diffuse erythroderma with flaky exfoliation after resolution of redness
Other	Hypo- and hyperthyroidism, decrease in vitamin K-dependent coagulation factors, severe myalgias

Hepatotoxity

At normal doses, few chemotherapeutic drugs cause significant hepatotoxicity on a regular basis (Table 52-5). However, with high-dose chemotherapy, venoocclusive disease (VOD) of the liver does become an issue. VOD rarely occurs with drugs at conventional doses, the antimetabolites being the one exception. With high-dose chemotherapy for bone marrow transplantation, there is an incidence of VOD of up to 20 percent. The symptoms include jaundice, hepatomegaly or right-upper-quadrant pain, and ascites or unexplained weight gain. It resembles Budd-Chiari syndrome clinically, with out-of-proportion hyperbilirubinemia and then transaminase elevation. The VOD begins about 10 days after bone marrow reinfusion. When this condition is severe, patients can die by day 35 posttransplant. In contrast, graft-versus-host disease (GVHD) begins after day 20 postreinfusion. There is also a late-onset version of VOD, which can present as severe abdominal pain and mimic an abdominal catastrophe. Drug effects and sepsis can minic VOD. This is a clinical diagnosis, since biopsy is usually contraindicated in these coagulopathic and thrombocytopenic patients. A liver ultrasound will reveal increased mean hepatic artery resistive index or reversal of portal venous flow. Care is primarily supportive, but there are case reports of resolution of VOD after treatment with tissue plasminogen activator.

Sepsis Syndrome

Many biologicals (interleukins, tissue necrosis factor, interferon) are in use or under investigation. They all share the same side effect profile, probably from the "cytokine cascade." High-dose interleukin-2 (IL-2) produces a sepsis-like capillary leak syndrome typical of biological agents. This syndrome can lead to hypotension and cardiovascular collapse. It usually resolves soon after treatment with IL-2 has been completed. Arrhythmias, myocardial infarction, and CNS toxicity can also be seen with the biologicals and resolve soon after treatment is completed (Table 52-6).

For a more detailed discussion, see Chap. 69 in *Principles of Critical Care*, 2d ed.

Chapter 53

BONE MARROW AND STEM CELL TRANSPLANTATION AND GRAFT-VERSUS-HOST DISEASE

CHANKANOK KUAGOOLWONGSE

SCOTT BUDINGER

Bone marrow transplantation (BMT) is increasingly used as therapy for a wide range of malignant and nonmalignant disorders. Donor stem cells are harvested from either the marrow or peripheral blood of the patient (autologous), an identical twin (syngeneic), matched donor (HLA-matched), or unrelated donor (HLA-mismatched) and reinfused into the patient's peripheral blood after high-dose cytotoxic chemotherapy, total body irradiation, or both.

BMT is associated with a high morbidity and mortality, resulting from toxicity of the induction regimen, profound immunosuppression, and a peculiar form of rejection—graft-versus-host disease (GVHD). Approximately 40 percent of BMT patients require admission to an intensive care unit (ICU). As most ICU admissions result from pulmonary complications, these are discussed first, followed by complications of the induction regimen and GVHD (Table 53-1).

Pulmonary Complications of Transplantation

Pulmonary complications, especially infectious pneumonia, are a major cause of morbidity and mortality in BMT patients (Table 53-2). Upon recognition of a pulmonary complication, appropriate empiric therapy should begin immediately.

TABLE 53-1 Selected Complications of Bone Marrow Transplantation

Complication	Diagnosis	Treatment
Hypoxemic respiratory failure	Blood, urine, stool culture, nasopharyngeal swabs, +/− bronchoscopy; consider chemotoxicity, cardiac dysfunction	Antibacterial and antifungal therapy
Focal infiltrates < 30 days	Bronchoscopy with BAL	Antibacterial/antifungal and specific therapy based on bronchoscopy
Hepatic VOD	Hepatomegaly, ascites, edema, increased LTFs < 2 weeks after transplant	Supportive
CMV pneumonia	CMV in BAL fluid, urine, or blood with new infiltrate, or lung biopsy	Ganciclovir + CMV immune globulin
VZV	Isolation from BAL fluid or skin lesion	Acyclovir + VZV immune globulin

HSV	Isolation from BAL fluid or skin	Acyclovir
RSV, parainfluenza virus	Isolation from nasopharynx or BAL fluid	Inhaled ribavirin
Pneumocystis carinii pneumonia	Isolation from BAL fluid	TMP/SMX or pentamadine; prophylaxis indicated
Idiopathic pneumonia syndrome	Infiltrates and hypoxemia in the absence of an identified etiology	Supportive
Acute GVHD (< 3 months)	Dermatitis, hepatitis, and enteritis (diarrhea); biopsy confirmation required	Increased immunosuppression; treatment of coexisting infection
Chronic GVHD (> 3 months)	Dermatitis, hepatitis, and enteritis	Increased immunosuppression
Bronchiolitis obliterans	Increasing dyspnea, fixed airflow obstruction on PFTs	Increased immunosuppression

ABBREVIATIONS: VOD, venoocclusive disease; CMV, cytomegalovirus; VZV, varicella zoster virus; HSV, herpes simplex virus; GVHD, graft-versus-host disease; BAL, bronchoalveolar lavage; LFTs, liver function tests; PFTs, pulmonary function tests; TMP/SMX, trimethoprim/sulfamethoxazole.

TABLE 53-2   Incidence of Common Etiologies
for Pulmonary Infiltrates after BMT

Complications	Approximate Incidence, %
COMPLICATIONS WITHIN 100 DAYS	
Pulmonary edema syndromes	0–50
Infectious pneumonia	20–30
Bacterial	2–30
Fungal	4–13
Viral	4–10
Protozoal	< 5
Idiopathic pneumonia	7–12
Pulmonary venoocclusive disease	Rare
COMPLICATIONS AFTER 100 DAYS	
Bacterial bronchopneumonia	20–30
Idiopathic pneumonia	10–20
Viral pneumonia	0–10
Obliterative bronchiolitis[a]	2–11

[a]Obstructive airflow among marrow recipients with chronic graft-versus-host disease.

Expeditious use of invasive diagnostic testing may establish a specific diagnosis, allowing for tailoring of empiric therapy to avoid toxicity. However, the benefits of invasive diagnostic testing must be weighed against the increased risks of complication in these patients (e.g., thrombocytopenia and impaired oxygenation).

The time after transplant when a pulmonary complication develops can be helpful in narrowing the differential diagnosis (Table 53-2). Infectious pneumonias can occur at any time after transplantation; however, the spectrum of pathogens changes over time, with bacterial and fungal infections predominating early and opportunistic pathogens occurring later. Pulmonary edema and pulmonary venoocclusive disease (VOD) are complications of chemotherapy and tend to develop early. Obliterative bronchiolitis, the histopathologic hallmark of GVHD in the lung, occurs late after transplantation.

DIAGNOSIS

Not all patients who develop diffuse infiltrates within 30 days of BMT require fiberoptic bronchoscopy, which has a low yield in this setting. Initial empiric treatment with antibiotics, correction of coagulopathy, diuresis, and salt restriction are appropriate in most patients. Blood cultures, including cultures through the central line, should be obtained. Culture of the nares for viruses should be considered. Nasopharyngeal swabs documenting colonization by *Aspergillus fumigatus* may decrease the threshold for empiric antifungal therapy. Fiberoptic bronchoscopy should be considered if there is clinical uncertainty about the diagnosis, failure to improve despite empiric therapy, focal infiltrates on chest x-ray, or toxicities of empiric therapy.

More than 30 days after transplantation, brochoscopy with bronchoalveolar lavage (BAL) and possibly transbronchial biopsy should be performed in most patients, as atypical infections are common. Video-assisted thoracoscopic lung biopsy should be considered for patients with a nondiagnostic bronchoscopy.

TREATMENT

Bacterial Pneumonia

Empiric antibiotics should include adequate coverage for gram-negative rods including *Pseudomonas*. Failure to respond or isolation of gram-positive organisms should prompt early addition of agents to cover nosocomial gram-positive agents.

Fungal Pneumonia

Prolonged neutropenia, failure to respond to antibacterial therapy, or isolation of fungus from any site should prompt addition of amphotericin B. Amphotericin B should be continued until the neutrophil count has recovered, steroids have been discontinued, and the infection has resolved. Itraconazole or fluconazole are generally not adequate to treat active fungal infections in neutropenic patients. However, they may be considered for patients with sensitive organisms and contraindications to amphotericin B or as continued therapy after an initial course of amphotericin B.

Viral and Other Pneumonias

Cytomegalovirus (CMV) is an important pathogen in BMT recipients. Definitive diagnosis often requires open-lung biopsy, but isolation of CMV from BAL fluid, blood, or urine in the setting of new pulmonary infiltrates warrants empiric therapy. Intravenous ganciclovir and CMV immune globulin should be given for at least 2 weeks. Clearance of viremia should be documented before discontinuing therapy to prevent relapse and drug resistance. In ganciclovir-resistant cases, foscarnet has been used alone or with combinations of other antiviral agents.

Herpes simplex virus (HSV) and varicella zoster virus (VZV) should be treated with acyclovir. Respiratory syncytial virus and parainfluenza virus should be treated with inhaled ribavirin and intravenous immunoglobulin. The treatment of *Pneumocystis carinii*, *Legionella* spp., and *Nocardia* infections is the same as for other immunocompromised patients.

PROPHYLAXIS

A protective environment with filtered laminar airflow to reduce airborne contamination may decrease nosocomial infection and help prevent the development of GVHD. Strict handwashing and isolation guidelines should be enforced. Ill health care workers should be sent home.

The incidence of *P. carinii* pneumonia is dramatically reduced with prophylactic daily oral trimethoprim/sulfamethoxazole administration 2 weeks prior to BMT and twice weekly after engraftment. Intravenous or aerosolized pentamidine or dapsone is less effective but can be used in sulfa-allergic patients who cannot undergo desensitization.

CMV-seronegative recipients should receive only CMV-seronegative blood products. Ganciclovir prophylaxis in seropositive recipients significantly reduces the incidence of CMV pneumonia. Prophylactic acyclovir is effective in reducing reactivation of HSV infection and CMV.

IDIOPATHIC PNEUMONIA SYNDROME

This diagnosis is made when other causes of pulmonary infiltrates are excluded. The presentation is identical to that of other causes of acute lung injury and/or acute respiratory distress syndrome (ARDS). Treatment is primarily supportive, although some advocate corticosteroids. Mortality is high.

BRONCHIOLITIS OBLITERANS

Bronchiolitis obliterans is thought to represent GVHD in the lung (see below). Clinically it presents as slowly progressive dyspnea on exertion with cough. Spirometry reveals fixed airflow obstruction. Treatment includes increased immunosuppressive therapy and bronchodilators. Unfortunately, most patients progress to respiratory failure and death.

Complications of the Induction Regimen

SEPSIS

Immunosuppression, use of central venous catheters with total parenteral nutrition (TPN), and prolonged neutropenia increase the risk of infection with and dissemination of bacteria and fungi. Treatment of preexisting infections prior to transplantation, adherence to strict infection control policies, and early empiric antibiotic therapy can decrease the rate of life-threatening infections.

DIRECT EFFECTS OF CHEMOTHERAPY/RADIATION THERAPY

The complications of chemotherapy are legion. It is important for the intensivist to consider these complications in patients with respiratory or other organ failures after BMT. Importantly, high-dose cytarabine may result in ARDS, Guillain-Barré syndrome, and peripheral neuropathies. High-dose cyclophosphamide has been associated with cardiac dysfunction, hemorrhagic cystitis, and tumor lysis syndrome.

HEPATIC VENOOCCLUSIVE DISEASE (VOD)

Hepatic VOD is thought to result from endothelial cell damage secondary to high-dose chemotherapy and especially radiation therapy. Histopathology reveals a hemorrhagic, obliterative terminal venulitis resulting in perivenular hepatocellular injury. Clinical symptoms and laboratory abnormalities develop in the first 2 weeks after BMT (earlier than GVHD). Patients develop progressive weight gain and peripheral edema, jaundice, painful hepatomegaly, ascites, and elevated liver function tests. Metabolic encephalopathy and hepatorenal syndrome may ensue. The diagnosis is made clinically after exclusion of cardiac causes of hepatic congestion, hepatic vein thrombosis, invasive fungal disease, and septicemia. Mortality is about 30 percent and there is presently no effective treatment.

Late Complications of BMT

COMPLICATIONS OF IMMUNOSUPPRESSION

Corticosteroids, cyclosporine, and methotrexate, used to prevent rejection in allogeneic BMT recipients, result in an increased risk of opportunistic infection. Aggressive diagnostic evaluation is necessary in all post-BMT patients.

RELAPSE OF UNDERLYING DISEASE

Relapse rates after BMT are about 20 percent for early-stage leukemic patients and increase to 50 to 70 percent in advanced leukemia. Most relapses occur with host cells indicating ineffective chemotherapy. Second transplantation is associated with substantially higher mortality.

GVHD

GVHD is a unique complication in allogeneic BMT. It results from an immune response of donor lymphocytes to alloantigens on the recipient's cells. Patients who receive genetically identical transplants or autologous stem cell reinfusion do not develop GVHD. It can be divided into acute and chronic forms.

Acute GVHD

Acute GVHD generally presents within the first 3 months of BMT with dermatitis, enteritis (diarrhea), and hepatitis. A specific diagnosis must be made by biopsy (often multiple) of affected organs, usually the skin, liver, or rectum. Histology demonstrates lymphocytic infiltration of the epidermis, liver, or gastrointestinal tract. Coexisting infections and drug reactions are the rule in these patients.

Supportive care is often complicated by malabsorption due to gut involvement, necessitating prolonged TPN with its attendant complications. Gastrointestinal hemorrhage may also result from gut involvement, but alternative possibilities must be excluded.

Treatment includes high-dose corticosteroids and antithymocyte globulin, with continued methotrexate and cyclosporine, but this is often ineffective and mortality remains high. Breakdown of mucosal barriers with concomitant immunosuppression results in a high rate of fatal nosocomial infection.

Chronic GVHD

GVHD is said to be chronic when it occurs or persists 3 months after BMT. Chronic GVHD is seen in 20 to 50 percent of allogeneic BMT recipients. Patients, often with a history of acute GVHD, present with a variable combination of characteristic dermatitis consisting of skin pigmentation and sclerosis, elevated liver enzymes, mucositis, and airflow obstruction reflecting bronchiolitis obliterans. Treatment is similar to that for acute GVHD and is unfortunately often ineffective.

For a more detailed discussion, see Chap. 68 in *Principles of Critical Care*, 2d ed.

Chapter 54

ACUTE RENAL FAILURE

PATRICK CUNNINGHAM

Initial Evaluation

Acute renal failure (ARF) is extremely common in the critically ill patient. Determination of its cause should always include several initial pieces of information. A thorough history and physical is always necessary, especially with regard to the patient's hemodynamics and volume status; when these data are confusing, invasive monitoring of hemodynamics may be helpful. It is imperative to measure urine output carefully; thus a Foley catheter is necessary. This will also give information pertaining to possible urinary obstruction.

Urine sodium concentration and urine osmolality can often help categorize the cause of the renal failure into either a prerenal or intrinsic renal cause, as described below. Last, examination of urine sediment is of underappreciated importance, especially when considering an intrinsic renal disease.

Causes and Therapy

One of the most common causes of ARF in the intensive care unit (ICU) setting is prerenal azotemia. Decreased perfusion of the kidneys of any cause will lead to a rise in creatinine. Thus, the management of this state will overlap with the management of shock. Volume depletion from hemorrhage, diuretics, diarrhea, or vomiting can be responsible, but so can decreased renal blood flow from cardiogenic or septic shock. The state of septic shock causes massive systemic vasodilation, so that, although the cardiac output is increased, blood is shunted everywhere but the kidney. The hemodynamics of advanced liver failure are very similar to this; in both states, circulating inflammatory mediators may actually cause renal vasoconstriction, only worsening the kidneys' perfusion. An extreme example of this is hepatorenal syndrome, in which this vasoconstriction becomes severe and *irreversible,* despite maximization of renal blood flow. True hepatorenal syndrome is usually seen only in advanced liver disease associated with hypotension, synthetic dysfunction, and ascites.

Besides the history and physical examination, several laboratory measurements may help confirm a diagnosis of the prerenal state. Urine sodium concentration and urine osmolality will be low and high, respectively, as the underperfused kidney attempts to resorb maximal sodium and water to maintain perfusion. Calculation of the fractional excretion of sodium, or FE_{Na}, helps correct the urine sodium concentration for the degree of water resorption in the urine and is more accurate than the urine sodium concentration alone. It is calculated as follows:

$$FE_{Na} = (\text{urine [Na]})(\text{serum creatinine}) / (\text{serum sodium})(\text{urine creatinine})$$

A value under 1 percent is consistent with prerenal azotemia, a value over 1 percent with tubular dysfunction associated with acute tubular necrosis (ATN). Several important caveats are in order, however, as this index is often overused (Table 54-1).

Also seen in prerenal azotemia is an elevation of the BUN-to-creatinine ratio above 20, because of increased urea absorption in the kidney, as it follows avid sodium resorption. Other causes of preferentially increased BUN—such as

TABLE 54-1   Limitations of Fractional Excretion of Sodium (FE_{Na})

Condition	Explanation
Diuretics	Increases urine sodium excretion
Chronic renal insufficiency	Limits ability to fully reabsorb sodium
Metabolic alkalosis	Bicarbonaturia obliges high urine sodium excretion
Urine output > 1 L/day	Value of FE_{Na} unconfirmed
Obstruction	Many other disorders associated with low sodium excretion
Acute glomerulonephritis	
Contrast dye	
Rhabdomyolysis or hemolysis	

steroids, hypercatabolism, or gastrointestinal bleeding should be considered, however. Also the *pattern* of creatinine increase helps guide the diagnosis: an inconsistent, more gradual rise is more consistent with prerenal azotemia, or various other causes, as opposed to the steady, rapid (>1 mg/dL per day) rise seen in ATN.

Obstructive, or "postrenal" causes of ARF are important to diagnose because they are often reversible. It should be emphasized that obstruction must be complete and bilateral to cause true acute renal failure. There are relatively few situations that will cause this. Most common is prostatic obstruction, classically occurring in an elderly male after receiving opiates or alpha agonists or after removal of a Foley catheter. Another common cause is an atonic bladder, seen in neuropathies such as diabetes or spinal cord lesions. Malignancies above the level of the bladder may cause some degree of obstruction but rarely bilaterally; cervical cancer can be seen in a position capable of obstructing both ureters. Last, obstruction can occur surprisingly often with a catheter in place if it is plugged or malpositioned and may not be recognized readily in a sedated or obtunded patient.

Diagnosis of obstruction can be suspected based on history and confirmed by finding an enlarged, tender bladder on examination and a large postvoid residual of urine. Another helpful clue is hyperkalemia out of proportion to the degree of renal failure; obstruction impairs the tubules' ability to excrete potassium. Ultrasound is generally required to either confirm the diagnosis or quantitate the chronicity of the obstruction. Although ultrasound is specific, it should be realized that in cases of very early obstruction, volume depletion, or encasement by tumor it may fail to show hydronephrosis.

When history, physical, and laboratory information do not clearly point to prerenal azotemia or obstruction, an intrinsic renal process must be suspected. Although there is a great variety of possible renal diseases, relatively few can cause truly acute renal failure ensuing over a period of days. Overwhelmingly the most common is ATN. It is caused by renal ischemia, such as severe and prolonged prerenal azotemia from hypovolemia, cardiogenic shock, or sepsis or by a variety of toxins, such as aminoglycosides, cisplatin, contrast dye, or myoglobin or hemoglobin from rhabdomyolysis or intravascular hemolysis. It is characterized by an acute, rapid, and progressive rise in BUN and creatinine, a FE_{Na} usually over 1 percent because of tubular necrosis and inability to reabsorb sodium, and lack of the ability to concentrate the urine.

Urinalysis may show many granular "muddy brown" casts as well as free tubular cells and tubular cell casts. If the initial insult is acute, recovery can be expected in 1 to 2 weeks, but it may take considerably longer if there is repeated or sustained hypotension or toxicity. In general, the process of ATN may be "patchy," and some nephrons may continue to function and be responsible for some urine production with a calculated FE_{Na} of less than 1 percent despite widespread tubular injury. Maximization of perfusion, with volume and vasoactive drug support, along with removal of nephrotoxic agents will improve the chance of renal recovery. In addition to the above, drugs that may affect renal function are listed in Table 54-2. Early alkalinization of urine with a bicarbonate infusion may help minimize toxicity from rhabdomyolysis or hemolysis. However, there is otherwise no clear therapy to speed recovery, and care must be supportive. Often, in the recovery phase, a brisk diuresis ensues; intravascular volume should be maintained during this period to avoid imposing further injury on the recovering kidney.

Other causes of intrinsic ARF are much less common than ATN. Interstitial nephritis is basically an allergic drug reaction affecting the kidneys. The most common offenders are cimetidine, ciprofloxacin, penicillins, or any drug with a sulfhydryl group, including furosemide and trimethoprim/sulfamethoxazole. It may be associated with rash, fever,

TABLE 54-2   Drugs That Affect Renal Function

Angiotensin converting enzyme inhibitors, angiotensin blockers, cyclosporine, tacrolimus	Decrease renal function, hyperkalemia
Nonsteroidal anti-inflammatory drugs	Decrease renal function
Cimetidine, trimethoprim	Spuriously raise creatinine by inhibiting its tubular secretion

or peripheral eosinophilia. Urinalysis may show white blood cells, white blood cell casts, and eosinophils, although the last test is poorly sensitive. ARF is best treated by removing the offending agent, and occasionally with steroids.

Atheroemboli to the kidney may result from instrumentation of the aorta or renal arteries. They cause irreversible decline in renal function of a variable extent. Atheroemboli may be associated with clinical evidence of emboli in the extremities, peripheral eosinophilia, and low serum complement levels.

Uric acid nephropathy may occur in the setting of tumor lysis syndrome or massive tissue necrosis. This usually requires a uric acid level over 15 to 20 mg/dL. The uric acid will precipitate in the tubules and cause them to be obstructed. This can be prevented with allopurinol and vigorous alkaline hydration of the urine to prevent precipitation. Despite very high serum uric acid levels, nephropathy does not occur in the setting of marked prerenal disease because in this case the uric acid is not being excreted into the tubules.

The vast majority of the many glomerular diseases do *not* progress to renal failure rapidly but instead do so over months to years. Even rapidly progressive glomerulonephritis (RPGN) goes on to renal failure over days to weeks—more slowly than ATN. This can be suspected by an active urine sediment with red blood cells and red blood cell casts and by mild to moderate proteinuria. A clinical setting of constitutional symptoms, rash, joint pain, and an elevated erythrocyte sedimentation rate may be seen. This category includes pulmonary-renal syndromes with hemoptysis, such as Goodpasture disease and Wegener granulomatosis as well as microscopic polyangiitis, fulminant lupus nephritis, and others. These diseases may respond well to pulse steroids and cyclophosphamide.

Hemolytic-uremic syndrome or thrombotic thrombocytopenic purpura are diseases in a spectrum of illness in which endothelial abnormalities cause plugging of small vessels with platelet thrombi. Diagnosis requires thrombocytopenia and intravascular hemolysis with schistocytes; there may also be fever and mental status changes. Urinary sediment may be benign. It may be a primary idiopathic syndrome or associated with various medications, hemorrhagic gastroenteritis, or human immunodeficiency virus. It often improves with steroids and plasmapheresis.

Renal vein thrombosis should be suspected in the setting of hypercoagulable states, especially nephrotic syndrome. It will cause true renal failure only if it is bilateral or superimposed on chronic preexisting disease. It may present with flank pain, hematuria, and proteinuria and improve with anticoagulation.

Renal failure may result from multiple myeloma due to deposition of light chains within the tubules. This is often initiated by dehydration. Urinalysis will be bland but light chains will be present in the urine. Quantitative proteinuria may be large despite a negative urine dipstick for protein, which picks up only amyloid. This may be improved by rehydration and alkalinization of the urine with intravenous bicarbonate and may also improve to an extent with chemotherapy and plasmapheresis, which decrease the level of the toxic light chains.

In addition to the limited specific therapies listed above, general supportive care of the patient with ARF is important. Medication dosages should be adjusted and intake of fluid, potassium, and phosphorus should be limited. Nutrition should be optimized. High intravenous doses of diuretics may help optimize fluid balance but do not hasten recovery of renal function. Low-dose dopamine may have a diuretic function but does not improve recovery from ARF or appear to be protective of renal function. Dialysis will be necessary if function is sufficiently impaired (see Chap. 55). However, the very best therapy is prevention: situations that are harmful to renal function must be avoided by patients with preexisting renal impairment.

For a more detailed discussion, see Chap. 70 in *Principles of Critical Care,* 2d ed.

DIALYSIS IN THE INTENSIVE CARE UNIT

PATRICK CUNNINGHAM

Indications

Although patients with established end-stage renal disease should continue to get their regular dialysis treatments in the intensive care unit (ICU) there are relatively few indications for emergent dialysis (Table 55-1). Hyperkalemia can lead to fatal wide-complex ventricular arrhythmias if not corrected. Severe metabolic acidosis may also merit correction via dialysis if there is evidence that it is contributing to hemodynamic instability or imposing an excess ventilatory load. Pulmonary edema refractory to other medical measures in an acutely dyspneic patient is another indication for dialysis. Other rarer indications for emergent dialysis include drug intoxications and severe hypothermia. Malignant hypertension in the setting of renal failure will often improve with volume removal via dialysis, but this is unpredictable. The first step in such cases is aggressive pharmacologic control, including a sodium nitroprusside drip if necessary (see Chap. 32). Symptomatic uremia is an indication for initiation of dialysis, but its manifestations—such as encephalopathy, platelet dysfunction, immunosuppression, or pericarditis—should not be expected to resolve immediately after one dialysis session.

When emergent dialysis is indicated, it must be realized that some time is necessary to achieve access, prepare the machine, etc., and all available measures to correct hyperkalemia, acidosis, or pulmonary edema should still be pursued in the meantime. It is all too easy at times to attribute acute shortness of breath in the setting of renal failure to pulmonary edema when other entities such as cardiac ischemia, tamponade, pulmonary embolism, or sepsis have not been adequately excluded.

TABLE 55-1   Indications for Emergent Dialysis

Hyperkalemia
Metabolic acidosis
Uremic symptoms (bleeding, seizures)
Pulmonary edema
Drug intoxications (salicylates, phenobarbital, lithium, methanol,
    ethylene glycol)
Severe hypothermia

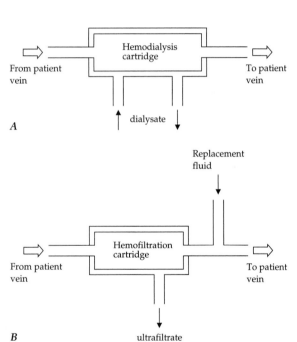

FIGURE 55-1   *A.* **Intermittent hemodialysis. As venous blood is pumped past dialysate, its solute composition changes by osmosis. Pressures can be manipulated to gradually remove volume as well.** *B.* **Continuous venovenous hemofiltration (CVVH). As venous blood is pumped through a more porous chamber, a large amount of serum is filtered out and discarded. The composition and volume of replacement fluid are varied to control the patient's chemistries and volume status.**

Modalities

Standard or intermittent hemodialysis involves circulation of the patient's blood past one side of a semipermeable membrane while a dialysate solution passes on the other side (Fig. 55-1). Solutes such as urea and potassium pass across the membrane by diffusion in the direction of their concentration gradient, and a variable but limited amount of water and solutes can be squeezed across the membrane by convection as well. This process is generally done in 4 h. Heparin is helpful but not mandatory to prevent clotting of the dialyzer.

There is at least theoretical concern that rapid volume and electrolyte changes are poorly tolerated in a critically ill patient. Because of these concerns, continuous venovenous hemofiltration (CVVH) is often more suitable in certain patients. Its principle is different: it pumps blood past a highly permeable membrane and removes water and solutes by convection at rapid rate, while the patient is continually given a replacement solution designed to optimize electrolytes. This process clears the blood only by convention, not diffusion, and is therefore slower. However, because it is run continuously over a period of days, it will achieve better and also more gradual clearance of waste products and volume. It is preferable to intermittent dialysis in hypotensive patients, especially if they are massively volume-overloaded. Its disadvantages include its burden on nursing staff due to the need to carefully monitor the volume of replacement fluid and the very frequent clotting of the dialyzer that occurs when heparin cannot be used. If even higher clearances are required, dialysate can be circulated on the other side of the membrane, adding solute removal by diffusion at the expense of a more complicated setup; this is known as continuous venovenous hemodiafiltration (CVVHD).

Peritoneal dialysis (PD) exploits the patient's peritoneum as a semipermeable membrane and removes solutes and volume by periodically instilling a hyperosmotic glucose-containing solution into the patient's peritoneal cavity via a catheter. Its relatively gradual rate of waste-product and volume removal can be either an advantage or disadvantage, depending on the situation. However, PD provides poor metabolic clearance in shock states, where the peritoneum is poorly perfused.

Complications

It is important to realize that dialysis is not an entirely benign procedure. In patients without preexisting hemodialysis access, complications frequently relate to the placement of the intravenous catheter. As with other lines, bleeding is a concern. Any catheter is a potential source of infection and should be left in no longer than necessary. After several days, catheters commonly develop thrombi on their tips, often leading to poor function and occasional embolic phenomena. With time, the use of catheters may cause venous stenosis. These complications guide selection of the catheter's site. Femoral catheters are simpler to place, with less bleeding risk, but anecdotal experience suggests that they carry a greater risk of infection compared with cleaner upper extremity sites. Subclavian dialysis catheters should be avoided because of their greater association with eventual stenosis. Any catheter should be removed and replaced if line sepsis is suspected, ideally after a few days to clear any bacteremia.

Ideally, hemodialysis is done with a heparin infusion via the dialysis machine to prevent clotting of the dialyzer and promote effective dialyzer function. This can be withheld in patients with significant bleeding risks. Continuous dialytic therapies have a much greater chance of clotting and are usually not feasible if the patient cannot receive heparin. At the end of dialysis, catheters are instilled with high-dose heparin to prevent them from clotting; when they are used for lab draws without withdrawal of their contents, spurious coagulation values will result, and infusion through them essentially boluses the patient with heparin.

The process of dialysis is frequently associated with some degree of hypotension, which is concerning in critically ill patients with already borderline perfusion. This results from the relatively abrupt removal of volume as well as possible effects relating to the dialysis membrane. This may worsen cerebral, cardiac, or gastrointestinal ischemia and may also retard the recovery of renal function in acute renal failure.

For a more detailed discussion, see Chap. 72 in *Principles of Critical Care*, 2d ed.

Chapter 56

SEVERE ELECTROLYTE DISTURBANCES

PATRICK CUNNINGHAM

Hyponatremia

It must be emphasized that hyponatremia has almost nothing to do with how the kidney handles sodium but instead with how it handles free water. Hyponatremia is normally prevented despite a large free water intake by the kidney's formation of a dilute filtrate in the loop of Henle; if antidiuretic hormone (ADH) can be turned off, this dilute urine can be excreted. When these two steps are impaired, hyponatremia results.

Pseudohyponatremia should always be considered initially (Fig. 56-1). It may occur with highly elevated triglycerides or serum protein levels. In this case, plasma osmolality will not be low, as in true hyponatremia, but normal. If the plasma osmolality is high, pseudohyponatremia due to hyperglycemia or mannitol infusions is likely responsible, as the osmotic activity of these compounds pulls water out of cells into the serum and dilutes the sodium concentration. Serum sodium will fall by 1 meq/L for each 62 mg/dL elevation of glucose.

The next step in diagnosis is measurement of urine osmolality. If the kidney functions normally, it should be under 100 mOsm/L in the setting of hyponatremia. Thus, a value below this would imply psychogenic polydipsia as the cause. Once this is excluded, a free water excretion problem must be present. Assuming renal function is normal and there is no evidence of hypothyroidism or hypoadrenalism, ADH must be present. The next question is whether it is "appropriate" or not. Effective volume depletion is a physiologic and therefore appropriate stimulus for secretion of ADH. This will be seen in true volume depletion as well as in states of decreased

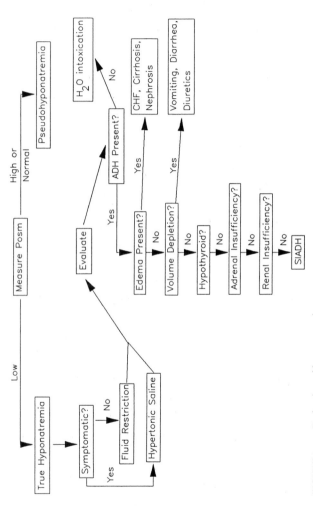

FIGURE 56-1   Evaluation of hyponatremia.

TABLE 56-1   Common Causes of the Syndrome
of Inappropriate Antidiuretic Hormone

CNS disorders (tumor, stroke, hemorrhage, infection)
Pulmonary disorders (pneumonia, abscess)
Carcinoma (lung, GI)
Psychosis
Severe pain
Severe nausea/vomiting
Drugs (neuroleptics, cyclophosphamide, chlorpropamide,
   carbamazepine, vincristine)

---

perfusion, such as heart failure, liver failure, or nephrotic syndrome. Inappropriate ADH is deemed to be present when there is no evidence of hypoperfusion. SIADH can be caused by a wide variety of conditions (Table 56-1). This can be supported by a fractional excretion of sodium (FE_{Na}) greater than 1 percent, where

$$FE_{Na} = \text{(urine [Na])(serum creatinine)} / \text{(serum [Na])(urine creatinine)}$$

A FE_{Na} under 1 percent supports a state of decreased effective circulating volume.

Symptoms of hyponatremia are due to cerebral edema as the extra water enters the brain. It can cause headache, nausea, or lethargy and may lead to seizures or coma when severe. Patients with serious neurologic symptoms or a sodium concentration less than 110 to 115 meq/L need an initially rapid correction until symptoms resolve or a safer level is reached. The goal should be to correct the serum sodium concentration at a rate of 1.5 to 2.0 meq/L per hour. This can be accomplished by giving hypertonic (3%) saline, with furosemide if needed to avoid volume overload. The amount to be given to reach a serum sodium of 120 meq/L can be calculated by the sodium deficit:

$$\text{Na deficit (milliequivalents)} = 0.5 \times \text{lean body mass (kilograms)} \times (120 - \text{serum [Na]})$$

A solution of 3% saline contains 513 meq Na/L, and an amount corresponding to this deficit should be given. Hyponatremia of lesser severity need not be corrected as fast. In fact, overly rapid correction, especially if the hyponatremia was chronic, may cause permanent neurologic injury. Patients with SIADH or an edematous state such as congestive heart failure, liver failure, or nephrotic syndrome should be restricted to less than 1 L of water per day, while true volume depletion should be repleted with 0.9% saline. A rate correction of 0.5 meq/L/h should be the goal. Whatever the initial rate of correction, it should be limited to no faster than 12 meq/L in 24 h.

Hypernatremia

Hypernatremia is usually a problem of excessive free water loss. The body normally defends against this with the powerful mechanism of thirst, but in sick patients unable to drink, hypernatremia will develop. Water may be lost via insensible losses, such as sweating and skin evaporation, which can be massive in patients with extensive burns. Free water may also be lost in the stool; normal diarrhea is not a cause of this, but osmotic diarrhea as in malabsorption and with lactulose or other laxatives may cause this. The most common source of free water loss is in the urine. This will occur with an osmotic diuresis, as with hyperglycemia, mannitol, and in the polyuria associated with recovery from acute renal failure, which is largely due to urea. Loop diuretics cause excretion of a hypotonic urine. Diabetes insipidus (DI) will also cause excretion of an inappropriately dilute urine. It may be caused by a failure to secrete ADH or a resistance to its action at the kidney (Table 56-2). Patients with chronic renal insufficiency will also be unable to maximally concentrate their urine, which could be considered a form of nephrogenic DI. Again,

TABLE 56-2   Causes of Diabetes Insipidus

Central	Nephrogenic
Idiopathic	Congenital
Anoxic encephalopathy	Lithium
Pituitary surgery	Hypercalcemia (> 11.00 mg/dL)
Hypothalamic tumor	Hypokalemia (< 3.0 meq/L)
Sheehan syndrome	

thirst usually allows these patients to maintain sodium concentration in the high normal range, but illness may cause hypernatremia to develop rapidly if fluid intake is impaired.

Sodium bicarbonate is a common cause of hypernatremia in critically ill patients when given excessively.

Diagnosis can be guided by measurement of urine osmolality. It will be high (> 700 mOsm/L) in insensible losses, diarrhea, or sodium overload. It will be low (< 300) in cases of complete central or nephrogenic DI. Partial cases of DI or urinary losses from an osmotic or pharmacologic diuresis will have intermediate values. These can be further delineated by performance of a water-restriction test (with close monitoring) and observing the response to exogenous desmopressin, an ADH analogue.

Hypernatremia can cause lethargy, seizures, and coma through osmotic shrinkage of brain cells and may even cause subarachnoid hemorrhage by tearing cerebral veins. Serious neurologic sequelae can result from correcting the sodium concentration too rapidly; correction should not exceed 12 meq/L in 24 h. This can be estimated with the calculation of the free water deficit:

$$\text{Free water deficit (liters)} = 0.5 \times \text{lean body mass (kg)} \times (\text{serum [Na]}/140 - 1)$$

This gives only the current water deficit; correction will fall short if ongoing insensible and urinary losses of free water are not also replaced. This also does not indicate the amount of volume depletion, only the amount of water necessary to correct the sodium concentration. Physicians should not let concern of pulmonary edema keep them from giving what may seem like a large amount of fluid by this estimate; two-thirds of the water will be taken up by cells. It is often best given orally. Last, the underlying cause of excess free water loss should be corrected; this may require desmopressin or other measures with DI.

Hypokalemia

Because normal kidney function can limit the amount of potassium excreted to very low levels, poor oral intake of potassium will rarely cause hypokalemia alone. Shift of potassium into cells may be seen in various conditions, such as in exchange for hydrogen ions in metabolic alkalosis, with excessive catecholamine release as in delerium tremens, head trauma, nebulizer treatments, or postarrest settings. Also, insulin drives potassium into cells, as is commonly seen in treatment of severe hyperglycemia. Severe hypothermia may also cause potassium to shift intracellularly. A spuriously low potassium may be seen with a leukocyte count over 100,000, as myelocytes may take up potassium if the blood sample is not run in timely fashion.

If hypokalemia cannot be entirely explained by transcellular shift, potassium loss must be responsible. This commonly occurs with diarrhea, vomiting, or drainage of gastrointestinal secretions. Sweating must be severe to account for hypokalemia. Also common is chronic or acute loss of potassium in the urine, most often from loop or thiazide-type diuretics. Any cause of excessive polyuria may cause excessive potassium loss in the urine, such as an osmotic diuresis with hyperglycemia or mannitol, recovery from acute renal failure, or even diabetes insipidus. In vomiting, most potassium loss is actually in the urine, as bicarbonate is wasted in the urine and potassium follows to preserve electroneutrality. Potassium reabsorption is impaired by amphotericin or cisplatin. Hypomagnesemia is a common reversible cause of potassium wasting in the urine. Renal tubular acidosis, either type I or II, is a rare cause of potassium loss in the urine. If these disorders do not adequately explain the potassium loss in the urine, a high aldosterone state must be expected. This may be caused by an adrenal adenoma or hyperplasia, Cushing's syndrome (although not iatrogenic Cushing's), or renal artery stenosis.

Calculation of the transtubular potassium gradient (TTKG) can suggest urinary potassium wasting. It is given by

$$\text{TTKG} = (\text{urine } [K])(\text{serum Osm}) / (\text{serum } [K])(\text{urine Osm})$$

It is unreliable in dilute urine or if urine sodium is low (< 25 meq/L). A TTKG over 7 in the setting of hypokalemia supports abnormal tubular handling of potassium.

The most concerning side effect of hypokalemia is cardiac arrhythmias. Electrocardiographic (ECG) changes can include QT prolongation, T-wave flattening, ST depression, and U waves. It can precipitate ectopy and arrhythmias, especially in those patients on digoxin. Severe hypokalemia (< 2.5 meq/L) may cause severe muscular weakness and even rhabdomyolysis. Hypokalemia has several effects on kidney function and can cause transient nephrogenic DI as well as an increase in ammonia synthesis sufficient to precipitate hepatic encephalopathy in patients with liver failure.

Besides correcting the underlying condition, hypokalemia is often best corrected with oral potassium chloride. It must be realized that the vast majority of potassium is stored intracellularly; supplements will transiently increase serum levels but are quickly taken up by cells. Only when the intracellular deficit (which may be several hundred milliequivalents if potassium is under 3.0) is finally repleted will serum levels increase significantly.

Hyperkalemia

It is almost impossible for elevated potassium intake to cause hyperkalemia without some defect in potassium excretion by the kidney. Sources of intake that may contribute include tissue necrosis, such as trauma, bleeding, hemolysis, or tumor lysis syndrome. Hyperkalemia may also result from transcellular shift. In metabolic acidosis, potassium may shift out of cells in exchange for hydrogen ions. Since insulin drives potassium into cells, insulin deficiency may cause hyperkalemia. Pseudohyperkalemia may be seen with extremely elevated leukocyte or platelet counts as potassium is released from cells during clot formation; this may be avoided by running a plasma and not a serum level.

Nevertheless, hyperkalemia usually results from a defect in urinary excretion. Potassium is normally excreted in the distal nephron under the stimulus of aldosterone in exchange for sodium or in parallel with hydrogen; a good distal urine flow encourages this process. Renal insufficiency or decreased urine output from a prerenal state will decrease distal flow enough to cause hyperkalemia. Deficiencies in aldosterone release or action will also cause hyperkalemia. These deficiencies include primary (not secondary) adrenal insufficiency, potassium-sparing diuretics including angiotensin converting enzyme inhibitors and angiotensin blockers, heparin, nonsteroidal anti-inflammatory drugs, sulfa-trimethoprim, and cyclosporine or tacrolimus. Some forms of renal tubular acidosis may also cause hyperkalemia via decreased aldosterone action. The TTKG will be low if there is a problem with aldosterone action. A value under 5 in the setting of hyperkalemia suggests a secretory defect.

The main consequence of hyperkalemia is cardiac arrhythmias. The severity of ECG changes correlates better with the need to intervene than does the plasma level alone. First seen is T-wave peaking. Eventually the P wave is lost and the QRS becomes widened. The danger of ventricular tachycardia becomes significant once QRS widening is observed. The sensitivity of the heart to hyperkalemia is increased with rapidity of rise and hypocalcemia and is worse with transcellular shift than with simple retention. Muscle weakness may also result from severely high levels. Treatment with intravenous calcium gluconate 1 to 2 ampules works most quickly to reduce the chance of arrhythmias but has the most short-lived effect. Intravenous sodium bicarbonate, 1 to 2 ampules, and 10 U intravenous insulin with 1 ampule of D50 will drive potassium intracellularly, but this effect wears off after several hours. Nebulized albuterol is also a useful therapy. Sodium polystyrene sulfonate (Kayexalate) 30 to 60 g orally or as an enema will actually remove potassium from the body; it is a resin that exchanges a sodium load for the potassium. It should be avoided if there is concern of bowel ischemia or severe ileus. Diuretics will cause significant potassium loss only if they also can induce a brisk urine output. Last, hemodialysis can correct hyperkalemia if above measures are insufficient.

Hypocalcemia

Hypocalcemia must be interpreted relative to the plasma albumin concentration; a useful approximation is for every 1.0 mg/dL that the albumin is below 4.0, the calcium is lowered by about 0.6 mg/dL. Alkalemia will cause more calcium to bind to albumin and will drop ionized calcium further. It is the free or ionized calcium that is physiologically relevant. Hypocalcemia may be due to vitamin D deficiency or to hypoparathyroidism. Measuring PTH levels as well as the concurrent phosphate level will often guide diagnosis. Vitamin D deficiency may result from malnutrition and poor sunlight exposure, malabsorption, drugs such as phenytoin and phenobarbital that impair its hepatic metabolism, or renal failure. Hypoparathyroidism may be postsurgical or idiopathic. Hypomagnesemia impairs PTH release. Severe pancreatitis or rhabdomyolysis can cause hypocalcemia via uptake by necrotic tissue. Severe sepsis may cause profound hypocalcemia by impairing the action of PTH. Severe hypocalcemia may cause tetany, including laryngospasm, mental status changes and seizures, and ECG changes such as QT prolongation, which may lead to arrhythmias. There is evidence that calcium administration in the critically ill may cause hypoxic cell damage, so calcium should be corrected in this setting only if the patient is symptomatic. When indicated, treatment of symptomatic hypocalcemia should include two intravenous ampules of 10% calcium gluconate with frequent monitoring of serum levels as well as correction of underlying cause. It is crucial to ensure that hypomagnesemia is corrected, as this may potentiate the tendency to tetany and arrhythmias.

Hypercalcemia

The most common cause of severe hypercalcemia is malignancy, via either extensive bony involvement or by ectopic production of a PTH-like hormone. The second most common cause is hyperparathyroidism, either primary or secondary (associated with renal failure). Other causes include vitamin D toxicity or sarcoidosis. Manifestations of hypercalcemia include lethargy and mental status changes, vomiting, reversible nephrogenic diabetes insipidus, renal insufficiency, and ectopic calcifications. ECG changes include shortening of the QT interval; hypercalcemia potentiates digoxin toxicity. The fastest treatment of hypercalcemia is increasing urine output with saline (not water) diuresis, followed by loop diuretics once euvolemia is restored. Pamidronate or similar drugs effectively drive calcium into bone but require days to work. Glucocorticoids inhibit both bony resorption and gastrointestinal uptake.

Hypophosphatemia

Some degree of hypophosphatemia may result from poor oral intake or phosphate-binding antacids. Any cause of vitamin D deficiency will cause decreased absorption of phosphate. Losses with diarrhea are usually modest but can contribute. Shift of phosphate intracellularly occurs with insulin or respiratory alkalosis. Phosphate can be briskly taken up by cells when malnourished patients are refed. Phosphate may be lost in the urine with polyuria, as in uncontrolled hyperglycemia, and urinary phosphate wasting can also be seen with a type II renal tubular acidosis. Urinary wasting can also be seen with hyperparathyroidism unless the patient has renal failure. Adverse effects of hypophosphatemia include muscular and diaphragmatic weakness, heart failure and arrhythmias, confusion, and even rhabdomyolysis when severe. Hypophosphatemia is best treated with oral supplements. Intravenous sodium or potassium phosphate (0.08 to 0.16 mmol/kg of sodium phosphate in 500 mL 0.45 normal saline over 6 h) should be given with caution only if phosphate is below 1.0 mg/dL.

Hyperphosphatemia

Hyperphosphatemia usually requires some degree of renal failure, although it may result from severe tissue necrosis even in people with normal renal function. Laxatives such as Fleet's phosphosoda contain large amounts of phosphate. Increased intestinal absorption is seen with vitamin D intoxication. Decreased phosphate excretion will be seen with hypoparathyroidism. Shift of phosphate out of cells can occur with respiratory acidosis and uncontrolled hyperglycemia. Chronic hyperphosphatemia contributes to bone disease; severe acute toxicity can result in ectopic calcification as well as hypocalcemia, with its adverse effects. Treatment consists of dietary restriction and phosphate binders when mild and may require dialysis if severe. If the calcium-phosphate product is over 70, aluminum-containing binders should be used, as calcium-containing binders may lead to ectopic calcification. Saline hydration or acetazolamide may help in those without renal failure.

Hypomagnesemia

Hypomagnesemia can result from malnutrition and chronically decreased body stores, diarrhea, or urinary wasting, as seen with alcoholism, diuretics, cisplatin, or amphotericin. It can lead to cardiac arrhythmias, which are further worsened by the renal potassium wasting that hypomagnesemia induces. It may also cause hypocalcemia via decreased parathyroid hormone release and action. Tetany or laryngospasm may result when hypomagnesemia is severe. Correction of hypomagnesemia may require large doses to replete body stores. Oral magnesium is often poorly absorbed. Intravenous magnesium is best retained when given slowly over several hours.

Hypermagnesemia

Hypermagnesemia usually occurs in the setting of renal insufficiency. This is worsened by intake of large amounts, as may occur with laxatives or antacids. It may result in lethargy, weakness, and hyporeflexia and, when severe, bradycardia, heart block, and hypotension. It can be corrected with hydration and loop or thiazide diuretics if the patient urinates or dialysis if he or she do not. Intravenous calcium will antagonize its cardiovascular effects.

For a more detailed discussion, see Chap. 73 in *Principles of Critical Care*, 2d ed.

Chapter 57

ACID BASE DISORDERS IN THE INTENSIVE CARE UNIT

EDWARD BOTTEI

Acidemia exists when the blood pH is less than normal; the process causing the acidemia is called *acidosis*. Likewise, alkalemia exists when the blood pH is higher than normal; the process causing the alkalemia is *alkalosis*.

It is critical to find and treat the cause of the acid-base disturbance, not to treat the numbers. There are many causes of acid base disorders that are mild and do not need treatment.

Physiologic Effects

ACIDEMIA

Cardiovascular

Mild acidemia causes a tachycardia from sympathetic stimulation. Severe acidemia leads to bradycardia because of direct myocardial effects. Acidemia decreases the ventricular fibrillation threshold but has little to no effect on converting ventricular fibrillation to sinus rhythm. There is a proportional decrease in contractility with degree of acidemia—the effects from respiratory acidemia happen faster than those from the metabolic form. Acidemia causes a sympathetic adrenal surge; but when severe, the acidemia causes a decreased responsiveness of adrenergic receptors to catechols. Despite these competing effects, there is, in general, increased cardiac output with mild acidemia and decreased cardiac output with vasodilation when the acidemia is severe.

Neuromuscular

Acidemia produces a marked increase in cerebral blood flow. These changes in pH need to be acute, because when chronic,

P_{CO_2} can be tolerated into the 100s. A P_{CO_2} in the 60s produces confusion and headaches; in the 70s patients lose consciousness and can seize. The effects are likely secondary to pH changes and not from the CO_2. Hypercarbia causes decreased diaphragm contractility and decreased endurance time. Metabolic acidemia probably causes decreased respiratory muscle contractility.

Electrolytes

Acidemia from inorganic acids increases serum potassium, but with organic acids the potassium is the same or lower. Clinically the hyperkalemia is due to something other than a direct pH effect. Both respiratory and metabolic acidemia cause hyperphosphatemia.

Experience with permissive hypercapnia has shown that its effects seem to be well tolerated. No changes in systemic vascular resistance, pulmonary vascular resistance, cardiac output, or oxygen delivery are seen. This is likely for three reasons: (1) the degree of acidemia is modest (CO_2 of 50 to 70 and pH of 7.15 to 7.30), (2) the acidemia develops slowly, and (3) those patients being treated with permissive hypercapnia are carefully chosen and monitored.

ALKALEMIA

Cardiovascular

Alkalemia increases myocardial contractility, but there is a slight decrease in contractility as pH becomes greater than 7.7. There is no change in ventricular fibrillation threshold. Alkalemia causes generalized vasodilation, which is maximal at pH 7.65. It does produce regional vasoconstriction, specifically of the cerebral and coronary circulation, which can lead to spasm in the coronary arteries.

Neuromuscular

Respiratory alkalosis decreases cerebral blood flow, the maximum effect at a P_{CO_2} of 20 with a 50 percent decrease in flow. The effect lasts only 6 h. Respiratory alkalemia produces confusion, mental status changes, asterixis, and myoclonus. Seizures can occur. There is possibly a slight increase in respiratory muscle contractility.

Electrolytes

Metabolic alkalemia decreases serum potassium and phosphorus. There is a slight increase in the lactate level and slight fall in ionized calcium. Paresthesias, carpal-pedal spasm, and tetany are likely direct effects of hydrogen ion concentration in the nerves.

Pulmonary

A deterioration of $\dot{V}/\dot{Q}$ matching is caused by alkalemia, which leads to a decreased P_{O_2}.

Oxygen Delivery

An increased hemoglobin afinity for oxygen occurs at an alkalemic pH. This effect is usually not important, but the physician needs to be aware of it if the patient has ongoing hypoxemia and is alkalemic.

Metabolic Acidosis

Characterized by a decreased serum bicarbonate with compensatory respiratory decrease in CO_2, the acidosis occurs because of either loss of bicarbonate or increase in hydrogen ion. It is customary to divide types of metabolic acidosis into those with or without an anion gap. The anion gap is defined as $[Na^+] - [Cl^+] - [HCO_3^-]$. A normal gap is 8 to 14 meq/L. This normal value can be variable depending on the laboratory's instrumentation. A non-gap acidosis arises when bicarbonate is lost through the kidneys and GI tract or by the addition of an acidifying substance as its chloride as its counter ion. The most common ICU non-gap acidoses are from diarrhea and renal tubular acidosis. The most common gap acidosis is lactic acidosis. See Table 57-1 for the differential diagnosis of gap and non-gap acidoses.

Ketoacidosis occurs when an increase in the production of fatty acid leads to their conversion into ketones. The body is in a state of low insulin and high glucagon. This is most commonly seen in diabetic, alcoholic, and starvation ketoacidosis.

Poisoning is an uncommon but important cause of gap acidosis. Any time there is a gap acidosis not clearly caused by ketones or lactate, a hunt for possible toxic ingestion

TABLE 57-1   Metabolic Acidosis

Increased anion gap
  Renal failure
  Ketoacidosis
    diabetic
    alcoholic
    starvation
  Lactic acidosis
  Toxins
    toluene
    salicylates/indocin
    methanol
    ethanol
    ethylene glycol
    paraldehyde
  Phenformin
  Hyperosmolar nonketotic coma
  Indoles/Isoniazid
  Iron
  Inborn errors of metabolism
    maple syrup urine disease
Normal anion gap
  GI bicarb loss
    diarrhea
    urinary diversion
    fistulas (small bowel, pancreas, biliary, surgical drains)
    anion exchange resins
    cholestyramine
  Renal bicarb loss
    renal tubular acidosis
    hypoaldosterone
    hyperparathyroid
    chronic renal insufficiency
    carbonic anhydrase inhibitors
    mafenide acetate
    posthypocapnic
    recovery from DKA
  Acidifying compounds
    arginine HCl, lysine HCl,
    sulfur, TPN with excess cationic amino acids
    HCl, NH_4Cl, $CaCl_2$, $MgCl_2$,
  Miscellaneous
    Dilutional acidosis

---

should be sought. It is important to remember that a fair number of toxins can cause a lactic acidosis. Laboratory diagnosis of poisonings is slow and therefore the physician needs to suspect a poisoning and look for other clues. One quick screening test is to calculate the osmolal gap. This can tell the physician if there is an osmotically active substance in the blood, many of which are toxins. The serum osmolality is $2 \times [Na^+] + [BUN]/2.8 + [glucose]/18 + [ethanol]/4.6$. The measured serum osmolality, when measured directly in the laboratory, should be no more than 10mOsm/L higher than the calculated value. If there is an osmolal gap, this should raise the suspicion that there has been a toxic ingestion. Of note, the absence of an osmolal gap does not preclude the ingestion of osmolol gap–producing poisons. See Chapter 67 for further discussion of the osmolal gap.

Of note, the exact identification of the ion causing a gap acidosis in the intensive care unit (ICU) patient might not always be as easy as it would seem from the short list of possibilities.

TREATMENT

In general, the underlying cause of the acidosis should be determined and appropriate treatment for the cause undertaken. This is to avoid the practice, common 15 or so years ago, of empirically giving bicarbonate to all acidemic patients. Empiric bicarbonate therapy can be complicated by intracellular acidosis and rebound alkalemia. If there is ongoing bicarbonate loss from a renal tubular acidosis (RTA) or there are gastrointestinal losses, replacement with sodium bicarbonate in amounts equal to the losses is indicated.

Lactic Acidosis

Lactic acidosis is the most common cause of metabolic acidosis found in the ICU. Usually defined as a lactate level greater than 5mmol/L with a pH less than 7.35, it can arise from a diverse group of conditions and diseases. While there is not a direct correlation between lactate level and mortality, there is a trend toward higher mortality in ICU patients with increasing lactate levels.

The causes of lactic acidosis are many, but the majority of lactic acidoses in the ICU come from shock (sepsis, cardiogenic shock, or hypovolemia), hypoxia, seizures, local ischemia (mesenteric ischemia, compartment syndrome), or toxic ingestions (see Table 57-2).

Aside from lactate's direct effects on pH, lactate also decreases the responsiveness of neutrophils and adipose cells to β-adrenergic stimuli; in animal models it decreases myocardial contractility.

Treatment is once again directed at detection and treatment of the underlying disorder causing the lactic acidosis. Therapy directed at correction of the lactic acidosis itself, if used at all, should be used only as a temporizing measure until the underlying problem is corrected.

Bicarbonate administration causes an increase in CO_2 production, which CO_2 must then be excreted through increased minute ventilation. Increasing the minute ventilation might not be possible for patients at a maximal minute ventilation already. If the patient can have the minute ventilation increased to eliminate CO_2, the pH can be raised without bicarbonate. Bicarbonate can also cause a paradoxical fall in intracellular pH as the increased CO_2 diffuses into the cells. It has also been shown to cause an increase in the lactate level in some studies. Bicarbonate has not been shown to be any more beneficial than saline injections with regard to improving hemodynamics in acidemia.

Carbicarb, 0.33M sodium carbonate and 0.33M sodium bicarbonate, has not yet been shown to be of benefit in patients with metabolic acidosis.

Dichloroacetate (DCA) is a chemical that increases the activity of pyruvate dehydrogenase (PDH). Increased PDH activity feeds more pyruvate into the tricarboxylic acid (TCA) cycle. This, in turn, increases the conversion of lactate to pyruvate. In studies of patients with severe lactic acidosis, DCA was found statistically to change the patients' lactate levels and serum pH. However, these changes were not found to be clinically significant.

Dialysis can help with lactic acidosis primarily by removing lactate from the serum, and secondarily by allowing for large quantities of bicarbonate to be administered without causing fluid overload.

All in all, there is little good evidence of clinical benefit in promoting the use of Carbicarb or DCA. The few data

TABLE 57-2   Lactic Acidosis

Increased oxygen consumption
  Grand mal seizure
  Severe asthma
  Neuroleptic malignant syndrome
  Pheochromocytoma
  Strenuous exercise
Decreased oxygen delivery
  Decreased cardiac output
  Sepsis
  Severe anemia
  Severe hypoxia
  Regional ischemia
    Mesenteric compartment syndrome
Changes in cellular metabolism
  Thiamine deficiency
  Hypoglycemia
  Diabetes out of control
  Leukemia/lymphoma
  Severe alkalemia
  Sepsis
Toxins and drugs
  Carbon monoxide
  Alcohols (ethanol, methanol, ethylene glycol)
  Salicylates
  Cyanide/nitroprusside
  Isoniazide, strychnine, xylitol,
  papaverine, acetaminophen,
  streptozocin, nalidixic acid,
  fenformin/biguanides, ritodrine,
  terbutaline, norepinephrine,
  epinephrine, albuterol, fructose,
  sorbitol
Congenital enzyme deficiencies
  Glucose-6-phosphate
D-lactate from bacterial overgrowth
Decreased lactate clearance
  Liver failure

---

available about bicarb administration seem to warn more about the problems caused by its administration then to show any consistant clinical benefit.

Metabolic Alkalosis

Characterized by a primary increase in serum bicarbonate with compensatory increase in P_{CO_2}, this comes about by processes that either elevate serum bicarbonate (acid loss from the stomach or kidney) or cause an increased renal bicarbonate reabsorption (hypovolemia with chloride deficit, hypokalemia, increased mineralocorticoid activity). The etiologies of the most common causes of metabolic alkalosis in the ICU are listed in Table 57-3. If the cause of a patient's metabolic alkalosis is not readily clear even after a careful search of the medications, total parenteral nutrition, and blood products given to the patient, a trial of volume with chloride replacement and correction of hypokalemia is warranted. If this fails to correct the problem, a search for increased mineralocorticoid activity might prove useful.

Treatment first consists of correction of the underlying disorder. Continued diuresis in the face of a metabolic alkalosis can be helped by acetazolamide (with potassium supplementation) to increase urinary bicarbonate excretion. If it is desired to correct a metabolic alkalosis rapidly, then 0.1 or 0.2N HCl is the drug of choice. It should be infused through a central vein at a rate of 20 to 50 meq/h.

Respiratory Acidosis

Respiratory acidosis is characterized by a primary increase in P_{CO_2} with compensation first by tissue concentration of bicarbonate, and later by renal retention of bicarbonate. Tissue buffering can, at most, buffer 4 to 5 meq/L acutely, therefore it is possible to become severely acidemic with a quick rise in P_{CO_2}. The etiology of respiratory acidosis can be divided into (1) CNS causes (drive to breathe), (2) chest wall and respiratory muscle causes (strength to breathe), and (3) disorders of the lung and upper airway (workload of breathing). The most common cause of respiratory acidosis in the ICU is intrinsic lung disease. Etiologies are listed in Table 57-4.

Treatment includes attempts to identify and correct the underlying cause of the respiratory acidosis. It is not uncommon that because of the effort to correct problems in all three areas (drive, strength, load) the patient develops a respiratory alkalosis.

TABLE 57-3   Metabolic Alkalosis

Chloride responsive (UrCl < 10 meq/L)	Chloride resistant (UrCl > 20 meq/L)

Hypovolemic states
  Vomiting, NG suction, villous
    adenoma of the colon,
    congenital chloride diarrhea
  Diuretics
Posthypercapnea with volume depletion
Nonreabsorbable anionic antibiotics (penicillins)
Cystic fibrosis
Alkali administration
  Acetate (TPN), citrate (transfusions),
    nonreabsorbable alkali (antacids,
    milk-alkali syndrome, exchange resins),
    bicarbonate, lactate
Hypochloremia
	Primary hyperaldosteronism
	Secondary hyperaldosteronism
	  Cushing's syndrome
	  Drugs with mineralocorticoid
	    activity
	  Bartter syndrome
	  Cirrhosis and ascites
	  Renin-secreting tumor
	  Congestive heart failure
	Severe hypokalemia
	Licorice poisons (glycyrrhizic acid)
	Refeeding after starvation
	Nonparathyroid hypercalcemia
	  (multiple myeloma, bone
	    metastases)

Key: Urinary [Cl⁻] = urinary chloride concentration.

705

TABLE 57-4 Respiratory Acidosis

Decreased respiratory drive	Neuromuscular diseases
Drugs/toxins	Myasthenia gravis
Narcotics, sedatives,	ALS
alcohols, anesthetics,	Tetanus
anticholinesterases	Guillain-Barré syndrome
CNS lesions	Poliomyolitis
Sleep apnea	Botulism
Myxedema	Multiple sclerosis
	Cervical spinal cord injury
Lung disorders	Muscular dystrophy
COPD/asthma	Brainstem injury
Severe pneumonia	Severe hypokalemia
Severe pulmonary edema	Severe hypophosphatemia
Pneumothorax/hemothorax	Familial periodic paralysis
ARDS	Diaphragmatic paralysis
Interstitial lung disease	
Upper airway obstruction	Chest wall disorders
Foreign bodies/aspiration	Kyphoscoliosis
Laryngospasm/laryngeal edema	Morbid obesity
Obstructive sleep apnea	Flail chest
Tracheal stenosis	Circumferential chest wall
	burns

ABBREVIATIONS: CNS, central nervous system; COPD, chronic obstructive pulmonary disease; ARDS, acute respiratory distress syndrome; ALS, amyotrophic lateral sclerosis.

Respiratory Alkalosis

Respiratory alkalosis is a primary reduction in P_{CO_2} with compensation first by buffering with tissue proteins and then by decreased renal acid excretion with increased renal bicarbonate excretion. Hyperventilation occurs commonly in the ICU for many reasons, ranging from the benign (anxiety) to the life-threatening (sepsis and pulmonary embolism). The etiologies of respiratory alkalosis are listed in Table 57-5. Treatment is directed at the underlying disorder. It is rare that respiratory alkalosis itself needs to be treated.

Diagnostic Approach to Acid Base Disorders

Acid base disorders can be difficult to sort through because they are frequently mixed disorders (respiratory and meta-

TABLE 57-5   Respiratory Alkalosis

Central Stimulation	Peripheral Stimulation
	Lung disease
Anxiety and pain	Pneumonia
Fever	Pulmonary embolism
Sepsis	Pulmonary edema
Liver disease	Restrictive lung disease
Hyperthyroidism	Pleural effusion
CNS disease	PTX
CVA	Bronchospasm
Tumor	
Infection	Hypoxemia
Trauma	High altitude
Drugs	Interstitial lung disease
Salicylates	Severe anemia
Progesterone	Asphyxiation
Medroxyprogesterone	ARDS
Catecholamines	
Xanthines	Miscellaneous
Nicotine	Mechanical ventilation
Pregnancy	Voluntary hyperventilation
Exercise	Heat stroke

ABBREVIATIONS: CNS, central nervous system; CVA, cerebrovascular accident; PTX, pneumothorax; ARDS, acute respiratory distress syndrome.

bolic derangement occurring at the same time) and the patients also have underlying chronic disease.

1. Look at serum pH—is patient acidemic (pH < 7.35) or alkalemic (pH > 7.45)
2. Look at the P_{CO_2} and $[HCO_3^-]$—is the main disturbance metabolic or respiratory

    acidemia: $P_{CO_2} > 45$ mmHg identifies a respiratory acidosis $[HCO_3^-] < 20$ mmol/L identifies a metabolic acidosis

    alkalemia: $P_{CO_2} < 35$ mmHg identifies a respiratory alkalosis $[HCO_3^-] > 28$ mmol/L identifies a metabolic alkalosis

3. If there is a primary respiratory disturbance, is it acute? expect $\Delta pH = -0.08(\Delta P_{CO_2}/10)$
4. If there is a nonacute primary respiratory disturbance, is there appropriate renal compensation?

for acidosis expect: early (6 to 24 h) $\Delta[HCO_3^-]$ =
$(1/10) \times \Delta P_{CO_2}$
late (1 to 4 days) $\Delta[HCO_3^-]$ =
$(4/10) \times \Delta P_{CO_2}$

for alkalosis expect: early (1 to 2 h) $\Delta[HCO_3^-]$ =
$(2/10) \times \Delta P_{CO_2}$
late (2 days) $\Delta[HCO_3^-]$ =
$(5/10) \times \Delta P_{CO_2}$

*If not, then there is a superimposed primary metabolic distur-
bance, or compensation is not yet complete.*

5. If there is a metabolic acidosis, is the anion gap increased?
6. If there is a metabolic disturbance, is there an appropriate
   respiratory compensation?
   for acidosis expect: $P_{CO_2} = (1.5 \times [HCO_3^-]) + 8 \pm 2$
   for alkalosis expect: $P_{CO_2} = (0.7 \times [HCO_3^-]) + 21 \pm 1.5$
   *If not, then there is a superimposed primary respiratory distur-
   bance hidden in the numbers.*

   If actual P_{CO_2} > expected P_{CO_2} → then there is a hidden primary respiratory acidosis
   If actual P_{CO_2} < expected P_{CO_2} → then there is a hidden primary respiratory alkalosis

7. If there is an increased anion gap acidosis, look for other
   metabolic disturbances by examining whether the parameter $\{[HCO_3^-] + (gap - 12)\}$ is nearly normal (i.e.,
   24 meq/L in a patient who does have a chronic respiratory acid-base disorder).

*If this parameter is not nearly 24, then there is a second superim-
posed metabolic abnormality hidden in the data:*

   if the parameter < 24 → then there is another, hidden non-
   gap acidosis
   if the parameter > 24 → then there is another, hidden
   metabolic alkalosis

For a more detailed discussion, see Chap. 74 in *Principles of Critical
Care*, 2d ed.

Chapter 58

ENDOCRINE EMERGENCIES

BABAK MOKHLESI

Diabetic Ketoacidosis, Hyperosmolar Nonketotic Diabetes, and Hypoglycemia

Diabetes mellitus (DM) is a common disease afflicting at least 5 percent of the U.S. population. Most patients can be classified as having either type I diabetes (insulin-dependent, or ketosis prone) or type II diabetes (non-insulin-dependent, obesity-related). Its major life-threatening complications, diabetic ketoacidosis (DKA), hyperosmolar nonacidotic diabetes (HNAD), and hypoglycemia may precipitate or complicate critical illness. DKA occurs as a result of severe insulin deficiency with an excess of counterregulatory hormones such as glucagon and epinephrine. This is more common in DM type I, but it may occur in any diabetic who is sufficiently stressed. HNAD, also known as hyperosmolar hyperglycemic nonketotic coma (HHNC) typically presents as a complication of DM type II. *HNAD* is a preferable term over *HHNC*, since clinical states with hyperosmolarity, dehydration, and electrolyte derangement can exist without neurologic symptoms. Though there is considerable overlap between DKA and HNAD, the prognosis of DKA tends to be better, since patients with HNAD often have significant associated illnesses.

DIFFERENTIAL DIAGNOSIS

DKA and HNAD are easily recognized when considered (Table 58-1). Development of DKA tends to be rapid, occurring within hours to days. Patients are often lethargic, have a fruity odor (acetone), and breathe with a Kussmaul pattern. They may complain of nausea, vomiting, and severe

TABLE 58-1 Signs and Symptoms of Glucose
Metabolism Disorders

Uncontrolled diabetes
  Polyuria
  Polyphagia
  Vaginitis
  Nocturia
  Weight loss
  Skin infection
  Thirst
  Blurred vision
  Fatigue
  Polydipsia
  Dizziness
  Malaise
Diabetic katoacidosis
  Dyspnea
  Normotension
  Hypo- and hyperthermia
  Nausea
  Tachycardia
  Lethargy to coma
  Vomiting
  Tachypnea
  Fruity breath
  Abdominal pain
  Abdominal tenderness
  Orthostasis
  Cerebral edema
Hyperglycemic hyperosmolar nonketotic coma
  Dehydration
  Hypo- and hyperthermia
  Stupor to coma
  Dehydration
  Focal neurologic signs or seizures
  Shallow respiration
  Hypotension to shock

---

abdominal pain. Most patients are significantly volume-
depleted even if they are normotensive.

HNAD develops over a period of days to weeks and patients are usually brought to medical attention because of al-

tered mental status. They typically have profound dehydration with hypotension and may manifest focal neurologic deficits. Often there is no acidosis, so dyspnea (tachypnea) is not a prominent presenting feature; patients may even exhibit depressed ventilation.

The sine qua non of DKA is a metabolic acidosis due to ketoacids. The two ketoacids produced in DKA are β-hydroxybutyrate and acetoacetate as well as the neutral ketone, acetone. In severe DKA β-hydroxybutyrate is the predominant ketone. The nitroprusside reaction commonly used to detect ketones does not react with β-hydroxybutyrate, thus it is possible to have a negative serum nitroprusside reaction in the face of severe ketosis. One readily available index for unmeasured anions in the blood, the "anion-gap," may overcome this limitation. The serum glucose level is usually about 500 mg/dL, although DKA with euglycemia has been described. The arterial pH is commonly less than 7.3 and can be as low as 6.5. There may be some evidence of mild hyperosmolarity, but usually less than 330 mOsm/L.

The sine qua non of HNAD is hyperosmolarity, generally greater than 350 mOsm/L. The glucose concentration will usually be greater than 600 mg/dL. In pure HNAD there is no significant metabolic acidosis or anion gap, but occasional patients have mild to moderate ketonemia and acidosis. Mild hyperosmolarity in DKA and mild ketonemia in HNAD may make the distinction more difficult; in fact, these disorders often coexist.

Other measures of anion-gap metabolic acidosis in face of hyperglycemia should be considered, such as lactic acidosis, starvation and alcoholic ketoacidosis, uremic acidosis, and toxic ingestions.

THERAPY

The optimum management of DKA and HNAD has been the subject of considerable controversy over the past half century. A general approach is outlined in Table 58-2.

Fluid deficits on the order of 5 to 10 L are common in DKA and HNAD. With signs of significant volume depletion, 1 L of normal saline should be administered over the first hour

TABLE 58-2 Treatment of Severe Disorders
of Glucose Metabolism

Diabetic ketoacidosis
Fluids (usual deficit, 5–10 L)
  If hypotensive: 1 L normal saline in the first few minutes; repeat
    as needed to restore the circulation, and consider invasive
    hemodynamic monitoring
  If normotensive: 1 L 0.45% NaCl in first hour
  In subsequent hours:
    Match urine output with 0.45% NaCl; in addition, provide
      100–500 mL/h 0.45% NaCl
    Calculate free water deficit and replajce 50% over 12 h with
      5% dextrose in water
    After glucose reaches 250–300 mg/dL, add dextrose to IV
      fluids (~100 g per 24 h)
Insulin
  10-U IV bolus
  0.1 (U/(kg·h), IV or IM
  Check glucose hourly and adjust drip to decrease glucose by
    100 mg/(dL·h) to a level of 250 mg/dL
Potassium (usual deficit, 200–1000 meq)
  Establish that the patient is not oliguric
  ECG monitoring for hyperkalemia and hypokalemia
  If hyperkalemic, follow hourly
  If normokalemic, 10–20 meq/h
  If hypokalemic, 20–40 meq/h
  Administer half as chl oride and half as phosphate salts
Bicarbonate
  None is generally indicated
  Some would consider administering $NaHCO_3$ 1 meq/kg IV for
    pH < 6.9
  May be useful for treatment of hyperkalemia
Search for underlying cause
Monitor:
  ECG
  Vital signs
  Hourly: glucose and electrolyte levels
  Every 2–4 h: calcium, magnesium, phosphate
  Every 6–24 h: BUN, creatinine, ketones
Hyperglycemic hyperosmolar nonketotic coma (HHNC)
  HHNC should be treated like DKA, though patients will
    generally require more fluids and less insulin.

---

and 200 to 500 mL/h in the subsequent hours until adequate circulation is maintained. At this point the fluid administration should be changed to 0.45 percent saline at a rate of 150 to 250 mL/h with monitoring of inputs and outputs. With the osmotic diuresis induced by hyperglycemia, the water deficits exceed sodium deficits. The water deficit can be calculated using the corrected sodium and should be replaced over a period of 24 to 48 h. Once the serum glucose level reaches 250 to 300 mg/dL, fluids should be changed to those that contain 5 percent dextrose, with a goal of maintaining the serum glucose in that range for 24 h. This will allow slow equilibration of osmotically active substances across all membranes. At least 100 g of dextrose per 24 h must be given to prevent ketogenesis if the patient is taking nothing by mouth. In general, patients with HNAD present with more profound dehydration and require more IV fluids than patients with DKA.

Insulin is the mainstay of therapy for DKA. The subcutaneous (SC) route is inappropriate in critically ill patients. Rather, a priming dose of insulin (10 U) should be given intravenously, followed by an infusion of 0.1 U/kg per hour. After the glucose level reaches 250 mg/dL, it is prudent to decrease but not stop the insulin infusion. Once systemic perfusion is restored and ketones are cleared (usually 12 to 24 h), the insulin can be given subcutaneously.

Potassium replacement is a fundamental part of DKA management. Most patients with DKA present with high normal or elevated blood potassium level but are deficient in total-body potassium. Insulin treatment promotes cellular uptake of potassium and phosphate. As treatment for DKA progresses, one may see a rapid fall in serum potassium and phosphate levels. Supplemental potassium should be administered when the serum level is less than 5.5 meq/L if renal function is normal and there are no electrocardiographic (ECG) signs of hyperkalemia. Replacing the potassium deficit with half potassium chloride and half potassium phosphate should replete phosphate stores.

The use of bicarbonate in DKA is highly controversial. No benefit of bicarbonate has been demonstrated in clinical trials. Its use should be restricted to those patients with a pH less than 6.9, hemodynamic instability and a pH less than 7.1, or ECG findings of hyperkalemia, but even in these patients bicarbonate is unlikely to be beneficial.

Even in severe cases of DKA, there is usually no role for mechanical ventilation. The ventilator can almost never achieve the reduction of Pa_{CO_2} of a spontaneously breathing patient. Mechanical ventilation in the presence of a high minute ventilation and hypovolemia can lead to iatrogenically induced shock.

TABLE 58-3   Causes of Hypoglycemia

Fasting hypoglycemia
  Hypersecretion of insulin or increased levels of insulin-like
  growth factors
    Insulinoma
    Nesidioblastosis
    Certain carcinomas (sarcoma, hepatoma, others)
  Hyposecretion of counterregulatory hormones
    Growth hormone deficiency
    Cortisol deficiency
  Hepatic failure
    Toxic (especially alcohol-induced)
    Infectious
    Congestive
    Shock-induced
    Caused by an inborn error of metabolism
  Starvation
    Uremia
    Pregnancy
    Severe protein-calorie malnutrition
  Autoimmune disorder (antibodies to insulin or insulin receptors)
Postprandial hypoglycemia
  Idiopathic
  Alimentary
  Early type II diabetes mellitus
Factitious or drug-related hypoglycemia
  Insulin
  Sulfonylureas and other sulfa compounds
  Salicylates
  β blockers
  Pentamidine
  Antiarrhythmic agents
  Glucose consumption in test tube by leukocytes

HYPOGLYCEMIA

Hypoglycemia can be a major complication of critical illness such as hepatic failure, drug overdose, or sepsis. It may also occur as a complication of therapy for diabetes. The causes of hypoglycemia are outlined in Table 58-3. The symptoms of hypoglycemia result from sympathoadrenal responses and consist of palpitations, anxiety, tremulousness, diaphoresis, and hunger. It can progress to confusion, seizures, coma, or death. The therapy is outlined in Table 58-4. The goal is to establish and maintain modest hyperglycemia.

Thyroid Disease

EUTHYROID SICK SYNDROME

Alterations in thyroid function tests (TFTs) are very common in critically ill patients, and knowledge of these abnormalities is necessary to avoid errors in diagnosis and therapy. Euthyroid sick syndrome (ESS), also known as nonthyroidal illness (NTI), refers to the reduction in serum T3, T4, and thyroid-stimulating hormone (TSH) associated with profound illness or malnutrition. These abnormalities are associated with a reduction in 5'-deiodinase activity, the enzyme that converts T4 to T3. Thus there is less T3 production with

TABLE 58-4   Treatment of Hypoglycemia

Consider the diagnosis

Determine capillary glucose concentration

Confirm with measurement of serum glucose (and insulin, C-peptide, and sulfonylurea screen if cause unknown)

Give oral calories if patient is conscious

Reassess; if glucose < 100 mg/dL, *then* administer 50 mL 50% dextrose

Reassess; if glucose < 100 mg/dL, *then* give infusion of 10% dextrose to maintain glucose level > 100 mg/dL

Reassess; if glucose < 100 mg/dL, *then* give infusion of 10% glucose + 100 mg/L hydrocortisone + 1 mg glucagon

Reassess; if glucose < 100 mg/dL, *then* add infusion of diazoxide and/or continuous enteral feeding

---

increased synthesis of the metabolically inactive reverse T3 (rT3). The perturbations of the hypothalamic-pituitary-thyroid axis in critically ill patients is less well understood. The basal TSH can be normal or low, but the response of TSH to thyrotropin releasing hormone (TRH) is usually attenuated. Several drugs such as dopamine and glucocorticoids may inhibit TSH secretion.

The interpretation of TFTs and the recognition of hypothyroidism in the ICU setting is challenging (Table 58-5). The strongest evidence for primary hypothyroidism in this population is an elevated TSH level associated with a normal or low rT3 levels. Patients with renal failure are an exception. Since the results of rT3 or T4 levels by equilibrium dialysis or radioimmunoassay (accurate measures of T4 levels) are not readily obtained, these tests add little to early decision making. Since only severe primary hypothyroidism requires emergency treatment, its recognition will depend upon some degree of TSH elevation, prior history of thyroid disease, and physical findings compatible with hypothyroidism. As to whether patients with low levels of thyroid hormone in the face of catastrophic NTI should receive hormonal replacement, the limited data available suggest that T4 therapy is not beneficial and may lead to earlier mortality. Therapy is not indicated unless signs of hypothyroidism such as hyporeflexia, hypothermia, macroglossia, or goiter are present (Table 58-6). If the decision is made to treat, the drug of choice is T3, which is very expensive and is available only in oral form.

TABLE 58-5   Interpretation of Thyroid Function Tests

Diagnosis	T_4 Level	T_3 Level	TSH Level	rT_3 Level
Primary hypothyroidism	↓	↓ or N	↑	↓ or N
Central hypothyroidism	↓	↓	N	↓
NTI	↓ or N	↓	N or ↓	↑ or N

ABBREVIATIONS: ↓, decreased; ↑, increased; N, normal.

TABLE 58-6   Indications for Thyroid Hormone Treatment in Patients with Severe NTI

Increased serum TSH concentrations
History of radioactive iodine treatment
Hypothermia
Macroglossia
Goiter
History of thyroid disease
Hypercholesterolemia
Hyporeflexia
Unexplained pleural or pericardial effusions
Increased serum creatine phosphokinase level

MYXEDEMA COMA

Myxedema coma is caused by marked and prolonged deple-tion of thyroid hormone and is associated with defective ther-moregulation, abnormal mental status, and an identifiable precipitating event (Table 58-7).

The usual features of myxedema are coarse skin and hair, jaundice, macroglossia, hoarseness, obtundation, delayed deep tendon reflexes, and hypothermia. There is little evidence to

TABLE 58-7   Common Precipitating Factors of Myxedema Coma

Exposure to cold
Infection
Surgery
Strokes
Occult gastrointestinal bleeding
Trauma
Drug overdose
    Sedatives
    Tranquilizers
    Narcotics
    Anesthetics
Congestive heart failure

support the contention that severe hypothyroidism alone causes coma or shock.

The laboratory findings are listed in Table 58-8. The common TFT abnormality is low T4 and high TSH. Depressed hypoxic and hypercapnic ventilatory drive can result in alveolar hypoventilation and arterial blood gas abnormalities. This may be exacerbated by a reduced central nervous system drive to breathe and decreased respiratory muscle activity. The cardiovascular complications include accelerated atherosclerosis, cardiomyopathy, and pericardial effusion, which rarely causes tamponade. The management of myxedema is outlined in Table 58-9.

Myxedema coma is potentially fatal in approximately 50 percent of the patients, although complete recovery can occur. Treatment is continued as long as serum TSH remains elevated. Reduction of TSH is the earliest indicator of response to therapy. The ultimate goal of successful therapy is complete clinical recovery.

THYROTOXICOSIS

Thyroid storm or thyrotoxic crisis is a life-threatening though rare complication of severe thyrotoxicosis. Table 58-10 points out the cardinal features of thyroid storm and thyrotoxicosis. The distinction between these two entities may not be clinically relevant in an intensive care unit (ICU) setting.

TABLE 58-8   Laboratory Findings in Myxedema Coma

Hypoglycemia
Hyponatremia
Hyperkalemia
Hypercortisolemia
Anemia
Leukocytosis with a left shift
Serum creatinine level > 2.0 mg/dL
Increases P_{CO_2} in arterial blood
Decreased P_{O_2} in arterial blood

TABLE 58-9   Management of Myxedema Coma

Endocrine
1. Thyroid hormone
   - T4 500 mg IV initially followed by 50 to 100 μg/day. Goal: normal T4 in 24 to 48 h.
   - T4 500 mg IV followed by 25 μg of T3 every 6 h through nasogastric tube. Goal: recovery (hypoadrenalism present in 5 to 10% of patients with myxedema)
2. Corticosteroids
   - Hydrocortisone 50 mg every 6 h IV
   - Can taper if a normal pituitary-adrenal axis is confirmed
   - Alternatively dexamethasone 2 mg IV followed by a 1-h ACTH stimulation test

Supportive care
   - Early intubation and mechanical ventilation
   - Passive warming for hypothermia, avoid external warming
   - Adjust drug dosing because of decreased metabolism
   - Avoid water intoxication or excessive diuresis
   - Correction of anemia
   - Search for infection

TABLE 58-10   Cardinal Features of Thyroid Storm and Thyrotoxicosis

Thyrotoxicosis	Thyroid Storm
Cardiovascular	Cardiovascular
Tachycardia	Congestive heart failure
Hypertension	Arrhythmia
Widened pulse pressure	
Atrial fibrillation	
Neuromuscular	Neuromuscular
Tremor	Agitation
Weakness	Delirium
Emotional lability	Seizures/Coma
Thermoregulation	Thermoregulation
Warm/moist skin	Fever
Gastrointestinal	Gastrointestinal
Increased intestinal	Diarrhea
Motility	Jaundice

TABLE 58-11 Laboratory Findings in Thyroid Storm

Elevated levels of T_4 and free T_4
Elevated T_3 level
Hyperglycemia
Leukocytosis with left shift
Anemia
Hypercalcemia
Hypokalemia
Abnormal liver function test findings
Hypercortisolemia

The laboratory findings are listed in Table 58-11. In entertaining a diagnosis of thyrotoxicosis, one should determine whether the patient has a previous history of thyrotoxicosis, thyroid hormone ingestion, or recent use of an iodine-containing agent. The presence of exophthalmos, goiter, or previous thyroid surgery can also be helpful. Factors that can potentially precipitate thyroid storm are listed in Table 58-12.

TABLE 58-12 Factors Precipitating Thyroid Storm

Surgery
Infection
Acute psychiatric illness
Congestive heart failure
Diabetic ketoacidosis
Pulmonary embolism
Bowel infarction
Parturition
Trauma
Vigorous palpation of thyroid gland
Withdrawal of antithyroid medication
Drugs
    Sympathomimetic drugs such as pseudoephedrine
    Amiodarone
Radioactive iodide therapy
Iodine-containing contrast agents
"Health food" preparation containing seaweed or kelp

The principles of therapy are to reduce serum thyroid hormone levels, reduce the action of thyroid hormone on peripheral tissues, prevent systemic decompensation, and treat precipitating events. A combination of drugs to inhibit thyroid hormone synthesis and secretion is recommended. To inhibit synthesis of T4, propylthiouracil (PTU) or methimazole (MMI) is used. PTU offers an advantage over MMI by also inhibiting synthesis of T3 in peripheral tissue. PTU is administered in 200- to 250-mg doses every 6 h; MMI is administered in 25-mg doses every 6 h. Each has side effects of rash, agranulocytosis, and hepatic toxicity. The addition of stable iodine, such as Lugol's solution or a saturated solution of potassium iodide (ssKI), 2 drops orally every 2 h, provides blockade of hormone secretion. Antithyroid drugs should be administered at least 1 h before iodine to establish blockade of hormone synthesis. This treatment plan should normalize hormone levels in 1 to 5 days. Corticosteroids and propranolol decrease the peripheral conversion of T4 to T3 and can be used to further reduce serum T3 concentration. Propranolol 1 mg can be administered every 5 min until pulse rate slows. A total daily dose of 300 mg of propranolol is often required. It should be used with caution in the elderly, or in patients with asthma or heart failure.

Cardiovascular collapse can be prevented by antipyretics, volume infusion, and propranolol. Treatment of congestive heart failure is supportive. Because of accelerated metabolism, administration of 100 mg of hydrocortisone every 8 h may be useful in preventing relative hypoadrenalism. Medication dosing should be adjusted accordingly.

Finally, a scrupulous search for the precipitating factor should be performed. Empirical use of broad-spectrum antibiotics is recommended pending culture results.

ANESTHESIA AND SURGERY

The stress of surgery can precipitate thyroid storm in any thyrotoxic patient. The preoperative therapeutic goal of normalizing thyroid function using antithyroid drugs often takes 3 to 7 days. If this wait is unacceptable, an alternative approach is to block the sympathomimetic effects of thyroid hormone.

Propranolol is the most commonly used drug in doses of 40 mg every 6 h.

LEVOTHYROXINE OVERDOSE

In the United States, 2000 to 5000 episodes of levothyroxine (L-T4) overdose occur annually. Despite the high frequency, no deaths have been reported. The symptoms begin as the L-T4 is converted to T3 approximately 24 h after ingestion. Treatment includes gastrointestinal decontamination using gastric lavage, followed by the administration of charcoal. Cholestyramine will increase fecal elimination of the drug by preventing hepatic portal circulation. Prednisone, PTU, and propranolol can also be used as needed.

Adrenocortical Insufficiency

Adrenocortical insufficiency is an uncommon finding in the ICU and a high index of suspicion is required to make the diagnosis. It is classified as primary (Addison disease) when it results from direct involvement of the adrenal gland, secondary when it results from deficient pituitary adrenocorticotropic hormone (ACTH), and tertiary because of deficient hypothalamic corticotropin releasing factor (CRF). Previous use of glucocorticoids is the most common cause of adrenocortical hypofunction and is an example of secondary adrenocortical insufficiency. The incidence of adrenal insufficiency is less than 2 percent in critically ill patients, but it can be higher in certain subpopulations. In one series of severely septic patients, 10 percent had a subnormal response to ACTH stimulation.

Autoimmune adrenalitis is the most common cause of primary adrenocortical insufficiency (Table 58-13). It often occurs in young white females in association with other autoimmune disorders. *Mycobacterium tuberculosis* is the second most common cause of primary adrenal insufficiency. Other important causes include fungal infection, metastatic cancer as of the lung or breast, melanoma or lymphoma, and sepsis-induced adrenal hemorrhage. Patients with acquired

TABLE 58-13   Etiology of Primary
Adrenocortical Insufficiency

Autoimmune (idiopathic) (80%)
Mycobacterium tuberculosis ($< 20\%$)
Miscellaneous ($< 1\%$)
  Hemorrhage (sepsis, anticoagulants, coagulopathy, history of
    thromboembolic disease, prior surgery, trauma, "difficult"
    pregnancy, burns, leukemia, metastatic carcinoma, pancreatitis,
    vasculitis, postadrenal venography)
  AIDS (fungal, mycobacterial, or cytomegalovirus infection;
    Kaposi's sarcoma)
  Fungal infection (histoplasmosis, coccidioidomycosis,
    paracoccidioidomycosis, cryptococcosis, blastomycosis,
    candidiasis, torulopsis)
  Metastatic carcinoma
  Lymphoma
  Drugs (rifampin, ketoconazole, barbiturates, phenytoin,
    aminoglutethimide, mitotane, metyrapone, trilostane,
    etomidate, cyproterone actetate, *o,p*-DDD, fluorouracil)
  Bilateral adrenalectomy
  Irradiation
  Sarcoidosis
  Amyloidosis
  Hemochromatosis
  Congenital conditions

---

immunodeficiency syndrome (AIDS) may develop adrenal
insufficiency because of opportunistic infection, Kaposi sarcoma, or drugs.

Secondary adrenocortical insufficiency occurs because of
diminished secretion of ACTH by the pituitary gland. There
are many potential etiologies (Table 58-14), but chronic glucocorticoid therapy is by far the leading cause. Most patients
entering an ICU with secondary adrenocortical insufficiency
are receiving glucocorticoids or have received them in the
prior year. A reasonable guideline is to consider all patients
who have received 40 mg/day of prednisone or its equivalent for a period greater than 2 to 3 weeks as adrenally compromised, especially if they have a cushingoid appearance.
All such patients should have their adrenal function evaluated and be considered for stress doses of corticosteroids.

TABLE 58-14   Etiology of Secondary
Adrenocortical Insufficiency

Glucocorticoid therapy
Tumors (pituitary adenoma, craniopharyngioma, meningioma,
   glioma, hamartoma, pinealoma, metastatic carcinoma [breast,
   lung, gastrointestinal], lymphoma, leukemia)
Vascular
   Pituitary apoplexy (almost always related to acute hemorrhagic
      infarction of a primary pituitary tumor)
   Sheehan's syndrome (from postpartum hemorrhage, hypotension)
   Intracranial aneurysm
   Cavernous sinus thrombosis
   Diabetes mellitus
   Vasculitis
   Sickle cell disease and trait
   Arteriosclerosis
   Eclampsia
Pituitary surgery
Irradiation (to nasopharynx, sella turcica)
Head trauma
Infection (tuberculosis, fungal disease, syphilis, malaria, brucellosis,
   nocardiosis, actinomycosis, abscess, viruses)
Autoimmune disorders
Sarcoidosis
Histiocytosis X
Hemochromatosis
Lipid storage diseases
Isolated ACTH deficiency
Congenital conditions
Transient ACTH deficiency of critical illness

CLINICAL FEATURES

A high index of suspicion is required in order to diagnose
chronic adrenocortical insufficiency in patients who present
in hypoadrenal crisis because of some superimposed stress
(Table 58-15). Weakness, fatigue, anorexia, hypotension,
and hyperpigmentation are usually present in primary
adrenocortical deficiency. Fever is common, even without
underlying infection. Hyperpigmentation is not a feature of

TABLE 58-15   When to Consider the Diagnosis of Adrenocortical Insufficiency

History of treatment with glucocorticoids (within the past year) or presence of cushingoid features
Hypotension (systolic blood pressure < 100 mmHg) with a chronic history of weight loss and weakness
Unexplained hypotension or volume depletion, gastrointestinal signs and symptoms, delirium, or fever, in a patient with a
  history or clinical evidence of tuberculosis, malignancy, AIDS, polyendocrine deficiency, vitiligo, a condition predisposing
  to adrenal hemorrhage, use of a drug known to precipitate adrenocortical insufficiency, or a disorder of the anterior
  pituitary or hypothalamus
Hyperkalemia and hyponatremia, especially in the absence of chronic renal failure
Hypotension with hypoglycemia or eosinophilia
Hypotension with hyperpigmentation
Hypotension with the absence of axillary or pubic hair in a female
Unexplained hypotension unresponsive to aggressive fluids and vasoactive drugs

secondary adrenocortical insufficiency. The absence of classic laboratory findings cannot be used to exclude the diagnosis (Table 58-16). Most laboratory abnormalities are nonspecific, but hypoglycemia, eosinophilia, and hypotension should immediately raise the possibility of this diagnosis.

DIAGNOSIS

The two most useful screening tests are the serum cortisol level and the rapid ACTH stimulation test. A random cortisol level greater than 20 μg/dL makes the diagnosis very unlikely. On the other hand, in the setting of shock, a cortisol level less than 20 μg/dL is highly suggestive and should prompt a rapid ACTH stimulation test. This test measures the response of the adrenal gland to stimulation by exogenous ACTH. After drawing baseline cortisol, aldosterone, and ACTH levels, 250 μg of synthetic ACTH (cosyntropin) is administered intravenously. Blood for cortisol and aldosterone is then redrawn 30 and 60 min later. A stimulated cortisol level greater than 20 μg/dL is a sufficient single criterion for normal adrenal function. A clearly normal response eliminates the possibility of primary insufficiency and makes the diagnosis of secondary adrenocortical insufficiency less likely.

TABLE 58-16   Laboratory Features of Chronic Primary Adrenocortical Insufficiency

Finding	% of Patients[a]
Hyponatremia	88
Hyperkalemia	64
Prerenal azotemia	NA
Hypoglycemia	NA
Hypercalcemia	6
Anemia	NA
Eosinophilia	NA
Lymphocytosis	NA

[a]NA, no data available.

Rare patients with secondary adrenocortical insufficiency show a normal response; because the rapid ACTH stimulation test occasionally gives a false-positive result, the test results should be verified when the patient's condition stabilizes. The "gold standard" is the standard or prolonged ACTH stimulation test.

MANAGEMENT

Figure 58-1 offers a flow diagram for the diagnosis and management of adrenocortical insufficiency.

Preexisting or Presumed Adrenocortical Insufficiency

Patients who are known to have adrenocortical insufficiency or who have a history of significant glucocorticoid treatment in the previous year should be given "stress doses" of corticosteroids during severe intercurrent illness or during surgical procedures. Hydrocortisone 100 mg IV every 6 to 8 h effectively treats the possibility of adrenocortical insufficiency. Hydrocortisone should be promptly tapered to maintenance levels once the acute illness has resolved.

The Hemodynamically Stable Patient

Measurement of plasma cortisol and a rapid ACTH stimulation test should precede initiation of stress doses of steroids. Hypovolemia should be treated with a glucose-containing saline solution. If the diagnosis is confirmed, hydrocortisone, 100 mg every 6 to 8 h, should be given.

The Hemodynamically Unstable Patient

Acute adrenal insufficiency is life-threatening and requires prompt and aggressive therapy. In addition to vigorous volume repletion with a glucose-containing solution, dexamethasone 4 mg should be given intravenously at once. It does not interfere with the assay for cortisol and will not

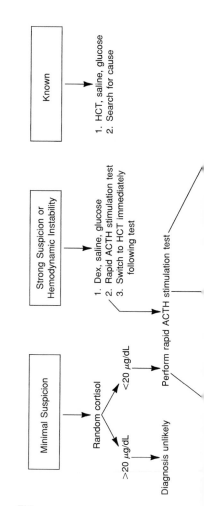

Minimal Suspicion

Random cortisol

>20 μg/dL → Diagnosis unlikely

<20 μg/dL → Perform rapid ACTH stimulation test

Strong Suspicion or Hemodynamic Instability

1. Dex, saline, glucose
2. Rapid ACTH stimulation test
3. Switch to HCT immediately following test

→ Perform rapid ACTH stimulation test

Known

1. HCT, saline, glucose
2. Search for cause

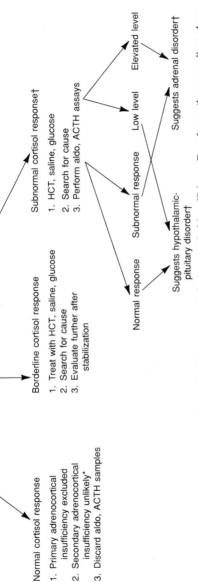

Normal cortisol response

1. Primary adrenocortical insufficiency excluded
2. Secondary adrenocortical insufficiency unlikely*
3. Discard aldo, ACTH samples

Borderline cortisol response

1. Treat with HCT, saline, glucose
2. Search for cause
3. Evaluate further after stabilization

Subnormal cortisol response†

1. HCT, saline, glucose
2. Search for cause
3. Perform aldo, ACTH assays

Normal response   Subnormal response   Low level   Elevated level

Suggests hypothalamic-pituitary disorder   Suggests adrenal disorder†

FIGURE 58-1 Flow diagram for the diagnosis and management of adrenocortical insufficiency. Dex, dexamethasone sodium phosphate, 4 mg IV; ACTH, adrenocorticotropic hormone; HCT, hydrocortisone sodium succinate, 100 mg IV every 6 to 8 hours; Aldo, aldosterone. (*If the possibility of secondary adrenocortical insufficiency still is entertained seriously, treat as borderline cortisol response. †Verify after stabilization.)

preclude performance of the rapid ACTH stimulation test. Although dexamethasone lacks any mineralocorticoid activity, vigorous hydration should allow the physician the 1 h needed to perform the ACTH stimulation test. Once the diagnostic tests are concluded, hydrocortisone should be substituted for dexamethasone because of its mineralocorticoid activity. The precipitating cause of adrenal decompensation, especially infection, should be sought.

For a more detailed discussion, see Chaps. 75, 76, and 77 in *Principles of Critical Care*, 2d ed.

Chapter 59

GASTROINTESTINAL HEMORRHAGE

DAVID T. RUBIN

Mortality from gastrointestinal hemorrhage has remained at approximately 10 percent, despite improvements in diagnosis and therapy, owing to a shift to care of sicker patients. The rate of bleeding determines the symptoms and signs as well as the outcome. However, it is important to identify the patient in a higher-risk group or the patient at risk of recurrent or ongoing bleeding in order to implement earlier surgical intervention and reduce mortality (Table 59-1).

Initial Management

The initial management of a gastrointestinal hemorrhage is the same regardless of the site or etiology of the bleeding (Table 59-2). Resuscitation and hemodynamic stabilization must be assured before the diagnostic workup begins. During resuscitation, blood transfusions must accompany crystalloid in order to maintain oxygen-carrying capacity and to reduce the chances of myocardial or mesenteric ischemia (the goal is HCT > 30 percent). If exsanguination is occurring and type-matched red cells are not available in a timely fashion, non-cross-matched blood should be used. Monitoring in an intensive care unit (ICU) environment and the use of central venous pressure or pulmonary artery catheters may be useful during resuscitation, especially in certain subgroups of patients (suspected variceal bleeding or coexistent respiratory or cardiac disease). Bleeding diatheses should be corrected.

Although nasogastric suction is performed routinely for diagnostic purposes, it has an estimated 14 percent false-negative rate and does not influence initial management. If there is a risk of emesis or aspiration, nasogastric suction is critical

TABLE 59-1 Mortality from Gastrointestinal Hemorrhage

Age > 60 = 30% higher mortality (13.4 vs. 8.7%)

CHF, arrhythmias = increased mortality (but angina and hypertension $\neq$ increased mortality)

CNS disease (encephalopathy or CVA) = increased mortality

Liver disease (even with nonvariceal bleeding) = increased mortality

Coexisting pulmonary, neoplastic, or renal disease = increased mortality

Bleeding that develops while hospitalized = worse mortality ($> 30\%$) than bleeding which is occurring at presentation

Black vs. brown stool does not worsen outcome or indicate need for specific therapies

Red stool with positive gastric aspirate = poorer outcome (30% mortality vs. 8%)

Bright red nasogastric aspirate = worse mortality, morbidity, and need for surgery than coffee grounds or clear aspirate

Esophageal variceal hemorrhage = 30% mortality

Mallory-Weiss tear = $< 5\%$ mortality

TABLE 59-2 Initial Management for Severe Gastrointestinal Bleeding

---

1. Maintain two large-bore (> 16 g) IV catheters.
2. Resuscitate with crystalline fluid to restore blood pressure.
3. Transfuse packed red cells early to maintain hematocrit $> 30\%$.
4. Use platelets and fresh frozen plasma transfusions as needed to correct thrombocytopenia or coagulopathy. Goal is platelets > 50 K and prothrombin time < 2 s above normal.
5. CVP or Ppw monitoring may be helpful if bleeding from varices is suspected or if the patient has coexistent respiratory or cardiac disease. A CVP < 10 mmHg helps prevent recurrent variceal bleeding.
6. A nasogastric tube should be inserted if the patient has hematemesis.
7. Use somatostatin or octreotide therapy if variceal hemorrhage is suspected. Vasopressin should be used only in young patients accompanied by a nitroglycerin patch.
8. Perform diagnostic and therapeutic endoscopy early, but only after hemodynamic stability has been achieved.
9. Obtain surgical consultation.

---

and endotracheal intubation for airway protection should be considered. Esophagogastroduodenoscopy (EGD) is the first procedure performed once the patient is hemodynamically stable, whether the presentation involves hematemesis or hematochezia.

Upper Gastrointestinal Bleeding

Most patients with gastrointestinal hemorrhage above the ligament of Treitz will present with melena, although 17 percent have bright red blood per rectum, which is associated with a poorer outcome. More than 50 percent of patients with upper gastrointestinal (UGI) hemorrhage will have hematemesis and most will not have abdominal pain.

DIAGNOSIS OF UPPER GI HEMORRHAGE

EGD is successful at diagnosing the source of an UGI bleed more than 85 percent of the time. Although prompt performance of EGD may lead to a prompt diagnosis and earlier etiology-specific therapy, this does not alter mortality or the need for surgical intervention. Early EGD may identify patients at higher risk for rebleeding and in high-risk patients may affect management and therefore indirectly limit mortality (Table 59-3). Evaluations of the benefits of early endoscopic therapy have not been performed yet.

Contraindications to EGD include hemodynamic instability (SBP < 100 mmHg or pulse > 120 beats per minute), suspected or impending perforation, carcinoma, trauma, or emetogenic injury and esophageal rupture (pneumomediastinum or subcutaneous emphysema). One of the risks associated with EGD is hypoxia, which will be worse if there is underlying pulmonary disease and may be further complicated by the hypoventilatory effects of sedation and physical obstruction by the endoscope. Cardiac arrhythmias including sinus tachycardia and premature ventricular contractions (PVCs) will be more likely if there is a history of underlying cardiovascular disease. Patients with valvular heart disease probably should receive prophylactic antibiotics, and patients with artificial valves should definitely receive antibiotic prophylaxis.

TABLE 59-3   Indications for Early
Esophagogastroduodenoscopy

Age > 60
Diagnosis of chronic liver disease
Bright red blood or maroon stool per rectum with hypotension or orthostasis
Patients who require more than 4 U of blood in 6 h

Patients with a clean, nonbloody ulcer have a 10 percent rebleeding rate. If there is an adherent clot or a nonbleeding visible vessel, there is a 50 percent chance of rebleeding. Actively bleeding lesions generally signify a need for surgical intervention, and in patients with bleeding peptic ulcers, earlier surgery results in less blood requirements and lower mortality. If EGD is negative or unrevealing due to retained blood or food products, it should be repeated 6 to 12 h later while supportive care is continued. Repeat EGD has a 70 percent success at identifying the cause of UGI hemorrhage.

If massive bleeding is continuing and EGD is negative, angiography is used in order to visualize extravasated contrast material in the gastrointestinal tract. The sensitivity of angiography is 0.5 to 1 mL/min. Brisk UGI bleeds are from the left gastric artery 85 percent of the time. Because angiography images varices during the venous phase of the circulation, visualization of varices does not guarantee that this is the source of bleeding; in fact, 40 percent of UGI bleeding in alcoholics is from a nonvariceal source.

Technetium-labeled red blood cells may detect acute bleeding at rates of < 0.5 mL/min. An advantage of using Tc-labeled blood is that the bleeding patient may be imaged for 1 to 2 days after injection; sensitivity is therefore > 90 percent in selected patients. This diagnostic test is helpful to localize an anatomic region for repeat endoscopy or surgery, but it does not provide information about the etiology of the bleeding.

THERAPY OF VARICEAL HEMORRHAGE

Variceal hemorrhage is associated with 30 percent mortality, and therapy is generally supportive. Pharmacologic therapy

for variceal hemorrhage is limited by unclear survival benefits; in most cases, it is supportive only until more definitive
endoscopic or surgical therapy can be instituted. Somatostatin
(synthetic analog, octreotide) decreases splanchnic blood flow
by inhibiting vasointestinal peptide release. Although this
medication controls hemorrhage, a mortality benefit has not
been shown. It is recommended to use somatostatin (octreotide) for the first 5 days of therapy to reduce the risk of
rebleeding. The recommended dosing of somatostatin is a
250-μg bolus IV followed by 250 μg/h IV and, if necessary, a
repeat bolus of 250 μg. Octreotide is administered as a 50-μg
bolus IV, followed by a continuous infusion of 25 to 50 μg/h.

The potent vasoconstrictor vasopressin has been used to
control gastrointestinal hemorrhage in the past, but its side
effects make this medication less desirable than somatostatin
and octreotide (abdominal pain, nausea, vomiting, hypertension, cardiac arrhythmias, heart failure, myocardial infarction,
pulmonary edema, intracerebral hemorrhage, and mesenteric
ischemia). Mortality benefit has not been shown, but bleeding does decrease. If it is used, it should be in conjunction
with nitrate administration, at a bolus of 20 U via central venous access followed by infusion of 0.4 to 0.6 U/min for no
more than 24 h, after which the infusion should be slowly
(over 24 h) tapered.

Chronically, beta blockers have been shown to reduce portal pressure and protect against recurrent bleeding, but beta-
blocking agents should *never* be used during acute variceal
hemorrhage and should be held in the event of bleeding.

Endoscopic sclerotherapy (ES) is a first-line therapy for
the control of esophageal variceal hemorrhage acutely as well
as for the prevention of rebleeding. It acts by causing thrombosis of the submucosal vessels, with subsequent tissue necrosis and eventual fibrosis. It is not indicated for gastric or duodenal varices owing to higher pressure in these vessels. When
active bleeding from a varix is identified endoscopically, ES
can control it 95 percent of the time. Rebleeding remains a
significant problem, however, and may occur between 20 and
74 percent of the time. ES may be more effective if it is performed earlier in the patient's presentation and should be
attempted prior to the use of a tamponade tube. ES has a
cost benefit when compared with portosystemic shunt, but

outcomes of both therapies in a patient with cirrhosis are similar.

Once ES is initially successful, it must be repeated several more times over the ensuing weeks until all varices are obliterated, but it should not be performed more than twice in the first 3 days. Successful obliteration of varices leads to long-term lower rebleeding rates and improved survival. The careful endoscopist must exclude other sources of bleeding before initiating ES on nonbleeding varices, since the complications of ES outweigh benefit in nonbleeding varices.

Endoscopic variceal ligation (EVL), which is the use of small elastic O rings for actively bleeding esophageal varices, is as effective as endoscopic sclerotherapy and has a lower complication rate. This procedure appears to have a favorable mortality reduction as well as fewer instances of pneumonia and esophageal strictures, and it requires fewer repeat sessions to achieve variceal obliteration. It is currently limited by endoscopist experience but is expected eventually to replace ES.

Hemorrhage that fails pharmacologic or endoscopic therapy may require balloon tamponade. This therapy is indicated for active hemorrhage that is severe enough to cause hemodynamic instability or lead to aspiration. In order to reduce the risk of aspiration, airway protection with an endotracheal tube is generally recommended prior to placement of a tamponade tube. Two types of tamponade tubes are commonly available. The Sengstaken-Blakemore (S-B) tube has a double-balloon system that allows for compression of gastric and esophageal varices with simultaneous gastric lavage and suction through a central lumen. Placement of an S-B tube mandates additional placement of a nasogastric tube above the esophageal balloon in order to minimize the risk of aspiration. The other type of tamponade tube is the Minnesota tube, which is similar to the S-B tube but has an additional lumen for esophageal suction.

In order to achieve hemostasis and minimize the risk of esophageal perforation, an S-B or Minnesota tube requires careful placement nasally or orally to full insertion. The gastric balloon is inflated with 100 mL of air and its correct position is comfirmed radiographically. Then, the gastric balloon is fully inflated (to 250 to 500 mL, depending on the balloon). The tube should be snugged up against the gastroesophageal junction and fixed to an external device, which usually halts bleeding. If bleeding continues, the esophageal balloon is subsequently inflated to a pressure of 35 mmHg, which exceeds the intravariceal pressure.

The esophageal balloon should be deflated for 15 min every 12 h in order to minimize the risk of ischemia. Compression of the varices is performed for no longer than 48 h because of a risk of local ischemia of the esophageal wall. After deflation, the tamponade tube should be left in place for 24 h in the event of rebleeding. Balloon tamponade is 90 percent effective, but the success is often temporary, with early rebleeding occurring as often as 25 percent of the time. Therefore it is important to have definitive therapy available at the time of deflation.

Transjugular Intrahepatic Portosystemic Shunt (TIPS)

TIPS should be considered a therapeutic option in the patient in whom attempts to control active bleeding have failed or when there is rebleeding despite sclerotherapy or ligation therapy. Transjugular intrahepatic portacaval shunts reduce hepatic capillary pressure and successfully decompress esophageal and gastric varices. Experienced angiographers have a 90 percent success rate placing the metallic stent in the hepatic parenchyma. TIPS placement may improve renal function in liver failure and reduce ascites but may worsen hepatic encephalopathy.

Surgery

Surgery should be considered if a patient with Child's class A or B cirrhosis has bleeding after 48 h of attempted pharmacotherapy, endoscopic therapy, or balloon tamponade. Surgical portosystemic shunting has a 50 percent mortality, higher in Child's class C cirrhosis. Patients with their third acute variceal hemorrhage despite previous variceal therapy and patients with acute variceal hemorrhage after noncompliance with sclerotherapy scheduling should also be considered for surgical therapy.

Although surgically placed portosystemic shunts decrease rebleeding rates, overall survival of patients with cirrhosis is not improved. Additional surgical approaches to variceal bleeding include esophageal and gastric devascularization, but these procedures are limited by the experience of the surgeon and the severity of the patient's illness.

Extrahepatic portal venous obstruction in the absence of cirrhosis may also cause variceal bleeding. Patients with this etiology for their hemorrhage may have less mortality and more favorable outcomes than cirrhotic patients. Gastric or duodenal varices in the absence of esophageal varices suggest the presence of splenic vein thrombosis; confirmation by celiac angiogram followed by splenectomy is the appropriate surgical therapy.

THERAPY OF NONVARICEAL HEMORRHAGE

Nonvariceal hemorrhage is characterized by a better prognosis than variceal bleeding owing in part to the self-limited nature of such hemorrhage. Most upper gastrointestinal hemorrhage is caused by peptic ulcer disease. Despite the effectiveness of modern pharmacologic therapies for peptic ulcer, these therapies do not stop ulcer-related bleeding or rebleeding. Identification and treatment of *Helicobacter pylori* is important for the prevention of recurrent disease, but the role of therapy for this ulcer-associated bacterium in the presence of acute bleeding is not known.

Endoscopic therapy involving bipolar electrocautery or injection is indicated when nonbleeding, oozing, or pulsating vessels are identified. When appropriately performed, thermal therapy or injection of hemostatic agents results in decreased rebleeding rates, fewer transfusions, and shorter hospital length of stay. Risks of injection therapy include a small risk of perforation when ethanol is used and a small risk of hypertensive crisis or ventricular tachycardia when epinephrine is used.

When endoscopic therapy fails to achieve hemostasis, angiographic therapy can be attempted. This is performed by either intraarterial infusion of vasoconstrictive drugs or embolization. Although intravenous vasopressin does not appear to affect nonvariceal bleeding, angiographic intraarterial infusion of vasopressin is therapeutically effective. If intraarterial vasopressin fails to achieve hemostasis, embolization with Gelfoam should be attempted. Embolization therapy may result in necrosis of the stomach, duodenum, gallbladder, liver, or spleen, especially if there was previous surgical resection. Recent studies have suggested a benefit to intravenous somatostatin and octreotide for acute nonvariceal hemorrhage, but this is not yet standard care.

Surgical therapy for bleeding peptic ulcers should be considered when hemorrhage has failed to respond to medical and endoscopic therapies and in patients in whom medical management has failed to heal bleeding ulcers or prevent recurrence of such ulcers. In addition, patients who are noncompliant with ulcer therapy and continue to suffer from bleeding complications should undergo elective surgery. When indicated, surgical therapies should be performed in the hemodynamically stable, nonbleeding patient. Prior to going to the operating room, the patient should have a corrected volume status, blood transfusions, correction of any coagulopathy, and protection from aspiration. Under controlled circumstances, selective vagotomy with pyloroplasty or antrectomy is performed. If the patient is actively bleeding at the time of surgery, morbidity and mortality are greatly increased and the bleeding site is oversewn, followed by truncal vagotomy and pyloroplasty. Postoperative wound infection is the major complication of these surgeries.

A Mallory-Weiss tear is most often self-limited and rarely requires more than supportive therapy. When bleeding from a suspected Mallory-Weiss tear continues, endoscopic confirmation followed by electrocautery or injection therapy is attempted. If more than 10 U of packed red cells are required, surgical oversewing should be performed.

Hemorrhagic gastritis is commonly seen in alcoholic patients and in patients undergoing physiologic stress; it may account for 25 percent of cases of UGI bleeding. It usually stops spontaneously. When therapy is needed, it should be primarily nonsurgical.

Acute Lower Gastrointestinal Bleeding

When acute gastrointestinal bleeding occurs below the ligament of Treitz, EGD is still the first diagnostic test. The color of blood is not predictive of the location of the bleeding, since brisk right colonic and small intestinal bleeding may appear bright red. The average age of patients with lower gastrointestinal (LGI) bleeding is 65, and most have coexistent cardiac and respiratory disease.

If the patient is orthostatic and the source of blood loss is below the ligament of Treitz, it is more likely that this source is from a vascular site (usually owing to diverticulosis or angiodysplasia) rather than a mass or polyp, and prompt resuscitation is necessary.

Angiodysplasia is most often in the right colon, cecum, or distal small bowel of the elderly patient, but it may occur congenitally and present in younger patients. Nonvascular LGI bleeding occurs rarely and may be from small bowel or colonic ulcerations. Hemodynamic instability is rare in these cases. In the younger patient, massive bleeding suggests a Meckel diverticulum, which may be diagnosed by a Meckel scan (with ^{99m}Tc pertechnetate), which has a 75 percent sensitivity.

DIAGNOSIS OF LGI HEMORRHAGE

Evaluation of the suspected LGI bleed depends on the suspected etiology. Vascular bleeding is usually intermittent, so angiography should be performed promptly when active bleeding is suspected based on ongoing hypotension, orthostasis, or tachycardia. Superior or inferior mesenteric angiography may localize bleeding sites in 70 percent of patients. Angiographic therapy or site-specific surgical resection can then be performed.

Colonoscopy in the emergent, unprepped patient is usually nondiagnostic and impractical. If a bleeding patient can be prepped with a clearing solution, emergent endoscopy may yield a diagnosis 75 percent of the time. In fact, early colonoscopy in a patient with diverticulosis may identify the source of bleeding when it would otherwise be missed if the procedure were not performed until bleeding has stopped. In addition, when an actively bleeding site is identified by colonoscopy, endoscopic therapy may be attempted, with electrocoagulation of an angiodysplastic lesion or lavage with epinephrine. Intraoperative endoscopy may be indicated to identify an intermittent source of bleeding that has not been located by routine methods or to more specifically limit resection of small bowel in such diseases as Peutz-Jeghers syndrome. Intraoperative endoscopy can be performed orally, with passage of the endoscope (pediatric colonoscope) aided by pleating of the small bowel over the end of the scope while the surgeon looks for transilluminated angiodysplastic lesions. It may also be performed with a sterile endoscope passed via an enterostomy site, but there is an increased risk of contamination of the peritoneum. An additional risk is prolonged ileus due to overinflation of intestines during the exam, but these complications may be minimized by teamwork between the endoscopist and surgeon.

Radionuclide scans are less specific but more sensitive than angiography for LGI bleeding. This type of scan should be used to localize bleeding to specific sites of the GI tract that can then be identified by endoscopy or angiography prior to surgical therapy.

THERAPY OF LGI HEMORRHAGE

In most episodes, LGI bleeding stops spontaneously and only supportive therapy is required until diagnosis. Surgical resection of the bleeding area is required in most patients with massive bleeding, although nonsurgical therapy may obviate the need for surgery or allow for nonemergent surgery. Surgical resection of bleeding bowel is indicated for bleeding that requires more than 6 or 8 U of packed red cells in 24 h. When aggressive diagnostics are unrevealing, blind resection may need to be performed. In elderly patients, this usually involves a subtotal colectomy and ileoproctostomy, with resultant debilitating diarrhea. Owing to the high percentage of left-sided diverticulosis as a site of LGI in elderly patients, blind hemicolectomy is sometimes performed. This, however, is associated with a high rebleeding rate, partly because angiodysplasia may be confined to the terminal ileum or involve the terminal ileum in addition to the cecum. Angiography that demonstrates a cecal lesion may fail to identify the small bowel lesion, so empiric resection of 30 to 60 cm of ileum should accompany partial colectomy or intraoperative enteroscopy should be performed. When surgical resection is performed emergently, it is associated with a 40 percent mortality rate. Angiographic diagnosis may be accompanied by intraarterial infusion of vasopressin to stop bleeding temporarily prior to surgical resection. Endoscopic therapy of a visible bleeding site includes local application of vasoconstrictors and coagulation procedures.

Bleeding of Unknown Origin

Sources of occult acute bleeding include angiodysplasia as well as hematobilia. Angiodysplastic lesions of the upper gastrointestinal tract may be mistaken for nasogastric or endoscope trauma. In patients with chronic renal failure, gastric angiodysplasia may account for significant bleeding. Likewise, the cecum may harbor angiodysplastic lesions that will be identified only with careful inspection but may easily be missed during colonoscopy. Intraoperative endoscopy of the entire small bowel should be considered before blind resection of the colon for bleeding of unknown origin.

Hematobilia is a rare cause of gastrointestinal bleeding from the liver and bile ducts or from the pancreas through the ampulla of Vater. Aneurysms of hepatic or splenic arteries or trauma may cause hematobilia. This diagnosis should be suspected when melena occurs in conjunction with jaundice or after blunt trauma or pancreatitis. Diagnosis may be made using angiography or a side-viewing duodenoscope and therapy generally requires surgery.

If the patient with gastrointestinal bleeding of unknown origin has previously received a synthetic vascular graft, an aortoenteric fistula should be suspected, usually involving the fourth portion of the duodenum. Endoscopy or angiography confirms this diagnosis and therapy requires prompt resuscitation and surgery to prevent exsanguination.

Stress-Related Mucosal Damage (Stress Ulcers)

Some 5 to 20 percent of ICU patients may suffer from stress-related mucosal damage; this may cause major GI hemorrhage. Stress ulcer bleeding may present with overt hemorrhage and hypotension or bleeding may be occult, detected in stool guaiac only. The underlying illness and the difficulty of controlling such hemorrhage results in a mortality rate greater than 30 percent. Severe burns, sepsis, respiratory failure and prolonged ventilatory support, fulminant hepatic failure, prolonged hypotension, and renal failure are all associated with increased risk of stress ulceration and hemorrhage. Diagnosis is confirmed endoscopically, with diffuse erythema and slow oozing at one extreme and multiple gastric ulcerations and even visible vessels at the other.

Therapy is mostly supportive until the underlying critical illness is adequately treated. Acid blockade has little benefit in reversing stress ulceration, and angiographic or endoscopic therapies are also of questionable benefit, especially if there are multiple lesions diffusely. Surgery usually requires a near total gastrectomy, with resultant mortality greater than 50 percent.

Prophylaxis of stress ulceration is directed toward acid reduction, although the cause of stress ulceration is not excess acid but rather mucosal ischemia. Acid control may be obtained by hourly titration of antacid via a nasogastric tube with a goal of maintaining gastric pH > 3.5. Alternatively, continuous infusion of intravenous H_2-receptor antagonists may provide similar benefits, although this is somewhat controversial. The use of proton pump–inhibiting drugs and the resultant achlorhydria is under investigation but looks favorable. Sucralfate increases mucosal blood flow, mucus secretion, and local prostaglandin production to protect against ulcer formation and aid in the healing of stress ulcers. Because sucralfate does not inhibit acid production, the gastric milieu is less likely to harbor gram-negative bacteria and nosocomial pneumonia is less frequent than with H_2-receptor blocking drugs or proton-pump inhibitors. Combination therapy comprising sucralfate and H_2-receptor blocking drugs may be needed in the most critically ill patients.

For a more detailed discussion, see Chap. 79 in *Principles of Critical Care,* 2d ed.

Chapter 60

ACUTE AND CHRONIC HEPATIC DISEASE

DAVID T. RUBIN

Patients with severe liver disease make up two main groups: those with cirrhosis and those with fulminant hepatic failure. Both groups have a high risk of death from a variety of causes, many of which are complications of therapy rather than being due to the natural progression of their underlying disease or precipitants of admission. Therefore, intensive care unit (ICU) monitoring should be considered for any patient with fulminant hepatic failure or a complication of cirrhosis. Controlled, efficient therapy must be delivered in a coordinated manner involving the intensivist, gastroenterologist, hepatologist, and transplant surgeon.

Attention to infection surveillance, airway protection, coagulation, nutrition, the adverse effects of drugs, and the development of hepatic encephalopathy will minimize complications and improve survival.

General Supportive Measures

INFECTION

Infection is an extremely common complication of liver failure, and more than 25 percent of patients with liver failure and infection will not present with a fever or leukocytosis. Patients with liver failure have an impaired ability to fight infection at a cellular and molecular level, but their risk of infection is also increased owing to an impaired ability to protect their airway. Because of these compromised defense mechanisms, the consequences of infection in the presence of liver failure are severe. There is a significantly increased risk of the acute respiratory distress syndrome (ARDS) and death due to sepsis in patients with liver failure. Careful assessment of the patient's ability to protect their airway and meticulous investigation for sources of infection in the presence of fever, leukocytosis, or hemodynamic instability are vital to early and aggressive therapy. Empiric antibiotics should be administered when any signs of infection are identified.

AIRWAY MANAGEMENT

Airway assessment must be a daily part of the care of a patient with liver failure. Contributors to the risk of aspiration include gastrointestinal hemorrhage, infection, drug effect, development or progression of hepatic encephalopathy, and interventions such as endoscopy or placement of a tamponade tube. In addition, ARDS and the hepatopulmonary syndrome may compromise gas exchange and require ventilatory support. It is preferable to electively intubate under controlled circumstances when these risks are identified than to wait until ventilatory support is urgent or emergent. If cerebral edema or hemorrhage is present, care must be taken to avoid increasing intracerebral pressure during intubation.

COAGULOPATHY AND RISK OF HEMORRHAGE

Patients with liver failure often have a multifactorial coagulopathy that may precipitate their hospitalization or complicate other therapies. This tendency to bleed is caused by an underproduction of hepatic coagulation factors, but it may be complicated by malnutrition, thrombocytopenia, disseminated intravascular coagulation, or fibrinolysis. In addition, treatments of infection and hepatic encephalopathy may eliminate bacterial sources of vitamin K. Therapy for the multifactorial coagulopathy of liver disease depends on the indication. In general, fresh frozen plasma (FFP) and vitamin K (10 mg subcutaneously daily for three doses) are delivered to the hemorrhaging patient or to a patient needing an interventional procedure. Platelets may also be required, with a goal of maintaining platelet counts above 50,000.

Although vitamin K is routinely delivered, prophylactic administration of FFP or platelets does not prevent clinically significant bleeding. However, patients with cirrhosis and varices have an increased risk of bleeding due to anatomic and physiologic abnormalities; alcoholics have a higher incidence of peptic ulcers and gastritis; and all of these patients are at risk of stress-related mucosal injury. Therefore, efforts to reduce these bleeding risks are essential. Acid blockade with H_2 antagonists, proton-pump inhibitors, or antacids should be used to maintain a gastric pH above 5. Hemodynamically stable patients with esophageal varices should receive β-blocking drugs. Endotracheal intubation should be performed orally to avoid epistaxis, and experienced personnel should perform any interventional procedures.

NUTRITION

Institution of full nutritional support should be an early priority in the patient with liver failure. Patients with liver disease tend to be malnourished to begin with, and this is worsened when they are acutely ill and may have an increased metabolic demand. Profound and prolonged hypoglycemia may develop due to liver failure, and thiamine and folate deficiencies are common. Therefore, enteral feedings, if safe and tolerated, should be the first choice, but when this is not possible, total parenteral nutrition (TPN) should be delivered. There are some data suggesting that branched-chain amino acids may lead to improvement in hepatic encephalopathy and survival.

DRUG EFFECT

Administration of drugs to the patient with acute or chronic liver failure is complicated by decreased protein binding, decreased hepatic metabolism, and sometimes coexisting renal failure. Because of this increased risk of subtherapeutic serum levels or increased toxicity, all drugs administered to the patient with liver disease must be carefully monitored for efficacy and adverse side effects.

PORTOSYSTEMIC ENCEPHALOPATHY

The neurologic and psychiatric deterioration that accompanies liver failure is known as portosystemic encephalopathy (PSE) or hepatic encephalopathy. Its cause is not known, and there appears to be a difference between the PSE of chronic liver failure, which is generally reversible, and the PSE of fulminant hepatic failure, which does not respond well to therapy. Although ammonia levels are routinely obtained as a serum marker for PSE, they correlate poorly with the degree of neuropsychiatric abnormality; nonspecific EEG abnormalities or visual-evoked potentials may aid in the diagnosis of this syndrome. It is important to distinguish PSE from other causes of encephalopathy and coma. A toxicology screen should be obtained, drug effects (especially narcotics and ethanol) should be carefully considered, and hypoglycemia, subdural hematoma, meningitis, subclinical status epilepticus, hypoxemia, and Wernicke encephalopathy ruled out. In addition, due to a suspected relationship between this disorder and endogenous benzodiazepines, patients with PSE show a distinct response to the benzodiazepine antagonist flumazenil, which may aid in distinguishing PSE from other causes of neuropsychiatric deterioration. Sometimes PSE can be confirmed only by response to empiric therapy.

Manifestations of PSE range from subtle personality changes and sleep-cycle disruptions usually noted retrospectively (stage I); to drowsiness, lethargy, and asterixis (stage II); to delirium, disorientation, somnolence, and possibly seizures (stage III); to deep coma and decerebrate posturing with or without response to deep painful stimuli (stage IV). Rapid progression from stage I to stage IV is often seen in fulminant hepatic failure.

Management of PSE involves identification and treatment of any precipitating factors, protein restriction, and colonic cleansing (Table 60-1). When PSE deterioration is due to gastrointestinal hemorrhage, blood should be removed from the

TABLE 60-1   Precipitants of Hepatic Encephalopathy

Gastrointestinal hemorrhage
Spontaneous bacterial peritonitis
Systemic infection
Drugs (especially benzodiazepines and barbiturates)
Acute deterioration in liver function (e.g., hepatitis, hepatotoxin, transplant dysfunction)
Dietary protein load
Alkalosis
Diuretic therapy, especially with hypokalemia
Diarrhea or dehydration
Constipation
Azotemia

---

stomach and colon with orogastric suction and enemas. Non-absorbable disaccharides (i.e., lactulose) are effective cathartic agents (3o to 45 mL hourly and then titrated to three loose stools per day, or retention enemas delivered every 6 h). Neomycin (2 g every 8 h) is an alternative agent and may be additive with lactulose. Nutrition should not be abandoned during therapy for PSE. In fact, branched-chain amino acids may improve PSE and survival in hepatic failure.

Fulminant Hepatic Failure

Fulminant hepatic failure (FHF) is defined as the development of PSE within 8 weeks of presentation of liver-related symptoms. FHF may be a result of an acute viral infection or toxin exposure or the first presentation of a chronic compensated cirrhosis. Patients with FHF may have coagulopathies, cardiovascular instability, renal dysfunction, and serious infections. The definitive therapy for FHF is liver transplantation, so patients with FHF should be transferred to a transplant center as soon as possible.

ETIOLOGY

The causes of FHF are many (Table 60-2), although the exact etiology is not often understood. Hepatocellular necrosis is the pathogenetic mechanism seen in viral or drug-induced FHF, while microvesicular steatosis is seen in fatty liver of pregnancy, tetracycline toxicity, or Reye syndrome. The most common cause of FHF worldwide is viral infection, and hepatitis B is the most common viral cause. Coinfection with hepatitis D appears to increase the incidence of FHF, and coinfection with hepatitis D should be ruled out in a patient with chronic hepatitis B presenting with FHF.

Patients with FHF may present with a variety of symptoms, although the predominant ones are those related to PSE, such as asterixis, confusion, or obtundation. Other findings supportive of the diagnosis of FHF include fetor hepaticus, jaundice, fever, tachycardia, and hypotension, although their presence is variable. Likewise, laboratory abnormalities are not uniformly predictable and depend on the etiology of FHF. Dramatic elevation of serum aminotransferases may accompany hepatic necrosis and elevations in the prothrombin time

TABLE 60-2   Causes of Fulminant Hepatic Failure

Infections
    Hepatitis virus
        Types A, B, C, D, E, non-A, non-B, non-C
    Other viral infections (cytomegalovirus, Epstein-Barr virus)
    Tuberculosis
    Coxiella burnetti infection
Poisons, chemicals, and drugs
    Acetaminophen
    Amanita phalloides
    Ethanol
    Halothane and certain other, chiefly halogenated, hydrocarbons
    Herbal teas and remedies
        Chaparral
        Germander
        Jin bu huan
        Callilepis laureola
    Hydroxychloroquine
    Isoniazid
    Methyldopa
    Monoamine oxidase inhibitors
    Phenytoin
    Phosphorus
    Pirprofen
    Potassium permanganate
    Sodium valproate
    Tetracycline
Hepatic anoxia
    Hepatic vascular occlusion
    Acute circulatory failure
    Heatstroke
    Sickle cell disease
    Gram-negative bacteremia with shock
    Congestive cardiac failure
    Pericardial tamponade
Miscellaneous metabolic abnormalities
    Acute fatty liver of pregnancy
    Reye syndrome
    Jejunoileal bypass
    Wilson disease
    Galactosemia
    Hereditary fructose intolerance
    Hereditary tyrosinemia

and ammonia levels are not uncommon, although it is the presence of PSE with liver dysfunction independent of laboratory abnormalities that defines FHF.

COMPLICATIONS

Complications of FHF include cerebral edema and circulatory, metabolic, renal, and pulmonary derangements. Cerebral edema is present in 50 to 80 percent of FHF cases and may be the leading cause of death from FHF. Management of cerebral edema is challenging owing to its subtle initial presentation. Patients with cerebral edema may present with heightened muscle tone, abnormal pupillary reflexes, and, with higher levels of intracranial pressure (ICP), decorticate or decerebrate posturing. If ICP continues to rise, hypertension, bradycardia, and ultimately death may result. Computed tomography (CT) scans may aid in the diagnosis of increased ICP by demonstrating obliteration of sulci, narrowing of ventricles, and obscured gray-white junction, but invasive ICP monitoring is a more accurate and sensitive method of monitoring and treating increased ICP. Invasive ICP monitoring should be considered early in the course of FHF, especially in patients with stage III or IV PSE, although this is controversial, and patients with increased ICP have survived liver transplantation without neurologic sequelae. Transcranial Doppler monitoring or frequent serial neurologic exams may offer similar information about progressive changes in ICP.

Careful airway management is crucial in the patient with cerebral edema. Endotracheal intubation raises ICP, so experienced personnel should use mask hyperventilation followed by a rapid-sequence intubation using lidocaine and short-acting barbiturates. Mannitol (1 g/kg) should be first-line therapy for the cerebral complications of increased ICP. As an osmotic diuretic, it acts to increase cerebral blood flow and cerebral oxygen consumption but should not be used to create a serum osmolality > 320 mOsm. Hyperventilation to a P_{CO_2} of 25 mmHg also decreases ICP, but its effects are transient because of cerebrovascular and renal compensation. Mannitol and hyperventilation should be used concomitantly to titrate ICP less than 20 mmHg. Factors contributing to increased ICP or decreased brain blood flow—such as fever, agitation, or hypotension—should be aggressively treated.

Circulatory impairment and hypotension are extremely common in patients with FHF. Hemorrhage and infection are common, but 60 percent of hypotension is due to unknown causes. Patients with liver failure have an increased cardiac output and decreased peripheral resistance as well as impaired microvascular regulation and oxygen utilization.

Hepatocellular necrosis and depleted hepatic glycogen stores may dictate impressive parenteral dextrose administration in the patient with FHF. Patients who require as much as 1000 g of 10 percent dextrose have been reported. In addition, because of impaired lactate metabolism, a significant lactic acidosis may develop, although bicarbonate administration will only increase lactate production. Renal failure due to acute tubular necrosis or functional impairment is common in FHF. In addition, hypoxemia and pulmonary edema due to multiple causes may complicate the care of patients with FHF.

PROGNOSIS

Multiple factors contribute to the outcome in FHF, but the etiology of the liver disease may be the most important. Patients with FHF due to acetaminophen overdose and hepatitis A have the highest percentage of survival. Survival correlates with the severity of liver injury as measured by prothrombin time, ability to correct coagulopathy, metabolic acidosis, and hepatic encephalopathy. A spontaneous decrease in ICP is an early indicator of improvement from FHF. Artificial hepatic support offers a bridge to native liver recovery or to orthotopic transplantation, but no therapy is widely available yet. Indications for orthotopic liver transplantation (OLT) are not clear cut, but OLT should be considered in patients with progressive deterioration of hepatic function and liver disease due to drug-induced liver injury (other than acetaminophen), toxins, or non-A, non-B hepatitis. OLT has a survival rate in excess of 80 percent.

Chronic Liver Disease

Patients with chronic liver disease include those with cirrhosis, chronic active hepatitis, hepatic vein thrombosis, or nodular regenerative hyperplasia. Unlike FHF, in which the major complication is PSE and cerebral edema, patients with chronic liver disease who require ICU care suffer from variceal hemorrhage, spontaneous bacterial peritonitis (SBP), and the hepatorenal syndrome (HRS). Patients with these complications have a poor prognosis and require aggressive diagnostic and therapeutic interventions.

VARICEAL HEMORRHAGE

Gastrointestinal (GI) hemorrhage in the face of chronic liver disease is a frequent cause of death. Variceal hemorrhage accounts for approximately 70 percent of the GI bleeding in cirrhotics, and portal hypertensive gastropathy, peptic ulcer disease, and Mallory-Weiss tears account for other sources of hemorrhage. Esophagogastroduodenoscopy (EGD) must be performed as soon as the bleeding patient is hemodynamically stable, both to identify the specific site of bleeding for appropriate therapy as well as to implement certain endoscopic therapies.

Because GI bleeding is frequently intermittent but rebleeding is common, the absence of active bleeding during EGD must not delay the implementation of therapy. The choice of appropriate therapy will depend on the site of bleeding and on any previous therapies administered. There is an important difference between the therapies administered for esophageal varices (endoscopic therapy, transjugular intrahepatic portosystemic shunt (TIPS), surgical shunts) and those for gastric varices due to splenic vein thrombosis (splenectomy).

As described in Chap. 59, the initial management of GI hemorrhage (independent of its etiology) is supportive. Two large-bore (16 g or greater) intravenous catheters should be placed and aggressive crystalloid, plasma, and packed red cells administered to achieve hemodynamic stability. The prothrombin time must be corrected to within 2 s of normal, and the platelet count should be greater than 50,000. In patients with severe hemorrhage, central venous catheter monitoring may aid in resuscitation; in patients with coexisting pulmonary or cardiac abnormalities, placement of a pulmonary artery catheter should be considered. Simultaneously, the patient's airway should be assessed. If there is a risk of aspiration due to altered mental status or uncontrolled hemorrhage or if diagnostic or therapeutic instrumentation is necessary, elective endotracheal intubation should be performed. The use of neuroleptic drugs such as haloperidol or droperidol has been associated with torsades de pointes in variceal hemorrhage, so alternative agents such as propofol should be used.

The acute control of bleeding can be obtained through a combination of endoscopic sclerotherapy (ES), endoscopic variceal ligation (EVL), pharmacologic therapy, balloon tamponade, and transjugular intrahepatic portosystemic shunt (TIPS) procedures. Urgent diagnostic EGD and possible ES should be the first priority after initial stabilization of the patient and may achieve successful control of acute bleeding of esophageal varices in 90 percent of cases. Gastric varices on the lesser curve of the stomach or within a hiatal hernia may also respond to ES. Newer equipment makes EVL less technically demanding than ES, and it is associated with less rebleeding, less esophageal stricture formation, and less mortality; it is expected to replace ES once more endoscopists are competent in its use. Pharmacologic agents like somatostatin and its synthetic analog octreotide have replaced the historically used vasopressin because of improved efficacy and fewer side effects. Octreotide is generally given as a 50- to 100-μg IV bolus followed by 25 to 50 μg/h for 24 h. It is superior to vasopressin and equivalent to ES in terms of initial control of hemorrhage, incidence of rebleeding, units of blood transfused, hospital length of stay, and mortality. Balloon tamponade of varices controls bleeding in 85 percent of patients. Its use should be viewed as a bridge to more definitive therapy; the details of its placement are described in Chap. 59.

TIPS can be performed in the patient who continues to bleed or to prevent long-term rebleeding. It is 95 percent successful and can be performed in patients who will subsequently require OLT. Surgical portosystemic shunting (PSS) is generally used for patients who are not transplant candidates and have failed sclerotherapy. Its use is controversial because it has a high intraoperative mortality, exacerbates hepatic insufficiency, and makes subsequent OLT technically difficult, although it is the treatment of choice for patients with varices of the gastric fundus. Total-volume paracentesis reduces portal pressure and variceal size and is probably useful to prevent rebleeding, although its use during acute hemorrhage has not been studied.

Once acute bleeding is controlled, definitive therapy should be performed to prevent fatal rebleeding. Liver transplantation should be carefully considered, and continued ES or EVL, TIPS, or surgical portosystemic shunting (PSS) should be performed. Esophageal transection should be considered for patients who have failed ES, especially if they are transplant candidates, although rebleeding may occur. β-blockers have a role for prophylaxis in variceal bleeding, but they should never be used during acute hemorrhage or if definitive therapy has not been administered.

SPONTANEOUS BACTERIAL PERITONITIS

Patients with spontaneous bacterial peritonitis (SBP) may be asymptomatic or septic or present with worsened PSE. SBP is associated with an in-hospital mortality > 50 percent, although it is not entirely due to infectious complications. In addition, SBP is a marker of poor long-term prognosis in patients with liver disease; OLT should be considered in any patient with an episode of SBP. Diagnosis is confirmed by ascitic fluid with any of the following characteristics: polymorphonuclear (PMN) leukocyte count > 250/mm^3, pH < 7.3, lactate concentration > 25 mg/dL, or positive fluid culture. Polymicrobial infections are rare, and *Escherichia coli*, streptococci, and *Klebsiella* species are the most common organisms in SBP. Blood cultures may also be positive and should be obtained when SBP is suspected. Paracentesis is a rare cause of SBP. When SBP is strongly suspected or confirmed, antibiotic therapy with cefotaxime (2 g IV q6h) should be empirically administered until organisms are identified. Duration of therapy is 10 to 14 days, and therapy should be continued in the absence of positive cultures if the ascitic PMN leukocyte count is > 500/mm^3. Serial paracenteses may be required to confirm therapeutic efficacy. Prevention of SBP may be achieved with trimethoprim/sulfamethoxazole 1 double strength tablet daily or ciprofloxacin 750 mg once weekly.

Polymicrobial infections, lack of response to antibiotics, a rising ascitic fluid PMN leukocyte count, glucose < 50 mg/dL, fluid lactate dehydrogenase level > 225 mU/mL, or total protein concentration > 1 g/dL suggest a possible perforated viscus.

HEPATORENAL SYNDROME

Hepatorenal syndrome (HRS) is a functional renal failure in patients with liver disease, usually patients with tense ascites or those with recent medical intervention (paracentesis, diuresis, prostaglandin inhibitors) or critical illness (hypotension). The only effective therapy for HRS is OLT. Because HRS is an irreversible and poorly understood phenomenon, patients with liver disease who develop renal insufficiency should be evaluated carefully to identify and treat the reversible causes of renal disease. In order to distinguish prerenal azotemia from HRS, diuretics should be stopped and a fluid challenge of 500 to 1000 mL administered. In order to confidently rule out hypovolemia, a pulmonary artery catheter may be required. Acute tubular necrosis should be ruled out by careful analysis of the urine sediment for renal tubular casts. Although dialysis can treat the uremic patient, it does not improve the functional impairment seen in HRS and should be used as a bridge to OLT. There are some data to support the administration of fresh frozen plasma and prostaglandin E_1 analog in HRS, although this is not well understood.

HYPOXEMIA AND THE HEPATOPULMONARY SYNDROME

Hypoxemia in patients with chronic liver disease may be due to many causes, but the hepatopulmonary syndrome (HPS) is thought to be due to ventilation/perfusion mismatch and diffusion limitation due to vasodilation of small pulmonary vessels. Diagnosis may be supported by measurement of a diminished diffusing capacity in the presence of normal spirometry or contrast echocardiography showing passage of microbubbles across the pulmonary microcirculation. Often patients with HPS compensate by increasing cardiac output and hyperventilating, but this can be insufficient in the presence of critical illness. Increased inspired oxygen may be effective short-term therapy, but the only long-term therapy for the HPS is OLT.

For a more detailed discussion, see Chap. 80 in *Principles of Critical Care*, 2d ed.

Chapter 61
ACUTE PANCREATITIS
DAVID T. RUBIN

Pancreatitis in the intensive care unit (ICU) patient is challenging to diagnose and difficult to treat. It may be a self-limiting disease from which recovery is without complication, or it may be severe, complicated by multisystem organ failure and sepsis and a mortality rate as high as 40 percent; it may then require aggressive interventions.

Etiology

Acute pancreatitis may have many causes (Table 61-1). In the critically ill patient, hypoperfusion injury is probably the major pathogenetic mechanism causing acute pancreatitis, but thrombosis and microembolism are also postulated. Shock of any type may cause acute pancreatitis or may amplify an existing mild pancreatitis. Regardless of the etiology, the common pathway of destruction is due to the release of activated pancreatic enzymes and intense inflammation. Additional systemic and organ-specific complications include fluid and electrolyte loss, hypotension, renal and pulmonary complications, infections, sepsis, multisystem organ failure, and death.

Diagnosis

Acute pancreatitis should be suspected in patients with abdominal pain, nausea and vomiting, fever of uncertain origin, leukocytosis, or hypotension or hemodynamic instability of uncertain explanation. Prompt confirmation of the diagnosis of acute pancreatitis needs to be obtained in order to initiate appropriate supportive therapy, and aggressive surgical intervention must be undertaken to minimize the risk of multisystem organ failure and death.

TABLE 61-1   Acute Pancreatitis—Etiologic Factors

Metabolic	Obstructive—Mechanical	Infectious—Obstructive	Idiopathic	Hypoperfusion
Alcohol	Gallstones	Mumps	Familial	Vascular
Hypercalcemia	Afferent loop obstruction	Coxsackievirus infection		PAN and other collagen disorders
Drugs	Duodenal obstruction	*Mycoplasma* infection		Embolic
Hyperlipidemia	Periampullary tumors	Ascariasis		Low-flow states
	Duodenal ulcer	Clonorchiasis		
	Pancreas divisum			
	Trauma			
	Blunt			
	Penetrating			
	Postoperative			
	Post-ERCP			

ABBREVIATIONS: ERCP, endoscopic retrograde cholangiopancreatography; PAN, polyarteritis nodosa.

If acute pancreatitis is suspected in the workup of a critically ill patient, the diagnosis may be confirmed by finding
an elevated lipase level, which is more specific than amylase
levels, although both biochemical tests are sometimes unreliable. An important component of the evaluation in suspected
pancreatitis is imaging of the retroperitoneum by ultrasound
or computed tomography (CT), in addition to routine chest
and abdominal films. The presence of pleural effusions, localized jejunal or colonic ileus, a widened C loop of the duodenum, pancreatic calcification, gallstones, or obliteration of
psoas shadows and free intraperitoneal fluid may suggest
pancreatitis. Laparoscopic surgery may be necessary to confirm the diagnosis of pancreatitis, although this degree of intervention should be a last resort.

ULTRASOUND AND COMPUTED
TOMOGRAPHY IMAGING

Ultrasonography is the modality of choice for mild pancreatitis, although paralytic ileus and obesity limit its sensitivity. It is a helpful test in patients with suspected obstructive
pancreatitis and in follow-up of retroperitoneal phlegmon
that may progress to pseudocyst. It is also useful in the critically ill patient because it can be performed at the bedside.
CT is the most helpful tool for imaging the pancreas and
retroperitoneal space. Although there are risks involved in
transporting a patient to the CT scanner and administering
intravenous contrast material, these are balanced by the benefit of accurate images that aid in diagnosis and therapy. CT
is most useful for following complications such as pancreatic
abscesses and for diagnosing pseudoaneurysms.

SEVERITY OF DISEASE

Appropriate management of acute pancreatitis depends on
knowledge about the severity of illness. The classically reviewed Ranson's criteria provide some information about
prognosis but are not particularly helpful in the ICU patient
with other illnesses that also affect these parameters. Clinical assessment of the patient and serial CT scans are the best
predictors of disease severity and progression. The development of abdominal pain and tenderness, fever, leukocytosis,

hemodynamic instability, and CT changes within 1 to 2 weeks of the onset of pancreatitis provides the best assessment of the severe complications of the disease. Percutaneous aspiration of the retroperitoneum with microscopic examination and cultures can be helpful in the patient with sepsis and CT evidence of pancreatic necrosis.

Treatment

After hemodynamic stabilization and appropriate diagnosis, the treatment of acute pancreatitis depends on the etiology. If the pancreatitis is due to an obvious precipitating factor, therapy should be directed at the precipitating factor first. If it is due to a mechanical obstruction, endoscopic therapy and sphincterotomy or stent placement may be useful. If cholecystectomy is indicated, it should be performed as soon as possible.

When no obvious simple solution can be offered or when the inciting cause of the pancreatitis was a hypoperfusion injury, the ICU patient with acute pancreatitis requires supportive care and monitoring. Pulmonary and renal complications of pancreatitis should be identified and treated early and the local complications of necrotizing pancreatitis should be minimized. Serial lipase levels and measures of renal function, electrolytes, and hematologic values may be obtained in order to monitor deterioration or improvement. Serial imaging studies to monitor necrosis and retroperitoneal fluid may be necessary to obtain early surgical intervention. Careful collaboration between the intensivist and the experienced abdominal surgeon facilitates control of ongoing destruction.

One of the most important components of therapy for the patient with acute pancreatitis is the administration of fluids. Vomiting and retroperitoneal destruction may necessitate 8 to 10 L of isotonic fluid in the first 24 h. If hemodynamic instability persists after aggressive fluid replacement, vasoactive drugs may be required; in the patient with coexisting cardiac abnormalities, careful invasive monitoring may be required during this resuscitation. Elimination of hypotension is essential, since it may contribute to ongoing pancreatic damage. Retroperitoneal hemorrhage may necessitate blood product administration.

Pulmonary complications of acute pancreatitis in the critically ill patient may range from a sympathetic pleural effusion to development of the acute respiratory distress syndrome and need for prolonged ventilatory support. The aggressive fluid resuscitation necessary in acute pancreatitis may also result in high-pressure pulmonary edema.

There is no specific link between pancreatitis and renal failure, but the hypoperfusion that may cause acute pancreatitis may also cause the acute tubular necrosis sometimes seen concurrently. In addition, the large fluid shifts associated with pancreatitis may lead to renal insufficiency. Electrolyte abnormalities should be judiciously corrected, with the exception of hypocalcemia, the correction of which is somewhat controversial owing to the unclear contribution of hypercalcemia to the mechanism of pancreatitis. Hemodialysis may be necessary.

Nutritional support during the prolonged course of pancreatitis is thought to be helpful, although no specific benefit has been proven. Total parenteral nutrition (TPN) should be instituted early, although the long-term administration of TPN has risks such as line sepsis and opportunistic infections. Patients can be fed enterally if there is no paralytic ileus.

CONTROL OF PANCREATIC ENZYME SECRETION

Nasogastric suction, anticholinergic agents, H_2 receptor blockers, somatostatin, glucagon, and calcitonin do not effectively minimize pancreatic enzyme secretions, but nasogastric suction is still routinely used to decompress ileus and minimize vomiting.

LOCAL COMPLICATIONS OF NECROTIZING PANCREATITIS

Early hemodynamic stabilization may limit ongoing pancreatic injury and the development of local complications. When they do occur, complications such as intraabdominal hemorrhage, pancreatic necrosis, pancreatic abscess, and pseudocysts should be treated early and aggressively.

Intraabdominal hemorrhage may result in exsanguination and must therefore be treated aggressively. The development of retroperitoneal necrosis is associated with a high risk of morbidity and death. Peritoneal dialysis may lead to earlier improvement in some patients, although it has not been shown to decrease the likelihood of complications and death.

The presence of abdominal pain, leukocytosis, and fever several days to weeks after the onset of acute pancreatitis suggests the presence of pancreatic or peripancreatic necrosis. This may be confirmed by CT, which may show solid necrosis or liquefaction and abscess formation. However, it is difficult to know when the necrosis is of a mild degree and will resolve spontaneously and when it will inevitably progress to infection, sepsis, and death. The former, of course, requires supportive care and expectant management, while the latter requires early and aggressive resection and debridement. Needle aspiration may guide the intensivist and surgeon in their management. Because resection in the sterile situation may cause more harm than good, it is recommended to avoid surgery unless sepsis is confirmed, although sterile aspirates and a prolonged smoldering course may also require debridement.

Antibiotics should be administered to the patient with pancreatic necrosis with or without sepsis, although this therapy should not replace retroperitoneal debridement when necessary. Although evidence suggests improved survival in patients receiving early antibiotics, this is not without the complication of opportunistic infections.

The development of a connection from a ruptured pancreatic duct system to the lesser sac of the stomach or other abdominal organ results in a pseudocyst. Treatment is indicated when the pseudocyst grows quickly, becomes infected, bleeds, or ruptures. Percutaneous decompression may suffice in the enlarging or infected pseudocyst, but surgery is needed for hemorrhage and often for rupture, although the hemodynamically stable patient with pseudocyst rupture may be monitored expectantly. Waiting for the walls of a pseudocyst to mature before instituting drainage may be advisable if the patient remains stable.

For a more detailed discussion, see Chap. 81 in *Principles of Critical Care*, 2d ed.

Chapter 62

PRIORITIES IN MULTISYSTEM TRAUMA

JOHN P. KRESS

Mortality from multiple injuries follows a trimodal distribution. The *first peak* represents death occurring at the scene from injuries such as cardiac rupture or disruption of the major intrathoracic vessels and severe brain injury incompatible with life. Here, death usually occurs within minutes of the traumatic event. The *second peak* occurs from minutes to a few hours after trauma and is related to injuries that are immediately life-threatening, such as tension pneumothorax and cardiac tamponade. This is also a period during which appropriate resuscitative measures significantly affect outcome. The *third peak* occurs as a result of complications of the injury, such as sepsis or multiple system organ failure, and can be significantly affected by the type of intervention during the second phase.

The approach to multisystem trauma requires immediate identification of an experienced team leader, followed by identification and treatment of immediately life-threatening injuries. One must assure adequate oxygenation and perfusion. Early identification of findings needing immediate surgical treatment is imperative.

PRIORITIES

The order of priorities is a key feature for successful management of the multiply injured patient and should adhere to the following sequence:

1. Establishment of the airway, oxygenation, and ventilation with control of the cervical spine
2. Maintaining adequacy of perfusion
3. Providing hemorrhage control
4. Assessment and correction of neurologic abnormalities

763

5. Stabilization of fractures
6. Detailed systematic assessment and provision of definitive care

Steps 1 to 4 constitute the Advanced Trauma Life Support (ATLS) primary survey during which immediately life-threatening injuries are identified by adhering to the following sequence: A (airway), B (breathing), C (circulation and hemorrhage control), and D (neurologic disability). Adherence to this order of priorities allows assessment and resuscitation to occur simultaneously because injuries will be identified in the order in which they are likely to threaten the patient's life.

Airway, Oxygenation, Ventilation, and Control of the Cervical Spine

- Observe nares and mouth, listen for unobstructed passage of air.
- Airway obstruction? Causes: (1) loss of tone of the muscles supporting the tongue—treat with chin lift and jaw thrust, oral or nasal airway, (2) foreign material (including vomitus)—look for foreign objects in the oropharynx.
- If endotracheal intubation is necessary (not needed > 90 percent of the time), it should be performed promptly and expeditiously by the most experienced person. Avoid prolonged attempts (better to assure oxygenation and ventilation with a mask).
- Rarely, a surgical airway is needed. Cricothyroidotomy is preferred route because the cricothyroid membrane is superficial and avascular. Either large-bore (14-gauge) needle or a scalpel may be used. The landmarks are indicated in Fig. 62-1. Cricothyroidotomy allows 30 to 45 min of oxygenation without severe hypercapnea during which follow-up tracheostomy can be done.
- Always assume C spine instability: Use in-line immobilization to maintain neck in neutral position during airway manipulation. Full C spine x-ray (C1-T1) and/or computed tomography (CT) should be done to rule out unstable C spine. If there are clinical signs of spinal cord injury, assume that the C spine is abnormal.

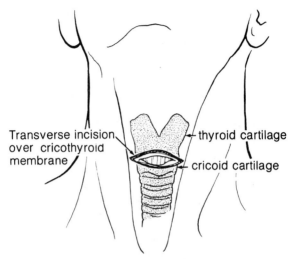

FIGURE 62-1 Landmarks for cricothyroidotomy.

- Assess adequacy of ventilation: (1) inspect patient for asymmetrical/paradoxical chest wall movement, and/or tracheal deviation and (2) auscultate and percuss chest for hyperresonance or dullness suggesting pneumothorax/ hemothorax; follow up with a chest x-ray. Suspicion of a tension pneumothorax requires immediate decompression without prior x-ray confirmation. Other thoracic injuries (cardiac tamponade, open pneumothorax, flail chest, ruptured thoracic aorta, massive hemothorax) should be evaluated with appropriate imaging studies if suspected clinically.

Adequacy of Perfusion

- Identify sources of major hemorrhage. Evaluate front and back sides of the patient, then cover to minimize heat loss/hypothermia. *Remember:* sympathetic discharge (vasoconstriction, tachycardia) may mask hypoperfusion, especially in the young. Sometimes massive blood loss may lead to vagally mediated bradycardia.

- Signs of hypoperfusion—weak pulses, cool, clammy skin color, delayed capillary refill. Tachycardia with cool extremities suggests hypoperfusion until proven otherwise. This is usually as a result of hemorrhage, although other causes of hypoperfusion (tension pneumothorax, cardiac tamponade, myocardial contusion, open pneumothorax, flail chest, and limb vascular injury) must be considered. Hemorrhage may be divided into classes I to IV (Table 62-1).

Hemorrhage Control

- Control the source of hemorrhage—direct pressure to visible bleeding sources without blind application of clamps or tourniquets.
- Venous assess—at least two large-bore (minimum 14- to 16-gauge) intravenous catheters. Vein selection priority: forearm, antecubital, saphenous, femoral, internal jugular, subclavian (chest x-ray to confirm central line placement). Use venous cutdown if necessary. After the patient is stabilized, replace unsterile central lines. Order a complete blood count, cross-matching of blood (4 to 10 U), coagulation, and toxicology screens. If normalization of blood pressure is not accomplished after ~50 mL/kg of crystalloid infusion, blood should be administered (un-cross-matched group O if necessary). Warm fluids and blood to avoid hypothermia.
- Once hemorrhage is controlled, the patient should be taken to the operating room, where visible bleeding can be definitively controlled.
- Covert bleeding sources include pelvic or extremity fractures, followed by the thorax or abdomen. The process of elimination usually determines the source of the hemorrhage. An intraabdominal bleeding source may require diagnostic peritoneal lavage, ultrasound/CT of the abdomen, and/or laparotomy for diagnosis. Covert blood loss may occur concomitantly with obvious sources.
- If massive fluid infusion does not restore hemodynamic stability, consider emergency thoracotomy, which allows

TABLE 62-1   Clinical Classification of Shock in a 70-kg Male[a]

	Class I	Class II	Class III	Class IV
Blood loss (mL)	Up to 750	750–1500	1500–2000	2000 or more
Blood loss (% blood volume)	Up to 15%	15–30%	30–40%	40% or more
Pulse rate	<100	>100 <120	>120 <140	140 or higher
Blood pressure	Normal	Normal	Decreased	Decreased
Pulse pressure (mmHg)	Normal or increased	Decreased	Decreased	Decreased
Capillary refill test	Normal	Decreased	Decreased	Decreased
Respiratory rate	14–20	20–30	30–40	>40
Urine output (mL/h)	30 or more	20–30	5–15	Negligible
CNS—mental status	Slightly anxious	Mildly anxious	Anxious and confused	Confused, lethargic
Fluid replacement	Crystalloid	Crystalloid	Crystalloid + blood	Crystalloid + blood

[a]3:1 Rule: Clinical signs in classes I and II are subtle, but diagnosis at this stage allows early fluid replacement before deeper levels of shock ensue. The 3:1 rule (estimated blood loss should be replaced by three times the volume of crystalloid) is a rough guideline, and the adequacy of perfusion of the patient is the true endpoint for determining adequacy of fluid resuscitation.

(1) identification and treatment of pericardial tamponade, (2) internal cardiac massage, (3) identification and control of intrathoracic hemorrhage, (4) cross-clamping of the thoracic aorta in order to maintain cerebral perfusion and coronary blood flow while decreasing bleeding from a subdiaphragmatic source, and (5) diagnosis and treatment of air embolism if present.

- Use vasoconstricting drugs (norepinephrine 5 $\mu g/min$) only after volume resuscitation or to temporarily stabilize the circulation during volume resuscitation; as soon as blood pressure and volume resuscitation are thought adequate, reduce the vasoconstricting drug dose to half to exclude persistent hypovolemia.

Neurologic Status

- A change in the level of consciousness is the hallmark of central nervous system (CNS) injury. A simple scale to define level of consciousness is as follows: (1) alert (A) level— patient responds appropriately to all commands and is completely oriented in all spheres, (2) V level— response to voice alone, (3) P level—responsiveness to pain, and (4) U level—unresponsiveness to stimuli. This simple grading of level of consciousness, in conjunction with the status of the pupils and any lateralizing signs, should be noted in the initial evaluation, and any change necessitates further investigation or surgical intervention if there is deterioration. More detailed assessments (e.g., Glasgow Coma Scale score) should be done after the primary survey.
- Brain hypoxia and hypoperfusion (often from uncorrected hypovolemia) commonly cause a depressed level of consciousness. Initial volume restriction to decrease intracranial pressure/cerebral edema is inappropriate in treating the hypovolemic head-injured patient.

Fracture Stabilization

- Fractures may appear dramatic but are not primarily life-threatening and are of lower priority.
- Early assessment of neurovascular integrity and the correction of any abnormality should be done to ensure limb

salvage and prevent rhabdomyolysis and compartment syndrome. Limb ischemia should initially be treated by reduction of the fracture and immobilization. Angiography is needed if reduction and immobilization do not restore perfusion. Keep limb ischemia under 4 to 6 h.

Detailed Systematic Assessment and Definitive Care

- Once the initial rapid assessment is complete, begin a more in-depth history and systematic, fully undressed physical exam. During this phase of the assessment, injuries that are likely to produce morbidity and require correction on a nonurgent basis are detected. Remember to examine the back, "log-rolling" the patient to protect the spine. Remember the rectal examination to assess the rectal integrity, identify blood in the gastrointestinal (GI) tract, detect extrarectal pelvic injury (bony as well as soft tissue—e.g., prostatic urethra) and assess sphincter tone, which may be abnormal in spinal cord injury.

- Consider x-rays of the thoracolumbar spine in unconscious patients or those with major torso trauma with or without neurologic deficit and those in whom the mechanism of injury suggests the possibility of spinal column injury. Until adequate radiologic assessment is complete, move patient by log-rolling only.

- Place nasogastric tube (*oro*gastric if basilar skull fracture is not ruled out) to decompress the stomach and monitor for evidence of upper GI hemorrhage.

- Place transurethral catheter for monitoring urine output unless contraindicated by the presence of a urethral injury (pelvic fracture, perineal/scrotal ecchymosis, bleeding through the urethral meatus, high-riding boggy prostate on rectal examination). If these signs are present, a urethrogram should be performed first.

- Reduce and stabilize uncomplicated fractures.

- Assess tetanus immunization status and give appropriate prophylaxis.

- At this point, consult subspecialities such as plastic surgery and otolaryngology if needed.

Repeated examination is important to detect and treat injuries that are not initially obvious. Stable patients involved in collisions with an associated fatality should be monitored carefully in an ICU setting, since it must be assumed that they have been exposed to the same force and energy transfer as the dead patient. Such patients may have temporarily contained hematomas of the spleen, liver, or retroperitoneum or around major vascular structures and can decompensate abruptly with sudden spontaneous hemorrhage. Slowly progressive tachycardia, hypotension, fall in hemoglobin, or worsening of abdominal findings (increasing pain or peritoneal signs) warrant aggressive investigation. Such patients should have 4 to 6 U of blood available at all times during their early hospital course. Respiratory deterioration may also be a sign of diaphragmatic rupture.

For a more detailed discussion, see Chap. 88 in *Principles of Critical Care,* 2d ed.

Chapter 63

TORSO TRAUMA

IVOR S. DOUGLAS

Torso Trauma

Consideration of chest and abdominal trauma as a single entity facilitates rational treatment strategies. Respiratory variation of diaphragmatic position implies substantial phase-dependent variation in the demarcation of the thoracic and abdominal cavities. Variable trajectories of blunt or sharp objects or forces make it virtually impossible to predict the extent and location of underlying injury based solely on the point of penetration. Two broad classifications of torso trauma are outlined in Table 63-1.

Integrative approaches to initial trauma management frequently require definitive control of intrathoracic or intraabdominal sources of hemorrhage as part of primary resuscitative measures. If the initial surgical intervention is to perform laparotomy and careful exploration suggests a potential intrathoracic source of bleeding, prompt and judicious reevaluation is required.

NECK INJURIES

Penetrating injuries to the root of the neck may injure vascular structures (resulting in hemorrhage or ischemia), the thoracic duct (resulting in chylothorax or pneumothorax), and the lung apex. Mandatory surgical exploration should be preceded by plain x-ray to determine depth of penetration, soft

TABLE 63-1   Classification of Torso Trauma

Blunt vs. penetrating trauma
Cardiorespiratory and hemodynamically unstable (immediate intervention) vs. stable

---

tissue air and hematoma, and airway deviation. Additionally, chest x-ray to exclude pneumothorax should be performed. Angiography is indicated for injuries between the angle of the mandible and the skull base (zone III), whereas this modality is more controversial for zone II injuries. The latter injuries, between the cricoid and the mandible, are effectively evaluated by surgical exploration. Additional modalities of endoscopy, contrast radiography, computed tomography (CT) and magnetic resonance imaging (MRI) assist in this evaluation. To avoid dislodgment of a clot due to excessive coughing, a nasogastric tube should be inserted only after endotracheal intubation. The thorax should be prepared and draped in the event that thoracic exploration becomes necessary during the neck exploration. Median sternotomy is preferred for optimal exploration.

Thoracic Injuries

IMMEDIATE INTERVENTION GROUP

Immediate resuscitative management is aimed at restoring an adequate circulating volume and correcting hypoxemia. These aims are accomplished by rapidly establishing airway patency and providing supplemental oxygenation and ventilation, large-bore high-flow vascular access, chest decompression to evacuate fluids and air, and pericardiocentesis. Tension and open pneumothorax, massive hemo- or pneumothorax, flail chest, traumatic air embolism, and aortic rupture require prompt stabilization and characterization. An approach to the diagnosis and management of these major traumas is presented in Table 63-2. Operating room facilities should be prepared while immediate resuscitative and emergency therapeutic interventions are performed. In the case of massive thoracic hemorrhage with an apparent inframammary right thoracic injury site, an upper midline laparotomy is indicated to manage liver lacerations with transdiaphragmatic penetration. Right anterolateral thoracotomy to repair lacerated intercostal arteries is indicated if the initial laparotomy is unrevealing.

Other surgical interventions are described in Table 63-2 and at the end of this chapter.

TABLE 63-2 Diagnosis and Management of Traumatic Torso Injuries Requiring Immediate Intervention

Definition	Pathophysiology	Clinical Diagnosis and Investigations	Emergent Therapy	Definitive Therapy
Tension pneumothorax Intrathoracic leak and air trapping in pleural space from one-way valve phenomenon.	Ipsilateral lung collapse, mediastinal shift to the contralateral thoracic cavity and kinking of major vessels → lethal compromise of venous return and gas exchange.	Hyperresonant chest, tracheal shift, tachypnea, dyspnea, ↓ breath sounds ↓ BP	Angiocath or scalpel: second intercostal space (IC) midclavicular line or fourth/fifth IC space anterior to midaxillary line.	• Intercostal chest tube drainage.[a] • Underwater seal.
Open pneumothorax Free pleural-cutaneous communication. Progressive lung collapse.	Similar to tension PTX. Lung collapse, mediastinal shift, and hemodynamic compromise.	As for tension + visible wound, audible sucking.	Supportive intubation and positive-pressure ventilation. Occlusive gauze dressing with three-side taping. ICD drain insertion through separate incision.	• Surgical debridement and closure.
Massive pneumothorax Large airway laceration with persistent PTX despite drainage.	Tracheobronchiopleural air leak and hemorrhage.	Persistent PTX despite large-bore ICD. Massive subcutaneous emphysema. Hypoxia and respiratory distress. • Confirm ICD functional.	Bronchoscopy— evaluate level of injury; selective bronchial intubation or balloon tamponade.	Thoracotomy • Direct repair. • Lung resection.

773

(Continued)

TABLE 63-2 Diagnosis and Management of Traumatic Torso Injuries Requiring Immediate Intervention (*Cont.*)

Definition	Pathophysiology	Clinical Diagnosis and Investigations	Emergent Therapy	Definitive Therapy
Massive hemothorax Major central vascular injury or intercostal artery laceration. (Aortic rupture—usually immediately fatal.)	Profound hypovolemic shock. Hypoxemia—lung collapse and $\dot{V}/\dot{Q}$ mismatch. Low-pressure pulmonary vessels usually stop bleeding with lung reexpansion.	$\downarrow$ BP; $\uparrow$ HR Percussion dullness Mediastinal shift to contralateral side. $\downarrow$ Neck veins ($\uparrow$ if blood causes mechanical obstruction to venous inflow).	Large-bore intercostal chest tube drain—1000–2000 mL.	Thoracotomy if ICD drainage > 100 mL/h and patient unstable. • Lung suture; lobectomy or pneumonectomy. • Rarely, aortic clamping and graft prosthesis.
Cardiac tamponade Intrapericardial fluid (and air) compromising cardiac function.	Reduced transmural filling pressure results in impaired right (and left) ventricular diastolic filling. Reduced cardiac output.	*Beck triad*: hypotension, jugulovenous distention; muffled heart sounds. Pulsus paradoxus > 10 mmHg • Exclude tension PTX – ? Needle aspiration. • Subxiphoid ultrasound.	Pericardiocentesis[a]—nonclotted blood.	Thoracotomy. • Repair cardiac and coronary artery laceration. • Deferred heart-lung bypass for formal coronary repair.

Traumatic air embolism Acute neurologic deficit after chest injury, after onset of positive-pressure ventilation.	Air-bubble absorption into negative pressure pulmonary venous circuit or ruptured aortic arch. Systemic venous embolism with patent foramen ovale. Cerebral embolization.	Acute focal or global neurologic deficit. Retinal arterial air bubbles. • Bubble in radial arterial blood. **High index of Suspicion.**	100% $F_{I_{O_2}}$ Immediate surgery. Thoracotomy. • Venting of intravascular air. • Lung suture, lobectomy, or pneumonectomy.
Flail chest Paradoxical chest wall movement with free-floating, discontinuous chest wall segment.	Multiple adjacent, bilateral rib fractures or two fractures on each of several adjacent, unilateral ribs. Hypoxemia and shock result from dyskinetic (flail) segment, underlying lung contusion, and pain.	Paradoxical flail movement on spontaneous ventilation (in with inspiration instead of out). Posterior injury, muscle spasm, and IPPV masks flail chest. • Chest x-ray—multiple, adjacent rib fractures.	Ipsi- or bilateral IC tube drainage. If ↓↓ Pa_{O_2}, intubate and IPPV; If stable, IV or epidural opiate analgesia. Surgical stabilization is controversial and rarely indicated. Liberation from IPPV *not* dependent on stabilizing of flail.

ABBREVIATIONS: PTX, pneumothorax; ICD, intercostal chest drain; IPPV, intubation and positive-pressure ventilation.
*Procedure detailed at end of chapter.

URGENT INTERVENTION GROUP—
STABLE PATIENTS

Table 63-3 describes the diagnosis and management of the second category of thoracic injuries. These are usually not immediately life-threatening but need urgent intervention to prevent further compromise and avert catastrophic complications.

Abdominal Trauma

GENERAL PRINCIPLES

In hemodynamically compromised patients with torso trauma, an abdominal source of blood loss is presumed if functional chest tubes demonstrate no free pleural blood or continued major air leakage. Thus rapid triage decisions about possible thoracic lesions can be made with chest x-ray and chest tube insertion. In the absence of pericardial tamponade or traumatic air embolism, laparotomy is indicated.

Features of abdominal penetration (by digital exploration), perforation (pain, tenderness, guarding, and rigidity), or hemorrhage (peritoneal irritation, shoulder tip pain, hypotension) are sought. Absolute indications for celiotomy are hemodynamic instability, major vascular injury (including devascularized solid organs), evisceration, peritoneal signs, pneumoperitoneum, evidence of diaphragmatic injury, neurologic injury with cord compromise, significant intraperitoneal blood (i.e., positive diagnostic peritoneal lavage (DPL), and evidence of hollow viscus perforation. Classic distributions of abdominal pain—epigastric/periumbilical (midgut), pelvic/iliac fossae (hindgut), boring midepigastric (foregut/pancreatic), and intrascapular pain (diaphragmatic peritoneal irritation)—assist somewhat in localizing pathology, Tympany—particularly loss of hepatic dullness—suggests hollow viscus injury, e.g., gastric distention from esophageal intubation or Ambubag. Percussion dullness suggests intraabdominal fluid or blood. Absent or hypoactive bowel sounds may imply mesenteric injury or a retroperitoneal process.

Knives, high- and low-velocity projectiles, and other implements result in differing patterns of penetrating abdominal

TABLE 63-3 Diagnosis and Management of Traumatic Torso Injuries Requiring Urgent Intervention

Definition	Pathophysiology	Clinical Diagnosis and Investigations	Emergent Therapy	Definitive Therapy
Lung contusion Localized lung hemorrhage extending to complete obliteration of lung.	Progressive hypoxemia with intrapulmonary shunt. Associated with flail segment.	Chest x-ray initially unremarkable. Consolidation apparent with hemorrhage and volume replacement.	Close monitoring, O_2 supplementation. *No fluid restriction;* Intubation and ventilation if severe hypoxemia or associated torso/ CNS injuries.	Thoracotomy only for management of associated massive hemo-pneumothorax.
Myocardial contusion Frequently subclinical; Chest pain, dysrhythmias.	Blunt sternum trauma (steering-wheel injury). Myocardial bruising, hemorrhage, rarely coronary artery injury or dissection.	Cardiac enzyme leak (CK and troponin T or I), echo-cardiographic wall motion abnormality. ECG changes; atrial or ventricular dysrhythmias, MI changes.	Management as for myocardial infarction. Emphasis on monitoring, O_2 and analgesia.	Inotropes. ? Angiography and coronary stenting for coronary dissection.

(Continued)

777

TABLE 63-3 Diagnosis and Management of Traumatic Torso Injuries Requiring Urgent Intervention (*Cont.*)

Definition	Pathophysiology	Clinical Diagnosis and Investigations	Emergent Therapy	Definitive Therapy
Aortic rupture Usually lethal at initial injury. Contained rupture may be silent.	Acceleration, deceleration, shear force injury at the ligamentum arteriosum (junction between fixed and mobile portions of thoracic aorta). Rupture contained by adventitial layer.	Thoracic bruit, arm:leg or left:right BP differences. • Chest x-ray: mediastinal widening, first/second rib fractures, pleural cap, left bronchus depression. • Transesophageal echo, CT/MRI; aortography definitive.	Prompt diagnosis. Cardiopulmonary resuscitation.	Thoracotomy. • Prosthetic graft.
Esophageal disruption Esophageal tear with leakage of gastric contents and air into the mediastinum.	Iatrogenic postendoscopy or instrumentation. Blunt abdominal trauma against closed glottis. Mediastinitis and hemopneumothorax.	Severe retrosternal pain. $\downarrow$ BP; $\uparrow$ HR. Clinical features of hemopneumothorax. • Chest x-ray: hemopneumothorax without rib fracture, mediastinal air. • $\downarrow$ pH; $\uparrow$ amylase; particulate pleural fluid. • Gastrograffin swallow/endoscopy.	Massive crystalloid volume infusion. Broad-spectrum antibiotics.	Thoracotomy. • Esophageal repair or diversion (if delayed).

778

Condition			
Diaphragm rupture Penetrating or blunt perforation with viscus herniation. Frequently silent.	Most frequently left-sided. Blunt trauma causes large, irregular lacerations with viscus herniation.	Frequently misinterpreted on chest x-ray as elevated left hemidiaphragm, gastric dilation, pneumothorax. NG tube position or peritoneal lavage fluid drainage through ICD.	*Early* laparotomy. • Allows exploration, hernia reduction, spleen and diaphragm repair. *Delayed* thoracotomy.
Rib fractures Localized chest wall and pleuritic pain.	Localized, direct blunt thoracic trauma. Minimal trauma in elderly or those with pathologic bone disease.	Localized chest pain. Crepitus, clicking on auscultation. Chest x-ray—exclude PTX. Bone scan.	Analgesia including regional blocks. Monitor ventilation.
Simple hemo-pneumothorax	See Table 63-2.	See Table 63-2. Usually no cardiovascular or ventilatory compromise.	Intercostal chest tube drainage.[a]

[a]Procedure detailed at end of chapter.

779

injuries. Only one-third of stab wounds penetrate the peritoneum while only half of intraperitoneal penetrating wounds require surgical intervention. More extensive soft tissue and organ injury is associated with gunshot wounds. Unlike stab wounds, 85 percent of abdominal wall gunshot wounds penetrate the abdominal cavity and 95 percent require a surgical procedure for correction. This results from direct obliteration of tissue in the direct path of the missile: missile fragmentation and shrapnel release *and* transient cavitation of surrounding soft, vascular and visceral tissues. That is, the missile's enormous kinetic energy is transferred into the tissues. Thus substantial injury is seen in tissues not directly in the bullet's path.

Intraperitoneal hemorrhage results in peritoneal signs and dysautonomic symptoms. Peritoneal and/or retroperitoneal hemorrhage and leakage of endoluminal fluids (chyme, bile, etc.) occurs from lacerated organs. Hemorrhage causes retroperitoneal nerve irritation and results in poorly defined and localized somatic pain. Penetrating foreign objects should not be removed in uncontrolled circumstances (e.g., outside the operating room), as this may precipitate massive hemorrhage from tamponaded vessels. To prevent further compromise, eviscerated abdominal organs should be secured with saline-moistened sterile gauze and taped prior to surgical cleaning.

Initial digital examination, diagnostic peritoneal lavage, and immediate ultrasound or CT scanning combine to assist in determining the need for laparotomy, particularly if clinical features are equivocal. CT scanning provides the most diagnostic utility but is costly and potentially destabilizing for critically compromised patients. The utility of DPL is reviewed in Table 63-4. Open, semiclosed and closed techniques are reviewed at the end of this chapter. Ultrasound is highly sensitive and specific for detecting free intraperitoneal fluid. It substantially enhances the utility of DPL. Preoperative antibiotics covering aerobic and anaerobic organisms must be commenced prior to skin incision and should be continued beyond 24 h if there is peritoneal fecal contamination. An upper midline incision provides optimal exposure and allows for extension into the thorax.

Details of abdominal organ injuries are described in Table 63-5. Of note is that multiple concomitant injuries are frequently encountered, particularly as a result of blunt trauma

TABLE 63-4 Utility of Diagnostic Peritoneal Lavage

Indications	Contraindications
1 Equivocal abdominal findings: e.g., rib, pelvic, or lumbar spine fractures frequently manifest with signs confused with intraabdominal pathology.	1. *Absolute:* Predetermined indication for laparotomy.
2. Masked abdominal signs: e.g., postintoxication or head injury.	2. *Relative:* Previous abdominal surgery (with adhesions); morbid obesity, coagulopathy, pregnancy (closed technique contraindicated).
3. Predicted prolonged intervals between sequential evaluations (e.g., orthopedic surgery).	
4. Severe extremity injury with concomitant abdominal trauma—to rule out intraabdominal source of blood loss.	

TABLE 63-5 Diagnosis and Management of Abdominopelvic Organ Injuries

Definition	Clinical Diagnosis	Investigations	Surgical Management
Stomach injuries	Epigastric and shoulder-tip pain (free perforation).	KUB: subdiaphragmatic free air Bloody NG aspirate.	• Complete gastric mobilization, debridement, and primary suture/anastamosis.
Duodenal injuries, usually second portion.	Frequently missed. Projectile vomiting with gastric outlet obstruction. Associated with other injuries of the upper abdomen.	AXR: Retroperitoneal free air.	• Isolated hematoma—conservative management. • Associated with other injuries—visualization of entire lesser sac/duodenum. Debridement with serosal patch, anastamosis or Roux-en-Y with duodenostomy.
Pancreatic injuries, blunt trauma.	Retroperitoneal—late peritoneal signs. Incidental at laparotomy or boring abdominal pain. Associated with high mortality and morbidity - (post injury pseudocysts).	Increasing amylase/lipase DPL[a]—frequently negative. Contrast upper GI series or abdominal CT.	• Simple contusion (no duct injury)—debridement and oversew. • Distal duct injury—enteroanastamosis. • Pancreaticoduodenal injury—conservative drainage initially. May require Whipple procedure or diverticulization procedure.

782

Intestinal injuries, ↑ postsurgical sepsis.	• Acceleration-deceleration injuries—fixed points (ligament of Treitz). • Blowout injuries anywhere. Abdominal contusions and features of peritonitis.	DPL,[a] US, CT	• Small bowel: Debridement, suture hemostasis and resection of devitalized tissues. • Large bowel: first degree anastomosis if early and minimal fecal soiling. Otherwise left colonic lesions—colostomy (± mucous fistula) and peritoneal irrigation. Rectal injury—proximal defunctioning colostomy.
Liver injuries, ↑ morbidity from blunt injury	Lower thoracic/upper abdominal contusions; rib fracture and ↑ hemidiaphragm. Signs of intraabdominal hemorrhage. Often seen only at surgery.	Positive DPL,[a] US, or CT features. Postop systemic inflammatory response syndrome is common. ↑ White count/bilirubin implies sepsis.	Surgical objectives: • *Control hemorrhage:* Initial packing and correct coagulopathy. Portal triad cross-clamping plus oversew, caval isolation, hepatic artery ligation. • *Resection of devitalized tissue.* • *Drainage of blood, bile, and tissue fluid* (T-tube drainage for biliary injury).
Spleen injuries	Left-upper-quadrant pain with rib fractures/contusions ± shoulder-tip pain. Hypovolemic shock and tense abdomen.	Positive DPL,[a] US, or CT features.	Surgical objectives after mobilization: • *Control hemorrhage:* Packing superficial—coagulation, fibrin glue, suture; Deep-short gastric vessel ligation, Dexon mesh compression. • *Splenic salvage:* Partial resection with pledget sutures. Splenectomy: postop Pneumovax.

TABLE 63-5 Diagnosis and Management of Abdominopelvic Organ Injuries (*Continued*)

Definition	Clinical Diagnosis	Investigations	Surgical Management
Biliary injuries, infrequent.	Usually asymptomatic. Hemobilia secondary to hepatobiliary injury.	Intraoperative—cholangiogram/ERCP. Postop cholangitis—bile Gram stain and antibiotic coverage.	Gallbladder—cholecystectomy. Extrahepatic bile duct anastamosis with T-tube drainage; choledoco- or cholecystoenterostomy.
Retroperitoneal hemorrhage	Hemodynamic instability in presence of pelvic fracture. Renal or pancreatic injury.	Pelvic x-ray, preop IVP, abdominopelvic CT.	Pelvic fracture: External fixation; no exploration. Angiography and embolization for persistent bleeding. Nonpelvic hematomas: • Nonpulsatile/expansile—no exploration. IVP and CT. • Pulsatile/expansile—surgical exploration with aortic cross clamp. Massive hemorrhage—peritoneal packing; correct coagulopathy; look again at 48 h.

| Genitourinary injuries | Hematuria—90–95%. Urethral meatus blood. Scrotal hematoma. Shock. 15% are major lacerations. Mortality from associated injuries. Blunt trauma—90% of injuries. Penetrating trauma—40% are major injuries. | Immediate US. Selective use of IVP, CT, pyelography.
• Micro/macrohematuria and shock.
• Hematuria with major abdominal injury.
• Possible penetrating renal injury even without hematuria.
• (Relative—one-shot IVP in unstable patient for possible nephrectomy).
Cystography/cystoscopy/ urethrography. | Goals: minimize morbidity; preserve renal function. Retroperitoneal approach—partial or complete nephrectomy, drainage.
• Most low-grade injuries can be treated conservatively.
• *Absolute indications for surgery:* Vascular (renal pedicle) injury. Shattered kidney. Expanding or pulsatile hematoma. Shocked polytrauma patient.
• *Relative indications for surgery:* Repair collecting system. Close capsule or use omental graft. Retroperitoneal drainage surgery only if patient is unstable despite aggressive volume resuscitation. |

ABBREVIATIONS: KUB, x-ray of kidneys, ureter, and bladder; NG, nasogastric; AXR, abdominal x-ray; DPL, diagnostic peritoneal lavage; US, ultrasound; CT, computed tomography; ERCP, endoscopic retrograde cholangiopancreatography; IVP, intravenous pyelogram.
^aProcedure detailed at the end of this chapter.

or high-velocity missile injuries. At laparotomy, the presence of dark blood may suggest liver injury, while bright red blood suggests arterial laceration. Rapid evisceration and packing assists in defining hemorrhage points. Lesions are approached in order of severity as opposed to the order in which they are encountered; brisk bleeding is staunched before closure of a small bowel laceration.

Radiologically guided percutaneous drainage is the most efficient management for localized postsurgical intraabdominal collections, pseudocysts, and abscesses. Rarely second-look laparotomy is required. Peritoneal soiling generally mandates open surgical wound packing to allow for healing by secondary intent. Wound-related sepsis is common.

ABDOMINAL COMPARTMENT SYNDROME

Massive visceral and/or vascular injury, aggressive volume resuscitation, mucosal leak, and ascites may result in vastly increased intraabdominal pressures, creating intraabdominal hypertension (IAH). IAH causes diaphragm shift, increasing peak airway pressures during mechanical ventilation and decreasing tidal volumes, compressing the inferior vena cava and renal veins, leading to decreased venous return and decreased renal and mesenteric perfusion. Tremendous tension along an abdominal wall repair may result. Monitoring of transvesical pressure through a Foley catheter placed in the urinary bladder attached to a pressure transducer allows for continuous assessment of IAH. Bladder pressure exceeding 30 mmHg indicates a need for reexploration for IAH when accompanied by the appropriate clinical signs and symptoms. However, a trend of increasing bladder pressures may be even more important. Temporary abdominal wall closures and leaving fascia open after exploration is an option, allowing for easy reexploration and control of IAH.

PROCEDURES

Diagnostic Peritoneal Lavage (DPL)

DPL may be performed via an infraumbilical or supraumbilical approach. The latter is used in pregnancy or when there has been a prior low-midline operation. After bladder and stomach catheter decompression, the insertion site is surgically prepared and anesthetized. A dialysis catheter is inserted by open, semiclosed, or closed techniques.

Open DPL

After skin incision, visualization and incision of the fascia, the parietal peritoneum is grasped and secured with a purse-string suture. Through this an incision is made and the dialysis catheter inserted toward the pelvis. In the semiclosed technique, the visualized fascia is punctured with a trochar needle and the procedure performed as per the closed technique.

Closed DPL

The skin is punctured and a guidewire introduced through a trochar needle. A dialysis catheter is then introduced by the Seldinger technique over the wire. Bowel penetration is excluded by gentle aspiration.

Once the catheter is secured and hemostasis diligently assured, initial aspiration is performed. Gross blood requires exploration, and the procedure is terminated with the catheter being withdrawn. If negative for blood, 10 mL/kg warm Ringer's lactate solution is infused rapidly, allowed to distribute for 5 min and then gravity-siphoned back out by placing the IV bag on the floor. Recovered fluid is analyzed for total and differential cell count, Gram stain, bilirubin, and amylase. Positive results (Table 63-6) are highly sensitive for major viscus injury. Since early postinjury DPL in relatively stable patients may not allow enough time for the white blood cell response to be mounted, low initial counts may not exclude viscus injury. Repeat lavage is indicated.

TABLE 63-6   Positive DPL Results

---

1. > 5 mL gross blood/enteric content
2. Nontranslucent (cannot read newsprint through tube)
3. Microscopy: $> 10^5$ red cells/microliter;
   > 500 white cells/microliter;
   bacteria or food fiber on Gram stain.

Pericardiocentesis

Urgent pericardiocentesis is indicated in cases of life-threatening tamponade. A long (6-in.) 16- or 18-gauge needle is attached to an empty 50-mL syringe and inserted below the xiphoid process at a 45-degree angle aimed cephalad toward the tip of the left scapula. An electrocardiographic lead is attached to the hub end of the needle and monitored for electrocardiographic evidence of myocardial injury. If the syringe is filled with clotting blood and the patient fails to improve hemodynamically, the myocardium may have been punctured, which could require operative repair. When tamponade is not immediately life-threatening, the pericardium should be drained with a pericardiostomy tube in the operating room.

Tube Thoracostomy

Ideally, the patient is positioned supine, with the arm on affected side draped up and over the head. The entire side of the chest is surgically prepped and draped.

1. If possible, give single dose of cefazolin 1 g IV before tube insertion.
2. Infiltrate 1 percent lidocaine into a large area of skin, soft tissue, and muscle around the fifth or sixth intercostal space in the midaxillary line. Infiltrate into the periosteum of the superior edge of the sixth or seventh rib. Important anatomic landmarks to remember are that intercostal arteries/nerves run beneath ribs; the spleen and liver lie well within the rib cage.
3. Make a 2-in. incision with a #10 or #11 blade scalpel through the skin and spread subcutaneous tissue with a clamp.
4. Slide the clamp down over the superior margin of the rib, pop through into the chest, and spread the clamp widely. In the case of tension pneumothorax, this is accompanied by a rush of air. Always place a gloved finger into the incision and feel the lung/pleura to be sure you are in the chest and not the subcutaneous tissues, liver, spleen, or peritoneum.

5. Cross-clamp the distal end of the chest tube. Grab the distal tip (Fig. 63-1) with a second clamp and slide it into the chest, directing it superiorly and posteriorly toward the apex of the chest. Ensure that all the holes on the tube are within the chest.

6. The skin incision is surrounded by a purse-string 3-0 silk suture.

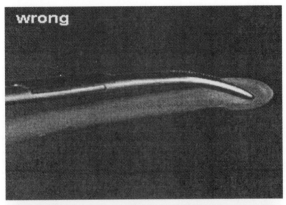

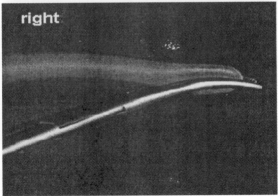

FIGURE 63-1 Correct clamp position for insertion of tube thoracostomy.

TABLE 63-7   Complications of Intercostal Tube Thoracostomy

---

1. Intercostal nerve/artery injury, splenic/hepatic injury, lung injury, and subcutaneous/abdominal injury.
2. Inadequate drainage from massive bleeding or major bronchus rupture: indicates second tube or emergent surgery.
3. Local wound sepsis or empyema—unusual.

---

7. Connect to underwater drainage system (Pleurovac) and only then release the distal clamp. A negative suction pump can be placed in line.
8. The purse string is drawn closed and tied tightly to the length of the tube. Two loosely tied vertical mattress sutures for later closing may be inserted on either side of the tube. Fix the tube onto the skin with gauze and a two-way helix of adhesive tape.
9. Chest x-ray for placement and lung reexpansion are mandatory postplacement.
10. The patient must cough vigorously while sitting up, as well as lying on his or her back and sides. This is important for early reexpansion of the lung and drainage of the free blood before coagulation occurs.

For patients on positive-pressure ventilatory support, the tube is often left in place until weaning can be accomplished. At times, more than one tube may be required, especially for patients with bullous disease or iatrogenic pneumothorax or in those with substantial volutrauma on ventilatory support. Complications of the procedure are reviewed in Table 63-7.

For a more detailed discussion, see Chap. 91 in *Principles of Critical Care,* 2d ed.

Chapter 64

HEAD INJURY AND INTRACRANIAL HYPERTENSION

STEVEN BAKER

Epidemiology

The annual incidence of traumatic brain injury in the United States has been estimated at 180 to 400 per 100,000. A bimodal age distribution is evident, with the highest peak incidence occurring between ages 15 and 24, and a secondary peak after age 70. Males are three times more likely than females to incur traumatic brain injury.

Deaths attributable to brain injury occur at a rate of 16 to 18 per 100,000. Motor vehicle accidents (57 percent), firearms (14 percent), and falls (12 percent) accounted for most fatalities in the 1980s; firearms have eclipsed motor vehicle accidents in many urban areas as the leading cause of traumatic brain injury.

Pathophysiology

Primary brain injury may occur with closed or with penetrating head trauma. Closed head trauma manifest by brief loss of consciousness and no apparent sequelae is termed a *concussion*. Hemorrhagic cortical contusion is the result of deceleration of the brain against the inner bony skull, occurs most often in the frontal and temporal lobes, and may result in delayed mass effect and intracranial hypertension if significant. Blunt trauma may result in linear, comminuted, depressed, or basilar skull fractures. Associated disruption of meninges and meningeal vessels can result in cerebrospinal fluid (CSF) leaks (rhinorrhea with frontal fractures; otorrhea

TABLE 64-1 Causes of Secondary Brain Injury

Hypoxia
  Hypoventilation
  Pulmonary shunt physiology (neurogenic
    pulmonary edema,
    aspiration of gastric contents)
  Systemic hypotension: infection, iatrogenic overdiuresis, diabetes
    insipidus, GI hemorrhage
  Regional hypoperfusion: intracranial blood; hypoosmolar edema
    (excessive volume resuscitation, SIADH); impaired venous
    drainage (neck kinked, excessive PEEP)
  Hypercatabolism (post-injury response, fever)
Infection
  Meningeal compromise, iatrogenic (device-related)
Coagulopathy
  DIC → recurrent bleeding, arteriolar thrombosis

ABBREVIATIONS: SIADH, syndrome of inappropriate antidiuretic hormone; PEEP, positive end-expiratory pressure; DIC, disseminated intravascular coagulation.

with petrous bone fractures), contiguous infection, or subarachnoid hemorrhage. Penetrating injury disrupts the scalp, skull, and meninges, allowing ingress of microorganisms.

    Secondary brain injury is caused by pathophysiologic processes set in motion by either the primary injury or by associated trauma to other organs (Table 64-1).

INTRACRANIAL PRESSURE—CONCEPTS

Intracranial volume includes brain (80 percent), CSF (10 percent), and blood (10 percent). Pathologic states that increase the volume of one compartment necessitate a compensatory decrease in the volume of another to maintain normal intracranial pressure (ICP) (Monro-Kellie hypothesis). The compliance curve in Fig. 64-1 illustrates intracranial pressure-volume relationships. Increases in intracranial volume have little effect on ICP initially; at a critical volume, compliance sharply worsens, such that even relatively small increases in volume result in large increases in ICP. The shape of the compliance curve is determined by a number of factors, including the location of the mass lesion, systemic mean arterial pressure (MAP), and Pa_{CO_2}.

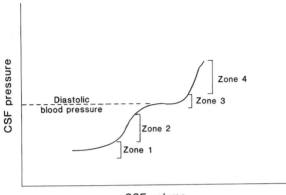

FIGURE 64-1   Relationship of CSF volume to CSF pressure. Initial increases in volume do not increase pressure greatly since compression of the venous system provides a "protective" factor preventing intracranial hypertension (zone 1). When this mechanism is no longer operative, further increases in CSF volume cause large increases in pressure (zone 2), until pressure rises above diastolic blood pressure. Further pressure rises are somewhat blunted by diminished arterial flow and blood volume (zone 3). Finally, as all vascular compartments have been maximally compressed, further increases in CSF volume cause very large increases in pressure (zone 4).

Cerebral blood flow (CBF) is constant at around 50 mL/100 g brain tissue as long as cerebral autoregulation of blood flow is maintained. Figure 64-2 illustrates the fact that autoregulation is normally intact at MAPs between 50 and 150 torr and Pa_{O_2}s between 50 and 150 torr. CBF is most sensitive to Pa_{CO_2}, varying almost directly at physiologic values. When ICP is normal, increases in CBF do not result in an increase in ICP because intracranial compliance is high.

Cerebral perfusion pressure (CPP) is determined by mean arterial pressure and intracranial pressure (CPP = MAP − ICP). Increases in ICP or decreases in MAP may result in a CPP at which autoregulation fails, CBF falls, and brain hypoxia worsens. This relationship becomes more complex in an injured noncompliant brain, when rapid increases in MAP

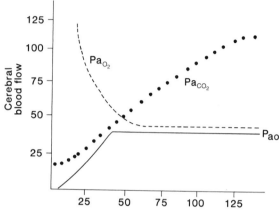

FIGURE 64-2   The relationship of CBF to Pa_{O_2}, Pa_{CO_2}, and mean aortic pressure (P_{ao}). Note that CBF rises sharply as Pa_{O_2} falls below 60 mmHg, a point at which small decrements in Pa_{O_2} are associated with large decreases in hemoglobin saturation and arterial oxygen content, due to the steep shape of the oxygen-hemoglobin dissociation curve. Note that decreases of Pa_{CO_2} from 40 to 20 to 25 mmHg are associated with an approximately 50 percent decrease in CBF. Finally, CBF remains constant over a wide range of P_{ao}, a phenomenon attributed to vascular autoregulation.

lead to increased cerebral blood volume and sharp increases in ICP. Autoregulation of CBF in the injured brain probably requires a global CPP of 70 mmHg, acknowledging that focal areas of injury/swelling have lower CPPs. Sustained ICPs of 20 to 25 mmHg indicate the loss of intracranial compliance (Fig. 64-1) and require therapy (Table 64-2).

Diagnosis

The mechanism of injury and change in level of consciousness since the injury are the two essential components of the history. Physical examination is used to gauge the level of consciousness, most commonly according to Glasgow Coma Scale criteria (Table 64-3), and to identify focal findings suggestive of the site and severity of injury. GCS scores of 8 or less constitute coma and account for most morbidity and mor-

TABLE 64-2   Medical Management of Increased Intracranial Pressure

---

Sustained ↑ICP (20–25 mmHg for 5–10 min)
↓
Ensure unimpeded jugular venous return (HOB at 30°, neck neutral)
Ensure adequate ventilation

↓ (continued elevation)
CT brain
(no surgically treatable cause)
↓
Moderate hyperventilation (P_{CO_2} 30–34 mmHg), avoiding excessive mean airway pressure
Sedation (morphine sulfate)
Antipyretic therapy if febrile

(continued elevation)
↓
Neuromuscular blockade

(continued elevation)
↓
Mannitol (0.5–1.0 g/kg as 20% solution, q2–6h, with volume replacement to maintain normovolemia)
Intermittent CSF drainage (ventricular drain required)
(continued elevation)
↓
Pentobarbital (10 mg/kg bolus over 30 min, then 1–3 mg/kg per hour, monitoring cardiac output and arterial pressure)

HOB = head of bed.

tality (Table 64-4). The four common ocular brainstem reflexes (pupillary light reflex, corneal reflex, oculocaloric reflex, and oculocephalic reflex) are used to assess brainstem function. Signs of associated skull fracture may be present. Physical signs of increased intracranial pressure are unreliable, but progressive drowsiness (as cerebral perfusion pressure falls) or rising blood pressure with falling heart rate (the Cushing response) are cause for concern when present. Computed tomography (CT) is essential to exclude intracranial hematomas, foreign bodies, occult skull fracture, and other

TABLE 64-3   The Glasgow Coma Scale Score

Finding	Score
Eye opening	
Spontaneous	4
To voice	3
To pain	2
None	1
Verbal response	
Oriented	5
Confused speech	4
Inappropriate words	3
Incomprehensible sounds	2
None	1
Motor response	
Obeys commands	6
Localizes pain	5
Withdraws	4
Abnormal flexion	3
Extension	2
None	1

intracranial lesions. Absent or minimal mass effect on CT suggests other causes of coma such as diffuse axonal injury, brainstem contusion, or anoxic injury.

Table 64-4   Acute Traumatic Subdural Hematoma: Mortality

Prognostic Factor	Mortality, %
Bilateral fixed pupils	64–93
One nonreacting pupil	48–68
GCS 3	90–100
GCS 3–5	60–84
GCS 6–8	36–46
Lucid interval	47–57
Immediate coma	76–83
ICP > 20	71

SOURCE: Adapted from Servadei F: Prognostic factors in severely head injured adult patients with subdural haematomas. *Acta Neurochir* 139:279–285, 1997.

Management

The goals of therapy are to rapidly identify surgically amenable lesions and to prevent secondary ischemic brain injury. The airway as usual comes first: the devastating effects of hypoxia and hypercapnia on ICP should be avoided. Patients with GCS scores ≤ 8 should be intubated and modestly hyperventilated to a Pa_{CO_2} of 30 to 35 mmHg. Endotracheal intubation should be performed by skilled personnel using a pharmacologic strategy designed to minimize reflexive increases in ICP. The acute use of glucocorticoids has no measurable benefit in either reducing ICP or improving outcome and may have significant adverse effects. Obvious signs of increasing ICP prior to imaging or ICP monitoring can be addressed with 20% mannitol, 1 g/kg.

MEDICAL MANAGEMENT

Therapy is directed at maintaining systemic and cerebral perfusion without increasing ICP. Correct assessment of volume status is critical, often difficult in patients who have multiple trauma, and usually requires central venous pressure monitoring. ICP monitoring is indicated in most head-injured patients with significant depression of consciousness (GCS score < 10) or who require heavy sedation, neuromuscular blockade, etc. Common ICP monitoring systems include fluid-filled intraventricular or subdural catheters and subarachnoid bolts. Catheters that transduce membrane-sensed pressure signals by fiberoptic light transmission are also commonly used. Subdural placement is associated with a lower infection and hemorrhage rate; intraventricular placement allows withdrawal of CSF. Subarachnoid bolts are prone to occlusion by brain, blood, or meninges. ICP is less than 10 mmHg in normals. In traumatic brain injury, ICPs less than 15 to 20 mmHg are associated with better outcomes. ICPs of 20 to 25 mmHg indicate marginal cerebral perfusion pressures, marginal intracranial compliance, and incipient loss of cerebral autoregulation; they call for and require evaluation and intervention. Localized cerebral edema (temporal lobe, posterior fossa) may result in compromise at lower ICPs.

Overvigorous attempts to reduce ICP, such as excessive diuresis or excessive hyperventilation ($Pa_{CO_2} < 25$) may do so at the expense of CPP. A cerebral perfusion pressure of 70 mmHg or greater is probably sufficient to overcome regional heterogeneity in ICP.

A general algorithm of medical management is outlined in Table 64-2. Mannitol (0.5 to 1.0 mg/kg in a 20% solution as a bolus, repeated q4–6h as long as $Osm_P < 320$ mOsm/L) remains the therapy of choice in normovolemic patients. Furosemide is probably synergistic with mannitol. Pentobarbital is a second-line agent requiring hemodynamic monitoring. It is given as an infusion (e.g., 10 mg/kg over 30 min, followed by 1 to 3 mg/kg per hour), may cause hypotension, and precludes assessment of ocular reflexes. As previously mentioned, no study to date has shown that the acute use of glucocorticoids, even in "megadoses," has any measurable benefit in either reducing ICP or improving outcome, in contradistinction to findings in acute spinal cord injury. Highly selected patients who fail to respond to medical measures may benefit from subtemporal decompression or decompressive craniectomy; the latter is more controversial.

ADJUNCTIVE MONITORING

Cerebral blood flow may be assessed by several other modalities. *Transcranial Doppler ultrasonography* is used to diagnose vasospasm [in subarachnoid hemorrhage (SAH)], hyperemic states, and brain death. *Jugular venous oximetry* ($S\bar{v}JO_2$ measurement), if less than 50%, is associated with poor outcomes; saturations greater than 75% suggest a hyperemic state or impaired central nervous system (CNS) oxygen extraction. *Radionuclide cerebral blood flow* measurements (xenon washout) are sometimes used in the assessment of brain death.

Evoked potentials (somatosensory, brainstem auditory, and visual) are useful in assessing heavily sedated/paralyzed patients and have prognostic value when used serially. *Electroencephalographic (EEG) monitoring* is useful in excluding nonconvulsive seizure activity; serial recordings may also have prognostic value.

ADJUNCTIVE THERAPY

Seizures: Prophylactic anticonvulsant therapy with phenytoin is usually undertaken; repeated seizures may result in additional brain ischemia. Therapy is continued for 6 to 12 months. The risk of late seizures (> 14 days after injury) is approximately 5 percent.

Nutrition: Early enteral nutrition is a priority; caloric requirements of head-injured patients approach those of patients with significant burn injuries. Parenteral nutrition should be used only if an absolute contraindication to the enteral route exists (visceral perforation, mechanical obstruction).

Fluid/electrolytes: Disorders of total body water are frequent. The syndrome of inappropriate antidiuretic hormone secretion (SIADH) is generally managed by water restriction. Cerebral salt wasting syndrome (CSWS), characterized by excessive natriuresis and hypovolemic hyponatremia, remains underrecognized despite the fact that it may occur at least as commonly as SIADH in some types of brain injury. Therapy consists of saline replacement. The distinction between the two is important, as inappropriate volume restriction in CSWS may lead to further decreases in cerebral perfusion pressure. Diabetes insipidus is managed with desmopressin, 1 to 2 μg IV tid to qid. Iatrogenic causes of excessive urine flow (mannitol, massive volume resuscitation) occur more commonly and need to be distinguished from diabetes insipidus with careful measurement of urine and serum osmolalities.

Mechanical ventilation: Positive pressure ventilation and positive end-expiratory pressure (PEEP) have the potential to increase ICP depending on intracranial and chest wall compliance, tidal volume, and the level of PEEP. In general, PEEP and other ventilatory strategies that increase mean airway pressure should be adjusted to avoid adversely raising ICP. However, if associated acute lung injury is present, PEEP should be used (in conjunction with ICP monitoring) to ensure adequate cerebral oxygen delivery.

Antithrombotic therapy: The stasis of bed rest and the thrombogenic properties of brain and other injured tissue are usually addressed with sequential compression devices applied to the lower extremities. Serial duplex studies of the lower extremities may signal the need for early and potentially lifesaving caval interruption.

Gastrointestinal ulcer prophylaxis: Gastrointestinal bleeding is more likely if respiratory failure or coagulopathy is also present. Gastric feedings in adequate volume are often sufficient prophylaxis; H_2 blockade or sucralfate are used otherwise.

Rehabilitation: Limb posture and range of motion should be maintained from admission to the ICU. Regular turning and skin care lessen the chance of pressure necrosis and ulceration. Progressive motor and cognitive exercises are tailored to the level of consciousness and should be started in the intensive care unit (ICU) as part of a comprehensive rehabilitation plan.

Prognosis

Mortality from severe brain injury ranges from 30 to 50 percent in most series. GCS score, age, and extent of trauma to other organ systems are major determinants of mortality. Uncontrollable intracranial hypertension occurs in 50 to 70 percent of those dying (Table 64-4). Regionalized systems of trauma care have been shown repeatedly to reduce mortality from CNS trauma. Their impact on functional outcomes are less demonstrable: available data suggest that at least 50 percent of patients with severe brain injury have limitations with self-care or with mobility. The extent of cognitive impairment and its impact are even less well known.

For a more detailed discussion, see Chap. 89 in *Principles of Critical Care,* 2d ed.

Chapter 65

MANAGEMENT OF BURNS

AVERY TUNG

Patients who survive thermal injury must navigate a clinical course filled with predictable obstacles. Although many of these obstacles can be anticipated, they remain life-threatening problems presenting difficult challenges to the critical care physician. Most problems complicating recovery from burns evolve directly from the three distinct physiologic phases that follow burn injury. The early postburn phase (0 to 36 h) is notable for dramatic tissue edema formation, hypovolemia, renal failure, life-threatening airway edema, compartment syndromes, and chest wall restrictive disease. The middle phase (36 h to 10 days) is marked by extreme protein-calorie catabolism, inflammatory lung disease in patients with inhalation injury, and moderation of edema formation. During this time skin grafting should be aggressively pursued in order to limit the infectious hazard of the open burn wound. In the late phase (10 days to wound closure), chronic open wounds propagate the catabolic state, act as a portal for infection, and mandate further surgery. Nutrition and rehabilitation issues also predominate. Although pneumonia is prominent in cases of inhalation injury, the primary cause of mortality in burn injury is sepsis, and careful attention to infection control may be the most important issue in securing good outcomes.

Burns: 0 to 36 Hours

AIRWAY AND BREATHING

Initial evaluation of thermal injury should always begin with an assessment of the airway and the degree of inhalation injury, which consists of three separate pathophysiologic processes presenting either singly or in combination. The first process is heat injury to the upper airway. Although hot, inhaled gases rarely retain enough heat to damage airway mucosa distal to the vocal cords, the oro- and nasopharynx can sustain significant damage. The result is marked upper airway swelling that peaks approximately 12 h postburn and may take 1 to 3 days to resolve. Clinical symptoms of upper airway heat injury include respiratory distress and difficulty talking or swallowing. Signs of airway damage include soot in the mouth or nose, blistering or redness of the tongue or hard palate, tachypnea, and inspiratory stridor. If *any* of these signs are noted in a patient with a history of exposure to fire in an enclosed space, intubation should be promptly performed to secure the airway. An upper airway damaged by heat can swell to nearly unrecognizable proportions in only 2 to 3 h, leading to complete airway closure and asphyxiation. Early recognition and treatment of this condition can be lifesaving. While the American Burn Association (ABA) recommends nasotracheal intubation as the procedure of choice, the route of intubation should be left to the discretion of the anesthesiologist or critical care physician performing the procedure.

The second process involved in inhalation injury is systemic toxicity from inhaled carbon monoxide and cyanide generated by incomplete combustion. Most fatalities occurring at a fire scene are due to asphyxiation or carbon monoxide poisoning, underscoring the rapidly lethal nature of these compounds. Although carboxyhemoglobin levels exceeding 30 percent are considered toxic, concurrent cyanide poisoning acts synergistically to lower the toxic threshold. Unfortunately, while routine blood gas analysis provides an assessment of carbon monoxide exposure, a rapid assay for cyanide is not widely available. Symptoms of carbon monoxide poisoning include headache and irritability. Signs of carbon monoxide poisoning include confusion or coma, vomiting, incontinence, tachypnea, and tachycardia. The "cherry red" appearance characteristic of high carboxyhemoglobin levels is rarely seen in burn patients. Arrhythmias, seizures, coma, or a persistent metabolic acidosis may suggest cyanide toxicity. Treatment of carbon monoxide poisoning involves prolonged administration of 100 percent inspired oxygen, which reduces the half-life of carboxyhemoglobin from 250 min in room air to less than 50 min. Coma persisting > 1 to 2 days often implies permanent brain injury. Treatment of cyanide poisoning is usually unnecessary because of metabolism of cyanide to thiocyanate in the liver. Patients with hypotension, arrhythmias, and acidosis despite appropriate hemodynamic management, however, may require empiric antidotal therapy with methylene blue, which induces conversion of endogenous hemoglobin to the cyanide scavenger methemoglobin; but such therapy may ultimately worsen oxygen delivery (Table 65-1).

The third process involved in inhalation injury is chemical irritation of the tracheobronchial tree. Hydrogen chloride, nitrogen and sulfur oxides, and aldehydes are present in smoke and can cause a severe inflammatory reaction in the lung parenchyma. Resulting pathophysiologic changes include small airway spasm, pulmonary edema, ulceration of the tracheal lining, bronchorrhea, and impaired ciliary activity. Signs and symptoms of this type of inhalation injury may be initially absent and include a rapid respiratory rate, use of accessory muscles, rales, wheezing, and hypoxemia. Definitive diagnosis of this "chemical burn" is difficult because symptoms may not become manifest for 24 to 48 h and no reliable test exists to predict the ultimate extent of injury. Although bronchoscopy has been recommended to follow the course of tracheobronchial injury, initial examination does not correlate with future injury. This type of inhalation injury, which nearly doubles the expected mortality from the burn wound alone, increases fluid requirements, requires aggressive ventilator management, and predisposes the patient to pulmonary infections.

CIRCULATION

Burn Shock

Major burn injury induces a severe inflammatory response in damaged tissue, causing cellular swelling and increased vascular permeability. Increased osmotic pressure in the burn wound as well as cellular swelling cause massive loss of intravascular volume into the burned tissue. Plasma proteins are also lost as a result of increased vascular permeability,

TABLE 65-1 Treatment of Carbon Monoxide and Cyanide Poisoning in Smoke Inhalation

---

Carbon monoxide poisoning[a]

FI_{O_2}	Half-life of COHb
21% at sea level	6–7 h
100% at sea level	1 h
100% at 2.5 atm	30 min

Cyanide poisoning[b]

Adults:

    Administer amyl nitrite inhaler for 30–60 s

    Administer sodium nitrite: 10 mL of 3% solution IV (30 mg/mL) at 2.5–5 mL/min (total = 300 mg).

    Administer sodium thiosulfate 50 mL of 25% solution IV (250 mg/mL) (total = 12.5 g)

    Keep methemoglobin level < 40%. May repeat sodium nitrite at half the original dose in 30 min if methemoglobin level < 20 or if levels are unobtainable.

    Rapid administration of sodium nitrite can cause hypotension.

Children:

    Administer amyl nitrite inhaler for 30–60 s

    Administer sodium nitrite 3% solution based on the following formula:

    Milliliters of 3% sodium nitrite = (hemoglobin)(weight in kilograms)/36

    Administer at 2.5–5 mL/min. Rapid administration can cause hypotension.

    Administer sodium thiosulfate 25% solution based on the following formula:

    Milliliters of 25% sodium thiosulfate = (hemoglobin)(weight in kilograms)/7.4

    Keep methemoglobin level < 30%.

---

[a]Because of synergistic toxicity between carbon monoxide and cyanide, treatment for carbon monoxide should be instituted whenever a history of CO exposure is elicited and continued until CO levels have normalized.
[b]Because induction of methemoglobinemia can be dangerous, treatment for cyanide poisoning should be administered only if both a strong clinical suspicion and a deteriorating clinical course are present.

leading to severe hypoproteinemia and a hypooncotic circulating volume. Large quantities of sodium are also lost into the burn wound, requiring replacement. Fluid and protein losses are maximal during the initial 6 to 8 h, reducing plasma protein levels by as much as 50 percent and causing dramatic hypovolemia. In patients with > 30 percent total body surface (TBS) burns, peripheral edema is noted even in unburned areas. Such generalized edema may be due to severe hypoproteinemia induced by thermal injury and worsens the loss of intravascular volume.

Although hypovolemia is the most important hemodynamic alteration observed during the first 36 h following a major burn, other cardiovascular changes also occur. Systemic vascular resistance is increased because of the catecholamines and other vasoactive mediators released by the burn injury. Cardiac output is depressed because of hypovolemia but may also be affected by contractile dysfunction, because of myocardial edema, in burns exceeding 40 percent of TBS. Tachycardia is common, driven by the high catecholamine state.

Initial Management of Burn Shock

The severe hypovolemia induced by thermal injury combined with depressed myocardial contractility and increased afterload lead to a syndrome of impaired end-organ perfusion in the presence of normal systemic blood pressures. The goal of hemodynamic management in the first 36 h following burn injury, therefore, is aggressive replacement of intravascular volume in order to maintain adequate end-organ perfusion. Intravenous access via peripheral vein catheter is preferable to central access; such a catheter should be placed in unburned tissue, if possible, to avoid infection. If intravenous access through unburned tissue is not possible, placement through burned tissue may be performed only as a temporary alternative. Because hypovolemia resulting from burn injury is predictable, monitoring of central pressures is usually necessary only in elderly patients or patients with severe cardiac disease for whom excessive fluid administration is problematic. Central lines should be removed as soon as they are no longer needed or rotated every 3 to 7 days to avoid infectious or thrombotic complications.

No one measure of end-organ perfusion is a completely reliable indicator of tissue oxygenation in the burn patient. While blood pressure and heart rate may be altered due to abnormal sympathetic tone, responses to hypovolemia still occur. A mean arterial pressure < 85 mmHg or heart rate > 120 beats per minute suggests hypovolemia even in the presence of increased intrinsic catecholamines. Arterial pH is often an extremely useful measure of tissue oxygenation. A metabolic acidosis or base deficit implies impaired tissue oxygenation due to hypoperfusion or carbon monoxide or cyanide poisoning. Massive administration of crystalloid can also induce a non-gap metabolic acidosis. Gastric mucosal pH may be monitored using gastric tonometry, although there are few data to correlate observed changes with therapy or outcome. Urine output (UOP) is perhaps the best indicator of end-organ perfusion in burn patients. UOP between 0.5 and 1 mL/kg per hour usually reflects adequate renal blood flow in the absence of osmotic agents. In order to avoid deleterious consequences of excess tissue edema, fluid administration should be decreased if UOP is consistently greater than 1 mL/kg per hour. Measurements of central venous and pulmonary capillary wedge pressure are usually low during this period even when organ perfusion is adequate. Overdependence on these monitors for resuscitation in the burn patient may lead to excessive fluid administration and consequently excess edema.

The most widely used resuscitation fluid in the resuscitation of thermal injury is lactated Ringer's solution. Other crystalloid solutions may be used provided that enough sodium is administered to replace that lost into the wound. As a result of the high volumes usually used in burn resuscitation, glucose-containing fluids should be avoided in order to prevent hyperglycemia. If hypertonic saline is used, the serum sodium level should not be allowed to exceed 160 meq/L. Because of increases in vascular permeability, colloid solutions may worsen edema in unburned tissue without any added effectiveness. Hetastarch, a 6 percent starch solution, can induce clotting abnormalities by altering platelet function when administered in volumes exceeding 1.5 L. Hemoconcentration is often seen in the early phase of burn resuscitation, obviating the need for blood transfusion. Fresh frozen plasma should be reserved for correction of documented clotting abnormalities.

Fluid administration should be titrated to end-organ perfusion. An initial rate can be estimated using the size of the burn and body weight, as below:

$$\text{Volume per 24 h in milliliters} = [4 \times (\% \text{ TBS burned}) \times (\text{body weight in kilograms})]$$

Give half of total in the first 8 h, half of total in subsequent 16 h.

Such a formula is an initial guide and must be adjusted to the individual patient. Once adequate urine output is established, an attempt should be made to titrate the infusion rate to the lowest level compatible with adequate organ perfusion.

Inotropic support is indicated if pulmonary edema resulting from excess fluid administration occurs before adequate organ perfusion is achieved. This problem is most common in elderly patients, patients with contractile dysfunction, or those requiring positive-pressure ventilation. Although low-dose dopamine (3 to 4 g/kg/min) is often used to improve urine output in these patients, there is little evidence to clearly support its use in the early resuscitation phase.

MANAGEMENT OF THE BURN WOUND

Although, in the first 36 h, the wound itself is not as important as maintaining adequate oxygen delivery, four issues need to be addressed during this period in order to preserve optimum long-term recovery: neutralizing the source of injury, assessing the burn, controlling heat loss, and preventing edema-related complications.

Neutralizing the Source of Burn Injury

The first step in management of thermal injury is neutralizing the source of burn injury. Removing burned clothing or other sources of heat from the patient is important to stop the burning process. Cooling of a fresh injury is appropriate if it halts spread of thermal injury, but it should not be applied to wounds that have already reached room temperature or to large (> 40 percent) burns because of the risk of hypothermia. Most chemical burns should be flushed with copious amounts of saline. Hydrogen fluoride burns should be neutralized with topical or subcutaneous administration of calcium gluconate, and topical phenol exposure should be neutralized by irrigation with polyethylene glycol solution. Concentrated sulfuric acid burns should be cautiously flushed with water because of the exothermic reaction that occurs when sulfuric acid and water are mixed together.

Assessing the Degree of Burn and Total Body Surface Area Percentage Affected

Burn injury is classified into three categories (first, second, or third degree), depending on the depth of burn injury. First-degree burns involve the outer epidermis only and resemble a sunburn on physical examination. The burned area will be painful, but healing should occur with minimal medical attention. Second-degree burns involve tissue destruction of the entire epidermis and partial but not complete destruction of the dermal layer. These wounds are characterized by a blanching, red appearance and are exquisitely painful. Burns that leave a large portion of viable dermis should heal with minimal scarring in 10 to 14 days, but burns that leave only a thin layer of viable dermis will require skin grafting to avoid severe scarring and disfigurement. Third-degree (or full thickness) burns involve complete destruction of both the epidermal and dermal layers. These wounds will have a waxy, white appearance and may demonstrate punctate red markings indicating hemoglobin that has been "fixed" by the heat. Such markings and the absence of pain imply thermal destruction of the dermis, dermal blood supply, and nerve endings. Third-degree burns will heal only by wound contraction and require surgical excision and skin grafting to avoid functional limitation. Often, differentiating deep second-degree burns from third-degree burns is difficult and may require observation for 24 to 48 h to allow the burn to evolve. Scald burns are particularly difficult to categorize and may require assessment by an experienced burn or plastic surgeon.

The percentage of total body surface (TBS) area burned may be estimated using the "rule of 9s." Under this system, the body is divided into zones, each with a multiple of 9 percent of body surface area. The head and each arm are considered to be 9 percent of TBS; the chest, abdomen, back, and each leg are estimated at 18 percent. Often, the patient's hand is estimated at 1 percent of body surface area and is used to mark off portions that do not neatly fall into the above groups. In pediatric patients, this formula should be modified, with each leg estimated at 14 percent and the head at 18 percent (Fig. 65-1).

Controlling Loss of Heat from the Burned Area

Because the skin represents an important barrier to heat loss, burned patients are at significant risk for hypothermia. Moisture from leakage of plasma into the burn wound, rapid administration of cold intravenous fluid, attempts to cool the patient, and topical antibiotic application all contribute to hypothermia during the initial 36 h of burn resuscitation. The burn patient should be transported to a warmed environment as soon as feasible and wet dressings should be removed from burned areas and replaced by dry dressings. External warming using heat lamps and forced air warmers should be applied. If possible, intravenous fluids should be warmed before administration. Because wound debridement and washing involve prolonged exposure of wet wounds, normothermia should be achieved before these activities are undertaken. Prolonged use of forced-air warmers over wet bandages will actually have a cooling effect secondary to evaporative heat loss.

Evaluating Edema-Related Complications

The consequences of excess edema are many. Chest wall edema or a circumferential third-degree chest wall burn can significantly decrease pulmonary compliance, leading to increased airway pressures, difficulty with mechanical ventilation, and hypercarbia. Treatment involves escharotomy of the chest wall. Two longitudinal incisions are made into the subeschar area in the midaxillary lines and a third incision is made across the lower chest wall connecting the longitudinal ones. Circumferential extremity burns are at high risk for compartment syndrome and compromise of neurovascular

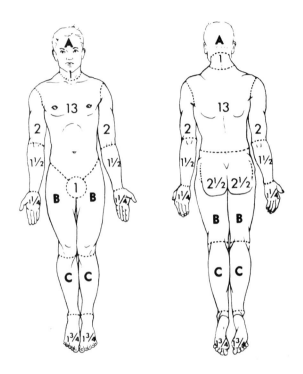

Relative Percentages of Areas Affected by Growth

	Age		
Area	10	15	Adult
A = half of head	5½	4½	3½
B = half of one thigh	4¼	4½	4¾
C = half of one leg	3	3¼	3½

FIGURE 65-1 Lund and Browder method of calculating the percent of the body surface area burned.

function secondary to tissue edema. Symptoms and signs of compartment syndrome include lack of palpable pulses or capillary refill, pain, and numbness or coolness in the affected extremity. Monitoring of extremities distal to circumferential second- or third-degree burns by palpation or Doppler examination of the distal extremity is recommended to avoid this complication. Escharotomies may be lifesaving in these patients also but should be placed with caution to avoid damage to vital nerve or vascular structures. Consultation with an experienced burn or plastic surgeon is imperative if finger escharotomies are contemplated. Complex burns classified by the American Burn Association (ABA) as "major" should be transferred to a comprehensive burn center as soon as stability is achieved (Table 65-2).

Care of the Burn Patient: Day 2 to Day 6

SUMMARY

The massive edema formation characteristic of initial burn resuscitation peaks at 8 to 10 h, moderating significantly by 36 to 48 h postburn. This reduction in edema formation ushers in a period of relative stability lasting 4 to 6 days. During this time the inflammatory, hypermetabolic state characteristic of

---

TABLE 65-2   American Burn Association Referral Criteria

---

1. Second- and third-degree burns of 10 percent or more of the body surface in patients under 10 or over 50 years of age
2. Second- and third-degree burns of more than 20 percent of the body surface area in other age groups
3. Third-degree burns of more than 5 percent of the body surface area in any age group
4. Second- and third-degree burns that involve the face, hands, feet, genitalia, perineum, or major joints
5. Electrical burns, including lightning injury
6. Chemical burns with serious threat of functional or cosmetic impairment
7. Inhalation injury
8. Coexisting medical problems
9. Combined blunt or penetrating trauma

---

the later stages of burn injury has not yet begun. Aggressive surgical excision and grafting of burn wounds is indicated during this period, as both operative risk and the likelihood of graft failure increase during later phases of burn injury. Parenchymal lung injury resulting from smoke inhalation peaks between days 3 and 5, however, and can limit the extent of burn surgery during this period.

PULMONARY MANAGEMENT

Both upper airway swelling and parenchymal lung injury may be present during this phase of burn care and require careful assessment before tracheal extubation is considered. Upper airway obstruction typically improves during this period, allowing assessment for extubation. Although no one preextubation measure can guarantee successful extubation, two tests are commonly used to evaluate for airway patency. Direct or indirect laryngoscopy can provide a subjective evaluation of both airway edema and ease of reintubation. Deflating the endotracheal cuff in an adult and determining airflow around the endotracheal tube also allow evaluation of airway edema. Once extubated, patients should be observed closely for 8 to 12 h in the event that redistribution of soft tissue edema after extubation causes delayed airway obstruction.

An inflammatory tracheobronchitis resulting from smoke inhalation, however, may prevent successful extubation by hindering adequate gas exchange. This reaction peaks during this period and can cause bronchorrhea, increased cough and mucus production, plugging small airways and predisposing to infection. Chest x-rays can reveal both diffuse and focal alveolar infiltrates. Hypoxemia and hypercarbia can result. Treatment for this syndrome is similar to that for acute respiratory distress syndrome (ARDS): judicious fluid management, aggressive treatment of infection, pulmonary toilet, and ventilator management directed at minimizing barotrauma. Although prophylactic antibiotics are not routinely administered, they can be useful in counteracting the diffuse, infectious bronchopneumonia that often results from airway mucosal damage and should be begun if signs of pulmonary infection are observed.

Repeated operative procedures and alterations in chest wall compliance or gas exchange resulting from either chest wall or pulmonary edema can also adversely affect pulmonary function. Anesthesia ventilators are unable to deliver the same inspiratory flows as critical care type ventilators in the setting of high airway pressures, resulting in intraoperative loss of functional residual capacity (FRC), atelectasis formation, hypercarbia, and increased oxygen requirements. Use of a critical care type ventilator in the operating room setting can often help to maintain FRC at preoperative levels, minimizing the impact of repeated surgical procedures. Pulmonary edema from burn-induced pulmonary capillary leak and aggressive fluid resuscitation is commonly present during this period and can significantly complicate the management of gas exchange and mechanical ventilation. Unfortunately, balancing the effects of ongoing fluid leakage into burn wounds, fluid shifts from operative interventions, and vascular redistribution resulting from burn-induced inflammation renders the assessment of fluid balance and adequate perfusion extremely challenging. In patients in whom adequate tissue perfusion cannot be maintained without pulmonary edema, echocardiography, pulmonary artery catheterization, or systemic pressors may assist management.

Reduced chest wall compliance secondary to burn tissue edema can also worsen pulmonary mechanics during this period. Although early excision of the chest wall can lessen this effect, return to normal compliance is not usually attained until wound healing is nearly complete. If decreased lung compliance results in unacceptably high airway pressures, permissive hypercapnia may reduce the incidence of barotrauma.

CIRCULATORY MANAGEMENT

Hemodynamic management during this period is characterized by difficulty maintaining intravascular volume, and by the transition to a hypermetabolic state that characterizes late recovery from thermal injury. The tachycardia, vasodilation, and increased oxygen consumption characteristic of this hypermetabolic state renders assessment of fluid balance difficult. In addition, thermally injured patients exhibit large ongoing fluid losses through the burn wound and require repeated surgical procedures—with massive blood loss. Further complicating the assessment of perfusion are hypolbuminemia from burn-induced hepatic dysfunction, anemia from depressed hematopoiesis, fever, tachycardia, and an increase in oxygen consumption which accompanies the hypermetabolic state. Urine output is the most commonly used indicator of adequate peripheral perfusion, although the absence of a progressive base deficit on arterial blood gas can also suggest adequate perfusion. Central monitoring should be used only if absolutely necessary because of the increased risk of line sepsis in burn patients and because the important endpoints (pulmonary edema, urine output) are clinical.

Because of decreased sodium loss into the burn during this period, hypotonic fluids are usually administered to replace intravascular volume. Potassium, magnesium, and calcium levels will be predictably low and will require daily replacement. Calcium replacement should be guided by measurement of ionized calcium, since correlation between total and ionized calcium levels is poor in burn patients. Red cell transfusion may also be necessary to maintain adequate oxygen delivery. A hematocrit between 30 and 35 percent is usually adequate.

NUTRITION

During this period a state of extreme protein catabolism develops, which, if not treated, can lead to poor wound healing, immune suppression, and breakdown of gut integrity. Increased cytokine, cortisol, and catecholamine levels induce marked gluconeogenesis from protein. Unlike other critically ill patients who convert to fat as the primary metabolic fuel during starvation, burn patients continue to utilize protein as a major fuel source until their wounds are closed. Glutamine levels are extremely low during the healing process, as glutamine is preferentially used by the gut as fuel and is the precursor to the antioxidant glutathione. Enteral feeds supplemented with vitamins should be begun as soon as possible after burn injury and continued until wounds are closed. Vitamins A, C, E, and zinc sulfate (220 mg bid) in particular should be aggressively replaced as they are utilized by the healing wound. Protein requirements are usually estimated between 1.5 and 2.0 g/kg per day, and nonprotein calories should be administered as 60 percent carbohydrate and 40 percent fat. Transferrin and prealbumin levels should be measured weekly to assess the adequacy of nutritional support. Transferrin levels > 100 mg/dL and prealbumin levels > 14 mg/dL suggest adequate nutrition (Table 65-3).

Although adequate nutrition will not prevent net protein loss in thermal injury, it can retard the catabolic process by as much as 50 percent and should be pursued aggressively. In patients who cannot tolerate gastric or duodenal feeds, total parenteral nutrition (TPN) should be considered, although its value is unclear in the critically ill and the risk of catheter infection is increased in burn victims.

CARE OF THE BURN WOUND

Toward the end of this period, an intense inflammatory response develops in the burn wound. Burn wound infection, rare in the first 6 days after a major burn, emerges as an issue between days 4 and 7, as bacteria repopulate an area initially sterilized by heat injury. Impaired cellular and humoral

TABLE 65-3   Nutritional Guidelines for Severe Thermal Injury[a]

Total calories	30–35 cal/kg per day
Protein	1.5–2.0 g/kg per day
Carbohydrate	60% of total calories
Supplements	
Vitamin A	10,000–15,000 IU/day
Vitamin C	1 g/day
Vitamin E	500–1000 IU/day
Zinc	220 mg bid
Carotene	50 mg/day
Selenium	100 μg/day
Optional	
Glutamine	30–40 g/day

[a]Measure transferrin and prealbumin levels weekly to assess adequacy of nutrition.

immune responses combine with loss of the outer epidermal barrier to increase the risk of infection during this period. Although topical antibiotics such as silver sulfadiazine (Silvadene) and mafenide actetate (Sulfamylon) are used to prevent wound infection, bacterial colonization of the burn wound is inevitable. In addition, some *Staphylococcus* species are resistant to Silvadene. Strict infection-control policies including frequent handwashing are critically important, because contamination of burn wounds by health care personnel moving between patients or from area to area on a single patient is a major source of wound infection.

While wound colonization involves bacterial growth in nonviable tissue and is ubiquitous, wound infection involves bacterial invasion of viable, living tissue. Burn wound infection is difficult to diagnose in the setting of burn-induced systemic inflammation and should be aggressively sought based on changes in the clinical condition. Although traditional markers of systemic infection such as fever, tachycardia, leukocytosis, and hyperglycemia are present in uninfected burn patients, an increase in the leukocyte count or frequency of fevers above baseline may suggest infection. Wound purulence is a poor indicator of infection.

The gold standard for tissue infection remains a biopsy of viable wound tissue. Greater than 10^5 bacteria per gram of tissue clearly indicates infection. Therapy includes upgrading topical antibiotics to increase activity or penetration, consideration of systemic antibiotics active against the bacteria, and surgical excision of the infected tissue. Often, the combination of topical and systemic antibiotics without surgical excision is effective in preventing wound infection from leading to systemic sepsis. The most common organism found in early wound infection is *Staphylococcus aureus,* while wound infections occurring > 1 week from injury are often caused by *Pseudomonas* or *Enterococcus* species. One complication of the aggressive use of powerful topical antibacterial agents such as mafenide is the development of fungal wound infection, most commonly with *Candida* species. Topical treatment for candidal wound infection includes nystatin cream, which can be combined with topical antibacterial creams. Because systemic candidal infection carries a high mortality, systemic antifungal agents are regularly added and wound excision is pursued more aggressively than in cases of bacterial wound infection in order to prevent systemic spread.

Perhaps the best strategy to prevent wound infection is early excision and grafting before the inflammatory response gains momentum. All wounds not expected to heal within 14 to 21 days should be excised and grafted at the earliest opportunity. In large burns (> 40 percent), a lack of donor sites may limit initial wound coverage. In this circumstance, alternatives to autologous skin such as allograft or synthetic substitutes may be used to cover the burn wound temporarily, allowing time for donor sites to regenerate. If insufficient skin is available to cover all wound surfaces, tracheostomy and central venous access sites should be covered first to facilitate the prolonged critical care that will be required to regenerate donor sites. Depth of excision can significantly affect the success of a skin graft. Excision only to subdermal fat before grafting produces a superior functional and esthetic result as compared with excision to fascia, but subdermal fat is relatively avascular, rendering a successful graft less likely.

Care of the Burn Patient: Day 7 to Wound Closure

SUMMARY

The primary goal during this period is closure of the burn wound. This goal is complicated by the inflammatory, immunosuppressed state characteristic of burn injury, which persists until approximately 60 to 70 percent of the patient's skin is closed. The most common cause of mortality during this period is multisystem organ failure (MSOF) due to sepsis and wound inflammation. Hypotension, renal failure, GI bleeding, and ARDS are common complications of sepsis during this period. Because the key to recovery from major thermal injury is wound coverage, the clinical agenda should be directed toward a successful series of operative skin graft procedures. To that end, vigilant surveillance for wound infection, aggressive nutritional support, maintaining end-organ perfusion, and preventing catastrophes such as GI bleeding or airway emergencies are the focus of critical care support during this period. As the patient becomes more alert, attention to pain control and rehabilitation also become important.

PULMONARY MANAGEMENT

Prolonged endotracheal intubation is typically required during this period both for patients with severe inhalation injury and patients (usually children) who require aggressive pain control for dressing changes. ARDS and frequent operative procedures may also require periods of intubation and mechanical ventilation. In children, tracheal stenosis resulting from endotracheal tube trauma can significantly complicate extubation and may necessitate tracheostomy or tracheal reconstruction.

The decision to perform tracheostomy in adults must be individualized. Tracheostomy decreases the requirement for sedation and simplifies pulmonary toilet, wound care, and weaning from mechanical ventilation. By removing the endotracheal tube from the mouth, tracheostomy can also simplify the care of face or lip burns. However, a fresh tracheostomy site can also be risky if it is located close to an unexcised wound or other infectious source. Also, tracheostomy ties can be irritating to neck burns and make skin grafting to the neck difficult. Consultation with a burn or plastic surgeon is recommended when such a procedure is planned.

INFECTION SURVEILLANCE

An uninfected, well-perfused wound bed is critical to a successful skin graft. As a result, patients should not be grafted until the wound is completely infection-free. Although increases in the white blood cell (WBC) count or frequency of fevers may suggest an infectious source, wound biopsy remains the gold standard for the diagnosis of burn wound infection. If systemic sepsis occurs in the presence of negative wound biopsy results, other sources of infection should be sought. Because of extensive bacterial wound colonization in burn patients, central line sites are at extremely high risk for infection and should be exchanged if line sepsis is contemplated. Nosocomial pneumonia is another common infectious complication, especially in patients with inhalation injury, and may be particularly difficult to diagnose in burn patients due to heavy use of systemic antibiotics for wound infection as well as preexisting abnormalities in WBC count and fever. The risk of aspiration from aggressive enteral feeds as well as altered mucociliary clearance due to inhalation injury contribute to an inceased risk of nosocomial pneumonia in this period. Treatment of nosocomial pneumonia in critically ill patients is detailed in Chap. 39.

FLUID AND NUTRITIONAL SUPPORT

Although some patients may still be volume-overloaded from their initial fluid resuscitation, fluid requirements continue to increase during this period. Operative procedures on large wounds can be extremely bloody and require extensive blood product administration, increasing intravascular volume. Sepsis complicated by hypotension may also require increases in intravascular volume to compensate for systemic vasodilation. Finally, increased insensible losses from open wounds and the baseline hypermetabolic state will usually mandate increased maintenance fluid requirements to avoid end-organ perfusion deficits. The role of volume expanders and vasopressors in the treatment of sepsis is discussed in Chap. 25.

Patients will continue to be severely catabolic during this period, necessitating aggressive nutritional support in order to minimize loss of nitrogen. In addition to protein replacement at two to three times the recommended daily allowance, adjunct agents such as human growth hormone and oxandrolone, an anabolic steroid approved by the Food and Drug Administration for restoration of muscle loss after severe injury, may be considered. The enteral route is strongly preferred over intravenous feeds and duodenal or jejeunal access should be aggressively sought if a gastric ileus prevents gastric feeds or if aspiration is a concern.

PAIN CONTROL AND REHABILITATION

If donor sites need to be harvested multiple times to cover an extensive burn, this period may last for several weeks and include multiple operative procedures. Although third-degree burns are generally not painful, second-degree burns can be exquisitely painful as the epidermis begins to regenerate.

TABLE 65-4 Recommended Pain Treatment Strategies

	Intubated	Extubated
Adults	*Narcotic* Fentanyl 1–5 µg/kg per hour IV Morphine 1–5 mg/h IV Methadone 10–30 mg PO bid Hydromorphone 0.2–2 mg/min IV *Benzodiazepine* Midazolam 0.5–7 mg/h IV Ativan 1–6 mg IV q4–6h IV *Hypnotic* Propofol 20–100 µg/kg per minute IV Begin with a combination of narcotic and benzodiazepine. Treat dressing changes with bolus doses of a rapid-acting agent such as fentanyl or propofol. If tolerance develops,	For dressing changes: *Narcotic* Fentanyl 50–100 µg/ IV bolus Morphine 2–10 mg IV bolus Methadone 10–30 mg PO bid *Benzodiazepine* Midazolam 2–4 mg IV bolus Lorazepam 2–4 mg IV bolus In patients who tolerate enteral feeds, Low-dose methadone and lorazepam PO often provides excellent baseline pain/anxiety control. Dressing changes should be medicated with bolus doses of narcotic as tolerated. Benzodiazepines are rarely necessary but may have an additional sedative effect.

820

	addition of propofol may be necessary. Continuous use of propofol for more than 24 h requires monitoring of triglyceride levels, particularly in children. See above.	The use of continuous infusions of narcotic, benzodiazepine, or propofol is not recommended in extubated patients. *Narcotic* Fentanyl 15–20 μg/kg oralet or 0.1 μg/kg IV bolus Morphine 0.1–0.15 mg/kg IV bolus *Benzodiazepine* Midazolam 0.05–0.15 mg/kg IV bolus Ativan 0.05–0.15 mg IV bolus *Ketamine* 5–7 mg/kg IM 10 mg/kg PO *Propofol* 1–3 μg/kg bolus Propofol should be administered to extubated patients only by trained anesthesiologists
Children	Continuous use of propofol for more than 24 h requires monitoring of triglyceride levels, particularly in children.	

Following a skin graft procedure, the donor sites will be the primary source of surgical pain, since the excised and grafted wounds are devoid of nerve endings. As a result, immediate postoperative pain in a bandaged, grafted extremity represents an abnormal finding and should be carefully evaluated for an ill-fitting splint or compressive bandage. The topical use of mafenide can also cause a burning sensation which is painful to some patients.

Ideally, control of pain should allow participation in physical and occupational rehabilitation. Pain therapy should be directed not only at chronic, ongoing discomfort but also at dressing changes, which occur every 12 to 8 h and can be significantly more painful. Although narcotics are typically employed, specialized pain techniques such as epidural nerve blockade with local anesthetic have also been used when side effects such as respiratory depression prevent adequate intravenous pain control. Because the period of healing can take weeks, tolerance to narcotics and benzodiazepines commonly develops and weaning of these medications should occur before transfer to rehabilitation (Table 65-4).

Rehabilitation should begin when a patient is alert enough to cooperate with physical therapy; it plays a crucial role in achieving optimal functional outcome. Attention should be given to splinting limbs in the appropriate position and maximizing range of motion. In addition, many patients become aware of their appearance during this period and may require psychiatric consultation or treatment with antidepressants to learn to cope with the life-transforming nature of thermal injury.

For a more detailed discussion, see Chaps. 94, 95, and 96 in *Principles of Critical Care*, 2d ed.

Chapter 66

IMMUNOTHERAPY AND ORGAN TRANSPLANTATION

EDWARD T. NAURECKAS

Improvements in immunosuppression as well as in transplant technique and case management, have resulted in a dramatic increase in the survival of transplant recipients and their grafts. This, in turn, has resulted in ever-increasing numbers of transplant recipients and of institutions participating in transplant programs.

Allograft Rejection

While the availability of immunosuppressive agents such as cyclosporine, tacrolimus (FK506), and mycophenolate mofetil have augmented the transplant physician's ability to prevent and treat rejection, it remains an ongoing problem, particularly in the form of chronic rejection. There are three types of allograft rejection. Hyperacute rejection is the result of performed alloantibodies and occurs soon after revascularization of the grafted organ. There is essentially no treatment for this form of rejection, which sometimes requires immediate removal of the transplanted organ. Chronic rejection is characterized by progressive vasculitis leading to graft ischemia, fibrosis and loss of function. This form of rejection is resistant to immunotherapy and is the most frequent cause of late graft failure. The greatest gains in transplant therapy have come from the prevention of acute rejection. This form of rejection is initiated predominantly by T lymphocytes responding to foreign major histocompatibility (MHC) antigens from the allograft.

Immunosuppressive Agents

Immunosuppressive agents, while effective in decreasing the incidence of acute rejection, have many side effects and predispose patients to infection. In order to avoid the toxicities of particular agents, immunosuppressive regimens are often modified. A number of immunosuppressive agents are listed in Table 66-1.

LYMPHOCYTE ACTIVATION INHIBITORS

The most commonly used agents in this category include cyclosporine and tacrolimus (FK506). These agents act by inhibiting the production of interleukin 2 (IL-2) by T lymphocytes, which, in turn, interferes with the development of expanded clones of effector cells against the transplanted organ. Cyclosporine, in combination with corticosteroids, is the mainstay of maintenance therapy. Administration is generally begun near the time of transplantation at 8 to 10 mg/kg per day divided into two daily oral doses. When it is necessary to give the drug by the intravenous route, the dose is one-third the oral dose. Higher doses are often required in children and in liver patients with external bile duct drainage due to enterohepatic circulation. Many drugs may interact with cyclosporine to raise or lower its serum level. A microemulsion of cyclosporine (Neoral) has increased bioavailability and avoids some of these issues. The most significant toxicity of cyclosporine is nephrotoxicity. Special regimens reduce the dose of cyclosporine or substitute other drugs until the posttransplant acute tubular necrosis (see below) has resolved, in order to minimize the impact of cyclosporine nephrotoxicity.

Tacrolimus is a macrolide antibiotic with immunosuppressive properties similar to those of cyclosporine. The side-effect profile of tacrolimus is similar to that of cyclosporine, the main concern being nephrotoxicity. Significant central nervous system (CNS) effects occur in approximately 10% of patients, but minor effects such as lethargy or delirium are frequently seen. Tacrolimus does not cause the gingival hyperplasia or hair growth seen with cyclosporine. The dose of tacrolimus is 0.1 to 0.3 mg/kg per day given as two divided

TABLE 66-1 Side Effects of Immunosuppressive Drugs in Clinical Use

Drug	Side Effects
Lymphocyte activation inhibitors	
Cyclosporine	Nephrotoxicity, neurotoxicity, hypertension, hyperkalemia, hirsutism, gingival hyperplasia
Tacrolimus	Nephrotoxicity, neurotoxicity, hypertension, hyperkalemia, diarrhea
Antiproliferative agents	
Azathioprine	Leukopenia, thrombocytopenia, anemia, hepatotoxicity
Mycophenolate mofetil	Leukopenia, diarrhea, gastritis
Antilymphocyte antibodies	
OKT3	Fever, rigors, headache, diarrhea, seizures, pulmonary edema, bronchospasm
ALG/ATG	Fever, leukopenia, thrombocytopenia, serum sickness
Corticosteroids	Hyperglycemia, osteopenia, delayed wound healing, cushingoid facies

825

doses in order to maintain a target serum level of 15 to 20 ng/mL immediately posttransplant and 5 to 10 ng/mL long-term.

PROLIFERATION INHIBITORS

Azathioprine and mycophenolate mofetile (MMF) interfere with DNA and RNA synthesis by inhibiting purine metabolism. These agents affect primarily rapidly proliferating cells. Azathioprine blocks the clonal expansion of T and B lymphocytes and their development into effector cells. Its role in immunotherapy has been reduced somewhat by the use of lymphocyte activation inhibitors, but it is often used in combination with cyclosporine and corticosteroids to reduce the doses of these drugs. A small subset of patients have markedly reduced metabolism of azathioprine, which can result in a marked severity of side effects. This genetic trait can be tested for in specialized centers such as the Mayo Clinic. Mycophenolate mofetil interferes with purine synthesis. As lymphocytes have a relatively deficient purine salvage pathway as compared with other cells, it is relatively lymphocyte-selective in its action. The main attraction of this agent is its lack of nephrotoxicity.

CORTICOSTEROIDS

Corticosteroids were among the original immunosuppressive agents used in transplantation. These agents, among their many effects, induce lymphopenia by triggering apoptosis in lymphoid cells. Corticosteroids also inhibit the phagocytotic function of macrophages and, at high doses, may inhibit neutrophil degranulation. Corticosteroids are often used in high doses for the induction of immunosuppression and the treatment of episodes of acute rejection. Smaller doses are used in multidrug regimens for the maintenance of immunosuppression.

The numerous side effects of corticosteroids are well known and are partially listed in Table 66-1. The most severe side effect of these agents is the nonspecific suppression of host immune defenses, leaving the patient susceptible to a number of infections. Corticosteroids may also mask and therefore delay the treatment of severe infections such as peritonitis and meningitis.

ANTILYMPHOCYTE ANTIBODIES

The first antilymphocyte preparation used in transplantation therapy was polyclonal antilymphocyte globulin (ALG). The only ALG preparation approved by the Food and Drug Administration that is currently available is ATGAM, produced from horse serum. A more frequently used mouse monoclonal antibody preparation is OKT3, which binds to CD3+ cells. Both of these agents can be used for either induction of immunosuppression or treatment of acute rejection. OKT-3 is given as a 7- to 14-day course at a dose of 5 mg/day. The long-term use of this class of agents is precluded by antiantibody formation. Toxicities include fever, chills, and hypotension and are attributed to an initial nonspecific activation of lymphocytes, leading to release of IL-2, IL-6, and tumor necrosis factor.

Infectious and Neoplastic Complications of Immunotherapy

The time courses of various infectious and malignant complications of immunosuppression are shown in Fig. 66-1.

TRANSPLANT RELATED MALIGNANCIES

Prior to the introduction of cyclosporine and tacrolimus, CNS lymphomas and skin cancer were the malignancies most often associated with transplantation. Currently the leading neoplasm is posttransplantation lymphoproliferative disorder (PTLD). This syndrome is characterized by proliferation of B lymphocytes infected with Epstein-Barr virus. The syndrome presents with varying severity, with some cases responding to a reduction in the degree of immunosuppression to highly malignant episodes. In these cases the prognosis is dependent on the patient's ability to tolerate withdrawal of immunosuppression.

BACTERIAL INFECTIONS

Defense against bacterial infections is mediated primarily by neutrophils, macrophages, and the humoral immune system. Thus agents that primarily affect T-cell function, such as

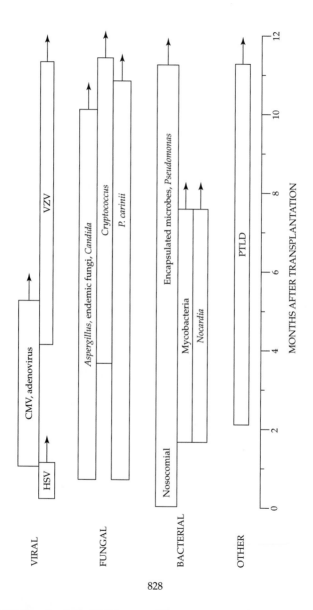

VIRAL

HSV

CMV, adenovirus

VZV

FUNGAL

Aspergillus, endemic fungi, Candida

Cryptococcus

P. carinii

BACTERIAL

Nosocomial

Encapsulated microbes, Pseudomonas

Mycobacteria

Nocardia

OTHER

PTLD

MONTHS AFTER TRANSPLANTATION

0   2   4   6   8   10   12

◀FIGURE 66-1 Usual time course of pulmonary infections following allogeneic organ transplantation. CMV, cytomegalovirus; VZV, varicella zoster virus; HSV, herpes simplex virus; PTLD, posttransplant lymphoproliferative disease. (From Duncan SR, Raffin TA: Immunosuppressive Diseases and the Lungs. In Murray and Nadel (eds): *Textbook of Respiratory Medicine*, 1994, page 2385. W. B. Saunders Company, Philadelphia, PA. With permission.)

tacrolimus and cyclosporine, are less likely to impair resistance to bacterial infections than corticosteroids and azathioprine. Bacterial infections are most often seen in the first month posttransplantation and reflect the flora of the transplantation site. Other sources of infection include the urinary tract, the respiratory system, and indwelling central venous catheters. It is also important to note that immunosuppression may mask the signs and symptoms of infections such as peritonitis and meningitis. A high degree of suspicion is required to diagnose these infections early in these patients.

FUNGAL INFECTIONS

Fungal infections usually occur within 1 to 2 months of transplantation and are more common with high-dose corticosteroid use. Repeated courses of broad-spectrum antibiotics, multiple operations, and prolonged stays in the intensive care unit (ICU) also predispose patients to fungal infections. *Candida* is the most frequent organism. Infections range from minor infections such as oral or bladder involvement, which can be treated with oral nystatin or amphotericin bladder irrigation, to invasive pneumonitis, fungemia, and intraabdominal infection. The more serious infections need to be treated with oral nystatin or amphotericin B therapy. Other fungi, such as *Aspergillus* and *Cryptococcus*, do not respond well to therapy and carry a high mortality.

VIRAL INFECTIONS

As most immunosuppressive therapies are targeted at T cells and defense against viral disease is primarily T lymphocyte–mediated, viral infections are a common problem in transplant patients. Cytomegalovirus (CMV) is the most important pathogen. Infection with this virus can be due to reactivation of CMV in a previously infected individual or to the transplantation of CMV-infected organs into an individual with no prior CMV exposure. Reactivation occurs within 1 to 4 months of transplantation and is usually milder than primary infection.

CMV may cause several different syndromes, including pneumonitis, hepatitis, nephritis, and gastrointestinal ulceration. The most common presentation, however, is fever and leukopenia, which often present with the additional features of thrombocytopenia and atypical lymphocytes. Diagnosis is confirmed by tissue invasion with nuclear inclusions seen on liver or lung biopsies.

The therapy of CMV infections depends on the severity of the disease. Many infections resolve with no treatment or with the reduction of immunosuppression. For more severe infections, the use of gancyclovir and CMV immune globulin is currently under investigation.

Many other types of herpesviruses are commonly seen in transplant recipients, including herpes simplex and varicella zoster (shingles).

PARASITIC INFECTIONS

Pneumocystis carinii pneumonia is the most common parasitic infection in the transplant recipient. This typically occurs several months after transplantation and should be suspected in any transplant patient presenting with a pulmonary infiltrate. Diagnosis can often be made with bronchoscopy with bronchoalveolar lavage. Intravenous trimethoprim/sulfmethoxazole (TMP/SMX) is the agent of first choice in treatment, but pentamidine may be used in case of allergy or other adverse reactions to TMP/SMX.

APPROACH TO PATIENTS WITH PULMONARY INFILTRATES

The most common serious infection occurring more than 1 month following transplantation is pneumonia. As pneumonia may progress rapidly in the immunocompromised host, pulmonary infiltrates need to be rapidly evaluated and treated. Infiltrates in these patients are usually diffuse and bilateral. Sputum culture is often nondiagnostic. In this case, presumptive coverage should be broadened by adding TMP/SMX to cover *Pneumocystis*. Bronchoscopy with bronchoalveolar lavage (BAL) should be performed, with transbronchial biopsy if possible. Often BAL is nondiagnostic; if so, an open-lung biopsy should be performed. This workup should be completed within 48 h of presentation.

Diagnosis and Treatment of Acute Rejection

Most rejection episodes occur within the first year after transplantation. In general, rejection episodes present with fever or symptoms and laboratory values suggesting inflammation or dysfunction of the graft. Biopsies should be used following the initial evaluation of graft function to diagnose rejection, as it can often be difficult to distinguish graft dysfunction due to rejection from dysfunction due to other causes. Initial therapy is usually high-dose corticosteroids followed by OKT3, ALG, or tacrolimus therapy if the presence of rejection is confirmed.

Organ-Specific Issues

RENAL TRANSPLANT

As renal transplant patients are generally hemodynamically stable following transplant, many of them may not require ICU admission following transplantation. As the posttransplant period may be marked by ATN, therapies with reduced nephrotoxicites are often chosen in renal transplantation. Specifically, ALG or OKT3 is often added to reduce the level of cyclosporine required. As it is free of nephrotoxicity, MMF is also often used. Rejection is rarely a cause of immediate post-transplant graft dysfunction, which is usually due to acute tubular necrosis (ATN), vascular occlusion, or obstruction of the urinary collecting system.

LIVER TRANSPLANT

Liver transplant is now the standard therapy for end-stage liver disease. As the decision to transplant is often prompted by acute complications of liver failure such as esophageal bleeding, critical care is often required in the pretransplant setting as well as in the perioperative period.

Liver transplant is a difficult and lengthy surgical procedure. Operative blood loss can be used as a means to quantify the magnitude of the surgical injury and correlates well with preoperative risk factors and postoperative prognosis. Postoperative therapy should be directed at the rapid withdrawal of invasive therapy in order to minimize iatrogenic complications. Postoperative complications include infection, encephalopathy, high-cardiac-output hypotension, pulmonary edema (both cardiogenic and noncardiogenic), and hepatorenal syndrome.

Following discharge from the ICU, the patient remains at high risk for vascular complications and cardiopulmonary decompensation. The risk of life-threatening infections persists post recovery.

Acute rejection in hepatic allografts is common and usually develops within the first month. Rejection is usually first detected by noting increases in serum values of ALT and AST. As other causes of hepatic dysfunction—such as vascular thrombosis, biliary obstruction, and cholestasis due to sepsis—can present in a similar fashion, a liver biopsy is usually performed early to confirm the presence of rejection.

LUNG TRANSPLANT

Single lung transplant is most common and is usually chosen for patients with end-stage fibrotic lung disease or chronic obstructive pulmonary disease (COPD). Double lung transplantation is still used for end-stage septic lung diseases such as cystic fibrosis, where a remaining diseased lung would infect a newly transplanted lung. In selecting donor lungs, the following criteria apply: Donor lungs must be normal by chest x-ray and must be capable of maintaining the donors Pa_{O_2} over 300 mmHg with a $F_{I_{O_2}}$ of 1.0 at a PEEP of 5 cmH_2O.

While it is advisable to have a fully primed bypass machine available during actual transplantation, cardiovascular bypass is required in only 20% of single lung transplants and can sometimes be avoided even in double lung transplants.

In the first 24 h following transplant, cardiovascular instability is often seen, along with high-cardiac-output hypotension. Pulmonary edema, both cardiogenic and from capillary leak, can also be seen. Following this initial rocky course, acute rejection can often be seen and is best diagnosed by transbronchial biopsy. In the setting of acute rejection, this demonstrates the histologic findings of perivascular lymphocytic infiltrates and varying degrees of peribronchial or bronchial mucosal inflammation.

Obliterative bronchiolitis is the major cause of late graft loss in lung transplantation and occurs most commonly in heart-lung transplants. Patients often present with malaise, dyspnea, and a progressive deterioration in FEV_1. This condition is also best diagnosed by transbronchial biopsy, which demonstrates fibrotic obliteration of the bronchioles.

HEART TRANSPLANTATION

Perioperative stability is determined in large part by donor characteristics. An ideal donor has the following characteristics: central venous pressure of 8 to 12 cmH$_2$O, systolic BP of > 100 mmHg, and inotropic support of < 10 μg/kg per min of dopamine. The physiologic response of the graft heart is influenced by its denervated state. Drugs such as atropine have no effect on the graft and the SA and AV nodal functions of digoxin are also abolished. As the rate response to stress is determined by circulating catecholamines, any increase in response to stress will be delayed and will show a persistence following resolution of the stress state. Sinus bradycardia is the most commonly seen arrhythmia posttransplant. As the transplanted heart may not be able to quickly increase rate to maintain cardiac output, cardiac output is closely linked to volume status. Isoproterenol is commonly used in these patients both for its chronotropic and inotropic effects.

Hypertension is very common following transplant. Due to the high sensitivity of these recipients to β blockers, these agents should be avoided in the treatment of this condition in favor of therapies such as salt restriction and diuretic therapy.

Approximately 50 to 60% of patients undergoing heart transplantation have an episode of acute rejection during the first 6 months. Acute rejection is diagnosed by endomyocardial biopsy, which is performed periodically for surveillance.

For a more detailed discussion, see Chap. 86 in *Principles of Critical Care,* 2d ed.

Chapter 67
TOXICOLOGY
EDWARD BOTTEI

Toxicology is a fascinating branch of medicine because of the numerous toxidromes (symptoms, signs, and laboratory findings specific to a particular toxin or poison) found in the discipline. While the majority of this chapter is dedicated to the management of specific toxins, the most important part of the poisoned patient's care is the general supportive management that all intensive care unit (ICU) patients receive.

Important General Principles

1. Supportive care is the basis of all care for the poisoned patient. Attention to the ABCs (airway, breathing, and circulation) of basic and advanced life support comes first. In a large number of poisonings, the exact poison is not immediately apparent to the physicians who initially assess and begin caring for the patient. Also, there are numerous poisons and toxins for which there are no specific antidotes.

2. The history and physical examination can provide a great many clues to the toxins/poisons involved—e.g., a history of industrial exposure or a suicide attempt. Getting collateral history from the patient's family and friends and from the police can be extremely helpful. Obtaining a history from someone who has attempted suicide can be difficult, especially when there is deliberate misinformation.

3. One must always suspect a coingestion of another poison or toxin until proven otherwise. Most patients who attempt suicide through overdose will use two or more poisons to achieve their goal. Just because the patient admits to taking an overdose of acetaminophen does not mean that he did not also take a handful of sleeping pills and washed all the pills down with rubbing alcohol.

4. Withdrawal from drugs—e.g., ethanol—can also be an-other toxicologic reason for the patient to be presenting to the ICU.

5. One must always suspect other, nontoxicologic causes for the patient's presentation. The patient who presents ine-briated with decreased mental status and a blood ethanol level of 180 mg/dL might also have a subdural hematoma from a fall, which is causing his stupor.

6. The regional poison control center should be contacted for assistance in diagnosing and treating any poisoning or overdose that is not completely familiar. Most centers are staffed around the clock with pharmacists, nurses, non-medical toxicologists, and physicians who are specially trained to deal with a tremendous variety of poisonings and exposures.

Helpful Initial Laboratory Testing

ANION GAP (AG)

The anion gap can be helpful in determining the etiology of metabolic acidosis. Calculated as $[Na^+] - [HCO_3^- + Cl^-]$, the normal value for the AG is about 12 ± 4 meq/L. This normal value can be somewhat variable depending on the sensitiv-ity of the equipment in the clinical laboratory. Also, the AG decreases by 2.5 meq/L for every 1 g/dL the patient's serum albumin is lower than 4.0 g/L. While there are many causes for an increased AG (see Chap. 57), the physician should sus-pect occult poisoning in all patients with an unexplained el-evated AG.

OSMOLAL GAP (OG)

The serum osmolality is calculated by $2 \times [Na^+] + [BUN]/2.8 + [glucose]/18 + [EtOH]/4.6$. The directly measured serum osmolality should be no more than 10 mOsm/L higher than the calculated value. If the measured value is substan-tially higher (i.e., the osmolal gap is elevated), an unex-pected low-molecular-weight compound may be present in the patient's serum, potentially indicating a toxic ingestion.

TABLE 67-1   Commonly Ingested Poisons Causing
an Increased Osmolal Gap

Mannitol	Chloroform
Trichloroethane	Chloral hydrate
Salicylates	Glycerol
Methanol	Glycine
Ethanol	Sorbitol
Isopropanol	Radiocontrast media
Acetone	
Ethylene glycol	
Paraldehyde	

Table 67-1 lists commonly ingested poisons that produce an elevated osmolal gap. The lack of an osmolal gap does not rule out poisoning by osmolal gap–producing toxins.

ARTERIAL SATURATION GAP

A standard blood gas analyzer calculates the arterial oxyhemoglobin saturation based on the Pa_{O_2}, the sample's temperature, and a standard oxygen-hemoglobin dissociation curve. Pulse oximetry, on the other hand, uses light absorption to measure the oxygen saturation; but since only two wavelengths of light are used, only two species (oxyhemoglobin and deoxyhemoglobin) can be measured. The most accurate determination is carried out by a co-oximeter, which directly measures the percentages of oxyhemoglobin, deoxyhemoglobin, carboxyhemoglobin, methemoglobin, and sulfhemoglobin. A disparity between the pulse oximetric saturation and the value reported by a standard blood gas analyzer is called an *arterial saturation gap*. When this gap is greater than 5 percent, co-oximetry is indicated to determine the concentration of abnormal hemoglobin species. In a patient with methemoglobinemia (not breathing supplemental oxygen), the pulse oximetry saturation will be lower than the calculated blood gas saturation. Conversely, patients with carbon monoxide, cyanide, and hydrogen sulfide poisoning will have a higher pulse oximetric saturation than the blood gas calculated value.

Toxicologic Screening from Urine and Blood

A rapidly acquired urine drug screen can be helpful in the diagnosis of poisonings. However, few routine urine toxicologic screens contain all the possible drugs and poisons of interest. It is important to know which drugs are not included on the drug screen run at any given hospital.

Serum levels for some more commonly encountered poisons (cyclic antidepressants, methanol, acetaminophen) are readily available at most hospitals. Other serum levels (ethylene glycol, cyanide, serum cholinesterase) need to be sent to reference laboratories, and it may take several days for the results to return. The diagnosis of many of these poisonings can be made on clinical grounds, and the treatment of such poisonings should begin promptly. Treatment should not be delayed until the test results return—the results should only confirm the previously made diagnosis.

Coma Cocktail

Initial management of any patient who presents with decreased mental status involves the administration of the "coma cocktail." This is made up of three relatively innocuous medications that can rapidly reverse common causes of mental status changes:

Dextrose: 50 mL of D_{50} W IV push
Thiamine: 100 mg IV push
Naloxone: 0.2 to 0.4 mg IV push. The dose can be repeated up to 10 mg total

Drug Elimination

Throughout the rest of the chapter, various methods for enhancing drug elimination are presented with respect to specific drugs.

GASTRIC LAVAGE (GL)

This works well if done within the first hour after ingestion. It can also be beneficial in the case of delayed gastric empty- ing [tricyclic antidepressants (TCAs) and opiates] and sus- tained release preparations. GL should not be performed when the patient cannot protect her or his airway, when the patient has already aspirated, or when the ingested material is either a caustic or a hydrocarbon. Some of the aspirated material must be sent to the laboratory for analysis.

SYRUP OF IPECAC (SOI)

This is used mainly for children rather than for adults—and only if the ingestion occurred in the recent past (1 to 2 h), and there is no doubt that the patient will continue to be able to protect her or his airway while vomiting. SOI is dosed as 30 mL followed by 16 oz of water.

ACTIVATED CHARCOAL (AC)

Given orally, and usually with a cathartic, AC acts as a non- specific adsorbent to bind any free toxin left in the lumen of the gastrointestinal (GI) tract or passing through the entero- hepatic circulation. The airway must be protected by the pa- tient's reflexes or an endotracheal tube, since aspiration of AC can lead to severe pneumonitis. AC is dosed as 1 g/kg.

WHOLE-BOWEL IRRIGATION (WBI)

This is performed as a way to cleanse the GI tract of toxins. It is especially helpful when the poison is a sustained-released form of a medication and in people who are transporting or hiding drugs from law enforcement officers. WBI must not be performed in those patients with ileus, bowel perforation, or GI hemorrhage. It is dosed as magnesium sulfate, 10% so- lution, 2 to 3 mL/kg; sorbitol, 70% solution, 1 to 2 mL/kg; or polyethylene glycol, 1 to 2 L/h.

URINARY PH CHANGES AND FORCED DIURESIS

These measures are recommended for toxins with extensive renal tubular reabsorption or renal excretion. They are of unproven benefit and can potentially cause harm via fluid and electrolyte shifts and imbalances. Alkalinization with sodium bicarbonate can cause alkalemia, hypernatremia, volume overload, and hypokalemia. The hypokalemia can prevent alkalinization of the urine because the kidney will exchange H^+ for K^+ in the distal nephron. Acidification of the urine can potentiate the detrimental effects of myoglobinuria. Table 67-2 lists drugs whose elimination is increased via manipulation of urinary pH. Alkalinization is achieved by 1 to 2 meq/kg of 8.4% $NaHCO_3$ every 3 to 4 h.

HEMODIALYSIS (HD)

HD works well with water-soluble, non-protein-bound toxins. It is also beneficial when there are accompanying acid/base disorders or renal failure. Maximum clearance of the toxin via HD is approximately 10 mL/min.

HEMOPERFUSION (HP)

This method is much better at removing toxins then HD. It works by direct contact between the patient's blood and AC filters. It can therefore remove both water and lipid soluble toxins at a clearance rate of 200 to 400 mL/min.

TABLE 67-2 Drugs Whose Elimination Is Increased by Acidic or Alkaline Urine

Alkaline Urine	Acidic Urine
Fluoride	Amphetamines
Isoniazid	Bismuth
Methotrexate	Ephedrine
Phenobarbital	Flecanide
Primidone	Nicotine
Quinolone antibiotics	Phencyclidine
Salicylic acid	Quinine
Uranium	

HEMOFILTRATION (HF)

HF can remove larger molecules, up to 6000 daltons, and may be of benefit when the toxin has a large volume of distribution or is highly bound in the tissues.

Specific antidotes for specific poisons are shown in Table 67-3.

Treatment of Specific Toxicities: Acetaminophen (N-Acetyl-p-Aminophenol, APAP)

MECHANISM

APAP is metabolized by the cytochrome P450 oxidase system into a quinone radical. It is normally detoxified by conjugation with glutathione, but when the ingestion is massive,

TABLE 67-3 Specific Antidotes for Specific Poisons

Toxin	Antidote
Methanol and ethylene glycol	Ethanol and 4-methylpyrrazole
Iron	Desferoxamine
Fluoride	Calcium gluconate
Cyanide	Sodium nitrite, amyl nitrite, and sodium thiosulfate
Acetaminophen	*N*-acetylcysteine
Organophophate insecticides	Atropine and pralidoxime
Opiates	Naloxone
Benzodiazepines	Flumazenil
Digoxin	Digoxin-specific antibodies (FAB)
β-Blockers and calcium-channel blockers	Glucagon, calcium gluconate, or chloride
Neuroleptic malignant syndrome	Dantrolene
Isoniazid	Vitamin B_6 (pyridoxine)
Warfarin	Vitamin K
Methemoglobinemia	Methylene Blue
Dystonic reactions	Diphenhydramine
Sulfanyl ureas	Diazoxide
Methotrexate and trimethoprim	Folinic acid

the radical conjugates with hepatic proteins, leading to hepatocyte death.

SIGNS AND SYMPTOMS

Phase One—First 24 Hours

Nausea, vomiting, diarrhea, anorexia, malaise, pallor, and diaphoresis are typical early symptoms. However, these symptoms can be masked by coingestants.

Phase Two—24 to 72 Hours

Nausea and vomiting resolve but malaise can persist. Right-upper-quadrant pain and tenderness develop; there can also be elevation in the transaminases and total bilirubin and prolongation of the prothrombin time.

Phase Three—72 to 96 Hours

Hepatic necrosis leading to hepatic encephalopathy, jaundice, disseminated intravascular coagulation (DIC), and, rarely, hemorrhagic pancreatitis, myocardial necrosis, and oliguric renal failure may be seen. Transaminase levels usually peak in this phase.

Phase Four—4 Days to 2 Weeks

If the patient does not die of liver failure in phase three, he or she can experience either a return to normal function of the liver or progressive destruction of liver parenchyma with lowering of enzymes but increasing ammonia, PT, and bilirubin.

RUMACK-MATTHEW NOMOGRAM
(FIG. 67-1)

This nomogram allows a stratification of risk for hepatotoxicity based on serum acetaminophen levels compared with time after ingestion. If any value falls above the lower line of the nomogram, a full course of oral N-acetylcysteine (NAC) is indicated. Note that levels drawn prior to 4 h after ingestion are uninterpretable, since the body has not fully absorbed and distributed the ingested APAP. Also, patients in phases two and three may have no APAP detectable in their serum.

HEPATOTOXIC DOSE

In most healthy adults, the potentially hepatotoxic ingestion of APAP is considered to be in the range of 8 to 10 g. In chronic alcoholics, people taking drugs that induce the cytochrome P450 system, and chronic APAP users, the potentially toxic dose can be as small as 5 to 6 g. Hepatotoxic levels are 200 μg/mL at 4 h postingestion or 50 μg/mL at 12 h.

TREATMENT

GL should be conducted if possible within 4 h of ingestion. AC is effective in binding residual APAP but can also bind NAC. Therefore administer the AC at least 2 h before oral NAC. HP effectively removes APAP from the serum but is not used on a regular basis, since the specific antidote *N*-acetylcysteine (NAC) is so effective.

NAC is proven very effective at repletion of the liver's glutathione stores and thus prevention of liver damage if administered within the first 8 to 10 h after ingestion. After 12 to 16 h, NAC is less effective at preventing hepatic injury but may limit the degree of injury sustained when administered even as late as 24 h postingestion.

Oral therapy is currently the main route of treatment in the U.S.A. (supplied as a 10% or 20% solution, but diluted to 5%):

Initial loading dose: 140 mg/kg
Maintenance dosing: 70 mg/kg q4 h for 17 additional doses

If vomiting prevents administration of the NAC, high-dose metoclopramide (1 to 2 mg/kg IV) can be tried.

The maintenance dosing can be discontinued after six doses if there is no evidence of hepatotoxicity and the serum APAP level is zero. There are shorter courses for oral administration of NAC (48 h) and intravenous protocols [not yet approved by the Food and Drug Administration (FDA)] that have been shown to be safe and effective.

Alcohols

MECHANISM

Methanol (MeOH) and ethylene glycol (EG) are metabolized by alcohol dehydrogenase into formic acid and formaldehyde

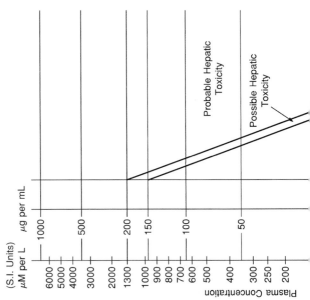

FIGURE 67-1 The Rumack-Matthew nomogram for predicting acetaminophen hepatoxicity. This nomogram allows for stratification of patients into categories of probable hepatic toxicity, possible hepatic toxicity, and no hepatic toxicity based on the relationship between acetaminophen level and time after ingestion. When this relationship is known, n-acetylcysteine therapy is indicated for acetaminophen levels above the lower nomogram line. N-acetylcys-

(for MeOH) or oxalic and glycolic acids (for EG). These metabolites have direct toxic effects on various organ systems, causing a severe metabolic acidosis, which can lead to death. Isopropanol (ISOP) is metabolized into acetone, which acts directly as a central nervous system (CNS) and cardiovascular depressant.

SIGNS AND SYMPTOMS

Methanol

There is usually a latent period of 12 to 24 h between the time of ingestion and the onset of symptoms. The most common

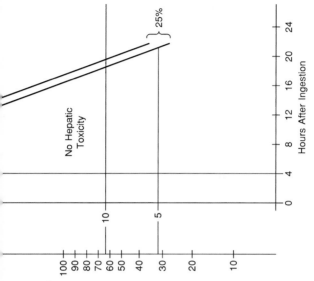

teine should also be given if there is $> 5\,\mu g/mL$ acetaminophen and an unknown time of ingestion (but < 24 h) and if there is a history of overdose and a serum acetaminophen level is not immediately available. Serum levels obtained prior to 4 hours postingestion are uninterpretable because of ongoing absorption and distribution of the drug. *(From Rumack BH: Pediatric Clin North Am 33:698, 1986, with permission.)*

symptoms include visual loss, optic nerve swelling, pancreatitis, seizures, and coma. Laboratory data reveal a severe metabolic acidosis with an anion gap and an osmolal gap.

Ethylene Glycol

The latent period between ingestion and symptoms appearing is approximately 1 to 12 h. The earliest symptoms include the appearance of inebriation, the notable absence of a smell of alcohol on the breath, and gastritis with vomiting. The patient can develop cerebral edema leading to lethargy, seizures, and coma. Laboratory data reveal a severe anion gap metabolic acidosis with an osmolal gap. The degree of hypocalcemia can be astounding and leads to arrhythmias and tetany. Urinalysis commonly but not always finds calcium oxalate crystalluria. If untreated, the patient develops progressive end-organ involvement in the first 1 to 2 days with arrhythmias and conduction disturbances, myocardial dysfunction, and pulmonary edema. By day 2 to 3, the kidneys fail.

Isopropanol

There is a rapid onset of symptoms after isopropanol ingestion, usually within 1 h. The most notable finding is ketonemia, leading to a fruity-smelling odor on the breath. Other early symptoms include hemorrhagic gastritis, peripheral vasodilation, pinpoint unreactive pupils, and mental status changes including slurred speech, ataxia, stupor, and coma. Laboratory studies reveal a mild anion gap metabolic acidosis with an osmolal gap. Urinalysis detects the presence of ketones. If left untreated, this will progress to hypotension, respiratory arrest, and finally death.

Lethal Dose

MeOH: 1 to 5 g/kg (= 1.3 to 6.3 mL/kg of 100% solution). Lethal serum level: 80 to 100 mg/dL

EG: 1.5 g/kg (= 1.4 mL/kg of 95% solution). Lethal serum level: 200 mg/dL

ISOP: 1.1 to 2.2 g/kg (= 2 to 4 mL/kg of 70% solution). Lethal serum level: 400 mg/dL

Treatment

The primary goal of therapy for MeOH and EG poisoning is to inhibit the conversion of the parent compound into its toxic organic acid metabolites. This is achieved with ethanol, which competes with the other alcohols for the alcohol dehydrogenase enzyme. The ethanol is metabolized and the other alcohols are either excreted unchanged or dialyzed. The target serum ethanol concentration is 100 to 150 mg/dL. The formula for loading and maintaining ethanol therapy listed below presumes that the patient started with a serum ethanol level of zero. Higher maintenance doses are needed for the chronic alcoholic and also for the patient on dialysis.

Load: 0.6 to 0.9 g/kg (7.5 to 11.2 mL/kg of 10% solution) IV
Maintenance: Nonalcoholic: 66 to 130 mg/kg per hour (= 0.85 to 1.625 mL/kg per hour of 10% solution) IV
Alcoholic: 100 to 154 mg/kg per hour (1.25 to 1.93 mL/kg per hour of 10% solution)
Double the above maintenance doses when the patient is on HD.

Complications of ethanol therapy include hypoglycemia, hyponatremia, and dehydration. Because ISOP is not metabolized into an organic acid, ethanol therapy is *not* indicated for ISOP intoxications.

Hemodialysis is very effective and is usually employed when the patient has evidence of end-organ involvement (coma, hypotension, renal failure), the osmolal gap is greater than 10, or serum levels are greater than 40 mg/dL for MeOH, greater than 50 mg/dL for EG, or greater than 400 mg/dL for ISOP.

4-Methylpyrazole is a chemical inhibitor of alcohol dehydrogenase that has fewer side effects than ethanol therapy, especially with regard to central nervous system (CNS) depression. It is currently FDA-approved only for EG intoxications. There are two dosing regimens:

Orally: 20 mg/kg per day
IV: 9 mg/kg q12h

Treatment with calcium, NaHCO$_3$, thiamine, folate, and pyridoxine can potentially hasten the patient's recovery, as these compounds serve as metabolic cofactors for the detoxification and elimination of the alcohol.

Amphetamines

MECHANISM

Amphetamines cause CNS stimulation, catecholamine release and inhibition of reuptake, and monoamine oxidase (MAO) inhibition.

SIGNS AND SYMPTOMS

The most common effects of amphetamine use and overdose are agitation, anxiety, tremor, euphoria, agitation, irritability, and confusion. The patient may also display mydriasis, tachycardia, arrhythmias, hypertension, hyperreflexia, hyperthermia, rhabdomyolysis, renal failure, myocardial ischemia, seizures, coagulopathy, and cerebral bleeds.

TOXIC DOSE

In general, the toxic dose is only slightly higher than the therapeutic dose. Toxic doses can be higher in patients with a tolerance to these drugs.

TREATMENT

Calming the patient is the first concern; it is usually achieved pharmacologically. The drugs of choice for agitation are benzodiazepines or phenothiazines. If calming the patient does not sufficiently bring hypertension under control, phentolamine and nitroprusside can be used. Esmolol or propanolol can be used to treat persistent tachycardia.

Use of AC can be helpful in decontamination of the GI tract if any pills remain.

SOI is contraindicated because of the possibility of seizures. HD and HP are not effective.

Barbiturates

MECHANISM

Barbiturates directly depress the CNS through enhanced gamma-aminobutyric acid (GABA) activity. Hypotension occurs through inhibition of central sympathetic tone and myocardial depression.

SIGNS AND SYMPTOMS

The most pronounced symptoms from barbiturate ingestion are a decreased sensorium, slurred speech, and ataxia. The patient may develop hypothermia, hypotension, bradycardia, flaccid hyporeflexia, coma, and apnea if not treated. Laboratory data reveal a mixed metabolic and respiratory acidosis. An interesting finding includes barbiturate-related skin blisters that result from tissue hypoxia and local pressure.

LETHAL DOSE

The lethal dose is somewhat variable but is approximately 5 to 10 times the normal hypnotic dose. Patients with tolerance to barbiturates will need larger doses to produce toxicity.

TREATMENT

Treatment is primarily supportive. GL and AC can decrease absorption. HP can remove the barbiturate from the serum but is usually reserved for severe overdoses with persistent hypotension. Alkalinization of urine increases urinary elimination of phenobarbital but none of the other barbiturates.

Benzodiazepines (BDZs)

MECHANISM

BDZs exert their effect by enhancing the inhibitory effect of GABA in the CNS.

SIGNS AND SYMPTOMS

The patient with a BDZ overdose can present with slurred speech, hyporeflexia, hypothermia, small to midrange pupils, lethargy, coma, and respiratory arrest.

LETHAL DOSE

Large oral doses (15 to 20 times the therapeutic dose) can be tolerated fairly well, but intravenous administration can produce toxicity at relatively small doses.

TREATMENT

GL and AC are effective in treating BDZ overdoses. SOI is contraindicated in ingestions of short-acting BDZs because of the possibility that the patient will rapidly go into a coma.

Forced diuresis, HD, and HP are ineffective in removing BDZs from the patient's system.

Flumazenil, a BDZ antagonist, can be both diagnostic and therapeutic, but there is always a concern of precipitating seizures in a patient who has coingested another drug that can lower the seizure threshold. Because of the greater possibility of inducing seizures in patients who are chronic BDZ users, flumazenil is not recommended for the chronic BDZ user.

Flumazenil is administered as 0.2 mg IV push, then 0.3 mg IV push after 30 s if there has been no response, then 0.5 mg IV push every 30 to 60 s up to a total of 3 mg. A small minority of patients will respond to doses greater than 3 mg. The dose of flumazenil used should be lowered in patients with hepatic dysfunction.

After treatment with flumazenil, the physician must monitor for resedation. If this happens, flumazenil is restarted at the initial dosing regimen given above. If the patient persistently needs redosing of the flumazenil to reverse the symptoms, an intravenous infusion at 0.1 to 0.5 mg/h can be substituted for intermittent boluses.

Carbon Monoxide (CO)

MECHANISM

CO is a colorless, odorless, tasteless, nonirritating gas commonly encountered in victims exposed to smoke, fumes from heaters that are poorly ventilated or do not completely burn fossil fuels, and car exhaust.

CO binds reversibly to and inhibits various cellular enzymes, especially cytochrome oxidase. A second mechanism of toxicity is to displace oxygen from hemoglobin with an affinity for hemoglobin 240 times that of oxygen's. Its affinity for fetal hemoglobin is even higher than that for adult hemoglobin.

SIGNS AND SYMPTOMS

The patient's presentation will depend on the concentration of CO inhaled, the duration of exposure, and the patient's minute ventilation. While carboxyhemoglobin levels in the blood correlate poorly with severity of toxicity, some generalizations can be made with regard to carboxyhemoglobin level and symptoms:

Up to 5% (as seen in heavy smokers) is well tolerated.

5 to 10% can produce headaches and mild dyspnea.

10 to 30% presents with severe headaches, dizziness, weakness, dyspnea, irritability, and cardiac ischemia.

At levels > 50%, coma, seizures, and cardiovascular collapse are seen.

Pulse oximetry tends to overestimate the true arterial oxyhemoglobin saturation in patients with CO poisoning because the CO creates an "arteriolization" of the venous blood, which results in the cherry-red color of the blood. The pulse oximeter interprets this very red-colored blood as oxygenated hemoglobin, not carboxyhemoglobin, and gives a high saturation percentage. When a blood sample is sent through a co-oximeter, there will be a normal or high Pa_{O_2} and a low oxyhemoglobin percentage because of the CO bound to hemoglobin. Of note, venous blood can accurately predict the arterial carboxyhemoglobin level.

LETHAL LEVEL

Death is imminent if the carboxyhemoglobin level is 80%. This corresponds to an atmospheric concentration of about 1900 ppm (parts per million). Immediate threat to life and health occurs at 1500 ppm.

TREATMENT

The first priority is to remove the victim from the exposure area. Treatment with oxygen hastens the elimination of CO from the body. Carboxyhemoglobin's half-life is 4 to 6 h on room air but falls to 40 to 60 min with 100% $F_{I_{O_2}}$. With hyperbaric oxygen (HBO), half-life falls to 15 to 30 min.

HBO produces a Pa_{O_2} of 2000 torr in the arterial blood and tissue tensions of 400 mmHg. Although the literature is conflicting as to whether there is a long-term benefit from HBO, most experts would recommend at least one HBO treatment provided that it is available in an expeditious and safe manner. There is also a debate about whether patients should receive one versus multiple treatments.

The majority of patients recover within 2 to 3 days, but despite appropriate treatment as many as 30 percent will develop delayed neurologic sequelae of hypoxic brain injury, sometimes permanently. There is currently no way to predict which patients will develop these problems. These delayed symptoms include persistent vegetative state, parkinsonism, memory deficits, behavioral changes, and hearing loss.

Cocaine

MECHANISM

Cocaine works via direct CNS stimulation and through inhibition of neuronal reuptake of catecholamines. Because of this, cocaine intoxication can present very much like amphetamine overdose.

SIGNS AND SYMPTOMS

Central nervous system: Euphoria, anxiety, agitation, psychosis, delirium, seizures, ischemic cerebral infarction, intracerebral hemorrhage, SAH.

Seizures induced by cocaine intoxication can be complicated by hyperthermia, rhabdomyolysis with myoglobinuria and CPKs > 10,000 U/L, hepatic dysfunction, renal failure, and disseminated intravascular coagulation (DIC). These complications portend a very poor prognosis.

Cardiovascular: Cardiac arrhythmias (supraventricular and ventricular), chest pain, congestive heart failure, pulmonary hypertension, endocarditis, aortic dissection, tachycardia, hypertension, vasospasm, and perhaps vasculitis.

Electrocardiographic (ECG) changes seen with cocaine use include LVH, ST- and T-wave changes, Q waves, and increased QRS voltage.

Although most patients with cocaine-induced chest pain probably do not have coronary artery disease, there are no validated means for stratifying the risk of underlying heart disease. Therefore all patients with cocaine use and chest pain should be evaluated for myocardial ischemia/infarction.

Pulmonary: Status asthmaticus, stridor from upper airway obstruction, barotrauma with pneumothorax or pneumomediastinum, pulmonary edema, and alveolar hemorrhage. An acute pulmonary syndrome can result from smoking crack cocaine; this involves dyspnea, diffuse lung infiltrates, and hemoptysis. It is thought to be a direct toxic effect on the lung parenchyma, which causes noncardiogenic pulmonary edema.

Other systems: Rarely ischemic colitis, renal infarction, nasal septum perforation, localized areas of skin necrosis, sinusitis, and botulism.

LETHAL DOSE

The lethal dose is somewhat variable but the maximum recommended dose for nasal anesthesia is 100 to 200 mg. Doses of 1 g or more tend to be lethal.

TREATMENT

Supportive treatment is paramount for the cocaine-intoxicated patient. BDZs can be used to treat the agitation and seizures. Haloperidol has not been shown to be of benefit for treating agitation. If seizures cannot be controlled with medications, paralysis (with electroencephalographic monitoring) might be necessary. Rapid cooling (cold water, fans, disrobing) should be employed to prevent complications from hyperthermia.

Chest pain can be treated with nitrates and calcium channel blockers. Tachycardia without myocardial ischemia or chest pain can be treated cautiously with beta blockers. However beta blockers alone leave the alpha stimulation unopposed and may exacerbate hypertension. If hypertension is not responsive to nitrates or calcium channel blockers, then nitroprusside with a beta blocker, phentolamine alone, or phentolamine with a beta blocker can be tried. All three regimens are reported to work well for HTN and myocardial ischemia.

Beta agonists and steroids effectively treat bronchospasm.

AC is recommended only if the patient is known or suspected to be carrying cocaine in the GI tract—i.e., a "packer" or a "stuffer." WBI with polyethylene glycol (not in the presence of ileus, perforation, or GI hemorrhage) is very effective

at clearing retained cocaine packages from the bowel. Endoscopic removal of cocaine packets is not recommended because of the risk of tearing the packets open. After it is believed that all of the cocaine packets have been flushed from
the patient's GI tract, a CT scan of the abdomen should be
performed for confirmation. Plain x-rays are neither sensitive
nor specific enough to exclude retained packets. Of note,
polyethylene glycol (PEG) displaces cocaine from AC.

HD and HP are not effective in cocaine intoxication.

Cyanide

MECHANISM

Cyanide (CN) binds to cytochrome oxidase and prevents aerobic oxygen utilization. The rhodenase enzyme in the liver
converts CN into thiocyanate (in the presence of sulfur),
which is then renally excreted.

SIGNS AND SYMPTOMS

There are four main modes of CN exposure: inhalation of hydrogen cyanide gas, oral ingestion of a salt form, sodium nitroprusside infusion, and cutaneous exposure. The mode by
which the patient is exposed to CN will determine the amount
and rate of absorption. These two factors, in turn, determine
how symptomatic the patient will be and how long he or she
must be observed.

If the patient is asymptomatic after an inhalational exposure, he or she will usually require no treatment and can be
discharged after observation. After oral ingestion, the patient
can develop symptoms either immediately or only after
several hours. Initial nitroprusside infusions rarely produce
rapid CN toxicity at infusion rates of less than 10 μg/kg per
minute. However, toxicity can begin at as low as 2 to 4 μg/kg
per minute after 3 hours of therapy. Therefore, CN and thiocyanate levels should be followed in any patient on a sustained nitroprusside infusion at a dose greater than this. Cutaneous exposures produce symptoms slowly.

At low levels of exposure, CN acts as a respiratory and
CNS stimulant. It can also produce anxiety, dyspnea,
headache, confusion, tachycardia, and hypertension. The clas-

sic sign of the scent of bitter almonds is present in only a minority of cases.

High concentrations of CN leads to a physiologically depressed state, with stupor, coma, seizures, fixed and dilated pupils, hypoventilation, hypotension, bradycardia, heart block, and ventricular arrhythmias. High-level exposures result in a severe lactic acidosis and high mixed venous oxygen tension with arteriolization of venous blood. Death results from coma and cardiovascular collapse.

Thiocyanate toxicity (levels greater than 50 to 100 mg/L), usually seen in patients with renal insufficiency, causes confusion, somnolence, seizures, and hyperreflexia.

LETHAL LEVEL

Immediate threat to life occurs at 50 ppm in the atmosphere. Ingestion of about 200 mg of the potassium or sodium salt is lethal. Lethal serum levels are generally 0.5 to 1.0 mg/L.

TREATMENT

The goal of treatment is to remove CN from cytochrome oxidase and convert it into the less toxic thiocyanate. Amyl and sodium nitrite are administered to induce methemoglobin. The methemoglobin acts as a scavenger of unbound cyanide. Amyl nitrite is supplied in capsule form, which is crushed and inhaled for 15 to 30 s with 30 s rest between inhalations. Sodium nitrite is infused as 300 mg IV over 3 min. The sodium nitrite dose can be repeated at half the initial intravenous dose after 2 h if needed. The goal is to achieve a methemoglobin level of 25 to 30 percent.

Sodium thiosulfate acts as a sulfur donor to rhodenase; 12.5 g (50 mL of 25% solution) is given intravenously. Half the initial intravenous dose can be repeated after 2 h if needed.

Oxygen is proven to help, but HBO is yet unproven.

Hydroxycobalamin (the vitamin B_{12} precursor) chelates CN to form the nontoxic cyanocobalamin. This drug is still relatively unknown with regard to its safety and efficacy. It can produce an acute allergic reaction and reddish discoloration of skin, mucous membranes, and urine. It can also produce slight hypertension and slight bradycardia. A one-time dose of 4 to 5 g is given intravenously.

Dicobalt ethylenediaminetetraacetate (EDTA) is a potent chelator of CN. 300 to 600 mg IV over 1 min is administered and followed by 300 mg again in 2 h if needed. This is also unproven in acute CN toxicity and can have the side effects of arrhythmias, nausea and vomiting, and allergic reactions.

Thiocyanate can be dialyzed effectively, but HD and HP are not beneficial in CN poisoning alone.

Cyclic Antidepressants

MECHANISM

Cyclic antidepressants (CAs) primarily affect the CNS by direct anticholinergic effects and by blocking reuptake of norepinephrine and serotonin. The cardiovascular system is affected by these same mechanisms but also by peripheral alpha blockade and as a cellular membrane depressant. The GI system is primarily affected by the anticholinergic effects.

SIGNS AND SYMPTOMS

Symptoms begin within 6 h after ingestion. If the patient is asymptomatic at 6 h, it is unlikely that he or she will develop any symptoms at all.

The anticholinergic symptoms commonly encountered are mydriasis, blurry vision, fever, dry skin and mucous membranes, lethargy, delirium, coma, tachycardia, ileus, myoclonus, and urinary retention.

Seizures are common and range from self-limited, short-term seizures to prolonged status epilepticus refractory to multiple medications. The muscle rigidity from these seizures can cause severe hyperthermia, rhabdomyolysis, brain injury, and death.

Cardiovascular manifestations are primarily electrocardiographic: tachycarda; prolonged QRS, QTc, and PR intervals; right bundle-branch block; various atrioventricular (AV) blocks; and rarely torsades de pointes. A limb-lead QRS duration greater than 0.12 s indicates serious CA intoxication. When the maximum QRS duration is less than 0.1 s, it is rare that the patient will develop seizures or ventricular arrhythmias. The QRS duration is usually a better indicator of severity than are the serum levels.

Pulmonary edema is common, as is hypotension refractory to fluid and vasoactive drug therapy. Concomitant metabolic or respiratory acidosis from any cause increases the amount of free drug in the serum and can worsen the patient's course and prognosis.

TOXIC DOSE

The usual doses causing toxicity are 10 to 20 mg/kg. Serious effects are seen when the total serum level of the parent compound and its metabolites reaches 1000 ng/mL.

TREATMENT

The major causes of mortality are arrhythmia, cardiovascular collapse, and intractable seizures. If the QRS is widened or the patient is hypotensive, sodium bicarbonate should be administered immediately. The dosing of $NaHCO_3$ is 1 to 2 meq/kg IV, and this can be repeated until the serum pH is in the target range of 7.5 or the QRS has returned to a normal duration. Even after correction of hypotension and ECG changes, the patient's ECG should be monitored for at least 48 to 72 h.

Advanced cardiac life support (ACLS) protocols should be modified in patients with CA poisoning: bretylium can cause or worsen hypotension; procainamide, quinidine, and disopyramide are not used because of added cardiac toxicity; lidocaine is the drug of choice for ventricular arrhythmias; phenytoin is recommended as a second-line antiarrhythmic, but support for its use is mainly from anecdotal reports. Physostigmine, previously recommended, is not used because of worsening or lethal effects on the conduction system.

When hypotension is refractory to intravenous fluid, preferred vasoactive drugs are norepinephrine and phenylephrine. These patients have depleted presynaptic stores of neurotransmitters, so dopamine is not effective. CAs inhibit reuptake of catechols and therefore enhance the pressor response to vasoactive drugs.

Seizures should be treated aggressively with BDZs. Phenytoin can be used cautiously in refractory seizures. Paralysis (with EEG monitoring) is indicated if the seizures persist.

HD and HP are not effective in CA overdose because a large fraction of the drugs is highly protein- and lipid-bound.

Digoxin

MECHANISM

Digoxin causes its toxic effects by increasing vagal tone, decreasing sinoatrial and atrioventricular nodal conduction, increasing Purkinje fiber irritability, and causing hyperkalemia. Digoxin has a long half-life, is highly tissue-bound, and is renally cleared. Anything that causes or worsens renal failure or alters digoxin's tissue binding (especially drug interactions) can precipitate digoxin toxicity.

SIGNS AND SYMPTOMS

Digoxin toxicity can cause fatigue, anorexia, nausea, vomiting, diarrhea, abdominal pain, blurry vision, visual color changes (the classic yellow halo around lights), headaches, dizziness, delirium, and cardiac arrhythmias (especially AV blocks). Massive ingestion causes hyperkalemia.

Toxicity is potentiated by hypokalemia, hypomagnesemia, myocardial disease, old age, hypothyroidism, hypoxemia, hypercalcemia, and hypernatremia. Serum levels correlate very well with toxicity.

LETHAL DOSE

Single ingestions of 3 mg or more usually result in death.

TREATMENT

Supportive measures for digoxin intoxication include correction of both hypokalemia and hyperkalemia. Calcium should not be used for the treatment of hyperkalemia as it can worsen ventricular arrhythmias. Cardiac pacing is indicated for severe bradycardia refractory to atropine. The antiarrhythmics of choice for ventricular arrhythmias are lidocaine and then phenytoin.

Gut decontamination with GL and AC can be enhanced by the administration of cholestyramine, which binds digoxin very well. HD and HP are not helpful in digoxin overdoses.

There are digoxin-specific antibodies that bind both free and tissue-bound digoxin, The antibody-digoxin complexes are then renally excreted.

After digoxin antibodies are administered, the total serum digoxin level (the test run by most laboratories) will be very high because both free and antibody-bound digoxin in the serum are being measured. Free digoxin levels, which correlate with symptoms and toxicity, are usually run at a reference laboratory.

Methemoglobinemia

MECHANISM

In methemoglobinemia (MetHb), the iron in hemoglobin is oxidized from its normal Fe^{2+} to Fe^{3+}, which is incapable of binding O_2. This oxidative change also shifts the oxyhemoglobin dissociation curve to the left. The congenital forms of MetHb include NADH cytochrome b5 reductase (also called methemoglobin reductase) deficiency, or hereditary hemoglobin M disease. MetHb is more often acquired from oxidant drugs (see Table 67-4). People with G6PD deficiency are more susceptible to MetHb when exposed to oxidants.

TABLE 67-4   Methemoglobin-Inducing Drugs/Chemicals

Amyl nitrite	Silver nitrate
Dapsone	Naphthalene
Lidocaine	Nitrous oxide
Nitroglycerine	Trinitrotoluene
Nitroprusside	Butyl nitrite
Phenacetin	Sulfonamides
Phenazopyridine	Aniline dyes
Prilocaine	Isobutyl nitrite
Chloroquine	Nitrophenol
Primaquine	Flutamide
Phenytoin	Metochlopramide
Benzocaine	Sodium chlorate
Foods with nitrates and nitrites	
Fire via direct oxidation	
Oral hypoglycemics	

SIGNS AND SYMPTOMS

At MetHb levels less then 15%, the patients are usually asymptomatic but look cyanotic. Between 20 and 50% MetHb, patients will experience fatigue, dizziness, weakness, dyspnea, and headaches. At levels greater than 50%, confusion, seizures, and death ensue.

MetHb classically gives the patient's blood a chocolate-brown color. When the MetHb level is approximately 20% or more, pulse oximetry will typically give a value of 82 to 86% saturation despite the patient's obvious cyanosis. This occurs because the oximeter interprets the chocolate brown color as a mixture of oxy- and deoxyhemoglobin corresponding to a saturation of 82 to 86%. Supplemental oxygen usually does not change the pulse oximeter's analysis. An arterial blood gas sample must be analyzed via a co-oximeter to measure the amount of MetHb directly.

TREATMENT

Definitive treatment involves removal of the offending agent and treatment to reduce the iron to its $^{+2}$ state. Methylene blue 1 to 2 mg/kg given intravenously should lead to a response within 30 to 60 min. This dose can be repeated every 30 to 60 min up to 5 to 7 mg/kg. At doses above 5 to 7 mg/kg, methylene blue can act as an oxidant and make the MetHb worse. Patients who fail to respond to methylene blue treatment are usually either undertreated or inadequately decontaminated. Other, rarer causes of failure to respond to methylene blue include chlorate poisoning, sulfhemoglobin, the hereditary forms of MetHb, and G6PD deficiency. In general, methylene blue is contraindicated in patients with G6PD deficiency because of the risk of hemolysis.

Therapy for patients who fail to respond to methylene blue includes HBO and exchange transfusion.

Opiates

MECHANISM

Opiates depress mental status and respiratory drive via opiate receptors in the CNS.

SIGNS AND SYMPTOMS

Common symptoms of opiate overdose include lethargy, coma, hypoactive bowel sounds, alveolar hypoventilation, respiratory arrest, and acute noncardiogenic pulmonary edema caused by an unknown mechanism. Noncardiogenic pulmonary edema can mimic aspiration pneumonia, a common occurrence in the obtunded patient. Pinpoint pupils are very commonly found, but lack of miosis does not rule out opiate intoxication.

Less common findings include hypotension and bradycardia, rhabdomyolysis, muscle flaccidity, hypothermia, and occasionally seizures (only with meperidine, propoxyphene, or dextromethorphan).

LETHAL DOSE

The lethal dose, based on the patient's tolerance of the drugs, is extremely variable.

TREATMENT

Naloxone, a central and peripheral opioid antagonist, is the drug of choice for narcotic overdose. The initial dose is 0.2 to 0.4 mg/kg IV. A lower dose should be used if the physician suspects opioid dependence or a stimulant coingestion. A dose of 1 to 2 mg IV can be repeated in 2 to 3 min if there was no response to the initial dose. If there is no response after a total of 10 mg, opiates can be excluded as a cause of the patient's problem. Naloxone's effects last 1 to 4 h, but redosing every 30 to 60 min is occasionally needed to prevent resedation. A naloxone infusion can be started at 0.4 to 0.8 mg/h if needed.

GL should be performed only if the obtunded patient's airway can be protected.

HD and HP are not effective in opiate overdose.

Organophosphates and Carbamate Insecticides

MECHANISM

Organophosphates (OP) irreversibly bind to and inhibit acetylcholinesterase (AChE). Carbamates differ in that they are reversible inhibitors of acetylcholine. This inhibition of AChE causes excessive accumulation of ACh at the neural end plates.

SIGNS AND SYMPTOMS

The symptom profiles for OPs and carbamates are virtually the same except that carbamates have no CNS toxicity because of their poor penetration into the CNS. Symptoms usually develop within the first 12 to 24 h but can occur rapidly with large exposures.

Muscarinic effects include the "SLUDGE" symptoms (excessive salivation, lacrimation, urination, defecation, GI-cramping, and emesis) and also vomiting, bronchospasm, bronchorrhea, miosis with blurry vision, and bradycardia. Nicotinic effects include muscle fasciculations, weakness, and tachycardia. CNS effects include dizziness, depressed mental status, anxiety, and psychosis.

Heart block and ST and T wave abnormalities, along with hyperglycemia, are also seen in OP poisoning.

TREATMENT

The most important point of treatment after the ABCs is decontamination. This is not only to protect the patient from ongoing poisoning but also to prevent health care workers from being poisoned also.

Atropine antagonizes acetycholine only at the muscarinic receptors but usually does not worsen fasciculations, hypertension, or tachycardia. Atropine is given as a 1 to 2 mg IV push every 5 to 10 min until mydriasis, dry mouth, and an increased heart rate are observed. Frequent redosing might be necessary to prevent recurrence until the OP is cleared. Doses of up to 100 mg or more in the first 24 h are not unheard of. A complete response with just 1 to 2 mg calls the diagnosis of OP poisoning into question.

Pralidoxime reactivates AChE and can also reverse the nicotinic effects. It is usually not needed in carbamate poisoning because of the reversible nature of enzyme inhibition. It must be given within 24 to 48 h of OP exposure to prevent aging (permanent binding) of the OP-AChE complex. Pralidoxime is given as a 1- to 2-g bolus over 10 to 20 min. This dose may be repeated once if needed. Then a continuous infusion is titrated to 200 to 500 mg/h until the desired effect is achieved.

HD and HP are ineffective in OP poisonings.

Phencyclidine

MECHANISM

Phencyclidine (PCP) works in the CNS as a dissociative anesthetic that produces decreased pain perception without altering the level of consciousness. It also produces a variety of anticholinergic, opiate, dopaminergic, and central alpha-adrenergic agonist effects.

SIGNS AND SYMPTOMS

The most notable sign in patients with PCP intoxication is the wide and rapid fluctuation in their behavior. The behavior can be bizarre, euphoric, violent, agitated, stuporous, cataleptic, lethargic, or even comatose. As the intoxication worsens, patients can display hallucinations, vertical and horizontal nystagmus, hypertension, muscle rigidity, rhabdomyolysis, fevers, focal or generalized dystonic reactions, athetosis, diaphoresis, bronchospasm, hypersalivation, urinary retention, apnea, grand mal seizures, and cardiac arrest.

TOXIC DOSE

Doses of about 10 mg will produce toxic psychosis and many of the behavioral changes noted above. Death occurs with doses of 150 mg or more.

TREATMENT

Immediate treatment goals include calming of the patient. The drug of choice for agitation is haloperidol. While large doses might be required, exceeding a total dose of more than 100 mg is not recommended. Haloperidol can cause tardive dyskinesia, extrapyramidal symptoms, neuroleptic malignant syndrome, prolongation of the QT interval and, most importantly, it lowers the seizure threshold. If further sedation is needed, a BDZ is the next drug of choice.

For hypertension not responding to sedation, nitro-prusside or labetalol can be tried. β blockers alone are to be avoided as they can leave the alpha stimulation unopposed.

Urinary acidification with NH_4Cl increases the urinary concentration of PCP, but has not been proven to enhance elimination. Also, urinary acidification can possibly worsen the effects of any rhabdomyolysis.

Salicylates

MECHANISM

Salicylates cause toxicity by stimulation of the respiratory centers in the CNS, uncoupling of oxidative phosphorylation, and disruption of glucose metabolism.

Toxicity can result from either acute or chronic ingestions.

SIGNS AND SYMPTOMS

The symptoms of acute ingestion include tinnitus, vertigo, nausea, vomiting, and diarrhea. More sever intoxication progresses to noncardiogenic pulmonary edema, centrally mediated fevers, mental status changes, seizures, coma, and death. Signs of acute ingestion include the characteristic acid-base disturbance of respiratory alkalosis (caused by direct CNS stimulation) and an anion gap metabolic acidosis (from uncoupling of oxidative phosphorylation). Both serum and CSF glucose levels can be quite low. Hypotension, coagulopathy, widening of the QRS, first- and second-degree AV block, ventricular arrhythmias, and oliguria can also develop.

Chronic intoxication usually presents with cerebral edema, noncardiogenic pulmonary edema, confusion and mental status changes, and elevation in the prothrombin time.

In the acute setting, symptoms usually develop with serum levels of 40 to 50 mg/dL. However, lethality of the overdose correlates poorly with serum levels. This is especially true for patients with chronic ingestions, multiple-dose ingestions, or the use of enteric-coated preparations.

LETHAL DOSE

Acute, single ingestions of 300 mg/kg or more, or chronic ingestions of 100 mg/kg per day will cause serious intoxication.

TREATMENT

Treatment in both acute and chronic toxicity is based on clinical symptoms more than on the salicylate versus time-since-ingestion nomogram.

All patients with salicylate ingestions should receive dextrose, since their glucose metabolism is abnormal.

Since most salicylates are weak acids, their distribution to various tissues is pH-dependent. Administration of sodium bicarbonate (bolus of 1 to 2 meq/kg and then infusion at 0.3 to 0.4 meq/kg per hour) until the serum pH is 7.45 to 7.50 can significantly decrease the CNS toxicity of salicylates. When urine pH is increased from 6.1 to 8.1, the renal clearance is increased 18-fold. Hypokalemia should be avoided, since this prevents alkalinization of the urine (K^+ is exchanged for H^+ in the distal nephron). Increased elimination carries added importance, since acute, large ingestions can double or triple the half-life of salicylate.

HD (with or without HP) is indicated when the serum salicylate level is greater than 100 mg/dL in acute ingestions or 60 mg/dL with chronic ingestions. HD can also be very beneficial when the patient has volume overload, noncardiogenic pulmonary edema, renal failure precluding the use of $NaHCO_3$, coma, seizures, depressed mental status, refractory acidemia, chronic ingestion, or when the clinical course is deteriorating.

Selective Serotonin Reuptake Inhibitors

MECHANISM

For the most part, selective serotonin reuptake inhibitors (SSRIs) are relatively innocuous medications. An overdose of an SSRI by itself usually produces few symptoms. SSRIs produce toxicity when combined with other drugs, specifically monoamine oxidase inhibitors (MAOI) or tryptophan. These combinations produce very high levels of serotonin and lead to the serotonin syndrome.

SIGNS AND SYMPTOMS

Serotonin syndrome is characterized by any combination of confusion, agitation, shivering, ataxia, sedation, hypomania, diaphoresis, flushing, fever, DIC, seizures, coma, muscle rigidity, myoclonus, hyperreflexia, involuntary movements, autonomic instability, nausea, diarrhea, orthostatic hypotension, rhabdomyolysis, hyponatremia, and rarely death.

TREATMENT

Treatment is supportive, since there is no conclusive evidence that serotonin blockers (methysergide and cyproheptadine) are safe or effective. GL, SOI, and AC are the mainstays of supportive treatment. HD and HP are not effective in the serotonin syndrome.

Theophylline

MECHANISM

The exact mechanism for theophylline toxicity is not understood but could be related to elevated cAMP levels, direct beta-adrenergic receptor stimulation, or release of endogenous catecholamines. There can be acute or chronic intoxication. In chronic intoxication, symptoms usually appear at lower serum levels than with acute intoxication.

SIGNS AND SYMPTOMS

Serious intoxication with theophyline can precipitate vomiting, tremor, anxiety, atrial and ventricular tachyarrhythmias, hypokalemia, hyperglycemia, hypomagnesemia, hypophosphatemia, hypercalcemia, respiratory alkalosis, status epilepticus with rhabdomyolysis, and cardiovascular collapse.

TOXIC DOSE

Single ingestions of 50 mg/kg can produce serum levels of 100 mg/L, the normal therapeutic range being 10 to 20 mg/L.

TREATMENT

There is no specific antidote for theophylline intoxication. AC is effective in binding theophylline, and multiple doses of AC can be given every 2 h to the awake and alert patient until the serum level is less than 20 mg/L. GL can be helpful, but the large size of sustained-release tablets can make GL difficult. WBI can be effective at table removal.

Seizures need to be controlled aggressively but frequently can be refractory to DBZ, phenytoin, and barbiturates.

SVTs and ventricular arrhythmias are frequently secondary to excessive adrenergic stimulation and should be treated with esmolol, metoprolol, or propranolol (these may be contraindicated in patients with asthma). Otherwise, regular ACLS protocols can be followed for ventricular arrhythmias.

A peripheral β_2-receptor effect is thought to be responsible for the hypokalemia and vasodilation and a beta-blocker can be used to treat these problems. Nausea can be refractory to most medications, but ondansetron seems to be somewhat efficacious.

Patients with seizures, arrhythmias, serum levels greater then 100 mg/L initially or 60 mg/L after 2 h, shock, chronic intoxication, respiratory failure, intolerance to AC, impaired metabolism of theophylline secondary to congestive heart failure, and hypoxemia should receive HD with HP.

For a more detailed discussion, see Chap. 99 in *Principles of Critical Care*, 2d ed.

Chapter 68 _____

CRITICAL CARE PHARMACOLOGY

MANU JAIN

Designing therapeutic regimens for critically ill patients is complicated by many factors. These include polypharmacy, altered handling of drugs by the body due to the effects of critical illness, as well as the substantial cost of these medications. Choosing an optimal regimen is crucial to the effective management of the critically ill patient. Errors in choosing a therapeutic regimen may actually contribute to worsening morbidity and mortality. In order to maximize the therapeutic benefit of drugs while minimizing the potential for harm, one must individualize the medication regimen for each critically ill patient, taking into account the issues mentioned above.

Before discussing critical care pharmacology further it is helpful to review a few definitions (See Table 68-1).

Pharmacokinetics

Intravascular administration generally results in 100 percent bioavailability. Other routes of parenteral (i.e., SQ or IM) and enteral (i.e., PO or PR) administration have bioavailabilities that are less complete and less predictable for the following reasons: patient factors, drug formulation properties, drug physicochemical properties, and first-pass metabolism. If one considers the body as a single homogenous compartment, then the volume of distribution (V_d) for an intravenous drug is calculated using the following equation:

$$V_d = D/C$$

where D = amount of drug administered, and
$\quad\quad C$ = concentration of drug once finished infusing.

TABLE 68-1   Definition of Terms

Term	Definition
Pharmacokinetics	Study of drug movement through the body ("what the body does to the drug")
Pharmacodynamics	Relationship of drug movement to pharmacologic response ("what the drug does to the body")
Bioavailability	Fraction of administered drug reaching systemic circulation
First-pass metabolism	Modification of administered drug by intestinal or liver enzymes
Zero-order kinetics	Elimination kinetics whereby a constant amount/time of drug is eliminated
First-order kinetics	Elimination kinetics whereby a constant fraction/time of drug is eliminated
Loading dose	First dose of drug administered that is intended to attain serum target levels rapidly

A multicompartment model of the body, which is a more accurate description, divides the body into central volumes and peripheral volumes. Central components are highly perfused tissues and peripheral components are less well perfused. The transition of a drug from the central volume to a final volume of distribution is quantified by the distribution half-life. This can influence the onset of drug effect as well as the duration of action. In considering drug elimination, it is important to remember the factors that prolong or shorten the serum half-life of a drug. A large volume of distribution or low clearance will prolong the half-life, whereas a small volume of distribution or high clearance will shorten the half-life. The term *clearance* refers to total-body clearance and reflects the sum of the clearances of the kidneys, liver, and other mechanisms.

Pharmacodynamics

The ability of a drug to produce its desired effect is dependent on many factors (Table 68-2), the most important of which is the concentration of drug present at the receptor site.

TABLE 68-2   Influences upon Drug Effects

Factor	Definition	Example
Concentration	Amount of total drug at site of action	Digoxin, theophylline, dilantin
Effect site	Tissue compartment of site of action (central vs. peripheral)	Lidocaine (central) Digoxin (peripheral)
Free drug	Drug unbound to serum protein	Dilantin (hypoalbuminemia)
Interindividual variability	Individual responses may vary to given drug level	Benzodiazopines (elderly), propranolol (Chinese)
Dose dependence	Effect of drug changes according to concentration of drug present	Dopamine

The tissue distribution of receptors for a drug will affect its onset and duration of action. If the receptors are located in tissues with rapid perfusion, there will be a short onset of action. In contrast, if receptors are located in tissue with slow perfusion, the onset of action will be longer. Many drugs have substantial protein binding, which limits the amount of free, active drug available at the receptor site. Any factor that influences the amount of free drug available, either up or down, will affect the pharmacologic response. Recognized increasingly as factors determining pharmacologic response are population and individual differences in sensitivity to drug action. Last, for certain drugs, the predominant pharmacologic response may change depending upon the dose administered.

Designing a Therapeutic Regimen

In optimizing a drug regimen for a critically ill patient, one must ask oneself a series of questions. After deciding which drug to administer, one must consider the route of administration. Intravenous (IV) administration is the preferred route in most critically ill patients for several reasons: more predictable bioavailability, more rapid onset of drug effect, and easier titration. Enteral bioavailability is unpredictable owing to factors such as gastrointestinal dysfunction, luminal conditions, and first-pass metabolism.

Managing critically ill patients often mandates initiating therapies that have a rapid onset of action. Drug concentrations do not reach steady-state levels for 3 to 5 half-lives of the drug. This delay may be unacceptable for drugs that have a prolonged half-life. One can reach the desired target level faster by administering a loading dose. Determinants of an appropriate loading dose are primarily the volume of distribution and the patient's body habitus and volume status. Critical illness is a catabolic process in which patients often retain massive amounts of third-space water. This makes estimating body habitus and volume status difficult and usually empiric. Certain pathologic states can also affect the loading dose. Uremia can reduce the apparent volume of distribution of drugs such as digoxin, methotrexate, and insulin. In contrast, edema-forming states such as sepsis, congestive heart failure, and cirrhosis can increase the volume of distribution for many drugs.

Once a loading dose has been given, one must decide on a maintenance regimen. The choice most commonly is between intermittent or continuous intravenous infusion. Considerations in this choice should include drug characteristics (half-life, therapeutic index), patient characteristics, desired pharmacologic effect, and cost/staffing considerations. Continuous infusion eliminates the peak-to-trough fluctuations in concentrations, which may improve therapeutic efficacy. It may eliminate failure to reach a continuous therapeutic concentration and counterregulatory effects during trough periods. An example of this phenomenon is a report that continuous loop diuretic infusions cause a greater natriuresis than equivalent intermittent dosing. Continuous infusions also allow rapid titration of effect, especially of short-acting agents such as esmolol. A corollary of rapid titration is the desired rapid disappearance of pharmacologic effects following discontinuation of the infusion. One exception is the use of sedatives such as midazolam (Versed). Intermittent bolus administration titrated to specific sedation parameters is less likely to lead to accumulation of active metabolites or saturation of clearance mechanisms and thus less likely to cause prolonged sedation. In addition, drugs that can induce tolerance (tachyphylaxis) may be more effective when administered intermittently. Otherwise escalating doses may be needed to maintain effect. Dobutamine and nitroglycerin are two common examples in the intensive care unit (ICU).

One must take into account the adequacy of clearance mechanisms in selecting a maintenance dose. Renal insufficiency, hepatic dysfunction, and shock may affect clearance of the parent drug or its active metabolites.

Renal Clearance

The glomerular filtration rate (GFR) and its effect on drug clearance can be estimated with reasonable certainty. Despite attempts to develop more accurate methods, estimating GFR by calculating creatinine clearance is still the most common. The equation for estimating creatinine clearance is as follows:

$$CrCl = \frac{(140 - age)(weight)}{72 \times [Cr]_s}$$

For women, multiply the above value by 0.85.

If GFR is found to be diminished using the above equation, dosage is adjusted by either increasing the dosing interval or decreasing the dosing amount. Increasing the interval is useful for medications that have long half-lives and a wide therapeutic range. Aminoglycosides exemplify such medications. Alternatively, in drugs with low therapeutic indices, the size of the individual dose should be reduced to minimize the chance of reaching toxic levels. Antiseizure medications should be adjusted in this manner. Hemodialysis and peritoneal dialysis may have effects on drug clearance as well. Both can eliminate drugs that have the following characteristics: high water-solubility, low molecular mass (< 500 Da; up to 5000 Da with "high flux" membranes), protein binding less than 90 percent, and a small volume of distribution.

As GFR falls, nonrenal processes become the predominant clearance mechanisms; among these, hepatic biotransformation is most important. The effect of acute renal failure on hepatic clearance mechanisms is not well understood and not easily predicted from studies of patients with chronic renal failure (CRF). Thus one must use caution in extrapolating data from CRF patients to the acute setting.

Drug-drug interactions may also impair renal clearance if two or more drugs compete for active tubular secretion. This takes place primarily via proximal tubular pumps, of which there is one for anionic compounds and one for cationic compounds. Cimetidine and trimethoprim compete for secretion with procainamide and some other drugs. Similarly, methotrexate and penicillin may compete for the same pump.

Hepatic Clearance

Most medications are lipophilic and are readily reabsorbed across renal and intestinal membranes. In order to be excreted efficiently, they must undergo biotransformation to more hydrophilic compounds. This process occurs predominantly in the liver in two steps. The first step, phase 1, is usually an oxidation and exposes a functional group. This step is catalyzed by the cytochrome p450 system, which consists of 12 families of enzymes.

The second step, phase 2, covalently links a polar side group to the compound (e.g., glucuronic acid, sulfate, acetate etc.). Once the linkage is complete, the compound can be eliminated by renal or biliary mechanisms. Biotransformation reactions generally inactivate a compound, but occasionally biotransformed metabolites will have pharmacologic activity.

Drug biotransformation may be enhanced or impaired by multiple factors. Increasing age will diminish biotransformation activity, perhaps due to age-related declines in hepatic size or hepatic blood flow. Gender, race, and individual genetic differences in drug elimination are being increasingly recognized. These differences relate most often to less active or absent biotransforming enzymes, both phase 1 and phase 2, in certain segments of the population. CYP2D6 belongs to the cytochrome p450 family and is responsible for metabolizing tricyclic antidepressants and many of the β blockers. Between 7 and 10 percent of Caucasians lack this enzyme and are prone to develop profound bradycardia with β-blocker therapy or severe drowsiness with psychoactive drug therapy.

The cytochrome P450 system can be induced or inhibited by many common drugs (Table 68-3). Inhibition of a particular biotransforming enzyme by one drug can allow one to lower dosage requirements of a second drug. Ketoconazole

TABLE 68-3   Drug-Drug Interactions Mediated by Enzyme Activity

Drug	Enzyme Inhibitor(s)	Enzyme Inducer
Theophylline	Cimetidine, ciprofloxacin, erythromycin	Omeprazole, rifampin
Phenytoin	Fluconazole, omeprazole	Phenobarbital, rifampin
Terfenadine	Macrolides, itraconazole	Dilantin, phenobarbital
Amiodarone	Fluconazole, verapamil	Tegretol, phenobarbital
Midazolam	Diltiazem, itraconazole	Dexamethasone, rifampin
Losartan	Diltiazem, itraconazole	Dexamethasone, rifampin
Propranolol	Ketoconazole, quinidine	Rifampin

is used to lower dosage requirements of cyclosporine in this manner. On the other hand, induction of biotransforming enzymes may reduce drug levels into a subtherapeutic range. Theophylline and rifampin are examples of this interaction.

Because hepatic dysfunction has profound effects on many aspects of drug elimination (Table 68-4), it is difficult to predict with certainty how a diseased liver will handle a particular drug. A prudent approach might be to begin at a low dose and titrate upward slowly, but this may not be possible in a critically ill patient. A reduction in dose is most likely to be needed for drugs that undergo extensive first-pass metabolism. In this situation, liver disease is likely to increase

TABLE 68-4   Effects of Liver Disease upon Pharmacokinetics

Effect of Liver Disease	Pharmacologic Effect
Increased or decreased biotransforming activity	Increased or decreased
Altered hepatic blood flow	Decreased
Hypoproteinemia	Increased or unchanged
Bowel edema	Decreased
Decreased glomerular filtration rate	Increased
Altered blood-brain barrier	Increased

TABLE 68-5   Measures to Reduce Adverse Drug Reactions (ADRs)

Recommendation	Example
Drug-patient interactions	Allergies, genetic factors
Drug-disease interactions	New organ dysfunction and impact on pharmacokinetics
Drug-drug interactions	Induction of hepatic enzymes
Drug-induced organ toxicity	Aminoglycoside-induced renal dysfunction
Discontinuation of unnecessary drugs	Stopping antibiotics after appropriate course completed

bioavailability as well as to decrease clearance. Careful therapeutic monitoring for drug levels that have a low therapeutic index is recommended in this case.

Disease states may have profound effects on drug clearance by the body. In shock states, hypoperfusion to the renal and hepatic circulation would be expected to impair normal clearance mechanisms. Sepsis without frank shock alters regional blood flow, which may affect drug handling. Actual data on these phenomena are limited and must be regarded with caution.

Adverse Drug Reactions

Adverse drug reactions (ADRs) are common in the ICU for many of the reasons highlighted above. ADRs can affect morbidity and mortality and present challenging diagnostic dilemmas. Some ADRs are not preventable and difficult to anticipate. Most preventable ADRs involve prescribing a drug to which a patient is allergic, the use of anticoagulants, failure to properly monitor drugs with low therapeutic indices, and not adjusting doses for renal failure. Accordingly daily review items in Table 68-5 has been put forward in an attempt to minimize ADRs.

For a more detailed discussion, see Chap. 100 in *Principles of Critical Care,* 2d ed.

Chapter 69

RHEUMATOLOGIC EMERGENCIES

ANNA LEE

Patients with rheumatic disorders admitted to the intensive care unit (ICU) often have problems not directly related to their primary disease. In some instances, however, the intensivist and the rheumatologist have to collaborate in the management of disease-specific complications, as in the following scenarios.

Systemic Lupus Erythematosus (SLE)

FEVER: IS IT LUPUS?

A febrile lupus patient prompts the question: Is this infection or lupus activity? Lupus fever is nonspecific; it may respond to antipyretics or require steroids. A shift to the left on peripheral smear or elevation of C3, C4, and C-reactive protein are more suggestive of infection. In the ICU setting, the febrile lupus patient is best considered infected and empiric treatment with antibiotics is warranted after appropriate cultures are obtained. Special infections include systemic *Salmonella* infection, endocarditis involving lupus-related valve lesions, and pneumococcal sepsis.

MYOCARDIAL INFARCTION IN THE LUPUS PATIENT: IS IT VASCULITIS?

The incidence of atherosclerosis is increased in SLE, probably because of chronic immune complex disease and corticosteroid administration. It is a major cause of ischemic heart disease in these patients. Vasculitis and antiphospholipid antibody (APLA) syndrome also cause myocardial ischemia. Vasculitis involving the coronary arteries is usually accompanied by clinical and serologic markers of lupus activity. High-dose corticosteroids are used for treatment with or without immunosuppressive agents and plasmapheresis. Anticoagulation is the treatment modality for the APLA syndrome. Patients in remission who have long inactive lupus should be treated like the nonlupus patient. Early cardiac catheterization may be helpful.

RENAL FAILURE: IS IT TREATABLE LUPUS NEPHRITIS?

SLE patients in the ICU often develop renal insufficiency from drugs, hypovolemia, or sepsis. Exclusion of these factors coupled to presence of glomerulitis, hypertension, and hypocomplementemia with elevated anti-DNA activity suggest active lupus nephritis requiring immunosuppression. A renal biopsy can be helpful. Overzealous administration of immunosuppressives in lupus patients with chronic renal disease should be avoided. Development of chronic renal failure leads to amelioration of extrarenal symptoms. Dialysis and transplantation have favorable results.

RESPIRATORY FAILURE: IS IT LUPUS PNEUMONITIS?

Lupus-related respiratory failure due to lupus pneumonitis or diffuse pulmonary hemorrhage is a diagnosis of exclusion. It is imperative to rule out infection. Bronchoalveolar lavage or lung biopsy is often needed. The presence of hemosiderin-laden macrophages suggests hemorrhage. Acute lupus pneumonitis can mimic pneumonia. Radiographs usually show bilateral and at least bibasilar disease. Diffuse alveolar hemorrhage is invariably associated with an acute drop in hematocrit and may present without hemoptysis in more than 50 percent of patients. Mortality is high and treatment should be aggressive. Pulse methylprednisolone or bolus cyclophosphamide are the usual drugs employed. Plasma exchange may be a temporizing measure during the interim.

BRAIN DYSFUNCTION: IS IT LUPUS?

CNS involvement in SLE usually presents early as an organic brain syndrome or seizures in young females with active multisystem disease. Distinguishing this from drug-induced psychosis with depressive symptoms, which usually occurs in patients on steroids at > 0.5 mg/kg per day can be difficult. Rapid steroid reduction may be required to differentiate between the two etiologies. Lupus-induced seizures are typically grand mal and are unlikely in patients in remission. Early onset of seizures associated with rapidly progressive multisystem disease has a poor prognosis. Conventional anticonvulsant therapy should be used, as there is little evidence that high-dose corticosteroids alone influence the course of the seizure disorder in SLE. Concomitant pulse steroids, alkylating agents, and plasma exchange have been tried.

Migraine headaches are common in these patients. Aseptic meningitis induced by nonsteroidal anti-inflammatory drugs (NSAIDs) and transverse myelitis due to APLA-associated thrombosis have been reported. Elevated serum antiribosomal P antibody levels have been found in lupus-induced depression or psychosis.

Scleroderma

PULMONARY HYPERTENSION: CAN ANYTHING BE DONE?

Pulmonary hypertension occurs in both diffuse scleroderma with pulmonary fibrosis and the limited CREST variant without parenchymal infiltrates. Endothelial proliferation and vascular occlusion with sparse inflammatory infiltrate are seen in both. Response to steroids and immunosuppressives is poor. Response to sequential doses of vasodilators with right heart catheter monitoring may identify a group of patients who will benefit from prostacyclin by continuous infusion. Lung transplantation may be the only hope for selected patients.

HYPERTENSIVE RENAL CRISIS

This often occurs early in the course of diffuse scleroderma and may be accompanied by end-organ dysfunction. Angiotensin converting enzyme (ACE) inhibitors are excellent drugs for this high-renin state. Diuretics may potentiate ACE inhibitor effect. Nipride must be used carefully in the setting of renal disease owing to risk of cyanide toxicity. Complete renal failure may occur, but recovery rate with the advent of ACE inhibitor use is a high as 50 percent.

Polymyositis/dermatomyositis (PM/DM)

De novo development of PM/DM in the ICU is unlikely and weakness with elevated creatine phosphokinase (CPK) is usually due to nonimmune causes, but the disease may be unearthed after admission for another reason. The skin lesions of dermatomyositis are diagnostic when accompanied by weakness and an increased CPK. DM may be associated with an underlying malignancy. Supportive evidence of active polymyositis includes proximal muscle weakness, myalgia, and elevated CPK or aldolase level. Electromyography (EMG) shows fibrillation potentials and is best done unilaterally to avoid confounding histologic changes related to needle artifact. An open biopsy may be needed for confirmation.

RESPIRATORY FAILURE

Diaphragm, intercostal, and accessory muscle weakness may precipitate respiratory failure. Steroids are the mainstay of treatment. Occasionally pulse steroids (500 to 1000 mg methylprednisolone IV daily for 3 days) may be warranted in the severely ill patient. A rise in maximum inspiratory pressure signals improvement. Second-line agents include methotrexate, azathioprine, and cyclophosphamide. Plasmapheresis and leukocytopheresis have been tried in refractory patients.

Rheumatoid Arthritis

METHOTREXATE PNEUMONITIS

The major toxicity of methotrexate is acute pneumonitis, with dyspnea, cough, and diffuse infiltrates. The mechanism is thought to be a drug hypersensitivity reaction. Some patients have been rechallenged without developing the syndrome. Symptoms occur with variable lengths of drug exposure even with low-dose methotrexate. Opportunistic infections must be ruled out aggressively. Treatment consists of oxygen, withdrawal of the drug, and corticosteroids. Most patients recover completely.

SUBLUXATION OF THE CERVICAL SPINE

Up to 80 percent of rheumatoid arthritis patients have arthritis of the cervical spine. Ligamentous laxity may lead to subluxation, particularly dangerous with C1 on C2, because the odontoid process of C2 may compress the anterior spinal cord with motion, as with neck hyperextension during intubation. If time allows, nasotracheal or fiberoptically guided endotracheal intubation is preferred. Diagnosis can be made by magnetic resonance imaging (MRI), myelogram, or cautious flexion/extension films of the cervical spine.

HYPERVISCOSITY SYNDROME

Visual disturbance, headache, and ischemia characterize this syndrome. The most common cause is Waldenstrom's macroglobulinemia, in which B-cell clonal expansion leads to monoclonal IgM production. Patients with seropositive rheumatoid arthritis often develop a similar syndrome related to circulating immune complexes. Treatment includes plasmapheresis, which acutely lowers levels of immune complexes, and cyclophosphamide therapy.

Outcomes of Patients with Rheumatologic Diseases in the ICU

In a bicentric retrospective French study of 69 patients, infection was the most common reason for ICU admission (26/69 patients), followed by acute exacerbation of the systemic rheumatic disease (19/69 patients). Mortality rate was 33 percent (23/69 patients), comparable to a nonselected population with similar acute physiologic scores and mainly caused by nosocomial infections. A 63 percent death rate was noted in mechanically ventilated patients. A study of 48 ICU admissions involving 36 patients with rheumatologic diseases at a tertiary care U.S. military hospital revealed a 22.9 percent death rate.

A total of 77.1 percent of ICU admissions survived and had eventual hospital discharge. The survivor and nonsurvivor subgroups had significantly different APACHE II and Therapeutic Intervention Scoring System (TISS) scores. Infection followed by gastrointestinal (GI) bleeding were the most common reasons for ICU admission.

Perplexing Cases: Is This a Rheumatic Disease?

FEVER OF UNDETERMINED ORIGIN: RHEUMATIC CAUSES

Classic causes of pyrexia such as infection, drugs, and malignancy should be considered in febrile patients with collagen vascular disease. Fever should be presumed infectious if accompanied by chills, hypotension, or leukocytosis with left shift. SLE, systemic necrotizing vasculitis, and adult Still's disease can present with high spiking or constant fevers. Rheumatoid arthritis, scleroderma, PM/DM, and polymyalgia rheumatica are not usual causes of significant fever. In the final analysis, a strong index of suspicion for a relentless, immunologically driven noninfectious inflammation may warrant empiric corticosteroid induction.

MULTIPLE AUTOANTIBODIES AND MULTISYSTEM INFLAMMATORY DISEASE: WHAT NAME DO I GIVE IT?

Sterile inflammation in multiple organs and multiple autoantibodies characterize the collagen-vascular diseases (Table 69-1). The overlap of features among the various diseases is great. Inability to assign specific diagnostic labels to patients with severe immunoinflammatory disease should not delay therapy, since treatment is not disease-specific.

THE ELDERLY PATIENT WITH AN ELEVATED SEDIMENTATION RATE: IS THIS TEMPORAL ARTERITIS?

Temporal arteritis is a granulomatous vasculitis affecting older (age > 60 years) patients with a tendency to affect extracranial vessels and branches of the aorta. The disease is insidious and rarely prompts admission to the ICU. Hallmarks are headache, polymyalgia rheumatica, visual disturbance, scalp tenderness, and jaw claudication. Temporal artery biopsy obtaining a large 4- to 5-cm piece with adequate cuts is the "gold standard" for diagnosis. Contralateral biopsy is often done if a first biopsy is negative. An empiric trial with steroids (40 to 50 mg/day of prednisone), which are highly effective for temporal arteritis, may be indicated in a classical clinical scenario.

ABDOMINAL PAIN AND ELEVATED ESR: IS THIS VASCULITIS?

Vasculitis may be a cause of an acute abdomen or massive GI bleeding. In patients with preexisting systemic vasculitis and a high ESR, early endoscopies with biopsy or contrast angiographies may be needed. Ultimately, diagnostic surgical exploration or arteriography may be required for patients with limited findings on examination.

High-dose steroids can mask physical findings of gut ischemia, even in the face of profound intraabdominal sepsis. Hepatic infarctions may occur in SLE and polyarteritis. Henoch-Schönlein purpura, polyarteritis, and mixed cryoglobulinemia can cause massive GI bleeding. Pancreatitis, profound protein-losing enteropathy, and acute bowel obstruction due to adhesive serositis have been reported. Less than 50 percent of endoscopically obtained biopsies will be helpful in the diagnosis of vasculitis involving the gut. More than 50 percent of patients with SLE and an acute abdomen will die. A vast majority of patients with polyarteritis nodosa die from extensive bowel ischemia, infarction, and perforation unless early surgical intervention occurs. Laparoscopies may obviate the need for laparotomy. Alkylating agents, steroids, and other aggressive therapies may be lifesaving.

LUNG INFILTRATES IN RENAL FAILURE: IS THIS AN IMMUNE-MEDIATED PULMONARY RENAL SYNDROME?

A young male presenting with renal failure, hemoptysis, and diffuse infiltrates should raise the suspicion of a pulmonary-renal syndrome. Causes include SLE, Wegener granulomatosis, advanced cardiac failure, polyarteritis nodosa,

TABLE 69-1 Serologic Tests in Rheumatic Diseases

Antibody	Disorder
Tests with high specificity[a] for collagen vascular disease:	
Anti-native DNA	SLE
	Rarely anything else
Anti-Sm (Smith)	SLE
Anti-Ro (SS-A)	Congenital heart block
	Antinuclear antibody-negative lupus
	Subacute cutaneous LE
	Primary Sjögren syndrome
	SLE
Anticentromere	Limited cutaneous variant of scleroderma (CREST)
Scl-70 (topoisomerase I)	Diffuse scleroderma, less commonly CREST
Antineutrophil cytoplasmic antibody	Wegener granulomatosis
	Microscopic polyarteritis nodosa
	Idiopathic crescentic glomerulonephritis
	SLE
Antribonucleoprotein	Mixed connective tissue disease

Anti-La (SS-B)	Undifferentiated connective tissue disease
	SLE
	Primary Sjögren syndrome
Tests with low specificity for collagen vascular disease:	
Antinuclear antibody	SLE
	Other autoimmune diseases
	Normals (usually low titer)
	Drug-induced
	Aging
Rheumatoid factor	Rheumatoid arthritis
	Mixed cryoglobulinemia
	Aging
	Subacute bacterial endocarditis
	Any cause of chronic antigenic stimulation
Anticardiolipin antibody	Anticardiolipin antibody syndrome
	Normals
	Viral illness
	SLE
	Other autoimmune diseases

[a]Unlikely to be found in normals, with aging, or as a nonspecific immune response to infection.

Henoch-Schönlein purpura, rapidly progressive glomeru-lonephritis, and Goodpasture syndrome. The approach to a patient with hemoptysis and renal failure should include close attention to maintenance of adequate pulmonary function, rapid acquisition of tissue (ideally renal biopsy), and appropriate immunopathologic analysis of biopsy specimens in parallel with serologic assays for circulating glomerular basement membrane (GBM) antibodies. Diffuse proliferative necrotizing glomerulitis with crescent formation is the characteristic histologic finding. Early treatment with plasma exchange and cytoreductive therapy improves prognosis. Effectiveness of therapy can be assessed by monitoring serial GBM antibody assays.

CNS DYSFUNCTION: IS THIS CEREBRAL VASCULITIS?

Rarely does CNS vasculitis cause psychosis or coma without focal neurologic signs. A skilled neurologist can be invaluable, especially in detecting focal lesions in a comatose or disoriented patient. MRI and CT scanning may reveal a lesion suggesting ischemia. Angiography is the gold standard but may be nondiagnostic in small-vessel vasculitis. The role for leptomeningeal biopsy is unclear. An empiric trial with steroids may be appropriate.

HYPERSENSITIVITY VASCULITIS: WHAT IS THE CAUSE?

Hypersensitivity vasculitis is the most common form of cutaneous vasculitis, typically manifesting as palpable purpura and sometimes as bullous disease and cutaneous ulcers. New-onset hypersensitivity vasculitis in the ICU is often due to drugs like thiazides, sulfa drugs, and penicillins. Skin biopsy revealing lymphocytic infiltration helps to support drug-induced disease. Clues to nondrug causes include digital involvement, nail-bed infarcts, ulcerative lesions, extracutaneous manifestations like glomerulitis, along with the presence of cryoglobulins or low complement levels.

ISCHEMIC DIGITS: IS THIS VASCULITIS?

Development of ischemic digits in the ICU is often related to hypotension, use of radial arterial lines, vasoconstrictors, or cholesterol emboli. Single extremity and isolated toe involvement or extreme symmetrical digital involvement are clues to noninflammatory vascular disease and diminished blood flow. Coexistence of a disease predisposing to vasculitis such as SLE or scleroderma, random involvement of multiple limbs, presence of nail-bed infarcts, and palpable purpura raise suspicion for vasculitis, as do extracutaneous markers like glomerulitis. Buerger disease (thromboangiitis obliterans) should be considered in male patients with a history of heavy smoking. Some connective tissue diseases may have APLA–related thrombosis and not true vasculitis. Biopsy of digits is impractical and may be hazardous. Amputation of a gangrenous digit should be accompanied by biopsy of the digital artery immediately proximal to the gangrene. In this setting, angiography often has nonspecific findings of small-vessel disease but may also reveal emboli or plaques.

LUNG INFILTRATES AND ELEVATED SEDIMENTATION RATE: IS THIS VASCULITIS?

Elevated ESRs often lead to an unrewarding workup for a secondary disease state. Common sense should prevail and more reasonable differential diagnoses should be entertained before launching into a workup for vasculitis. For example, a young female on steroids with a fever, rash, and pulmonary infiltrates should be considered to have infection or pulmonary embolism until proved otherwise.

Absence of extrapulmonary markers of vasculitis should make the diagnosis of primary pulmonary vasculitis suspect, since it very rarely is isolated to the pulmonary tree. Patients with APLA may develop a pseudovasculitic picture with pulmonary infiltrates from pulmonary artery thrombosis or pulmonary embolism. Anticoagulation in this case remains the primary therapy.

Interpretation of Rheumatology Lab Abnormalities in the ICU (Table 69-1)

ERYTHROCYTE SEDIMENTATION RATE (ESR)

This acute-phase reactant may be elevated in the setting of infection or active rheumatic disease. Female sex, age, end-stage renal failure, and normal pregnancy are associated with higher values. Monoclonal proteins and changes in erythrocyte morphology or number influence the ESR, which correlates imperfectly with disease activity. Markedly elevated ESRs (MESRs) with values > 100 mm/h are unlikely to be explained by the normal physiologic state alone. A MESR is seen with infection, malignancy, rheumatic disorders such as vasculitis, connective tissue disease, rheumatoid arthritis, and temporal arteritis as well as end-stage renal failure, nephrotic syndrome, and inflammatory bowel diseases.

ANTINUCLEAR ANTIBODIES

High titers of antinuclear antibodies (ANA) strongly suggest the presence of collagen vascular disease, in particular SLE. Lower levers may be explained by age, prior drug therapy, or a first-degree relative with lupus. An estimated 15 to 20 percent of normal, healthy individuals age > 60 have circulating ANA.

ANTICENTROMERE ANTIBODY

The antibody to the kinetochore of chromosomes is detected by a particular speckled pattern of immunofluorescence on Hep-2 cells, the only pattern detected on screening ANA useful for diagnosis. 44 to 98 percent of tested patients with the CREST variant of scleroderma have positive results. It is also seen less commonly in diffuse scleroderma and primary biliary cirrhosis with or without evidence of scleroderma.

ANTIBODIES TO DNA

Two major categories include those that react to antigenic determinants on the phosphate deoxyribose backbone of the DNA helix, called native double-stranded DNA antibodies, and those that react to determinants on the nucleotide bases, called single-stranded DNA antibodies. Antibodies to double-stranded DNA are more clinically useful, since they have great specificity for SLE and are found in 60 to 70 percent of lupus patients.

ANTIBODIES TO Sm

This antibody has great specificity but only 30 percent sensitivity for SLE and is rarely found with other connective tissue diseases. Sm is not to be confused with an antibody to smooth muscle (SM) found in patients with chronic liver disease, which is not a marker for collagen vascular disease.

ANTIBODIES TO NUCLEAR RIBONUCLEOPROTEIN (nRNP)

These antibodies may be seen in SLE, scleroderma, or overlap syndromes, often together with antibodies to Sm. The presence of overlapping clinical features and high titers of antibody to RNP defines a subset of patients with a condition referred to as mixed connective tissue disease (MCTD).

ANTIBODIES TO SS-A Ro AND SS-B La

These antigens are RNA-protein conjugates. SS-A and Ro have antigenic identity, as do SS-B and La. The Ro and La are cytoplasmic antigens, whereas SS-A and SS-B are nuclear antigens. They were first described in patients with Sjögren syndrome (SS) and SLE. SS-A/Ro is far more relevant clinically than SS-B/La. The Ro antibody is detected in 60 percent of so-called ANA-negative SLE and is seen commonly with congenital heart block and neonatal SLE. Other associated scenarios include subacute cutaneous lupus and C2 deficiency. Anti-Ro antibody occurs in 25 to 40 percent of unselected patients with SLE.

ANTINEUTROPHIL CYTOPLASMIC AUTOANTIBODIES (ANCA)

These antibodies are useful for the diagnosis and management of disorders characterized by systemic necrotizing vasculitis and glomerulonephritis, including Wegener granulomatosis, microscopic polyarteritis nodosa (PAN), and idiopathic crescentic glomerulonephritis. ANCA are found in 90 percent of patients with active generalized Wegener granulomatosis and 60 to 70 percent of those with limited disease. The titer can be used to monitor disease activity. ANCA can be found in 80 percent of patients with active pauciimmune necrotizing and crescentic glomerulonephritis. Two specific patterns of ANCA identified are cytoplasmic (cANCA) and perinuclear (pANCA). In general, patients with Wegener granulomatosis have cANCA, whereas those with idiopathic crescentic glomerulonephritis, polyarteritis nodosa, and Churg-Strauss vasculitis have pANCA. Patients with ulcerative colitis and Crohn's disease have been found to have pANCA as well. An overlap of patterns occurs. ANCA have been identified in Takayasu arteritis, SLE, relapsing polychondritis, and Behçet disease.

ANTIBODIES IN POLYMOYSITIS-DERMATOMYOSITIS

Jo-1 antibody can be found in 20 to 30 percent of patients with polymyositis and less commonly dermatomyositis. It correlates highly with associated interstitial lung disease. Some 25 percent of patients with dermatomyositis have antibodies to the nuclear antigen Mi, which is rarely seen with polymyositis. A small subset of polymyositis patients (10 percent), half of whom have features of scleroderma, have antibody to PM-1 or PM-SC1. Scleroderma without myositis may also have this antibody. Titers are not useful in monitoring the disease course of polymyositis/dermatomyositis.

RHEUMATOID FACTOR (RF)

RF are autoantibodies, usually IgM isotype, directed against antigenic determinants on the heavy chain of IgG. They are nonspecific and can be found in normal or disease states. A female preponderance is notable and levels vary directly with age. Significant titers may be found in bacterial endocarditis, granulomatous diseases, and most rheumatic diseases at some point in time. RF can also arise as an epiphenomenon during acute illness or chronic antigenic stimulation.

CRYOGLOBULINS

Cryoglobulins are thermally reactive immunoglobulins that precipitate with decreased temperatures and resolubilize with warming; they are commonly seen with infections and rheumatic disease. Plasma cryoglobulins are nonspecific and may simply reflect ongoing antibody-antigen complexing. They should not be used to make decisions on therapy. Cryoglobulins can be highly efficient complement activators. Crystallized cryoproteins interfere with automatic cell-counting procedures, leading to a pseudoleukocytosis and pseudothrombocytosis.

ANTIPHOSPHOLIPID ANTIBODIES

The family of antiphospholipid antibodies (APLAs) includes the anticardiolipin (ACL) antibodies, the lupus anticoagulant (LA), and biologic false-positive tests for syphilis. Clinical features of the APLA syndrome are recurrent venous and arterial thrombosis, thrombocytopenia, and recurrent fetal loss. Prolonged PTT is often noted because the LA inhibits the generation of prothrombinase by interfering with calcium-dependent binding of prothrombin and factor Xa to phospholipids.

APLAs can be detected via the enzyme-linked immunosorbent assay. The IgM isotype may arise from acute infections and drugs like phenothiazines, procainamide, phenytoin, hydralazine, quinidine, and streptomycin and are not associated with thrombosis. Risk of thrombosis or fetal loss is associated with higher levels of antibody and the IgG isotype. The presence of APLAs should not in itself prompt treatment.

Use of Corticosteroids, Immunosuppressives, and Anti-inflammatory Drugs in the Critically Ill Patient

Corticosteroids are the drug of choice for initial therapy of most acute, life-threatening rheumatic disorders. "Short-acting" glucocorticoids with little or no mineralocorticoid activity are preferred. Prednisone is the popular oral form and methyl-prednisolone its intravenous counterpart. The dose equivalency is 4 mg of methylprednisolone to 5 mg prednisone. For life-threatening problems, 1 mg/kg per day of prednisone is often the initial dose used. Pulse doses of 500 to 1000 mg daily of intravenous methylprednisolone have been used for 3 to 5 days, especially in the treatment of SLE.

Patients who have a positive reaction to purified protein derivative (PPD) and are about to undergo corticosteroid therapy (particularly with doses of prednisone of 20 mg/day or more) are at risk for reactivation of tuberculosis and should be considered for isoniazid (INH) prophylaxis (300 mg/day). Steroid therapy can cause a cutaneous anergy to the tuberculin skin test by inhibiting macrophage recruitment to the test site. This phenomenon is reversible on stopping the drug.

Acute adrenal insufficiency can occur in critically ill patients on chronic steroid therapy, especially patients receiving at least 20 to 30 mg/day of prednisone or its equivalent. Empiric therapy at 100 mg of hydrocortisone intravenously every 8 h is the usual "stress dose" used.

CYCLOPHOSPHAMIDE

Cyclophosphamide (CYTOXAN) is an alkylating agent used for suppression of severe autoimmune disease unresponsive to corticosteroids. It suppresses B- and T-cell function and inhibits antibody production. The drug is rapidly absorbed orally and metabolized to the active form by the liver. Some 60 percent of the drug is excreted in the urine in the form of active metabolites. Impaired renal excretion can potentiate the therapeutic and toxic effects of a given dose. The usual oral dose is 2 mg/kg per day. Alternatively, intravenous bolus cyclophosphamide therapy at 0.5 to 1.0 g/m^2 is used and is thought to reduce toxic effects. Onset of immunosuppressive activity is at 10 to 14 days after initiation of therapy. A predictable white blood cell count nadir 7 to 10 days after bolus therapy is a major side effect. Gross hematuria may signal the development of hemorrhagic cystitis or bladder cancer. Gonadal suppression, oncogenesis, pulmonary interstitial fibrosis, and hypogammaglobulinemia are other side effects of chronic therapy.

AZATHIOPRINE

Azathioprine is a steroid-sparing drug with mild to moderate immunosuppressive activity due to its reduction of natural killer cells. Onset of action is slow. Doses range from 1 to 3 mg/kg per day in oral or intravenous form. The drug interferes with purine biosynthesis and is ultimately metabolized by xanthine oxidase. In the presence of allopurinol, the azathioprine dose should be reduced by 50 to 75 percent to avoid risk of a drug overdose, as allopurinol inhibits xanthine oxidase.

METHOTREXATE

Methotrexate is a folic acid analog, clinically used as a folic acid antagonist, that can alter antibody production and cellular immunity. Low-dose oral methotrexate is now widely used in rheumatoid arthritis. Use of methotrexate in the critically ill rheumatic patient is currently limited to patients with polymyositis/dermatomyositis refractory to steroids.

For rheumatoid arthritis, initial doses are 5.0 to 7.5 mg gradually increased to levels of 25 mg/week. Intravenous methotrexate for myositis is given in doses ranging from 25 to 75 mg weekly. A dose of 1 mg/kg per week may be a reasonable first approach.

Toxicity is associated with advanced age, malnutrition, and impaired renal function. Nausea, vomiting, oral ulcers, rash, pancytopenia, and cirrhosis may occur. Toxicities of concern in ICU patients include leukocytoclastic vasculitis, opportunistic infections with Herpes zoster and *Pneumocystis carinii,* and hypersensitivity pneumonitis. Concurrent use of other antifolates increases toxicity. Folic acid, 1 mg daily, may help prevent adverse reactions. Leucovorin has been used in serious episodes of pancytopenia.

CYCLOSPORINE

Cyclosporine is rarely used emergently outside of clinical transplantation. It can be used for urgent therapy of fulminant psoriasis, inflammatory bowel disease, and idiopathic thrombocytopenic purpura with bleeding. An initial dose of 3 to 55 mg/kg per day orally is acceptable. One-third to one-fourth of the calculated oral requirement may be used as the intravenous dose to attain rapid therapeutic blood levels. The intravenous route is preferable in young children and patients with hypermotile or malabsorptive gastrointestinal disease. An empiric therapeutic trough level of approximately 200 ng/mL of cyclosporine in serum assays and 400 ng/mL in whole blood assays is recommended. Side effects include seizures, psychosis, systemic hypertension, and nephrotoxicity, which can be potentiated by certain drugs. Volume depletion increases the latter morbidity. Hyperuricemia from decreased renal excretion can precipitate gouty arthritis.

HIGH-DOSE INTRAVENOUS GLOBULIN

Although these expensive immunoglobulins have been used in many clinical settings, they are generally indicated for therapy-resistant immune-mediated thrombocytopenia with significant bleeding or when there is a need to transiently elevate platelets or prolong the half-life of transfused platelets before splenectomy. The usual dose is 0.4 g/kg.

For a more detailed discussion, see Chap. 101 in *Principles of Critical Care*, 2d ed.

Chapter 70

CRITICAL ILLNESS IN PREGNANCY

SANGEETA BHORADE

In the pregnant patient, a complex interaction between disease state and maternal/fetal physiology exists that is often incompletely understood. Thus, we rely on an approach that assumes optimizing maternal well being is usually best for the fetus. The following chapter details the normal physiology of the cardiovascular, respiratory, gastrointestinal, and renal systems of the pregnant patient and than focuses on the disorders that may result in critical illness of pregnancy. In addition, the determinants of fetal oxygen delivery are reviewed.

Adaptation of the Circulation

In pregnancy, numerous circulatory adjustments occur that ensure adequate oxygen delivery to the fetus (Table 70-1). Early in pregnancy, maternal blood volume increases, reaching a level 40 percent above baseline by the 30th week. This increase is due to a 20 to 40 percent increase in the number of erythrocytes and a 40 to 50 percent increase in plasma volume. This extracellular volume expansion results in a mild dilutional anemia as well as a decrease in serum albumin concentration. In addition, a 30 to 45 percent increase in cardiac output (CO) results from an increase in both stroke volume (SV) and heart rate (HR). The increase in SV is due to an increase in preload secondary to an increased venous return and to a decrease in afterload secondary to a fall in systemic vascular resistance (SVR). The fall in SVR is attributed to increased synthesis of prostacyclin and to arteriovenous shunting to the low-resistance placental bed. Pulmonary vascular resistance (PVR) falls are related to an increase flow through

TABLE 70-1 Circulatory Changes in Pregnancy

Parameter	Direction	Time Course
Heart rate	↑	1st and 2d trimesters
Blood pressure	↓	Falls in 1st and 2d trimesters, to return to baseline in 3d trimester
Cardiac output	↑	Increases to as much as 45% above prepregnancy value by 24th week
Stroke volume	↑	Increase peaks at 16 to 24 weeks
Systemic vascular resistance (SVR)	↓	Reaches nadir by mid pregnancy
Pulmonary vascular resistance	↓	20 to 30% decrease

a recruitable vascular bed. During the course of pregnancy, CO becomes dependent upon body position. The enlarged uterus may obstruct the inferior vena cava (IVC), thus reducing venous return. This effect is most prominent in the supine position and is decreased in the left lateral decubitus position. Blood pressure decreases early in pregnancy (16 to 28 weeks) because of peripheral vasodilation. Blood pressure then increases gradually, reaching prepregnancy levels shortly after delivery. In general, diastolic pressures of 75 mmHg in the second trimester and 85 mmHg in the third trimester should be considered the upper limits of normal.

Adaptation of the Respiratory System

Oxygen consumption ($\dot{V}_{O_2}$) increases during pregnancy by 20 to 35 percent of baseline levels and increases further to levels of 40 to 100 percent of baseline levels during labor. This increased $\dot{V}_{O_2}$ is associated with a 30 to 50 percent increase in carbon dioxide production ($\dot{V}_{CO_2}$). Alveolar ventilation is increased above the need to eliminate carbon dioxide, resulting in a P_{CO_2} of 27 to 32 mmHg throughout pregnancy. This augmented alveolar ventilation, presumably secondary to increased levels of progesterone, is due to an increase in tidal volume (TV) without a significant change in respiratory rate

(RR). Renal compensation results in a slightly alkalemic pH (7.40 to 7.45) with serum bicarbonate levels of 18 to 21 meq/L. Functional residual capacity (FRC) and expiratory reserve volume (ERV) are reduced by approximately 20 percent secondary to increased abdominal pressure from the enlarged uterus and decreased chest wall compliance. This decreased FRC and increased oxygen consumption makes the pregnant woman and fetus more vulnerable to hypoxia in the event of apnea—an important consideration during endotracheal intubation.

Adaptation of the Renal and Gastrointestinal Systems

Renal blood flow and glomerular filtration rate both increase early in pregnancy. These changes are reflected in creatinine levels that are lower than baseline prepregnant levels by approximately 0.5 to 0.7 mg/dL. Therefore, creatinine levels that may be normal in nonpregnant patients may indicate renal dysfunction in pregnant patients.

Lower esophageal sphincter (LES) tone decreases during pregnancy, perhaps as a result of increased plasma progesterone levels. This change, in combination with a gravid uterus displacing the stomach, may increase the risk of aspiration. In addition, labor and narcotic analgesics given during labor delay gastric emptying time, significantly increasing the risk of aspiration. Basal gastric acid secretion and pH remain unchanged during pregnancy.

Fetal Oxygen Delivery

Oxygen delivery to the fetal tissues depends on the oxygen content of uterine artery blood and uterine artery blood flow. The anemia of pregnancy reduces the oxygen content significantly; thus, oxygen delivery to the fetus is highly dependent on CO.

Several factors affect uterine artery blood flow. The uterine vasculature is maximally dilated under normal conditions and therefore unable to increase flow and oxygen delivery under conditions of stress. Fetal oxygen delivery may be decreased by uterine vasoconstriction. Exogenous or endogenous catecholamines, maternal alkalosis, and maternal hypotension may cause uterine vasoconstriction.

Several compensatory mechanisms are in place to maintain fetal oxygen delivery. Fetal hemoglobin has a higher affinity for oxygen than maternal hemoglobin, allowing aerobic metabolism under relatively hypoxic conditions. Redistribution of fetal blood flow to vital organs, decreased oxygen consumption in response to hypoxic stress, and the successful prolonged dependence of certain tissue beds on anaerobic metabolism aid in preserving fetal oxygen content.

Management of Critical Illness

Assessment of adequacy of perfusion must be made with the understanding that baseline flow is increased and that oxygen delivery is critically dependent upon CO. Diminished placental blood flow represents a threat to fetal well-being, especially in the presence of coexistent anemia or hypoxemia. In general, measurements of oxygen delivery and acid-base status in the mother (as opposed to the fetus) are the best measures of adequacy of oxygen delivery for mother and fetus. Labor represents a tremendous aerobic load to the mother; the clinician must decide if labor should be avoided or postponed when oxygen delivery is marginal. One effective way to reduce oxygen demand is to assume the work of breathing; early elective intubation and mechanical ventilation should be considered in selected patients.

Circulatory Disorders of Pregnancy

In pregnancy, circulatory impairment may be life-threatening due to the dependence of mother and fetus on CO for oxygen delivery. Circulatory disorders during pregnancy account for a significant percentage of maternal deaths related to pregnancy (Table 70-2).

Hypoperfused States

The initial approach to the critically ill hypoperfused pregnant patient is to distinguish between high- and low-flow states. While this differentiation may be made on the basis of

TABLE 70-2   Maternal Mortality[a] in the United States, 1980–1985

Cause	Percent
Embolism	20
Hypertensive disease	15
Ectopic pregnancy	12
Hemorrhage	11
Cerebrovascular accident	10
Anesthetic complications	8
Abortion complications	6
Cardiomyopathy	5
Infection	4
Hydatidiform mole	1
Other	8

[a]Direct maternal deaths.

SOURCE: From Hayashi R: Obstetric hemorrhagic and hypovolemic shock, in Clark SL, Cotton DB, Hankins GDV, Phelan JP (eds): *Critical Care Obstetrics.* Boston, Blackwell Scientific, 1991.

clinical and historical information, occasionally pulmonary artery (PA) catheterization may be needed to aid in the diagnosis. In these cases, an internal jugular or subclavian approach should be used. Femoral vein catheterization is relatively contraindicated secondary to possible obstruction of the vena cava by the uterus and the possible need for emergent delivery. In the healthy pregnant woman, right ventricular, pulmonary artery, and pulmonary capillary wedge pressures are unchanged from prepartum values, while the changes in CO, SVR, and pulmonary vascular resistance (PVR) during pregnancy are described above.

HEMORRHAGIC SHOCK

The common causes of hemorrhagic shock are listed in Table 70-3. Hemorrhage that occurs during pregnancy may be massive and is frequently associated with disseminated intravascular coagulation (DIC). Patients at increased risk of bleeding should be identified early and appropriate intravenous access and blood product support administered. Initial management includes the placement of two or three large-bore peripheral venous catheters (16-gauge or larger) and

TABLE 70-3 Etiology of Hemorrhagic Shock in Pregnancy

Early	Late (Third Trimester)	Postpartum
Trauma	Trauma	Uterine atony
Ectopic or abdominal pregnancy	Placenta previa or abruption	Surgical trauma
	Uterine rupture	Uterine inversion
Abortion	DIC	DIC
DIC[a]	Marginal sinus rupture	Retained placenta
Hydatidiform mole		

[a]Disseminated intravascular coagulation.

immediate volume resuscitation with crystalloid or colloid until blood is available. Blood replacement with packed red blood cells should begin immediately. Massive obstetric hemorrhage is one setting in which initial resuscitation with unmatched type-specific blood may be indicated. Evidence for coagulopathy, particularly DIC, should be sought in any case of massive bleeding. Platelet transfusion may be considered when counts fall below 50,000/mm^3. Fresh frozen plasma should be used to correct measured clotting abnormalities.

It is useful to position the patient in the left lateral decubitus position to assure that vena caval obstruction does not worsen already diminished venous return. In patients who are postpartum, uterine atony can be treated with uterine massage, intramuscular methylergonovine, and intravenous oxytocin. Methylergonovine should not be given if the patient is hypertensive. Alternatively, prostaglandins may be used to improve uterine contraction and decrease bleeding.

CARDIAC DYSFUNCTION

Hypoperfusion from cardiac dysfunction is most often caused by congestive heart failure due either to preexisting heart disease or to a cardiomyopathy arising de novo. Prior subclinical heart disease may manifest for the first time during pregnancy because of the cardiovascular changes described above. Patients with severe mitral or aortic stenosis have a moderate risk of death (5 to 15 percent), while those with

Eisenmenger syndrome, Marfan syndrome with aortic root involvement, or pulmonary hypertension have an even higher mortality rate (25 to 30 percent) during pregnancy.

Once the cause of cardiac dysfunction is determined, the initial management of the hypoperfused patient should focus on volume status. PA catheterization and echocardiography may be beneficial in determining the diagnosis and further management. If the patient is adequately volume-resuscitated but remains hypoperfused, the initial vasoactive medication that should be administered is dobutamine. Low doses of dopamine (2 to 3 μg/kg per min) have been advocated to preserve splanchnic and renal perfusion, but its use in pregnancy has been limited. Recent studies demonstrate that it does not benefit critically ill patients with sepsis syndrome. As a result, we do not advocate its routine use in the pregnant patient, but it may be beneficial in treating oliguria associated with preeclampsia. Intravenous furosemide may be beneficial when pulmonary edema complicates cardiogenic shock. Afterload reduction with intravenous sodium nitroprusside or nitroglycerin should be considered if cardiogenic shock persists. However, because of the risk of fetal cyanide poisoning with nitroprusside, the patient should be converted to oral medications including hydralazine as soon as possible. Angiotensin converting enzyme (ACE) inhibitors are absolutely contraindicated during pregnancy, as they have been associated with oligohydramnios and anuric renal failure in neonates.

The optimal method of delivery is an assisted vaginal delivery in the left lateral decubitus position. Epidural anesthesia may ameliorate tachycardia in response to pain and beneficially lower SVR. Since decreased SVR may lead to decompensation in patients with aortic stenosis, hypertrophic cardiomyopathy, or pulmonary hypertension, general anesthesia may be preferred in these patients. In general, cesarean sections should be reserved for obstetric complications and fetal distress.

TRAUMA

Death from trauma is a leading cause of nonobstetric maternal mortality. During pregnancy, shock may occur as a result of injury from motor vehicle accidents, falls, and assaults.

Some injuries are unique to pregnancy, including amniotic membrane rupture, placental abruption, uterine rupture, premature labor, and fetal trauma. In most cases, vaginal bleeding is present, although there have been occasional reports of the absence of vaginal bleeding following traumatic injury. DIC often complicates abruption and therefore should be monitored in all severely injured pregnant patients. Displacement of abdominal contents, including the bladder, increases the risk of visceral injury from penetrating trauma.

Initial management includes assessment and stabilization of cardiorespiratory function. If intubation is required, it should be performed by a skilled individual owing to the increased risk of aspiration during pregnancy. If hemorrhage is present, aggressive resuscitation, as discussed above, is appropriate. Hypovolemia may be initially difficult to evaluate because of tachycardia and supine hypotension attributable to pregnancy itself. Thus, when hypovolemia is clinically evident, blood loss may already be enormous. Once the cervical spine is cleared, the patient should be placed in the left lateral position. Pelvic examination should be performed provided that there is no overt vaginal bleeding. Nitrazine paper may identify amniotic fluid and confirm rupture of the amniotic membranes. Physical findings of peritoneal injury may be masked by pregnancy and peritoneal lavage may be positive in the absence of signs or symptoms of injury. Open peritoneal lavage, rather than needle paracentesis, should be performed to assess for blunt abdominal trauma. Ultrasound or computed tomography may be helpful in the diagnosis of pelvic or abdominal bleeding. Once the mother is stabilized, cardiotocographic monitoring of fetal cardiac activity and uterine activity should be performed for 4 h after the injury. Fetomaternal hemorrhage may be assessed by the Kleihauer-Betke test. If maternal death occurs despite aggressive resuscitation and the fetus is alive, postmortem cesarean section should be considered.

SEPTIC SHOCK

Septic shock is another important cause of hypoperfusion in pregnancy, accounting for up to 15 percent of maternal deaths. Since the diagnosis of sepsis in the febrile pregnant patient may be obscured by the normal hemodynamic changes of pregnancy, an awareness of the usual settings and patients at risk for sepsis will increase the chance of recognizing this life-threatening state. Caution must be used in interpreting the hemodynamic profile of a pregnant patient, because the three most useful signs of sepsis—tachycardia, hypotension, and low systemic vascular resistance—are present in both the pregnant and septic states. However, extreme values and rapid changes in hemodynamic parameters suggest infection. Pregnant patients may also have an increased susceptibility to the systemic effects of bacteremia and endotoxemia, perhaps owing to a decreased cell-mediated immune response.

Common causes of sepsis in pregnancy include septic abortions, antepartum pyelonephritis, chorioamnionitis, and postpartum infections (Table 70-4). Common bacterial pathogens that should be considered are presented in Table 70-5. Cesarean section, premature rupture of membranes, poor progress in labor, and prior instrumentation of the genitourinary tract increase the risk of postpartum sepsis. Complications of sepsis include pulmonary capillary leak with subsequent adult respiratory distress syndrome (ARDS) as well as DIC.

Thorough culturing and evaluation of pelvic sites should be performed. Empiric antibiotic therapy should include at least two antibiotics (a third-generation cephalosporin and clindamycin or semisynthetic penicillin) to cover the above organisms until specific bacteriologic cultures are available. If possible, it is best to avoid aminoglycosides owing to their potential fetal ototoxicities and nephrotoxicities. Surgical drainage of pelvic and abdominal sources may be required. If required, mechanical ventilation should be instituted early. In addition, pulmonary artery catheterization may guide therapy, owing to the risk of precipitating low-pressure pulmonary edema. Inotropic agents such as dobutamine may be of use in patients with abnormal ventricular function. However, in patients with an adequate cardiac output, inotropic agents are of less clear benefit and may decrease placental blood flow. Acetaminophen and a cooling blanket may be used to control elevated temperatures. Recent trials of new agents—including immunotherapeutic

TABLE 70-4   Bacterial Infections Associated with Sepsis in Pregnancy and after Parturition

Obstetric
  Postpartum endometritis
  Chorioamnionitis (intraamniotic infection)
  Septic abortion
  Septic pelvic thrombophlebitis
  Antepartum pyelonephritis
Nonobstetric
  Appendicitis
  Cholecystitis
  Pyelonephritis
  Pneumonia
Invasive procedures
  Abdominal wall or perineal incisions (necrotizing fasciitis)
  Amniocentesis/chorionic villus sampling (septic abortion)
  Infected cerclage (chorioamnionitis)

SOURCE: From Fein AM, Duvivier R: Sepsis in pregnancy. *Clin Chest Med* 13:709, 1992.

agents, corticosteroids, and naloxone—have not proven useful in septic shock and therefore should not be considered in the pregnant septic patient.

Preeclampsia–Eclampsia

Preeclampsia occurs in 5 to 10 percent of all pregnancies and is characterized by hypertension, proteinuria, and generalized edema. Importantly, these features may be mild and may not occur simultaneously. Hyperuricemia is almost invariably present in patients with preeclampsia. Risk factors for the development of preeclampsia include chronic hypertension, preexisting renal disease, diabetes mellitus, multiple gestation, hydatidiform mole, and antiphospholipid antibody syndrome.

Although the exact etiology of preeclampsia is unknown, increasing evidence suggest that arterial vasoconstriction, vasospasm, and microthrombi all contribute to its pathogenesis. Markers of disease severity that may increase the

TABLE 70-5   Pathogens Responsible for Severe Sepsis in Obstetric Patients

---

Gram-negative rods
  Escherichia coli
  Klebsiella-Enterobacter species
  Proteus species
  Serratia species
  Pseudomonas species
  Haemophilus influenzae
Anerobes
  Clostridium perfringens
  Fusobacterium species
  Bacteroides species
  Peptostreptococcus
Gram-positive cocci
  Streptococci, groups A, B, and D
  Pneumococcus
  Staphylococcus

NOTE: Infectious but nonbacterial pathogens (viruses, fungi, and mycoplasma) seem to be rare for extrapulmonary infections.
SOURCE: From Fein AM, Duvivier R: Sepsis in pregnancy. *Clin Chest Med* 13:709, 1992.

risk of complications include systolic blood pressure > 160 or diastolic blood pressure ≥ 110 mmHg, proteinuria greater than 2 g in 24 h or greater than 100 mg/dL in a random specimen, marked hemoconcentration, oliguria, or pulmonary edema. Especially worrisome signs and symptoms of preeclampsia include headache, blurred vision, scotomata, altered consciousness, clonus, epigastric or right-upper-quadrant pain, worsening renal failure, and microangiopathic hemolytic anemia. Maternal complications of severe preeclampsia include cerebral hemorrhage or edema; renal dysfunction; pulmonary edema; placental abruption with DIC; the HELLP (hemolysis, elevated liver enzymes, low platelets) syndrome; and hepatic infarction, failure, subcapsular hemorrhage, or rupture. Preeclampsia may progress to a convulsive state, termed *eclampsia,* without any preceding symptoms or warning signs. Both eclampsia and HELLP syndrome are associated with increased fetal and maternal morbidity and mortality.

Management of preeclampsia includes early diagnosis, close medical observation, and timely delivery. Once the diagnosis is made, further treatment is based on evaluation of mother and fetus. Delivery is curative in most cases; it is recommended in patients who are more than 34 weeks pregnant and in those with impending eclampsia, multiorgan involvement, or fetal distress. Early in gestation, conservative management with close monitoring to improve neonatal survival may be appropriate at tertiary perinatal centers. Antihypertensive therapy should be instituted to maintain mean arterial pressure between 105 to 126 mmHg and diastolic pressure between 90 to 105 mmHg to prevent cerebral complications. Hydralazine (5 mg IV, then 5 to 10 mg every 20 to 30 min) and labetolol (10 mg IV, then increasing every 10 to 20 min to 300 mg until blood pressure is controlled) may be administered. Other agents that may be used include calcium channel blockers and diazoxide in patients with refractory hypertension. Nitroprusside is relatively contraindicated, and ACE inhibitors are absolutely contraindicated in pregnancy. Diuretics may aggravate the reduction in intravascular volume and should not be used. Magnesium sulfate should be given to all women with eclampsia during labor and delivery and for a minimum of 24 h postpartum.

Cardiopulmonary Resuscitation (CPR)

Pregnancy may interfere with adequate CPR due to decreased venous return and aterial perfusion by the gravid uterus and increased intrathoracic pressure. These considerations have prompted the following modifications to the usual approach in the administration of CPR to the pregnant patient:

1. The pregnant patient should receive standard CPR while being place in the left lateral decubitus position to decrease aortocaval compression by the uterus.
2. If standard closed-chest compression cannot generate a pulse, especially in late pregnancy, open-chest massage and emergency cesarean section should be considered. To facilitate this plan, obstetric, medical, and anesthesia staffs must be notified quickly of any circulatory deterioration in the critically ill pregnant patient.

Respiratory Disorders of Pregnancy

VENTILATORY FAILURE

If ventilatory failure is imminent, intubation and mechanical ventilation should be performed electively. Indications for intubation are similar in pregnancy although considerations should be made for the normal P_{CO_2} of 27 to 32 mmHg in pregnancy. Several difficulties in airway management should be anticipated in the critically ill pregnant patient. These include increased upper airway edema, diminished airway caliber, propensity for hemorrhage, and increased risk of aspiration. Small endotracheal tubes (6 to 7 mm) may be necessary; nasotracheal intubation is best avoided because of upper airway narrowing. Accordingly, airway management should include early and elective intubation by a skilled individual whenever possible. Noninvasive mask ventilation has not been studied in pregnant patients and therefore should be used with caution.

Initial ventilator settings should be aimed at achieving eucapnea. Respiratory alkalosis should be avoided, since studies in animal models suggest that hyperventilation can reduce fetal oxygenation and decrease uteroplacental flow. Initial guidelines include tidal volumes (TV) of 10 mL/kg and respiratory rates (RR) of 15 to 18 breaths per minute. In the asthmatic, lower TV and RR minimize the development of intrinsic positive end-expiratory pressure (PEEP) (see Chap. 18). Patients with acute pulmonary edema should be ventilated with low TV and high RR to decrease the risk of barotrauma and worsening lung injury (see Chap. 15). When increased levels of oxygen are required because of a diffuse lung lesion, sufficient PEEP should be added to maintain oxygenation on a nontoxic fraction of inspired oxygen ($Fi_{O_2} \leq 0.6$). The use of PEEP, sighs, and alternating positions may minimize atelectasis. In unstable patients with severe lung lesions, muscle relaxation and sedation may decrease the oxygen requirement. Nondepolarizing neuromuscular blocking agents and narcotic analgesics are not associated with adverse fetal effects. Benzodiazepines increase the risk of cleft palate when used early in pregnancy. These agents all cross the placenta and may necessitate immediate intubation of the neonate if given near the time of delivery.

Pregnancy does not affect patients with marginal baseline ventilatory function, including cystic fibrosis, kyphoscoliosis, neuromuscular diseases, pulmonary fibrosis, and chronic obstructive pulmonary disease (COPD) to progress more rapidly to ventilatory failure. Severe reduction in lung volume (vital capacity of 1 L/min) does not preclude a successful conception and pregnancy. Patients with severe restrictive lung disease and progressive ventilatory insufficiency during pregnancy may benefit from nocturnal positive-pressure ventilation and oxygen administration. Pulse oximetry should be used to screen patients with marginal ventilatory function for nocturnal hypoxemia.

ASTHMA

The course of asthma in pregnant patients is variable: approximately one-third of pregnant patients do not have any change in their asthma; one-third have asthma that worsens; and one-third have asthma that improves. Adverse effects of asthma on maternal and fetal well-being are uncommon unless the asthma is poorly controlled. Thus, control of asthma and prevention of acute exacerbations are crucial to a good outcome. With a few exceptions, the management of the pregnant patient with status asthmaticus is similar to that of nonpregnant patients. Mild hypoxemia should be avoided because of its detrimental effect on the fetus. Oxygenation should therefore be assessed even in mild attacks. In addition, a P_{CO_2} of > 35 mmHg should alert the clinician to impending ventilatory failure.

Most drugs used to treat asthma are considered safe for use during pregnancy. Inhaled bronchodilator therapy has minimal side effects, while parenteral epinephrine may cause vasoconstriction of the uteroplacental circulation and should be used with caution. Terbutaline may inhibit labor and cause pulmonary edema if given near term. Heliox, a low-density mixture of helium and oxygen, may decrease the work of breathing and preclude intubation and mechanical ventilation. Theophylline is safe in pregnancy, with the only fetal risk being neonatal theophylline toxicity when the drug is given at the time of delivery. Pregnancy decreases theophylline clearance in the third trimester, so dose adjustment is necessary. Parenteral corticosteroids should be administered to patients who respond poorly to other therapy. Adverse fetal effects due to cortiocosteroids, including adrenal insufficiency, are rare.

Acute Hypoxemic Respiratory Failure (AHRF)

AHRF may be caused by a variety of disorders in the pregnant patient. These etiologies are presented in Table 70-6.

AMNIOTIC FLUID EMBOLISM

Although amniotic fluid embolism is rare, it is estimated to account for 11 to 13 percent of all maternal deaths. Risk factors include advanced maternal age, multiparity, amniotomy, cesarean section, insertion of an intrauterine fetal or pressure monitoring device, and term pregnancy in the presence of an intrauterine device. Amniotic fluid embolism may also be associated with first- and second-trimester abortions or trauma and may occur spontaneously at 20 weeks of gestation.

The classic presentation is the abrupt onset of severe dyspnea, tachypnea, and cyanosis during labor or soon after delivery. Cardiovascular collapse, hypoxemia, and seizures may complicate the course of the disease. Shock and bleeding are the initial presentation in 10 to 15 percent of cases. In addition, most patients have evidence of DIC. Pulmonary artery catheterization may reveal acute elevation of pulmonary artery and central venous pressure or isolated left ventricular failure.

The treatment is supportive and aimed at ensuring adequate oxygenation, stabilizing the circulation, and controlling bleeding. Intubation, administration of 100% oxygen, and mechanical ventilation with a low TV (8 mL/kg) and high RR (24 breaths per minute) should be instituted immediately. Sedation, muscle relaxation, and addition of PEEP to ensure adequate oxygenation at nontoxic levels of Fi_{O_2} ($Fi_{O_2} < 0.6$) may be required. Pulmonary artery catheterization may aid in the management of these patients. Pulmonary artery blood may be examined cytologically for evidence of abnormal amniotic

TABLE 70-6 Differential Diagnosis of Adult Respiratory Distress in Pregnancy

Disorder	Distinguishing Features	Chest Radiograph
Venous thromboembolism	Evidence of DVT, pleuritic chest pain, positive V̇/Q̇ scan, leg Dopplers, angiogram	Normal/atelectasis/effusion
Amniotic fluid embolism	Hemodynamic collapse, seizures, DIC	Normal/pulmonary edema
Pulmonary edema secondary to preeclampsia	Hypertension, proteinuria	Pulmonary edema
Tocolytic pulmonary edema	Tocolytic administration, rapid improvement	Pulmonary edema
Aspiration pneumonitis	Vomiting, reflux, fever	Focal infiltrate/pulmonary edema
Peripartum cardiomyopathy	Gradual onset, cardiac gallop	Cardiomegaly, pulmonary edema
Pneumomediastinum	Occurs during delivery, subcutaneous emphysema	Pneumomediastinum, subcutaneous air
Air embolism	Profound hypotension, cardiac murmur	Normal/pulmonary edema
Other: asthma, pneumonia, cardiac disease, ARDS	As for nonpregnant patient	As for nonpregnant patient

ABBREVIATIONS: DVT, deep venous thrombosis; V̇/Q̇, ventilation-perfusion; DIC, disseminated intravascular coagulopathy; ARDS, adult respiratory distress syndrome.

SOURCE: From Lapinsky SA, Kruczynski K, Slutsky AS: Critical care in the pregnant patient. *Am J Crit Care Med* 152:247, 1995.

fluid components, but this is not sufficient to make the diagnosis, as small numbers of fetal squamous cells are present in patients without clinical evidence of amniotic fluid embolism. Once DIC is established, appropriate therapy should be undertaken in conjunction with a hematology consultant.

TOCOLYSIS—ASSOCIATED PULMONARY EDEMA

Pulmonary edema has been associated with the intravenous administration of β-adrenergic agents, including ritodrine, terbutaline, isoxsuprine, and salbutamol to inhibit preterm labor. Associated risk factors include twin gestation and concurrent evidence of infection. Pulmonary edema typically occurs during tocolytic therapy or within 24 h after the discontinuation of these drugs. When pulmonary edema develops postpartum, the majority of cases occurs within 12 h of delivery. Clinical symptoms include chest discomfort and dyspnea with physical findings of tachypnea, tachycardia, and crackles on lung exam. A positive fluid balance is often noted in the hours and days preceding the onset of symptoms. The course of the disease is usually benign and treatment includes discontinuation of tocolytic therapy, oxygen administration, and diuresis. Rapid resolution of symptoms often occurs within hours of institution of therapy.

ASPIRATION

Factors that increase the risk of aspiration include the upward displacement of the gastric contents by the gravid uterus, relaxation of the lower esophageal sphincter, delayed gastric emptying, depressed mental status, and vocal cord closure from analgesia. A chemical pneumonitis typically results. Diffuse lung injury with the development of ARDS may occur early in the course. Evolution to bacterial pneumonia, which tends to be focal and polymicrobial, may occur 24 to 72 h after the event. Prevention should be the primary goal of all physicians assessing and managing the patient's airway. Once aspiration has occurred, treatment is supportive. Antibiotics should be given only if bacterial pneumonia develops.

VENOUS AIR EMBOLISM

Venous air embolism is rare but accounts for 1 percent of all maternal deaths. It may occur during normal labor, delivery with placenta previa, criminal abortions using air, orogenital sex, and insufflation of the vagina during gynecologic procedures. Symptoms include cough, dyspnea, dizziness, tachypnea, tachycardia and diaphoresis. Sudden hypotension is usually followed by respiratory arrest. A "mill-wheel murmur" or bubbling sound is occasionally heard over the precordium. Right heart strain, ischemia, and arrhythmias may be noted on the electrocardiogram. Patients who survive the initial cardiopulmonary collapse may develop noncardiogenic pulmonary edema. When venous air embolism is suspected, the patient should be placed in the left lateral decubitus position to direct air away from the right ventricular outflow tract. Aspiration of air from the right ventricular outflow tract can be attempted with a pulmonary artery catheter. The patient should be ventilated with 100% oxygen in an effort to decrease the size of the embolus by removing nitrogen.

RESPIRATORY INFECTIONS

The incidence of pneumonia in pregnancy may be increasing, reflecting a decline in the general health of a segment of the population of childbearing women and infection with human immunodeficiency virus (HIV). The spectrum of organisms that result in bacterial pneumonia is similar to that in the nonpregnant population. Viral pneumonia due to influenza and varicella zoster may also occur in the pregnant patient, though it is unclear whether pregnancy increases the risk for these infections or whether increased morbidity and mortality result when they occur during pregnancy. Coccidioidomycosis is the most common fungal infection associated with increased risk of dissemination during pregnancy, especially if contracted during the third trimester. Infection with *Mycobacterium tuberculosis* during pregnancy is a reemerging health care problem. With appropriate chemotherapy, the prognosis for pregnant women with tuberculosis is excellent. Pregnancy does not affect the response to tuberculin skin testing, and this test can be performed safely during pregnancy. *Pneumocystis carinii* pneumonia (PCP) may complicate pregnancy and may be especially virulent in this setting.

The choice of antibacterial agents to treat pneumonia should take into account potential fetal toxicity. The penicillins, cephalosporins, and erythromycin (except for the estolate, which increases the risk of cholestatic jaundice in pregnancy) are considered safe. Tetracycline and chloramphenicol are contraindicated, and sulfa-containing regimens should be avoided near term except for the treatment of PCP. Acyclovir is safe in pregnancy and should be started at the first sign of respiratory involvement in pregnant patients with cutaneous varicella infection. Amphotericin B should be used to treat disseminated coccidioidal infections in pregnancy, with ketoconazole reserved for cases of hypersensitivity due to amphotericin B. Active tuberculosis during pregnancy should be treated with isoniazid, rifampin, and ethambutol plus pyridoxine until drug susceptibility testing is complete. PCP should be treated with trimethoprim sulfamethoxazole with the addition of corticosteroids if clinically indicated.

Acute Renal Failure and Liver Failure

Acute renal failure may complicate preeclampsia, the HELLP syndrome, and acute fatty liver of pregnancy. In addition, acute cortical necrosis may be associated with placental abruption, septic abortion, prolonged intrauterine retention of a dead fetus, hemorrhage, or anmniotic fluid embolism. Idiopathic postpartum renal failure may occur days to weeks after a normal pregnancy. This type of renal failure may be a variant of hemolytic uremic syndrome (HUS) or thrombotic thrombocytopenic purpura (TTP).

In general, treatment is supportive, with the institution of dialysis as necessary. Renal dysfunction associated with preeclampsia and the HELLP syndrome should respond to delivery of the fetus, while TTP and HUS require plasmapheresis with fresh frozen plasma.

Acute liver failure rarely complicates pregnancy, with the differential diagnosis including hyperemesis gravidarum, intrahepatic cholestasis of pregnancy, biliary tract disease, drug-induced hepatitis, acute fatty liver, preeclampsia, HELLP syndrome, and viral hepatitis. Acute fatty liver is rare with risk factors of multiple gestations and a first pregnancy. The clinical presentation is nonspecific, with symptoms of nausea, vomiting, right-upper-quadrant pain, and anorexia. The treatment is delivery of the fetus. Maternal and fetal mortality is less than 20 percent and without sequelae.

Acid-Base Status

As previously discussed, pregnancy results in a compensated respiratory alkalosis. Although this condition is worsened by maternal hyperventilation, the resulting alkalemia does not significantly affect fetal oxygen delivery. However, respiratory alkalosis from excessive mechanical ventilation can cause fetal asphyxia in animal models owing to decreased uteroplacental blood flow. Close monitoring of maternal acid-base status should allow prevention or early correction of the alkalosis.

Acidosis may be detrimental to the fetus and should be avoided. Early intubation and mechanical ventilation are indicated in gravidas before hypercapnia and severe respiratory acidosis develop. While maternal acidosis that occurs in normal labor may pass rapidly to the fetus, this acidosis resolves over the first 60 min of neonatal life. The use of bicarbonate is controversial in both pregnant and nonpregnant patients with acidosis. Infused bicarbonate may increase acidosis intracellularly or in fetal tissue beds. Thus, treatment with bicarbonate in conditions of a significant metabolic acidosis is not recommended.

Gastrointestinal Hemorrhage

While pregnancy does not increase the risk of gastric acid secretion or of gastric mucosal ulceration, critically ill pregnant patients may develop gastric hemorrhage. There are some considerations for the use of prophylactic agents in pregnancy. Antacids and sucralfate may not provide adequate prophylaxis because of inadequate mixing and neutralizing of gastric contents owing to division of the stomach into antral and fundal pouches by the enlarged uterus. Histamine receptor blockers have had limited use in pregnancy but appear safe for life-threatening situations. Cimetidine has antiandrogen activity and may cause fetal feminization in animals. While no ideal agent is available, a safe approach may be to begin treatment with antacids or sucralfate with consideration of ranitidine if necessary.

Food and Drug Administration (FDA) Drug Classification

The following are the FDA use-in-pregnancy ratings:

Category A: Drugs that have undergone adequate controlled studies in pregnant women and have not demonstrated a risk to the fetus.

Category B: Drugs without evidence of fetal risk in human beings. (If animal studies demonstrate risk, human findings do not, or if human studies are inadequate, animal findings are negative.)

Category C: Drugs in which risk cannot be ruled out (human studies are lacking, and animal studies are either positive for fetal risk or lacking; still, potential benefits may outweigh risk).

Category D: Drugs with positive evidence of fetal risk by virtue of investigational or postmarketing human data (still, in critical illness, potential benefits may outweigh risks).

Category X: Drugs that are contraindicated in pregnancy.

Category D and X drugs include ACE inhibitors, tetracycline, acetylsalicylic acid, and warfarin. A more general table may be found in Chap. 102 or the main text.

For a more detailed discussion, see Chap. 102 in *Principles of Critical Care,* 2d ed.

Chapter 71

HYPOTHERMIA AND HYPERTHERMIA

SEAN FORSYTHE

Thermoregulation, the process of maintaining the body's temperature in the narrow range between 36.2 and 38.2°C, is very important to normal body function. Any change in heat production or loss results in any of three compensatory responses. The first response is heat exchange with the environment through radiation, convection, conduction, or evaporation. This response is further controlled through vasoconstriction or vasodilation of the splanchnic and cutaneous circulatory beds. The second response is a change in metabolic heat production through a change in the metabolic rate, shivering, or metabolism of brown fat in infants. The third is a behavioral response, such as putting on more clothing, moving out of the hot sun, or taking a cold bath. These compensatory mechanisms can be overwhelmed by extremes in temperature, metabolic derangements, or loss of the appropriate behavioral responses.

Hypothermia

The presentation of hypothermia can range from the obvious (cold water or outdoor winter exposures) to the more subtle (an elderly patient with decreased mental status) (Table 71-1). Diagnosis requires a high index of suspicion and a reliable measure of body temperature from two simultaneous sites, if possible. Mortality from profound hypothermia (< 28°C) can be as high as 70 percent. The organ system effects of hypothermia are shown in Table 71-2. Most of the organ system dysfunction of hypothermia is corrected with rewarming and requires no specific intervention.

TABLE 71-1   Clinical Presentation of Hypothermia

Clear instances of exposure
    Immersion
    Winter outdoor exposure
    Postoperative state
    Extensive burns or severe dermatologic disorders
Hypothermia complicating other disorders
    Elderly patients with diverse injuries
    Prolonged immobility, even indoors
    Drug use
        Alcohol
        Psychotropics
        Barbiturates
    Endocrinopathies
        Hypoglycemia
        Hyperosmolar coma and diabetic ketoacidosis
        Myxedema coma
        Hypoadrenalism
        Hypopituitarism
    Central nervous system disorders
        Traumatic injury
        Neoplasia
        Degenerative disorders
        Cerebrovascular accident
    Spinal cord injuries
    Sepsis
    Shock

The management of hypothermia consists of the initial resuscitation, rewarming, careful monitoring for the complications of rewarming, and a search for inciting or contributing factors. The initial resuscitation should consist of intubation unless the patient is alert and can protect his or her airway, ensuring adequate oxygenation and maintaining an adequate circulation. Pulse oximetry and noninvasive blood pressure monitoring can be very unreliable, and so an arterial line may be necessary. Arterial blood gases should not be temperature-corrected. A pulmonary artery catheter runs the risk of ventricular irritation and is not necessary unless one feels un-

TABLE 71-2   Organ System Effects of Hypothermia

CNS
  Reversible coma
Metabolic and endocrine disturbances
  Increased metabolic rate with shivering
  Oxygen consumption falls to 50% of normal at 26°C (78.8°F)
  Hyperglycemia
Respiration and acid-base disturbances
  Diminished minute ventilation
  Altered pH regulation
  Increased aspiration risk
Cardiovascular and renal disorders
  Dysrhythmias
  Peripheral vasoconstriction
  Typical ECG changes
  Diuresis
Hematologic and coagulation disorders
  Granulocytopenia
  Platelet dysfunction
  DIC?
Gastrointestinal disturbances
  Ileus
  Pancreatitis

---

comfortable with the volume infusions that are required. Rewarming is the most effective therapy and should be started immediately. If the patient's temperature is > 32°C, then passive rewarming (blankets, humidified inspired gases, and IV fluids warmed to 40–42°C) and supportive therapy are usually sufficient. If the patient is < 32°C, then active rewarming is necessary. The most effective active rewarming techniques include a warm air circulating system (BAIR hugger), body cavity (gastric, peritoneal, pleural, colonic, or bladder) lavage with 40–45°C isotonic solution, hemodialysis or hemofiltration using heated countercurrent dialysate, and cardiopulmonary bypass. Warm water immersion is slow and impractical, warming blankets and heating lamps are ineffective, and hot (> 60°C) inspired air can cause mucosal damage. The most serious complications of rewarming are cardiac arrhythmias and shock. Asystole is common at temperatures $< 20°C$. The heart is very irritable at temperatures 28°C to 32°C, and there is a high rate of ventricular fibrillation during rewarming. As antiarrhythmics (with the possible exception of bretylium) and transvenous pacing are ineffective, the correct response to ventricular fibrillation is immediate detection, electric conversion, and continued rewarming. Rewarming causes peripheral vasodilation and decreased venous return, and if not accompanied by aggressive volume resuscitation can result in shock unresponsive to ionotropes. The correct treatment is volume and continued rewarming.

Hyperthermia

Hyperthermia, defined as a body temperature of $> 38.2°C$, has a broad differential and is very common in the intensive care unit. Extreme hyperthermia, with a core temperature $> 42°C$, is much less common and can result in widespread damage at the cellular and subcellular level in a very short time. Prompt diagnosis and treatment are essential to limit the damage. The three main clinical syndromes that will be reviewed here are environmental hyperthermia, malignant hyperthermia, and neuroleptic malignant syndrome.

Environmental Hyperthermia

The inability to compensate for increased ambient temperatures through the normal thermoregulatory methods can lead to a spectrum of disease as shown in Table 71-3.

Classic heat stroke occurs during heat waves, when ambient temperature approaches or exceeds body temperature for prolonged periods of time. As the heat and humidity rise, the body's cooling mechanisms become less efficient and behavioral responses become more important. Those in whom these responses are blunted (the very old, the very young, and the disabled) are at the highest risk for injury. Other risk factors for classic heat stroke include chronic illness, low socioeconomic status, alcoholism, social isolation, diuretic use,

TABLE 71-3   The Spectrum of Environmental Heat Injury

Heat cramps: Muscular cramps associated with exertion at high
temperatures and consumption of large quantities of water;
hyperthermia often not present

Heat exhaustion: A syndrome of moderate severity, characterized by
variable neurologic symptoms (headache, dizziness, weakness,
euphoria), variable states of dehydration and electrolyte
disturbances, and modest hyperthermia (37–40°C)

Classic heatstroke: A syndrome primarily afflicting the elderly and
chronically ill, characterized by mental status changes (confusion,
stupor), severe dehydration, and hyperthermia

Exertional heatstroke: A syndrome associated with heavy exertion in
the setting of high ambient temperatures, characterized by
headache, dizziness, nausea, vomiting, dehydration, weakness,
and hyperthermia

and anticholinergic use. Meeting the criteria of temperature
> 42°C, altered mental status, and hot, dry skin in the ap-
propriate setting makes the diagnosis. Cessation of sweating
is a late finding and may not always be present. Organ system involvement is widespread (see Table 71-4), with shock,
rhabdomyolysis, renal insufficiency, coagulopathy, and coma
being especially common.

Exertional heat stroke primarily affects young, otherwise
healthy individuals who do strenuous exercise in very high
temperatures. Most of these individuals are not yet accli-
mated to the warm environment that they are in, and the combination of the high temperature and the heat production
from exercise overwhelms the body's compensatory mechanisms. The presentation is typically straightforward (a new
recruit or a high school athlete who collapses during warm
weather training) and the diagnosis is made clinically. Exertional heat stroke differs from classic heat stroke not only in
its epidermiology and patient populations, but also in its
higher rate of rhabdomyolysis and acute renal failure.

Treatment for environmental heat illness consists of removing the patient from the heat stress, cooling, rehydration,
and close monitoring for complicating factors. Rapid cooling

TABLE 71-4   Organ System Involvement of Heat Stroke

CNS
  Altered mental status
  Seizures
  Coma
  Cerebral edema
  Ataxia/dysarthria
  Aphasia
Cardiac
  Shock
  Myocardial dysfunction
  Myocardial infarction
Pulmonary
  Respiratory alkalosis
  Pulmonary edema
  Aspiration
  ARDS
Renal
  Acute renal failure
    Dehydration
    Acute tubular necrosis
    Direct thermal injury
  Rhabdomyolysis
  Proteinuria
  Uric acid nephropathy
Hepatic
  Hepatic cellular injury
  Jaundice
Gastrointestinal
  GI bleeding
  Ischemic bowel
  Pancreatitis
Hematologic
  Coagulopathy
    Platelet dysfunction
    DIC
    Impaired clotting factor production
    Clotting factor dysfunction
    Fibrinolysis
  Increased WBC
Electrolyte
  Potassium
    Hyperkalemia related to renal dysfunction and tissue necrosis
    Hypokalemia related to GI and sweat losses
  Hypocalcemia
  Hyperphosphatemia
  Hypoglycemia secondary to muscle consumption and liver
    dysfunction

is of the utmost importance. Methods of cooling include ice water immersion, cool circulating air, and cool gastric lavage. Ice water immersion appears to be most effective. Aspirin, NSAIDs, and acetaminophen should be avoided, as they do not help reduce the body temperature, and they potentially worsen the coagulopathy, renal insufficiency, and liver dysfunction. Cooling should be stopped when the body temperature reaches 39 to 40°C to prevent overshoot hypothermia. Patients with altered mental status who cannot protect their airways should be intubated. Patients may often need very large amounts of fluid hydration. Hypotension that persists after fluid resuscitation may require echocardiography or right heart catheterization to help guide further fluid management and to rule out intercurrent myocardial events.

Malignant Hyperthermia

Malignant hyperthermia is a clinical syndrome of increased temperature, muscle rigidity, increased carbon dioxide production, lactic acidosis, tachycardia, shock, and possible death. It can be triggered by certain anesthetic agents (depolarizing paralytics and inhalational anesthetics) and stress. The syndrome has an autosomal dominant inheritance pattern and is caused by a single point mutation in the ryanodine receptor, which is involved in calcium release from the sarcoplasmic reticulum. The deficiency results in increased calcium release, which leads to tonic muscle contraction and eventually anaerobic metabolism with the resultant production of heat, lactic acid, and carbon dioxide. The treatment consists of withdrawing the offending agent, volume resuscitation, intensive care unit monitoring, external cooling, and administration of dantrolene, a drug that prevents calcium release from the sarcoplasmic reticulum (Table 71-5). The patient should be monitored for the development of DIC, renal failure, and the recrudescence of malignant hyperthermia, which can occur up to 36 h after the initial episode.

Neuroleptic Malignant Syndrome

Neuroleptic malignant syndrome is a clinical syndrome that occurs 4 days to 2 weeks after the administration of neuroleptic

TABLE 71-5 Synopsis of Therapy
for Malignant Hyperthermia

---

1. Discontinue all anesthetic agents and hyperventilate the patient
   with 100% oxygen; call for HELP.
2. Administer dantrolene 2 mg/kg every 5 min (up to 10 mg/kg)
   until muscle rigidity diminishes and end-tidal carbon dioxide
   falls.
3. Intubate the trachea if this has not already been accomplished.
   Insert two large-bore IVs, an arterial catheter, and a urinary
   catheter. Patients with limited cardiovascular reserve may benefit
   from monitoring of central venous or pulmonary artery
   pressures.
4. Administer sodium bicarbonate 2–4 meq/kg.
5. Control temperature by whatever means are available, including
   iced fluids, surface cooling, cooling of body cavities (stomach,
   bladder, rectum) with sterile iced fluids, and heat exchanger with
   either a dialysis machine or pump oxygenator. Cooling should be
   halted when body temperature reaches 38–39°C to prevent
   accidental hypothermia.
6. Monitor urine output and blood gases to guide ventilation and
   fluid therapy.
7. Send blood to the laboratory for electrolytes, liver profile,
   BUN, lactate, glucose, PT, PTT, fibrinogen, fibrin split products,
   D-dimer, serum hemoglobin, and myoglobin. Send urine to the
   laboratory for hemoglobin and myoglobin.
8. Uncertainty about how to proceed may be dealt with by calling
   the MH hotline at (209) 634-4917 Index Zero, MH consultant.
9. Administer additional doses of dantrolene every 10 h after the
   initial episode for three doses.

SOURCE: Modified with permission from Gronert GA: Malignant hyperthermia.
Anaesthesiology 53:395, 1980.

agents (most commonly haloperidol or fluphenazine) or the
withdrawal of dopaminergic agents. It typically begins with a
fluctuating level of consciousness and then progresses to autonomic instability, muscle rigidity, and hyperthermia. Its cause
is thought to be decreased central nervous system dopaminergic activity. The most common complications of this disease are
rhabdomyolysis, acute renal failure, acute respiratory failure,
DIC, dysrhythmias, and shock. Management consists of with-

TABLE 71-6   Therapy for NMS

---

1. Cease administration of suspected trigger agent.
2. Assess oxygenation and ventilation. If either is compromised, intubate and mechanically ventilate patient.
3. If mental status is significantly depressed and airway reflexes are diminished, intubate to protect airway.
4. Cool patient with cooling blankets. Monitor hemodynamics as necessary.
5. Evaluate patient for other syndromes that may mimic NMS.
6. Initiate therapy with either bromocriptine 2.5–20 mg PO q8h or amantidine 100 mg PO q12h.
7. Consider nondepolarizing muscle relaxants and/or dantrolene therapy in patients who do not demonstrate adequate clinical response (diminished fever, muscle rigidity, improved mental status).

---

drawing the offending agent, volume resuscitation, intensive care unit monitoring, external cooling, administration of a dopaminergic agent (either bromocriptine 2.5–20 mg PO q8h or amantidine 100 mg PO q12h) and muscle relaxation with a non-depolarizing agent and/or dantrolene (Table 71-6).

For a more detailed discussion, see Chaps. 106 and 107 in *Principles of Critical Care*, 2d ed.

Chapter 72

WITHHOLDING AND WITHDRAWING LIFE-SUSTAINING THERAPY

MATTHEW TRUNSKY

Appropriate care of patients at the end of life may involve the withholding or withdrawing of life-sustaining therapy. This process occurs when a specific therapy is not offered (withheld) or taken away (withdrawn) because it is viewed as excessive, of low utility, and not in the patient's best interest as determined by the patient, his or her surrogate, and medical team. Examples of withholding therapy include a decision not to intubate a patient with severe chronic obstructive pulmonary disease (COPD) who is in acute respiratory failure or a decision not to perform cardiopulmonary resuscitation (CPR) on a patient with irreversible shock. An example of withdrawal is the removal of mechanical ventilation from a patient with end-stage COPD who cannot be successfully weaned. In each of these cases, the goal of providing end-of-life comfort and dignity through psychosocial, religious, and pharmacologic support supersedes artificial and technical support of biological life.

Ethical Aspects of Withholding and Withdrawing Life-Sustaining Therapy

Several essays regarding the ethical aspects of withholding and withdrawing life-sustaining therapy have been published. Perhaps the best known is the 1990 "Consensus Report on the Ethics of Foregoing Life-Sustaining Treatment in the Critically Ill" prepared by the Task Force of Ethics of the Society of Critical Care Medicine. In this report, withholding and withdrawing therapy were considered to be ethically the same. To cite a specific example, it can be argued that each breath delivered by mechanical ventilation is a separate intervention and that withdrawal from mechanical ventilation is, in effect, the same as withholding the next breath. The report also supported as ethically sound the practice of withdrawing a therapy that was added (i.e., not withheld) during the initial patient evaluation once this therapy was deemed inappropriate. Indeed, the report states that once an intervention (from intravenous fluids to CPR) has achieved its goal or is no longer able to achieve its goal, it may be stopped. Therapy that serves only to prolong the dying process should not be initiated or sustained.

This report also concluded that either patients (or their surrogates) or physicians may choose to forego or limit life-sustaining therapy when the goals of therapy are no longer achievable. When health care workers and patients or their surrogates agree that therapy should be limited, it should be. When patients or their surrogates decline recommended therapy, the physician should generally adhere to their wishes. When patients or their surrogates demand that therapy continue despite medical staff recommendations, it is helpful to review the goals of the patient or surrogate and to explain why these goals are no longer achievable. When common ground cannot be found, one option is to transfer the care of the patient to another physician. Physicians are not obligated to provide futile care. However, the statement fails to address the scenario in which an accepting physician cannot be found or the patient cannot be transferred safely, or whether the medical staff is obligated to provide futile therapy when the patient or surrogate demands such care and transfer cannot be effected. This statement also dose not address the role of hospital-based ethics committees and the impact of managed care on the physician-patient relationship.

Legal Aspects of Withholding and Withdrawing Life-Sustaining Therapy

The legal aspects of withholding and withdrawing therapy have influenced terminal care practice patterns in the intensive care unit (ICU). Several prominent cases illustrate various courts' opinion that (1) patients have the right to refuse treatment, (2) life is more than just a biological process that must be extended at any cost, (3) there is no distinction between withholding and withdrawing support, and (4) aggressive sedation and analgesia are appropriate to relieve pain and suffering even if terminal sedation hastens death from another cause.

In 1976, the New Jersey Supreme Court affirmed the principle of "substituted judgment," arguing that the father of Karen Ann Quinlan was most qualified to make decisions in her behalf. The court also supported the father's claim that Ms. Quinlan would have chosen to forego life-sustaining therapy, thereby recognizing the right of patients or their surrogate to refuse care. Furthermore, the court held that life was more than a biological process that must be supported indefinitely.

In *Barber v. Superior Court* (1983), the California Court of Appeals held that the physicians who discontinued mechanical ventilation, intravenous fluids, and nutrition (in agreement with the family) in a patient with irreversible coma had not failed to perform their duty to the patient and that they were not guilty of murder as charged by the district attorney. The court again upheld the belief that biological existence is not the same as sentient life. Also supported was the idea that there is no difference between categories of life support (e.g., mechanical ventilation versus nutrition), that family members generally serve as the best surrogates in cases of patient incompetence, and that prior judicial approval was not necessary if surrogates and physicians decided to limit care.

In *Cruzan v. Director, Missouri Department of Health* (1990), the U.S. Supreme Court upheld the state's claim that no one, not even parents, could refuse interventions (in this case tube feedings) on behalf of a patient unless there is clear and convincing evidence that the patient would have rejected such treatment. The court acknowledged that patients had a constitutional right to refuse life-sustaining therapy; however, the court also concluded that the constitution did not prohibit the state of Missouri from requiring evidence of a patient's wishes. This decision stresses the importance of advance directives to facilitate medical decision making during critical illness.

The case of Helen Wanglie (1991) concerns an elderly woman who had suffered a cardiopulmonary arrest during a prior attempt to wean from mechanical ventilation at a long-term-care facility. She was transferred to Hennepin County Medical Center in a persistent vegetative state. There, physicians recommended withdrawal of life-sustaining therapy. The family insisted that therapy be continued because it prolonged biological life and was therefore not futile. After failed attempts to transfer Mrs. Wanglie to another facility, the Hennepin County Medical Center asked a district court to appoint a conservator other than Mr. Wanglie, the patient's husband, to determine if mechanical ventilation was beneficial, and if not, whether it was required. The court refused to replace Mr. Wanglie, arguing that he was best able to represent his wife's interests. The court never ruled on whether mechanical ventilation was beneficial or whether physicians could override the family's wishes.

In the case of Catherine Gilgunn (1996), a Massachusetts district court absolved two physicians and the hospital for which they worked of liability when the physicians (in agreement with the patient's husband and two daughters) chose to withdraw life-sustaining therapy from a critically ill woman against the wishes of a third daughter who subsequently brought suit.

Two recent U.S. Supreme Court rulings (*Vacco v. Quill* and *Washington v. Glucksburg*) (1997) held that there is no constitutional right to physician-assisted suicide. However, the court did affirm the right to palliative care at the end of life, even if pharmacologic palliation hastened death from an underlying illness.

Scientific Aspects of Withholding and Withdrawing Life-Sustaining Therapy

Most data regarding the clinical practice of withholding and withdrawing life-sustaining therapy come from retrospective analysis. Surveys have shown that a majority of critical care physicians have withheld or withdrawn therapy at some time during their careers and that many do so frequently. Prospective studies conducted at two California hospitals revealed that the withholding or withdrawing of life support preceded

51 percent of deaths in 1988 and 1989 compared with 90 percent of deaths in 1992. A larger prospective trial of teaching hospitals demonstrated that support was withdrawn in 33 percent of ICU deaths, some form of therapy was withheld and no CPR given in 36 percent of deaths, and that 25 percent of patients died despite full ICU intervention and CPR (the remaining 6 percent of patients were brain dead).

Physicians generally cite two reasons for withholding or withdrawing therapy. First, that the patient or surrogate requests this option. Second, that continued treatment is deemed "futile," a word that unfortunately defies clear definition in modern ICU practice. Derived from Greek mythology, *futility* is understood to mean the uselessness of attempting to accomplish a task. Applied to individual patients, however, physicians use the word to mean little hope of survival or reversing a terminal process (i.e., low utility). To aid in such prognostication, several systems have been developed, including the well-known Acute Physiology and Chronic Health Evaluation (APACHE) system, which uses a scoring system to predict severity of illness and mortality rate. Although questionable when applied to individual patients, APACHE scores, along with other factors including the presence of a persistent vegetative state and multiple-system organ failure, have been used by physicians to guide end-of-life decisions. Clearly additional data are needed to facilitate these important decisions.

Survey data reveal that surrogates and physicians generally agree about withholding and withdrawing therapy, although family members may require days to come to terms with this recommendation. One-third of survey responders reported continuing care against the wishes of a surrogate decision maker, and 80 percent of physician responders reported that they had unilaterally withheld or withdrawn therapy in cases of medical futility.

The majority of patients receive sedation and analgesia during the withholding and withdrawing process. Most of the time a combination of a benzodiazepine and an opioid are used to relieve pain, suffering, anxiety, and air hunger at the time of death and to comfort families. Most physicians do not use terminal sedation/analgesia to hasten death. Indeed it is unclear what effect terminal sedation/analgesia has on the timing of death in most situations.

Practical Aspects of Withholding and Withdrawing Life-Sustaining Therapy

The following 12 suggestions are offered to help with the process of withholding and withdrawing life-sustaining therapy:

1. Schedule frequent meetings with the family during which prognosis and goals are discussed.
2. Present, whenever possible, a uniform opinion to the family.
3. Inform surrogates that they should make decisions representing the patient's wishes, not theirs.
4. Conduct frank, informative, and understandable discussions with the surrogate.
5. Recommend withholding or withdrawing therapy when appropriate. Do not ask surrogates to decide this issue in the absence of medical staff recommendation.
6. Focus the discussion on what can be done for the patient (e.g., palliation through pharmacologic, social, and religious means) rather than what will not be done (e.g., CPR).
7. Allow time for the family to process information and accept recommendations.
8. Consider patient transfer when common ground cannot be found regarding goals of therapy.
9. Allow family members to be present at the bedside, if they wish, at the time of withdrawal.
10. Ensure that social and religious needs have been addressed.
11. Review the specifics of withdrawal prior to proceeding. Will the endotracheal tube be left in place? What specific sedation/analgesia will be provided?
12. Remain accessible to family members during and after the death.

For a more detailed discussion, see Chap. 18 in *Principles of Critical Care,* 2d ed.

INDEX

Note: Page numbers followed by *f* indicate figures; page numbers followed by *t* indicate tables.